METHODS IN RENAL TOXICOLOGY

Edited by

Rudolfs K. Zalups
Lawrence H. Lash

CRC Press
Boca Raton New York London Tokyo

CRC Press
METHODS IN THE LIFE SCIENCES

Gerald D. Fasman - Advisory Editor
Brandeis University

Forthcoming Titles

Cellular and Molecular Neuropharmacology
Joan M. Lakoski, Advisory Editor

- Molecular Regulation of Conscious States, Ralph Lydic

Methods in Pharmacology
John H. McNeill, Advisory Editor

- Biochemical Techniques in the Heart, John H. McNeill
- Measurement of Cardiac Function, John H. McNeill
- Measurement of Cardiovascular Function, John H. McNeill
- Methods in Cardiac Electrophysiology, Michael J.A. Walker and M.K. Pugsley

Methods in Toxicology
Edward J. Massaro, Advisory Editor

- Molecular and Cellular Methods in Developmental Toxicology, George P. Daston
- Methods in Inhalation Toxicology, Robert F. Phalen
- PCR Applications to Molecular Toxicology, Jack Vanden

CRC Press
METHODS IN THE LIFE SCIENCES

Gerald D. Fasman - Advisory Editor
Brandeis University

Series Overview

Methods in Biochemistry
John Hershey
Department of Biological Chemistry
University of California

Cellular and Molecular Neuropharmacology
Joan M. Lakoski
Department of Pharmacology
Penn State University

Research Methods for Inbred Laboratory Mice
John P. Sundberg
The Jackson Laboratory
Bar Harbor, Maine

Methods in Neuroscience
Sidney A. Simon
Department of Neurobiology
Duke University

Methods in Pharmacology
John H. McNeill
Professor and Dean
Faculty of Pharmaceutical Science
The University of British Columbia

Methods in Signal Transduction
Joseph Eichberg, Jr.
Department of Biochemical and Biophysical Sciences
University of Houston

Methods in Toxicology
Edward J. Massaro
Senior Research Scientist
National Health Effects and Environmental Research Laboratory

Library of Congress Cataloging-in-Publication Data

Methods in renal toxicology / edited by Rudolfs K. Zalups and Lawrence H. Lash.
p. cm. -- (Methods in toxicology)
Includes bibliographical references and index.
ISBN 0-8493-3341-5 (alk. paper)
1. Nephrotoxicology--Methodology. I. Zalups, Rudolfs K. II. Lash, Lawrence H. III. Series: Methods in toxicology (Boca Raton, Fla.)
[DNLM: 1. Kidney--physiology. 2. Kidney--drug effects. 3. Kidney Function Tests--methods. 4. Toxicology--methods. WJ 301 M592 1996]
RC918.N45M48 1996
616.6′107--dc20
DNLM/DLC
for Library of Congress 95-41061
CIP

International Standard Book Number 0-8493-3341-5
Library of Congress Card Number 95-41061
Printed in the United States of America 1 2 3 4 5 6 7 8 9 0
Printed on acid-free paper

Preface

Numerous approaches and methods have evolved over the last few decades for the study of renal cellular, glomerular, and tubular structure, function, and biochemistry under physiological, toxicological, and pathological conditions. They range from noninvasive measurements of renal function in the whole animal (which has obvious potential clinical applicability) to a variety of *in vitro* preparations utilizing the intact kidney, portions of the kidney (such as isolated segments of the nephron or glomeruli), isolated renal epithelial cells, and subcellular and molecular approaches. Hitherto, however, these approaches and methods have not been compiled and covered in detail in a single, published volume, especially one with a focus on renal toxicology. Therefore, we felt that it was time to provide the renal investigator, especially the renal toxicologist, with a single, published resource covering the major experimental techniques and approaches that can be applied to the evaluation of chemically or pathologically induced renal injury. Although the focus of this volume is directed toward renal toxicologists, the information and methods presented should be of considerable interest and value to scientists in other fields of study, including physiology, pharmacology, pathology, and biochemistry as well as both clinical and experimental nephrology. Included in each chapter is a concise but detailed description of the methods and techniques — including historical perspectives, applications, procedural details, recipes, calculations, and advantages and limitations — pertinent to the topic.

The Editors

Rudolfs K. Zalups, Ph.D., is currently a professor in the Division of Basic Medical Sciences at Mercer University School of Medicine (MUSM) in Macon, GA and adjunct associate professor in the Department of Biology at Georgia State University in Atlanta. Dr. Zalups is head of the Histology and Cell Biology Group and coordinates education in nephrology in the problem-based curriculum at MUSM.

Dr. Zalups received a B.S. degree in mathematics in 1975 and a M.S. degree in biology (zoology) in 1978 from The State University of New York (SUNY) College at Brockport. He received a Ph.D. degree in anatomy and cell biology in 1981 from the University of Western Ontario in London, Ontario, Canada. He received postdoctoral training in the Departments of Physiology at The Mayo Clinic, Yale University School of Medicine, and The University of Maryland School of Medicine. After his postdoctoral work, Dr. Zalups received faculty appointments in the Department of Pharmacology at the University of Rochester and the Department of Anatomy at Oral Roberts University School of Medicine followed by a position with MUSM in 1988.

Dr. Zalups is a member of the Society of Toxicology and the American Physiological Society. He has served as a scientific editorial reviewer for the *American Journal of Physiology, Toxicology and Applied Pharmacology, Journal of Histochemistry and Cytochemistry, Life Sciences,* and the *Journal of Pharmacology and Experimental Therapeutics.* Currently, Dr. Zalups serves on the Editoral Board for the *Journal of Toxicology and Environmental Health* and is also a member of the Medical Advisory Board for the National Kidney Foundation of Georgia.

Dr. Zalups has presented close to 40 papers at national and international meetings and has been invited to numerous universities as a guest speaker at seminars. Dr. Zalups has received several grants from the National Institutes of Health and the American Heart Association. Currently, he recieves funding from two major grants from the National Institutes of Environmental Health Sciences to study mechanisms involved in the renal tubular transport of mercury and other heavy metals and to study the effects of reduced renal mass and chronic renal failure on the nephropathies induced by heavy metals. He ...o has research projects dealing with the cellular and molecular mechanisms involved ...pathophysiology of compensatory renal cellular hypertrophy and glomerular scle- ...Zalups has published more than 50 articles in peer reviewed journals and has ... several chapters to books.

Lawrence H. Lash, Ph.D., is associate professor of pharmacology in the School of Medicine at Wayne State University in Detroit, MI. Dr. Lash graduated with a B.A. from Case Western Reserve University, Cleveland, OH in 1980 and obtained his Ph.D. degree in biochemistry from Emory University School of Medicine, Atlanta, GA in 1985. He received postdoctoral training at the University of Rochester, Rochester, NY in pharmacology and toxicology from 1985 to 1988. Dr. Lash joined the Department of Pharmacology at Wayne State University in 1988 as an assistant professor and was promoted to his current position of associate professor of pharmacology in 1994.

Dr. Lash is a member of the American Association for the Advancement of Science, the American Society of Biochemistry and Molecular Biology, the American Society for Pharmacology and Experimental Therapeutics and its toxicology division, Sigma Xi, and the Society of Toxicology. Dr. Lash was elected as president-elect (1995–96) and president (1996–97) of the Michigan Chapter of the Society of Toxicology. Dr. Lash has served as an ad hoc reviewer for the National Institutes of Health and for approximately two dozen scientific journals. He was the recipient of the American Institute of Chemists Student Research Award (1984); a research grant from the Pharmaceutical Manufacturers Association Foundation (1988–89); and a National Research Service Award (1986–88) and a Research Career Development Award (1993–98) from the National Institutes of Health.

Dr. Lash has authored over 70 publications and is the co-editor of one other book. Dr. Lash's research is funded by the National Institutes of Health and the U.S. Environmental Protection Agency. His current research focuses on renal transport and metabolism of glutathione and its role in cellular mechanisms of nephrotoxicity and hepatotoxicity.

Acknowledgments

I wish to express my deepest gratitude to both my mother and father, who recently passed away, for their never-ending love and support throughout my pursuits in life. I would also like to thank my wife for her love and support during the preparation of this book.

Rudolfs K. Zalups

Contributors

Michael D. Aleo
Pfizer Central Research
Drug Safety Evaluation
Groton, Connecticut

Delon W. Barfuss
Department of Biology
Georgia State University
Atlanta, Georgia

Klaus Brendel
Department of Pharmacology
University of Arizona
Tucson, Arizona

Eduardo N. Chini
Departments of Physiology and Biophysics
Mayo Clinic and Foundation
Rochester, Minnesota

Deborah E. Devor
Office of Laboratory Animal Science
National Cancer Institute
Frederick, Maryland

Gary L. Diamond
Syracuse Research Corporation
Syracuse, New York

Bhalchandra A. Diwan
SAIC Frederick
National Cancer Institute
Frederick, Maryland

Thomas P. Dousa
Departments of Physiology and Biophysics
Mayo Clinic and Foundation
Rochester, Minnesota

Quintus Fernando
Department of Chemistry
University of Arizona
Tucson, Arizona

A. Jay Gandolfi
Department of Anesthesiology
University of Arizona
Tucson, Arizona

Carlotta E. Groves
Department of Physiology
University of Arizona
Tucson, Arizona

Peter J. Harvison
Department of Pharmacology and Toxicology
Philadelphia College of Pharmacy and Science
Philadelphia, Pennsylvania

Dean P. Jones
Department of Biochemistry
Emory University School of Medicine
Atlanta, Georgia

Franklyn Knox
Department of Physiology and Biophysics
Mayo Clinic and Foundation
Rochester, Minnesota

Jim Koropatnick
Department of Oncology
University of Western Ontario
London, Ontario, Canada

Paul J. Kostyniak
University at Buffalo
Toxicology Research Center
Buffalo, New York

Lawrence H. Lash
Department of Pharmacology
Wayne State University School of Medicine
Detroit, Michigan

Jytte Banner Lundemose
University Institute of Pathology
Aarhus Kommunehospital
Aarhus, Denmark

Niels Marcussen
University Institute of Pathology
Aarhus Kommunehospital
Aarhus, Denmark

Steven B. Miller
Department of Medicine
Washington University School of Medicine
St. Louis, Missouri

R. Rita Misra
Laboratory of Comparative Carcinogenesis
National Cancer Institute
Frederick, Maryland

Raymond F. Novak
Institute of Chemical Toxicology
Wayne State University
Detroit, Michigan

Carla R. Ramsey
Department of Physiology and Biophysics
Mayo Clinic and Foundation
Rochester, Minnesota

Gary O. Rankin
Department of Pharmacology
School of Medicine
Marshall University
Huntington, West Virginia

Rick G. Schnellmann
Department of Pharmacology and Toxicology
University of Arkansas for Medical Sciences
Little Rock, Arkansas

Sudhir V. Shah
Department of Medicine
University of Arkansas for Medical Sciences
Little Rock, Arkansas

Joan Tarloff
Department of Pharmacy and Toxicology
Philadelphia College of Pharmacology and Science
Philadelphia, Pennsylvania

Mary L. Taub
Department of Biochemistry
State University of New York at Buffalo
Buffalo, New York

Norishi Ueda
Department of Medicine
University of Arkansas for Medical Sciences
Little Rock, Arkansas

Michael P. Waalkes
Office of Laboratory Animal Science
National Cancer Institute
Frederick, Maryland

Jerrold M. Ward
Office of Laboratory Animal Science
National Cancer Institute
Frederick, Maryland

Kimberley J. Woodcroft
Institute of Chemical Toxicology
Wayne State University
Detroit Michigan

James S. Woods
Centers for Public Health Research and Evaluation
Battelle Seattle Research Center
Seattle, Washington

Siu-Pok Yee
Department of Oncology
University of Western Ontario
London, Ontario, Canada

Rudolfs K. Zalups
Division of Basic Medical Sciences
Mercer University School of Medicine
Macon, Georgia

Richard C. Zangar
Institute of Chemical Toxicology
Wayne State University
Detroit, Michigan

Table of Contents

1 Clearance Methods in Renal Toxicology 1
Joan B. Tarloff

2 Urinary Markers 19
James S. Woods

3 Histopathologic Methods in Renal Toxicology 35
Niels Marcussen and Jytte Banner Lundemose

4 The Isolated Perfused Kidney 59
Gary L. Diamond

5 Micropuncture and Microperfusion Techniques 79
Carla R. Ramsey and Franklyn G. Knox

6 Microdissection and Microanalysis of Specific Nephron Segments from Mammalian Kidney 97
Eduardo N. Chini and Thomas P. Dousa

7 Preparation and Use of Precision-Cut Renal Cortical Slices in Renal Toxicology 109
A. Jay Gandolfi, Klaus Brendel, and Quintus Fernando

8 *In Vitro* Perfusion of Isolated Nephron Segments: A Method for Renal Toxicology 123
Rudolfs K. Zalups and Delon W. Barfuss

9 Suspensions of Rabbit Renal Proximal Tubules 147
Carlotta E. Groves and Rick G. Schnellmann

10 Characterization and Use of Rabbit Renal Proximal Tubular Cells in Primary Culture for Toxicology Research 163
Michael D. Aleo and Paul J. Kostyniak

11 Use of Freshly Isolated and Primary Cultures of Proximal Tubular and Distal Tubular Cells from Rat Kidney 189
Lawrence H. Lash

12 Immortalized Cell Lines of Renal Cells 217
Mary L. Taub

13 Methods in Renal Carcinogenesis and Mutagenesis 237
R. Rita Misra, Bhalchandra A. Diwan, Deborah E. Devor, Jerrold M. Ward, and Michael P. Waalkes

14 Measurement of Reactive Oxygen Species, Oxidative Damage, and Antioxidant Systems in the Kidney 255
Norishi Ueda and Sudhir V. Shah

15 Mechanisms of Repair After Renal Injury 283
Steven B. Miller

16 Mitochondrial Toxicity in Renal Injury 299
Lawrence H. Lash and Dean P. Jones

17 Biotransformation and Membrane Transport in Nephrotoxicity 331
Peter J. Harvison and Gary O. Rankin

18 Methods to Evaluate Renal Cytochrome P450 as a Bioactivation System for Nephrotoxicants 353
Kimberley J. Woodcroft, Richard C. Zangar, and Raymond F. Novak

19 Molecular Methods in Renal Toxicology 377
Jim Koropatnick

20 Transgenic Animals 413
Siu-Pok Yee

Index 427

chapter one

Clearance Methods in Renal Toxicology

Joan B. Tarloff

1.1 General interpretation of renal clearance data 1
1.2 Measurement of inulin clearance in laboratory animals 3
  1.2.1 Surgical preparation 3
    1.2.1.1 Rats 4
    1.2.1.2 Rabbits 5
    1.2.1.3 Dogs 6
  1.2.2 Dosing regimens 6
    1.2.2.1 Rats 6
    1.2.2.2 Rabbits 7
    1.2.2.3 Dogs 7
1.3 Determination of GFR by plasma clearance of inulin 8
1.4 Determination of inulin in plasma and urine 10
  1.4.1 Diphenylamine assay 10
  1.4.2 Resorcinol assay 11
  1.4.3 Radiochemical assay 12
  1.4.4 Calculations 12
1.5 Determination of GFR using creatinine clearance 12
1.6 Determination of renal clearance of toxicants 15
1.7 Determination of the effects of toxicants on GFR 15
1.8 Conclusions 16
References 17

1.1 General interpretation of renal clearance data

Clearance methods may be useful in determining the effects of toxicants on glomerular filtration and for identifying the mechanism(s) involved in renal excretion of a toxicant. Simply defined, the renal clearance of a compound is the volume of plasma from which that compound is completely cleared by the kidneys per unit time.[1]

Renal clearance (Cl) of any compound (X) can be determined by comparing the urinary excretion rate or absolute excretion of compound X to the plasma concentration of compound X. The urinary excretion rate (milliliters per minute) is calculated as:

$$\text{Urinary Excretion Rate} = U_X \times V \tag{1}$$

0-8493-3341-5/96/$0.00+$.50

where U_X represents the concentration of substance X in urine and V represents the volume of urine collected per unit time (generally in ml min^{-1}). Thus, the clearance equation may be constructed:

$$Cl_X = \frac{U_X \times V}{P_X} \qquad (2)$$

where Cl_X is the clearance rate of compound X (in milliliters per minute) and P_X is the concentration of compound X in plasma (in mg ml^{-1}). Plasma concentration is usually measured at the midpoint of the urine collection interval. Alternatively, an average plasma concentration may be used in calculations by measuring the plasma concentration of compound X at the beginning and end of the urine collection interval. Generally, it is more convenient to infuse the compound to be measured over the collection interval, thereby achieving a steady state concentration of the compound in plasma. Analysis of plasma or renal clearance following a single injection of a compound may be more practical for determining the clearances of toxicants that may be available in limited quantities or that may be too toxic for prolonged infusion. More comprehensive reviews of the theories underlying clearance methods and assumptions involved in calculating renal clearances may be found in Vander and Valtin.[1,2]

Inulin serves as a marker for glomerular filtration rate (GFR) because of the following characteristics:

1. Inulin is freely filtered through the glomerular filtration barrier.
2. Inulin is biologically inert and is neither reabsorbed nor secreted following filtration at the glomerulus.
3. Inulin is nontoxic and easily tolerated when infused in quantities that permit quantification in plasma and urine. Inulin does not alter glomerular or renal function. In addition, inulin causes a mild osmotic diuresis that increases urine volume.
4. Inulin may be readily measured in plasma and urine either colorimetrically or by using radiolabeled inulin.

Since inulin is freely filtered and then is neither secreted nor reabsorbed, all of the inulin that appears in urine must have originated from plasma through the process of glomerular filtration. Thus, measurement of inulin clearance serves as a method for estimating GFR. Inulin clearance is regarded as the "gold standard" for measuring GFR.[3] Representative inulin clearances and urine flow rates for commonly used laboratory animals are listed in Table 1.

Table 1 Normal Values for Urine Flow Rate and Glomerular Filtration Rate in Laboratory Animals

Species	Urine flow	Inulin clearance	Ref.
Rats (n = 6)	2.76 ± 0.31 μl × min^{-1} × g $kidney^{-1}$	0.948 ± 0.078 ml × min^{-1} × g $kidney^{-1}$	30
Rats (n = 8)	3.0 ± 0.25 μl × min^{-1} × 100 g bw^{-1}	1.0 ± 0.05 ml × min^{-1} × 100 g bw^{-1}	10
Rabbits (n = 11)	0.44 ± 0.05 ml × min^{-1} × kg^{-1}	4.04 ± 0.24 ml × min^{-1} × kg^{-1}	12
Dogs (n = 105)	0.094 ± 0.009 ml × min^{-1} × kg^{-1}	3.56 ± 0.12 ml × min^{-1} × kg^{-1}	31
Dogs (n = 15)	0.058 ± 0.008 ml × min^{-1} × kg^{-1}	2.92 ± 0.26 ml × min^{-1} × kg^{-1}	15

The clearances of other compounds can be compared with inulin clearance to determine how the kidney functions in the elimination of a test compound. Typically, the renal clearances of a compound of interest (X) and inulin are determined. From these data, a clearance ratio is constructed by dividing the renal clearance of the test compound (Cl_X [milliliters per minute]) by the renal clearance of inulin (Cl_{inulin} [milliliters per minute]):

$$\text{Clearance Ratio} = \frac{\text{Renal clearance of test compound } (Cl_X)}{\text{Renal clearance of inulin } (Cl_{inulin})} \quad (3)$$

For example, if a substance has a clearance less than that of simultaneously administered inulin, then some of the test substance must be reabsorbed following filtration to account for the lower clearance relative to the clearance of inulin. Glucose is an example of a compound that is reabsorbed, and the clearance ratio for glucose ($Cl_{glucose}/Cl_{inulin}$) is always less than unity (Figure 1, left panel). Alternatively, if a test substance has a clearance greater than that of simultaneously administered inulin, then the test compound must be filtered and secreted by the renal tubules to account for the higher clearance relative to inulin. *p*-Aminohippurate (PAH) is an example of a compound that is secreted by the renal tubules, and the clearance ratio for PAH (Cl_{PAH}/Cl_{inulin}) is always greater than unity (Figure 1, right panel). In fact, secretion of PAH at low plasma PAH concentrations is extremely efficient, and the renal venous concentration of PAH is essentially zero. Therefore, at low plasma PAH concentrations, all of the PAH that enters the kidneys is cleared in a single pass, allowing investigators to use PAH clearance as an estimate of effective renal plasma flow.[1,2]

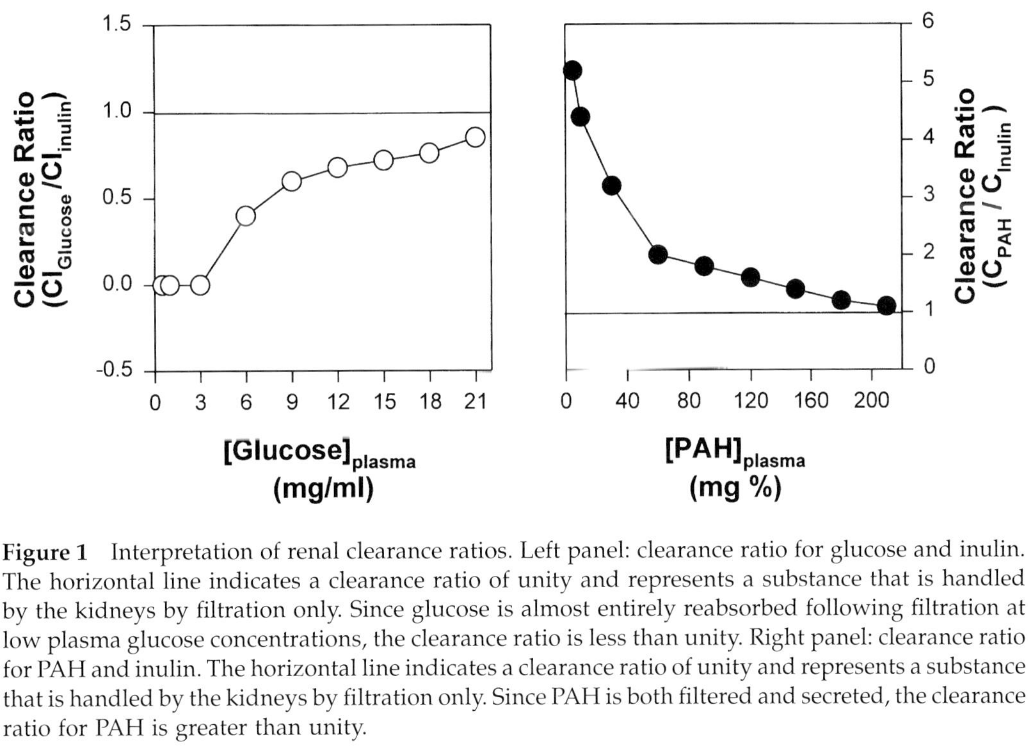

Figure 1 Interpretation of renal clearance ratios. Left panel: clearance ratio for glucose and inulin. The horizontal line indicates a clearance ratio of unity and represents a substance that is handled by the kidneys by filtration only. Since glucose is almost entirely reabsorbed following filtration at low plasma glucose concentrations, the clearance ratio is less than unity. Right panel: clearance ratio for PAH and inulin. The horizontal line indicates a clearance ratio of unity and represents a substance that is handled by the kidneys by filtration only. Since PAH is both filtered and secreted, the clearance ratio for PAH is greater than unity.

1.2 *Measurement of inulin clearance in laboratory animals*

1.2.1 *Surgical preparation*

Clearances are easily measured in small laboratory animals such as rats and rabbits. The limiting factor in any clearance measurement is the ability to collect sufficient plasma and urine for determination of the quantity of test substance. Clearance may be determined in chronically instrumented or anesthetized, surgically prepared animals. For the inexperienced investigator, clearance determinations in anesthetized, surgically prepared animals may be easier than trying to master techniques involved in preparing chronically instrumented animals.

1.2.1.1 Rats

For clearance determinations in rats, we anesthetize a rat with a mixture of ketamine (50 mg kg^{-1}), xylazine (5 mg kg^{-1}), and acepromazine (0.75 mg kg^{-1}). Pentobarbital (50 to 60 mg kg^{-1}) may also be used as an anesthetic agent, but we have had better success in maintaining anesthesia with ketamine. Pentobarbital has a fairly steep concentration–response curve, and overdosing the rat is easy. Inactin (100 mg kg^{-1} i.p.) is a long-acting thiobarbiturate that can also be used for clearance studies.

When the rat is fully anesthetized, we cannulate the carotid artery using PE-50 tubing (I.D. 0.023", O.D. 0.038") for collection of blood samples. Before cannulation, we fill vascular cannulae with heparinized saline, using about 100 U of heparin per milliliter of saline (arbitrarily selected). We prefer polyethylene tubing because of its rigidity, which helps threading the cannula into the respective arteries and veins. We usually cannulate the trachea using PE-240 polyethylene tubing (I.D. 0.066", O.D. 0.095") to ensure an unobstructed airway for the duration of the experiment. We implant a pediatric cannula (24 G, 3/4" Surflo IV catheter, Terumo Medical Corporation, Elkton, MD) into the tail vein for infusion of inulin and administration of additional anesthetic. For supplemental anesthesia, we use pentobarbital (10 to 20 mg kg^{-1}) i.v. until surgical anesthesia is restored. The jugular vein may be cannulated for infusion of inulin and administration of supplemental anesthetic agents if desired.

We catheterize the urinary bladder using PE-205 (I.D. 0.062", O.D. 0.082") or PE-240 polyethylene tubing. We flange one end of the catheter by heating the tubing and pressing the end against a flat surface such as a bench top (Figure 2). To catheterize the urinary bladder, we make a midline incision in the pelvic area and expose the bladder. We cut a small hole in the bladder and thread the catheter into the hole with the flanged end inserted into the bladder. The flange makes a lip that is convenient for tying the catheter into the bladder. The catheter is tied in place with surgical thread. It is possible to catheterize the ureters in a rat using PE-10 (I.D. 0.011", O.D. 0.024") tubing (Figure 3). However, in our experience, the ureters are quite fragile and easily torn during isolation so we catheterize the urinary bladder instead of the ureters. We place the rat in the lateral recumbent position so that the bladder catheter drains into the collection vial. We insert a rectal thermometer to monitor body temperature and place the rat on a heating pad that can be turned off and on in response to changes in body temperature as necessary.

Clearances may be determined in conscious, chronically instrumented rats. Briefly, 1 or 2 days before an experiment, a rat is anesthetized and a cannula is implanted in a jugular vein for administration of test compounds and/or blood sampling. The cannula is exteriorized by tunneling subcutaneously to exit at the base of the neck. The cannula is filled with heparinized saline to retard clotting and capped with a metal stylus to prevent bleeding. The cannula must be flushed with heparinized saline periodically to maintain patency. As with anesthetized rats, the tail vein may also be cannulated for administration of test compounds, although with this maneuver the rat will need to be restrained to prevent dislodging of the tail vein cannula. The use of conscious rats for clearance determinations offers several advantages over the use of anesthetized rats. First, since the rat is conscious during the clearance interval, no other drugs have been administered that may complicate detection of the compounds of interest. Second, there is some evidence that anesthesia alters renal blood flow and may alter glomerular filtration rate[4,5] so that anesthetized animals may not accurately reflect renal function in conscious animals.

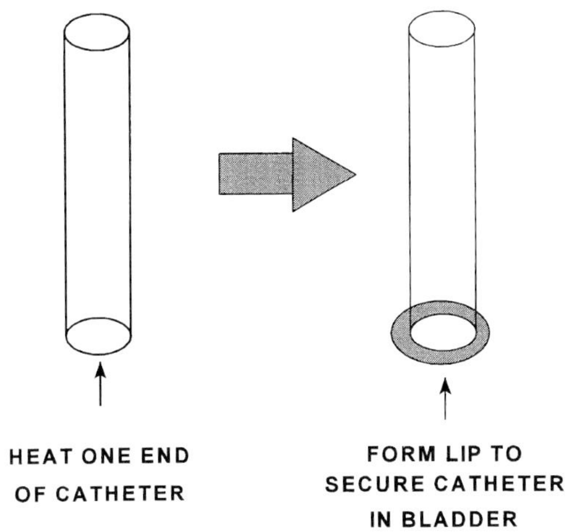

Figure 2 Schematic diagram of bladder catheter. The tip of a piece of polyethylene tubing is heated and pressed against a flat surface to form a lip (stippled ring). The lip is inserted into a hole cut in the urinary bladder and tied in place for urine collection.

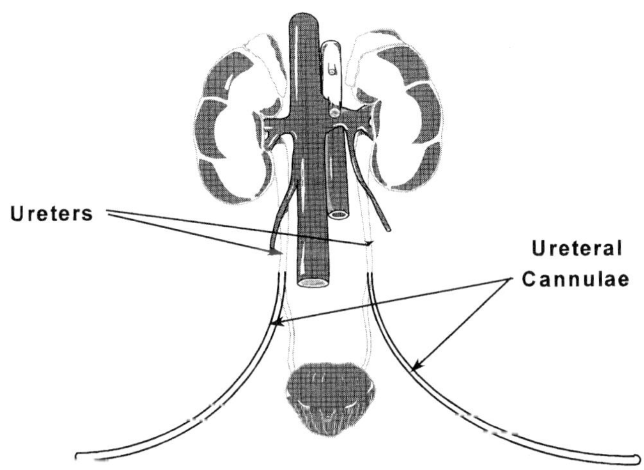

Figure 3 Schematic representation of placement of ureteral cannulae. Ureters may be catheterized using narrow polyethylene tubing. Generally, the catheter is inserted into the ureter about midway between the kidney and bladder. The catheter is advanced until it rests close to the renal pelvis and is then tied in place. (Drawing of the kidneys, bladder, and ureters courtesy of Corel Corporation, Ontario, Canada.)

However, there are several major problems with using conscious rats for determination of renal clearances. First, ensuring complete bladder evacuation is impossible; therefore urine collections may underestimate excretion of the test compound. Second, maintaining patency of a venous cannula for an extended period is difficult, since rat blood clots quickly. Third, infection may be a problem if the rat is to be kept alive for longer than a few days.

1.2.1.2 Rabbits

Similar procedures may be used for clearance determinations in rabbits. We anesthetize rabbits with a mixture of ketamine (50 mg kg^{-1}), xylazine (6 mg kg^{-1}), and acepromazine (1 mg kg^{-1}) given i.m. and supplement with the same mixture, given i.m. at half the original dosages. As with rats, a carotid artery or jugular vein is cannulated for collection of blood samples, and a cannula may be inserted into a marginal ear vein for infusion of inulin. We fill the vascular cannulae with heparinized saline (100 U ml^{-1}, arbitrarily selected). We use PE-90 tubing (I.D. 0.034″, O.D. 0.050″) for the carotid artery cannula and a butterfly infusion set (23 G 3/4″ with 12″ tubing, Abbott Laboratories, North Chicago, IL) for cannulation of the marginal ear vein. The urinary bladder of the rabbit may be exposed by a midline incision and a flanged catheter inserted for urine collection. Alternatively, the ureters may be cannulated with PE-10 or PE-50 tubing. We have not tried cannulating rabbit ureters directly and cannot comment on ease of cannulation. A third option for urine collection is by catheterization of the urinary bladder using a sterile Bardex Foley catheter (No. 8–10) as described by Babini and co-workers.[6]

As with rats, clearances may be determined in conscious rabbits that have been surgically prepared before an experiment. Again, a jugular vein may be cannulated in an anesthetized rabbit for administration of test compounds and/or blood sampling. The cannula must be exteriorized to a location inaccessible to the rabbit to prevent gnawing and disruption of the cannula by the rabbit. The same advantages and limitations mentioned previously for determination of clearances in conscious rats apply in rabbits.

1.2.1.3 Dogs

We have determined renal clearances in anesthetized dogs. Dogs received sodium pentobarbital (33 mg kg^{-1} body weight) slowly via the cephalic vein until the eyelid reflex was inhibited. The dogs were placed in the dorsal recumbent position for surgical preparation. Briefly, the trachea was cannulated to ensure an unobstructed airway. The left external jugular vein was cannulated with PE-260 tubing (I.D. 0.070″, O.D. 0.110″) connected to a constant infusion pump set to deliver 0.9% saline at a rate of 0.3 ml × kg^{-1} × min^{-1}. Supplemental doses of 2% sodium pentobarbital (20 to 40 mg) were given intravenously as required to maintain surgical anesthesia. The right or left femoral artery was cannulated with PE-260 tubing connected to a one-way metal stopcock. The femoral cannula was used for blood sampling and was filled with heparinized saline (4 U ml^{-1}) between collection intervals.

The ureters were exposed via a ventral midline incision and tied off close to the entrance to the bladder (Figure 3). The ureters were catheterized proximally to the ties with PE-190 (dead space of approximately 0.3 ml each) or PE-90 (I.D. 0.034″, O.D. 0.050″, dead space approximately 0.15 ml each) tubing. Body temperature was monitored with a rectal thermometer and maintained at 37 ± 1°C using a heat lamp. Dogs were allowed to recover for approximately 1 h following surgical manipulations.

Clearances may be determined in conscious dogs trained to rest quietly in slings. For such determinations, catheters may be placed in the saphenous vein and urinary bladder. Inulin is infused via the saphenous vein catheter, and urine is collected via the bladder catheter; the bladder is rinsed with sterile water after each collection. Blood is sampled by jugular vein venipuncture.[3]

1.2.2 Dosing regimens

1.2.2.1 Rats

A variety of dosing regimens have been reported for the determination of inulin clearance in rats. For example, Burtin and colleagues used a priming dose of 50 mg kg^{-1} followed by a continuing infusion of saline (0.8 ml × h^{-1} × 100 g body $weight^{-1}$) containing inulin (6 g l^{-1}).[7] Ohishi and co-workers administered a priming dose of inulin (188 mg kg^{-1}) followed by a continuous infusion of 235 mg inulin × kg^{-1} × h^{-1} at a rate of 5 ml × kg^{-1} × h^{-1}.[8] These dosing regimens are usually sufficient to maintain the plasma concentration of inulin constant over a 2- to 4-h time interval. Trial runs may be necessary when dealing with inulin clearance following administration of a toxicant, since these conditions may lead to rising plasma inulin concentrations if GFR has been altered by the toxicant. We allow a 15- to 30-min equilibration period before beginning our collections. For rats, we usually use a 30-min urine collection interval to obtain sufficient urine for analysis. We collect urine from the bladder catheter into a preweighed vial and determine urine volume by weight (assuming a specific gravity for urine of 1.0). We obtain a blood sample, usually 200 to 250 μl, from the carotid artery cannula at the midpoint of the urine collection period. Blood is allowed to clot, and serum is harvested following centrifugation.

Inulin may be detected following conjugation of a fluorescent tag. For example, Gekle and Silbernagl measured inulin clearance using fluorescein isothiocyanate (FITC)-inulin dissolved in Ringer's solution at a concentration of 2 mg ml^{-1} and infused at a rate of 50 μl min^{-1}.[9] FITC-inulin was determined fluorimetrically with an excitation wavelength of 480 nm and an emission wavelength of 520 nm.

Radioactive inulin (see below) may be used to determine inulin clearance. A typical dosing regimen would be a bolus i.v. dose of 10 μCi of [methoxy-^{3}H]-inulin (specific activity about 300 μCi g^{-1}) with a sustaining infusion of 10 μCi in a volume of 1.2 ml saline for 60 min.[10] Other investigators have omitted the bolus dose of inulin and used a sustaining infusion of [^{14}C]-inulin in saline (1 μCi ml^{-1}) at a rate of 1.2 ml h^{-1}.[11] A distinct advantage of using radiolabeled inulin is that much smaller blood samples are required for quantitation of inulin. Typically, 50 to 100 μl of blood or urine is sufficient for radiochemical detection.

1.2.2.2 Rabbits

Various dosage regimens are available for inulin administration to rabbits. For example, Pedrotti and colleagues used 1.8 to 3.0-kg rabbits and administered a priming dose of 125 mg ml^{-1} inulin followed by a sustaining infusion of Ringer solution containing 2.5 mg% inulin at a rate of 0.1 ml min^{-1} into the marginal ear vein.[12] Benabe and Cordova infused inulin at a dose of 25 mg ml^{-1} saline and a rate of 0.12 ml min^{-1}.[13] They allowed a 45-min equilibration period, then obtained urine for 10- to 20-min collection intervals. Hanslik and co-workers used [^{3}H]-inulin infused at a concentration of 0.1 μCi min^{-1} in saline (0.5 ml $\times$ min^{-1} $\times$ kg^{-1}) and allowed a 90-min equilibration period, after which they used urine collection intervals of 30-min, with blood drawn at the midpoint of the urine collection interval.[14]

1.2.2.3 Dogs

For determination of inulin clearance, dogs received inulin at a dose of 35 mg kg^{-1} body weight via the jugular cannula. Following administration of the bolus dose, inulin was infused via the jugular cannula at a dose of 1.10 mg $\times$ kg^{-1} $\times$ min^{-1} (infusion rate was 0.3 ml $\times$ kg^{-1} $\times$ min^{-1}). This dosage regimen was sufficient to maintain stable plasma inulin concentrations for 6 h. We collected urine for 10- or 30-min intervals and obtained a blood sample at the midpoint of the collection period. Inulin solutions were prepared by dissolving inulin in 0.9% saline.

In conscious, chronically instrumented dogs, inulin clearance was determined following intravenous administration of a 1.4-g inulin bolus dose followed by a continuous infusion of 0.015 g inulin per minute in 1 ml min^{-1} 5% dextrose. Dogs were allowed to equilibrate for at least 50 min, after which urine was collected for 30-min intervals, with blood sampling at the midpoint of the collection period.[15] In conscious dogs, inulin clearance was determined by administering a bolus dose of 0.27 μCi [^{14}C]-inulin kg^{-1} body weight followed by 0.002 μCi $\times$ min^{-1} $\times$ kg^{-1} as a maintenance infusion. Dogs were allowed to equilibrate for 40 min, then 20-min urine collections were made. Blood was sampled at the beginning and end of each clearance period.[3]

1.3 Determination of GFR by plasma clearance of inulin

As a fairly large molecule, inulin (mol wt 5000) distributes into extracellular fluid, but does not cross cell membranes to enter intracellular fluid. The only route of elimination of inulin is via urinary excretion. Therefore, the plasma clearance of inulin is a measure of GFR. For this analysis, an investigator may administer a large dose of inulin i.v. and monitor the plasma concentration of inulin over time. Collection of urine is not necessary and animals need not be anesthetized if an arterial or venous sampling port has been established. We have tried this method to determine inulin clearance in conscious rats, using a cannulated tail vein as our venous line. However, we have found that obtaining the blood sample at the correct time is not always possible and have abandoned this approach. We have had limited success in determining plasma clearance of inulin in anesthetized rats by cannulating the carotid artery for obtaining blood samples.

Lin and co-workers used a single injection of [^{14}C]-inulin (administered intra-arterially) at 6 mg kg^{-1} (specific activity 2.7 mCi g^{-1}) in male Sprague–Dawley rats and followed plasma concentrations of inulin to determine GFR.[16] They implanted cannulae in the right jugular vein for blood sampling and the left carotid artery for drug administration the day before inulin administration and allowed rats to recover from the surgical procedures. Time-averaged total body clearance of [^{14}C]-inulin was 11.3 ± 1.3 ml × min^{-1} × kg^{-1}, half-life was 20.7 ± 2.5 min, and apparent volume of distribution was 225 ± 17.3 ml kg^{-1}.[16] The value for total body clearance of inulin calculated by the single injection method was in good agreement with their estimates of GFR following an infusion protocol (loading dose of 5 μCi inulin kg^{-1} followed by continuous infusion of 0.0855 μCi min^{-1} yielding a chemical concentration of 31.66 μg min^{-1}).[16]

Figure 4 illustrates the plot we would expect following administration of inulin to a 300-g rat. We assumed that we could achieve a maximal plasma inulin concentration of 50 mg ml^{-1} and the concentration would decline according to GFR, assumed to be 10 ml × min^{-1} × kg^{-1}. Further, we assumed that the volume of distribution of inulin was approximately 250 ml kg^{-1} or about 75 ml in a 300-g rat. We assumed our initial dose of inulin was 12.5 g kg^{-1} (3.75 g in a 300-g rat) in order to achieve a maximum plasma concentration of 50 mg ml^{-1}. By standard pharmacokinetic analysis, the slope of the regression line is $-k_{el} \div 2.3$ where k_{el} = elimination rate constant (min^{-1}) and the half-life of inulin is $k_{el} \div 0.693$. The hypothetical values used to construct the curve illustrated in Figure 4 are given in Table 2. For these hypothetical concentrations, a linear regression analysis of time (X variable) vs. log [inulin]$_{plasma}$ (Y variable) yielded a slope of –0.0174.

$$\text{slope} = -k_{el} \div 2.303 \text{ so } k_{el} = -\text{slope} \times 2.303 = 0.0174 \times 2.303 = 0.04007 \text{ min}^{-1} \quad (4)$$

$$t_{1/2} = 0.693 \div k_{el} = 0.693 \div 0.04007 \text{ min}^{-1} = 17.3 \text{ min} \quad (5)$$

$$Cl_{plasma} = V_d \times k_{el} = 250 \text{ ml kg}^{-1} \times 0.04007 \text{ min}^{-1} = 10.0 \text{ ml} \times \text{min}^{-1} \times \text{kg}^{-1} \quad (6)$$

A value of 10 ml × min^{-1} × kg^{-1} for plasma clearance of inulin in a 300-g rat is quite close to the measured value of 1 ml × min^{-1} × 100 g body weight^{-1} measured by other investigators for GFR (see Table 1). More detailed considerations of simple pharmacokinetic analyses may be found in Welling[17] and Pratt and Taylor.[18]

Similarly, plasma clearance of inulin may be used to estimate GFR in conscious, restrained rabbits. For example, Babini and colleagues administered a bolus dose of 15 mg inulin kg^{-1} i.v. to conscious rabbits and obtained blood samples via a cannula in the central ear artery from 3 through 90 min following inulin administration.[6] They determined that inulin clearance was 2.27 ± 0.29 ml × min^{-1} × kg^{-1} in rabbits fed a diet containing a normal amount of salt.[6]

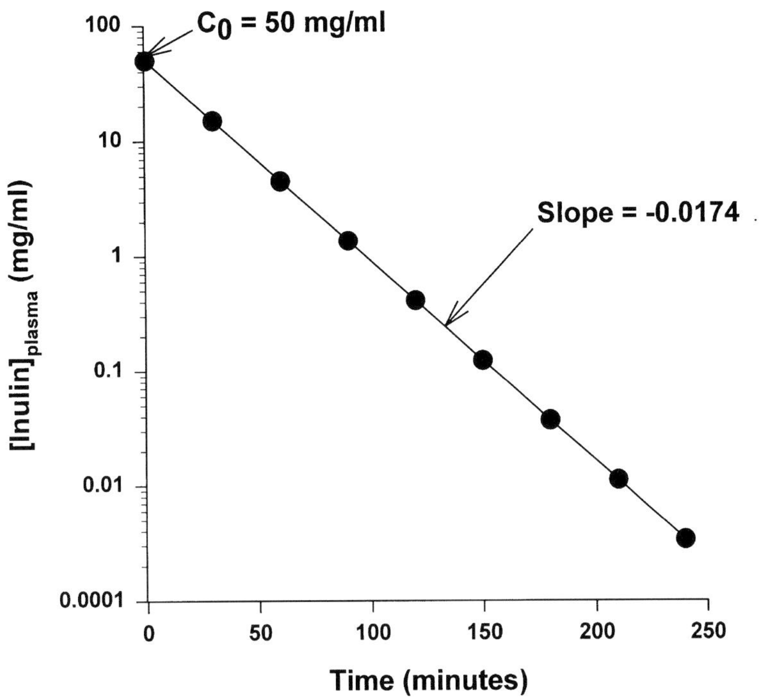

Figure 4 Plasma clearance of inulin (hypothetical). A 300-g rat received inulin sufficient to yield an initial plasma concentration of 50 mg ml^{-1}. Plasma inulin concentration was modeled to decline according to glomerular filtration rate. The data were plotted as log $[\text{inulin}]_{\text{plasma}}$ vs. time, and linear regression analysis yielded a slope of –0.0174.

Table 2 Theoretical Plasma Inulin Concentrations in a 300-g Rat

Time (min)	$[\text{Inulin}]_{\text{plasma}}$ (mg min^{-1})
0	50
30	15.039
60	4.524
90	1.361
120	0.409
150	0.123
180	0.037
210	0.011
240	0.003

Determination of GFR by measuring the plasma clearance of inulin is not without problems. For example, blood samples must be collected at short intervals during the first one or two half-lives (20 to 40 min in a rat), and small imprecisions in timing of blood collections may complicate interpretation of the data. As plasma inulin concentration declines, at some point the investigator is working with inulin concentrations at or below the limit of colorimetric detection, again complicating interpretation of the data. However, measuring the plasma clearance of inulin, particularly if radioactive inulin is used, is a quick and convenient method to determine if alterations in GFR have occurred following toxicant administration.

1.4 Determination of inulin in plasma and urine

Several methods exist for colorimetric determination of inulin. All methods involve hydrolyzing inulin by incubation with hot acid and developing the resultant fructose with various reagents. Colorimetric detection of inulin in plasma is not difficult, since infusion conditions are adjusted so that plasma inulin concentrations are maintained at 0.5 to 1 mg ml^{-1}, well within the detection range of most assays. Detection of inulin present in urine is more complicated because urine will generally need to be diluted to bring the inulin concentration into the desired range. Some calculations may be required in order to achieve the correct dilution. For example, normal glomerular filtration rate in rats is 1 ml × min^{-1} × 100 g body $weight^{-1}$, and urine flow rate is 3 µl × min^{-1} × 100 g body $weight^{-1}$ (see Table 1). For an average 300-g rat and a plasma inulin concentration of 1 mg ml^{-1}, the rate of inulin filtration will be about 3 mg min^{-1} (calculated as GFR × $[inulin]_{plasma}$). Over a 30-min collection period, urine will contain about 90 mg of inulin. The amount of urine collected from a 300-g rat over 30 min would be about 270 µl so that the concentration of inulin in urine would be about 333 mg ml^{-1}. In order to come into the range of the standard curves described below, the urine sample would require a 300- to 350-fold dilution. If urine flow rate is lower than normal, urine will need more dilution; whereas if urine flow rate is greater than normal, urine will require less dilution. It is advisable to estimate the amount of inulin filtered and the expected urinary inulin concentration based on the volume of urine collected in order to accurately dilute urinary samples for quantitation of inulin.

1.4.1 Diphenylamine assay[19]

Reagents

A. 0.75 *N* sodium hydroxide: 15 g NaOH in 500 ml ultrapure water
B. 4.8 *N* sodium hydroxide: 96 g NaOH in 500 ml ultrapure water
C. 6 *N* H_2SO_4: 7 ml concentrated H_2SO_4 plus 35 ml ultrapure water
D. $ZnSO_4$ in H_2SO_4: 25 g $ZnSO_4$ in 10 ml 6 *N* H_2SO_4; dilute to 250 ml with ultrapure water and heat to get into solution
E. Diphenylamine mixture (do under fume hood): glacial acetic acid, 200 ml; diphenylamine, 4 g; concentrated HCl (37%), 120 ml (completely dissolve diphenylamine in glacial acetic acid before adding HCl)

Standards

1. Prepare a working stock solution of inulin at a concentration of 10 mg ml^{-1}. This solution may be prepared by appropriate dilution of the inulin solution used for the priming and sustaining doses.
2. Working standards: dilute all solutions to 10 ml. Prepare a standard curve with concentrations of inulin ranging from 0.01 mg ml^{-1} to 1 mg ml^{-1}. For example, for a working standard containing 0.01 mg inulin ml^{-1}, dilute the 10 mg inulin ml^{-1} stock solution 1000-fold (e.g., 10 µl of 10 mg ml^{-1} stock solution diluted to 10 ml).
3. Use 100 µl of each standard as described in the assay procedure to construct a standard curve.

Procedure

1. Dilute 100 µl of plasma, standard, or urine (diluted as necessary) with 500 µl of ultrapure water.
2. Add 200 µl of zinc sulfate–sulfuric acid solution.
3. While vortexing, add 200 µl of 0.75 *N* sodium hydroxide solution.

4. Centrifuge mixture for 15 to 20 min at about 1000 rpm.
5. Transfer 0.5 ml of supernatant to fresh tubes. We generally use screw-top culture tubes.
6. Add 100 μl of 4.8 *N* sodium hydroxide solution and mix.
7. Cover tubes with cap and heat for 10 min at 100°C. We use a heating block for this step since it gives more reliable temperature control than a water bath.
8. Cool samples to room temperature.
9. Add 2 ml of diphenylamine mixture and mix.
10. Cap again and heat for 30 min at 100°C.
11. Cool samples to room temperature and read absorbance at 620 nm.

1.4.2 *Resorcinol assay*[20]

Reagents

A. Cadmium sulfate: 34.67 g $CdSO_4 \cdot H_2O$ plus 169 ml 1 *N* H_2SO_4 diluted to a final volume of 1 l with ultrapure water
B. 1.1 *N* NaOH: 22 g NaOH in 500 ml ultrapure water
C. Resorcinol solution: 100 mg resorcinol dissolved in 100 ml 95% ethanol
D. 30% HCl solution: 100 ml ultrapure water plus 22.4 ml concentrated hydrochloric acid

Standards

1. Prepare working standards as follows:

Standard No. 1	0.2 mg ml^{-1}	Use 100 μl for assay
Standard No. 2	0.4 mg ml^{-1}	Use 100 μl for assay
Standard No. 3	1 mg ml^{-1}	Use 20 μl for assay
Standard No. 4	4 mg ml^{-1}	Use 20 μl for assay

2. After pipetting the proper amount of standard, dilute to a final volume of 2.0 ml with ultrapure water.

Procedure

Plasma (final dilution of plasma is 1:15)

1. Pipet 500 μl of plasma into screw-top culture tube.
2. Add 5.0 ml ultrapure water.
3. Add 1.5 ml cadmium sulfate solution and 0.5 ml 1.1 *N* NaOH solution.
4. Place cap on culture tube and vortex mixture.
5. Centrifuge culture tubes for 10 min at about 1000 rpm.
6. Pipet 2 ml supernatant into clean screw-top culture tubes.

Urine

1. Dilute urine as necessary to come into range of standard curve.
2. Pipet 2 ml of dilute urine sample into a screw-top culture tube.
3. To all samples (blanks, standards, urine, and plasma), add 2.0 ml resorcinol solution.
4. To all samples, add 5 ml 30% HCl and vortex.
5. Place in 80°C water bath for 25 min. Cool in ice bath for 3 min. Read absorbance at 490 nm.

Note: Standards in this assay are used as references to check the reliability and reproducibility of the assay, not to construct a standard curve. Standards No. 1 and No. 3 should have approximately equal absorbencies. The absorbance of Standard No. 2 should be approximately twice that of Standards No. 1 and No. 3. The absorbance of Standard No. 4 should be approximately twice that of Standard No. 2.

1.4.3 Radiochemical assay

Particularly in rats, obtaining sufficient blood for colorimetric determination of inulin is often difficult. We often use radioactive inulin to ease detection, particularly when inulin concentrations in plasma or urine are low. We prepare a solution containing 1 to 10 μCi of radiolabeled inulin diluted with nonradiolabeled inulin to a concentration of 100 mg ml^{-1} and administer as an i.v. bolus dose. For determination of GFR, we use a single injection and measure the plasma clearance of inulin, as described above. We usually use carboxyl-[^{14}C]-inulin, commercially available from DuPont–New England Nuclear with a specific activity of 1 to 3 mCi g^{-1}. Generally labeled [^{3}H]–inulin and methoxy-[^{3}H]-inulin are commercially available from DuPont–New England Nuclear with specific activities of 100 to 500 mCi g^{-1}. Usually, for radiolabeled inulin, using a 50- to 100-μl aliquot of plasma or urine for liquid scintillation counting is sufficient.

1.4.4 Calculations

Inulin clearance is calculated as described below. It is not necessary to convert absorbancies or dpm data to concentrations since both plasma and urine inulin concentrations will be expressed in absorbance units or disintegrations per minute per milliliter of sample. It is necessary to account for any plasma or urinary dilutions made for colorimetric determination of inulin. The following formula describes the calculation of inulin clearance:

$$Cl_{inulin} = \frac{[\text{inulin}]_{urine}(\text{absorbance units per ml}) \times \text{dilution facor } \times \text{urine flow rate (ml per min)}}{[\text{inulin}]_{plasma}(\text{absorbance units per ml}) \times \text{dilution factor}} \quad (7)$$

Similarly, inulin clearance may be calculated using disintegrations per minute (dpm) sample $volume^{-1}$ as follows:

$$Cl_{inulin} = \frac{[\text{inulin}]_{urine}(\text{dpm per sample volume}) \times \text{urine flow rate (ml per min)}}{[\text{inulin}]_{plasma}(\text{dpm per sample volume}^{-1})} \quad (8)$$

1.5 Determination of GFR using creatinine clearance

Clearance of endogenous creatinine may also be used to measure GFR.[2,21] Creatinine has several advantages over inulin for the determination of GFR:

1. Since creatinine is present in serum, it does not require continuous infusion to achieve steady-state plasma concentrations.
2. Creatinine may be measured colorimetrically using commercially available kits or autoanalyzer methods.

However, measurement of creatinine clearance is not without drawbacks. Specific criticisms include:

1. Relatively large plasma samples (300 μl) are required for determination of creatinine by a commercially available method using alkaline picrate (Sigma Tech. Bull. No. 555).
2. Nonspecific chromagens in plasma and urine may interfere with the determination of creatinine, overestimating plasma and urinary concentrations.[21,22]

3. Creatinine may undergo tubular secretion in the kidney, thus overestimating GFR to the extent that tubular secretion occurs. Secretion of creatinine is readily apparent in humans, rats, and dogs.[21,23,24]
4. Plasma concentrations of endogenous creatinine are relatively low and may be at the lower limit of detection by the alkaline picrate assay method. In dogs, plasma creatinine concentrations ranged from 0.75 to 3.2 mg dl^{-1}, while in rats, plasma creatinine concentrations ranged from 0.2 to 0.3 mg dl^{-1}.[3,24] Standards provided in the alkaline picrate reaction kit (Sigma Tech. Bull. No. 555) range from 2.5 to 10 mg dl^{-1}.

Darling and Morris measured exogenous inulin clearance and endogenous creatinine clearance in female Lewis rats and observed that the mean control $Cl_{creatinine}/Cl_{inulin}$ ratio was 2.33 ± 0.83 (mean ± SD).[24] For these determinations, creatinine in plasma and urine was measured by a method employing fuller's earth to remove interfering substances. Following administration of probenecid to the same rats, $Cl_{creatinine}/Cl_{inulin}$ decreased to 1.26 ± 0.28, suggesting that a portion of creatinine clearance is due to tubular secretion.[24] When the same samples were analyzed by the less specific commercial assay (Sigma Tech. Bull. No. 555), the $Cl_{creatinine}/Cl_{inulin}$ ratio was not significantly different from unity (1.12 ± 0.41) and probenecid treatment significantly decreased the clearance ratio to 0.53 ± 0.12, suggesting that creatinine undergoes tubular reabsorption as well as tubular secretion in rats.[24]

Van Liew and co-workers compared endogenous creatinine clearance with inulin clearance in five strains of rats (Table 3).[25] Rats were anesthetized and surgically prepared for inulin infusion and blood and urine collection. Inulin was administered in isotonic saline at a rate of 0.02 ml min^{-1}, and saline contained 4 g dl^{-1} inulin. Urine collection intervals were 120 min and blood was taken from the tail vein at the beginning, middle, and end of the urine collection period. Creatinine concentrations in plasma and urine were measured following absorption and elution of nonspecific chromagens by chemical treatment of samples. Except in the Biobreeding strain of rats, creatinine and inulin clearances were not significantly different, suggesting that creatinine and inulin clearances are both suitable markers for GFR. In Biobreeding rats, creatinine clearance was significantly lower than simultaneously determined inulin clearance, suggesting that in this strain of rats, creatinine is filtered and reabsorbed by the kidneys and creatinine clearance underestimates GFR.[25] Thus, the interpretation of creatinine clearance data may be complicated by the detection method used as well as by competing processes of tubular secretion and reabsorption.

Table 3 Clearance of Inulin and Creatinine in Anesthetized Rats

Strain	Age (months)	Creatinine (ml × min^{-1} × g $kidney^{-1}$)	Inulin
Wistar (nephrotoxic nephritis, n = 9)	4	0.64 ± 0.06	0.68 ± 0.07
Wistar/Kyoto (n = 6)	3	1.14 ± 0.11	1.39 ± 0.08
Spontaneously hypertensive (n = 5)	17	0.39 ± 0.07	0.31 ± 0.05
Biobreeding			
Diabetic prone (n = 10)	7	0.55 ± 0.07[a]	1.08 ± 0.12
Diabetic resistant (n = 4)	7	0.57 ± 0.12[a]	1.04 ± 0.07

[a] Significantly different from inulin clearance.

Modified from Van Liew, J. B., Zamlauski-Tucker, M. J., and Feld, L. G., *Life Sci.*, 53, 1015, 1993.

Van Liew and colleagues also compared endogenous creatinine clearance with the plasma clearance of [^{3}H]-inulin. Conscious, restrained rats received 50 μCi of [^{3}-H-methoxy]-inulin (specific activity 42 mCi g^{-1}) via tail vein injection.[25] Blood samples (40 μl) were taken from the cut tail tip over 2 h with a total volume of 0.4 ml removed for analysis. In Wistar–Kyoto rats, values for 18-h creatinine clearance (in fed rats) were indistinguishable from clearance values calculated from a single injection of ^{3}H-inulin (Table 4), suggesting that determination of endogenous creatinine clearance was a reliable marker for GFR. In the Biobreeding strain of rat, endogenous creatinine clearance was lower than ^{3}H-inulin clearance, again suggesting that creatinine reabsorption occurs in this strain of rat.[25]

Table 4 Comparison of Creatinine Clearance and Plasma Clearance of Inulin in Conscious, Restrained Rats

Strain	Sex	Age	N	Creatinine	^{3}H-inulin
				(ml × min^{-1} × 100 g body weight^{-1})	
Wistar–Kyoto	M	3	6	0.81 ± 0.02	0.84 ± 0.03
Biobreeding diabetic prone	M	8	6	0.87 ± 0.04[a]	1.31 ± 0.12
	M	16	6	0.67 ± 0.04[a]	0.91 ± 0.04
	F	9	6	0.71 ± 0.04	0.99 ± 0.13
Biobreeding diabetic resistant	M	8	8	0.42 ± 0.02[a]	0.63 ± 0.03
	M	16	9	0.47 ± 0.01[a]	0.67 ± 0.03

[a] Significantly different from ^{3}H-inulin clearance.

Modified from Van Liew, J. B., Zamlauski-Tucker, M. J., and Feld, L. G., *Life Sci.*, 53, 1015, 1993.

Finco and co-workers compared clearances determined with [^{14}C]-inulin and creatinine infusions in conscious dogs.[3] Creatinine concentrations in plasma were determined by a specific enzymatic method, peroxidase–antiperoxidase (PAP)[26] as well as the standard Jaffe method (Sigma Tech. Bull. No. 555). For 111 measurements, mean ± SE clearance values were 2.34 ± 0.82 ml × min^{-1} × kg^{-1} for [^{14}C]–inulin, 2.40 ± 0.83 ml × min^{-1} × kg^{-1} for PAP creatinine, and 2.01 ± 0.59 ml × min^{-1} × kg^{-1} for Jaffe creatinine. The PAP creatinine-to-inulin clearance ratio was 1.03 ± 0.08 while the Jaffe creatinine-to-inulin clearance ratio was 0.88 ± 0.10, indicating that PAP creatinine clearance and inulin clearance agree well, but the Jaffe creatinine clearance significantly underestimates inulin clearance.[3] Finco and co-workers also determined 20-min and 24-h creatinine clearances with creatinine determined by the standard Jaffe method and the PAP method. In clinically normal dogs, 20-min PAP creatinine clearances were not significantly different from 24-h PAP creatinine clearances. Similarly, Jaffe creatinine clearances were not significantly different for 20-min or 24-h collections. However, PAP creatinine clearance values were significantly greater than Jaffe creatinine values for both 20-min and 24-h collection intervals.[3]

Hall and co-workers measured creatinine clearance in conscious rats by collecting urine for 24 h, with blood sampling at the end point of the collection interval.[27] In control rats, 24-h endogenous creatinine clearance was about 3 ml × min^{-1} × kg^{-1}, considerably lower than the values reported in Table 1 for inulin clearance in rats. Brooks and colleagues collected 24-h urine samples from conscious, unrestrained dogs, with blood sampling at the beginning and end of each 24-h clearance interval.[28] Using this method, 24-h endogenous creatinine clearance in the dogs averaged about 2.5 ml × min^{-1} × kg^{-1} (estimated from graph[28]), slightly lower than values reported for inulin clearance in dogs (Table 1).

1.6 Determination of renal clearance of toxicants

Standard clearance methods may be used to determine renal clearance of a particular drug or chemical. Incorporation of a reference marker such as inulin or creatinine into the experimental design simplifies interpretation of clearance data. The same surgical manipulations are used to obtain blood and urine samples, and the same calculations are done to estimate clearance of the chemical of interest and/or marker substance.

Lin and colleagues used simultaneous infusion of famotidine and [^{14}C]-inulin in rats to determine renal clearance of famotidine.[16] The data in Table 5 obtained from these experiments suggest that (1) famotidine is filtered and secreted by the kidney, accounting for fractional excretions (Cl_R/GFR) greater than 1.0, and (2) some famotidine may be reabsorbed, particularly at high filtered loads of famotidine, as suggested by fractional excretions less than 1.0. Total systemic clearance of famotidine was greater than renal clearance, suggesting that a portion of famotidine was cleared from plasma by nonrenal mechanisms, presumably by hepatic metabolism.[16] Thus, by comparing clearances of a test compound (famotidine) with a suitable marker substance (inulin), an investigator may identify renal mechanisms involved in urinary elimination of the test compound (filtration, reabsorption, and/or secretion) as well as the extent of nonrenal mechanisms in the plasma elimination of the test compound.

Table 5 Renal Clearance of Famotidine and Inulin in Rats

Famotidine				
Loading dose (mg kg^{-1})	Infusion rate (μg min^{-1})	Cl_R (ml × min^{-1} × kg^{-1})	GFR (ml × min^{-1} × kg^{-1})	Clearance ratio
0.25	3.6	35.4 ± 4.9	10.9 ± 1.6	3.25
0.5	7.2	42.2 ± 5.4	11.8 ± 2.1	3.58
1.25	18	29.5 ± 9.6	8.7 ± 1.4	3.39
2.5	36	43.0 ± 11.3	12.9 ± 2.9	3.33
5	72	30.8 ± 6.4	12.3 ± 2.3	2.50
10	140	11.9 ± 3.5	8.4 ± 1.6	1.42
20	290	11.8 ± 1.7	11.7 ± 0.6	1.01
30	433	9.23 ± 2.6	8.7 ± 3.3	0.72
45	576	7.89 ± 5.0	9.1 ± 4.6	0.87

Modified from Lin, J. H., Los, L. E., Ulm, E. H., and Duggan, D. E., *Drug Metab. Dispos.*, 15, 212, 1987.

1.7 Determination of the effects of toxicants on GFR

The ease of determining GFR, either as inulin clearance or as endogenous creatinine clearance, has facilitated comparison of GFR in drug-treated vs. control animals. Hanslik and co-workers induced severe end-stage renal disease, as assessed by histological examination, by administering saline (2 ml every 12 h) or gentamicin (60 mg kg^{-1} every 12 h) subcutaneously to male New Zealand rabbits.[14] After 7 days of treatment, rabbits were anesthetized and surgically prepared for clearance determinations. In these experiments, gentamicin treatment for 7 days resulted in a 55% reduction in GFR (from 5.79 ± 1.07 ml × min^{-1} × kg^{-1} in saline-treated rabbits to 3.23 ± 2.26 ml × min^{-1} × kg^{-1} in gentamicin-treated rabbits) and a 60% reduction in renal plasma flow (from 16.54 ± 2.69 ml × min^{-1} × kg^{-1} in saline-treated rabbits to 9.84 ± 7.97 ml × min^{-1} × kg^{-1}), measured as PAH clearance.[14] Despite the marked reduction in inulin clearance, glomerular morphology was normal. However, the authors observed massive and diffuse acute tubular necrosis involving medulla and cortex, indicating that gentamicin is nephrotoxic.[14]

In male Sprague–Dawley rats, treatment with gentamicin (40 mg kg^{-1} body weight day^{-1} s.c.) for 13 consecutive days caused a significant decrease in GFR (1.20 ± 0.07 ml × min^{-1} × g $kidney^{-1}$ in control rats vs. 0.33 ± 0.02 ml × min^{-1} × g $kidney^{-1}$ in gentamicin-treated rats) and a significant increase in urine volume (1.39 ± 0.14 µl × min^{-1} × g $kidney^{-1}$ in control rats vs. 3.49 ± 0.69 µl × min^{-1} × g $kidney^{-1}$ in gentamicin-treated rats).[11] Concurrent administration of superoxide dismutase or dimethylthiourea, a hydroxyl radical scavenger, partially prevented gentamicin-induced changes in inulin clearance and urine output.[11]

In male Wistar rats, daily administration of ochratoxin A (0.5 mg kg^{-1} i.p.) for 6 days resulted in a 64% decrease in GFR (measured as FITC-inulin clearance, 1.08 ± 0.06 ml × min^{-1} × g kidney $weight^{-1}$ in control rats vs. 0.69 ± 0.04 ml × min^{-1} × g kidney $weight^{-1}$ in ochratoxin A-treated rats) and a 49% decrease in renal plasma flow (measured as PAH clearance, 3.98 ± 0.18 vs. 1.97 ± 0.18 ml × min^{-1} × g kidney $weight^{-1}$ in control vs. ochratoxin A-treated rats, respectively). The parallel decreases in GFR and renal plasma flow suggested that ochratoxin A produced these effects through alterations in renal hemodynamics or by activating tubuloglomerular feedback mechanisms.[9] Blocking tubuloglomerular feedback by use of furosemide failed to protect rats from ochratoxin A-induced changes in GFR or renal plasma flow whereas inhibition of angiotensin II by enalapril, a converting enzyme inhibitor, or DUP 753, a specific angiotensin II receptor antagonist, ameliorated ochratoxin A-induced alterations in GFR and renal plasma flow. These studies demonstrate the importance of determining not only GFR but also renal plasma flow in order to rule out hemodynamic factors that may contribute to reductions in GFR.[9]

Amphotericin B nephrotoxicity is characterized initially by a decline in renal blood flow and GFR followed by severe damage to the distal tubule. By measuring endogenous creatinine clearance in conscious, unrestrained dogs, Brooks and colleagues demonstrated that treatment with 1 mg kg^{-1} day^{-1} of amphotericin B (i.v.) significantly decreased creatinine clearance with corresponding increases in serum creatinine concentrations from 2 through 4 days of treatment, from slightly greater than 2 ml × min^{-1} × kg^{-1} on the first treatment day to a low of about 0.5 ml × min^{-1} × kg^{-1} on days 3 and 4 of amphotericin B treatment (estimated from graphical data).[28] It is not entirely clear what values the authors used for plasma creatinine concentration in their calculation of creatinine clearance. Blood was obtained at the beginning and end, rather than the midpoint, of the urine collection interval so that technically, the values should have been averaged for the clearance calculation. Since glomerular filtration rate was falling, plasma creatinine concentrations were not at steady state, complicating interpretation and calculation of clearance values. However, even allowing for these ambiguities, determination of 24-h creatinine clearance was sufficiently sensitive to detect a 50 to 75% reduction following amphotericin B treatment.[28]

1.8 Conclusions

Determination of GFR, either as inulin or creatinine clearance, is relatively simple once surgical techniques are mastered. The procedure is inexpensive unless radiolabeled inulin is used. Clearance techniques are not routinely used in toxicological studies, and deterioration of renal function is usually assessed as increases in serum creatinine or blood urea nitrogen concentrations. However, alterations in serum creatinine or blood urea nitrogen concentration require a substantial loss of renal function;[29] therefore subtle toxicant-induced changes in GFR may be overlooked.

Measurement of renal clearance of a toxicant may be of more toxicological relevance than determination of GFR per se, particularly if the renal clearance of a toxicant is compared with the renal clearance of inulin. By this method, an investigator may obtain preliminary information concerning the mechanisms involved in renal elimination of the toxicant. For example, by comparing the clearances of toxicant and inulin, an investigator may be able to correlate nephrotoxicity with either reabsorption or secretion of the toxicant. By either reabsorption or secretion, renal tubular epithelial cells will be exposed to relatively high concentrations of a toxicant that may contribute to selective renal damage caused by the toxicant.

References

1. Vander, A. J., Renal clearance, in *Renal Physiology*, 3rd ed., McGraw–Hill, New York, 1983, chap. 3.
2. Valtin, H., Glomerular filtration, in *Renal Function*, 2nd ed., Little, Brown, Boston, MA, 1983, chap. 3.
3. Finco, D. R., Tabaru, H., Brown, S. A., and Barsanti, J. A., Endogenous creatinine clearance measurement of glomerular filtration rate in dogs, *Am. J. Vet. Res.*, 54, 1575, 1993.
4. Gagnon, J. A., Felipe, I., Nelson, L. D., and Butkus, D. E., Influence of thiopental anesthesia on renal sodium and water excretion in the dog, *Am. J. Physiol.*, 243, F265, 1982.
5. Walker, L. A., Buscemi–Bergin, M., and Gellai, M., Renal hemodynamics in conscious rats: effects of anesthesia, surgery, and recovery, *Am. J. Physiol.*, 245, F67, 1983.
6. Babini, R., Larose, P., Lécrivain, A., and duSouich, P., Furosemide dynamics: influence of dietary sodium and of saralasin, *Pharmacology*, 43, 282, 1991.
7. Burtin, M., Laouari, D., Kindermans, C., and Kleinknecht, C., Glomerular response to acute protein load is not blunted by high-protein diet or nephron reduction, *Am. J. Physiol.*, 266, F746, 1994.
8. Ohishi, K., Okwueze, M. I., Vari, R. C., and Carmines, P. K., Juxtamedullary microvascular dysfunction during the hyperfiltration stage of diabetes mellitus, *Am. J. Physiol.*, 267, F99, 1994.
9. Gekle, M. and Silbernagl, S., Mechanism of ochratoxin A-induced reduction of glomerular filtration rate in rats, *J. Pharmacol. Exp. Ther.*, 267, 316, 1993.
10. Wang, P., Ba, Z. F., Meldrum, D. R., and Chaudry, I. H., Diltiazem restores cardiac output and improves renal function after hemorrhagic shock and crystalloid resuscitation, *Am. J. Physiol.*, 262, 1435, 1992.
11. Nakajima, T., Hishida, A., and Kato, A., Mechanisms for protective effects of free radical scavengers on gentamicin-mediated nephropathy in rats, *Am. J. Physiol.*, 266, F425, 1994.
12. Pedrotti, A., Bonjour, J.-P., and Guignard, J. P., Protection from hypoxemia-induced renal dysfunction by the thiophosphate WR-2721, *Kidney Int.*, 41, 80, 1992.
13. Benabe, J. and Cordova, H. R., Effect of high-protein diet on renal concentration capacity in rabbits, *Am. J. Physiol.*, 263, F1051, 1992.
14. Hanslik, T., Blanchet, F., Nochy, D., Pirotzky, E., Guilmard, C., Seta, N., and Carbon, C., Effect of the platelet activating factor antagonist BN52021 in rabbits: role in gentamicin nephrotoxicity, *Toxicol. Appl. Pharmacol.*, 128, 111, 1994.
15. Woods, L. L., Mechanisms of renal vasodilation after protein feeding: role of the renin-angiotensin system, *Am. J. Physiol.*, 264, R601, 1993.
16. Lin, J. H., Los, L. E., Ulm, E. H., and Duggan, D. E., Urinary excretion kinetics of famotidine in rats, *Drug Metab. Dispos.*, 15, 212, 1987.
17. Welling, P. G., *Pharmacokinetics: Processes and Mathematics*, ACS Monograph 185, American Chemical Society, Washington, D.C., 1986.
18. Pratt, W. B. and Taylor, P., *Principles of Drug Action: The Basis of Pharmacology*, 3rd ed., Churchill Livingstone, New York, 1990.
19. Walser, M., Davidson, D. G., and Orloff, J., The renal clearance of alkali-stable inulin, *J. Clin. Invest.*, 34, 1520, 1955.
20. Schreiner, G. E., Determination of inulin by means of resorcinol, *Proc. Soc. Exp. Biol. Med.*, 74, 117, 1950.
21. Levey, A. S., Perrone, R. D., and Madias, N. E., Serum creatinine and renal function, *Ann. Rev. Med.*, 39, 465, 1988.
22. Narayanan, S. and Appleton, H. D., Creatinine: a review, *Clin. Chem.*, 26, 1119, 1980.

23. Bauer, J. H., Brooks, C. S., and Burch, R. N., Clinical appraisal of creatinine clearance as a measurement of glomerular filtration rate, *Am. J. Kidney Dis.*, 2, 337, 1982.
24. Darling, I. M. and Morris, M. E., Evaluation of "true" creatinine clearance in rats reveals extensive renal secretion, *Pharm. Res.*, 8, 1318, 1991.
25. Van Liew, J. B., Zamlauski–Tucker, M. J., and Feld, L. G., Endogenous creatinine clearance in the rat: strain variation, *Life Sci.*, 53, 1015, 1993.
26. Goren, M. P., Osborne, S., and Wright, R. K., A peroxidase-coupled kinetic enzymatic procedure evaluated for measuring serum and urinary creatinine, *Clin. Chem.*, 32, 548, 1986.
27. Hall, R. L., Wilke, W. L., and Fettman, M. J., Captopril slows the progression of chronic renal disease in partially nephrectomized rats, *Toxicol. Appl. Pharmacol.*, 80, 517, 1985.
28. Brooks, D. P., Mitchell, M. P., Short, B. G., Ruffolo, R. R., and Nichols, A. J., Attenuation of amphotericin B nephrotoxicity in the dog by the fenoldopam prodrug, SK&F R-105058, *J. Pharmacol. Exp. Ther.*, 257, 1243, 1991.
29. Berndt, W. O. and Davis, M. E., Renal methods for toxicology, in *Principles and Methods of Toxicology*, 2nd ed., Hayes, A. W., Ed., Raven Press, New York, 1989, 629.
30. Corman, B., Pratz, J., and Poujeol, P., Changes in anatomy, glomerular filtration, and solute excretion in aging rat kidney, *Am. J. Physiol.*, 248, R282, 1985.
31. Tarloff, J. B., Induction and Modification of the Nephrotoxicity of *S*-(1,2-dichlorovinyl)-L-cysteine in the Dog, Doctoral dissertation, Medical College of Ohio, Toledo, 1982.

chapter two

Urinary Markers

James S. Woods

2.1 Introduction 19
2.2 Enzymes 19
  2.2.1 Alanine aminopeptidase 20
  2.2.2 Alkaline phosphatase 20
  2.2.3 γ-Glutamyltranspeptidase 20
  2.2.4 *N*-Acetyl-β-D-glucosaminidase 21
  2.2.5 Cathepsin B 22
  2.2.6 Lysozyme 23
  2.2.7 Lactate dehydrogenase 24
2.3 Low molecular weight proteins 24
  2.3.1 β_2-Microglobulin 25
  2.3.2 α_1-Microglobulin 26
  2.3.3 Retinol-binding protein 27
2.4 Kidney-specific antigens 29
2.5 Kidney-derived porphyrins 29
2.6 Acknowledgment 29
References 29

2.1 Introduction

Renal injury resulting from exposure to drugs or environmental toxicants is a public health problem of major concern. The measurement of constituents excreted into the urine following injury to various segments of the nephron or collecting duct or other renal structures has proven to be highly useful in the clinical assessment of the site and severity of renal damage. Among the more important of these constituents are enzymes, low molecular weight proteins, kidney-specific antigens, and kidney-derived porphyrins. This chapter describes some of the more important techniques that have been developed in recent years to assess renal function by analysis of these constituents in the urine.

2.2 Enzymes

A number of enzymes have been employed as markers of renal tubular dysfunction and toxicity. The renal tubular brush border enzymes — alanine aminopeptidase, alkaline phosphatase, and γ-glutamyltranspeptidase — are excreted into the urine when released from the proximal tubular epithelium following tubular insult or injury. *N*-acetyl-β-D-

0-8493-3341-5/96/$0.00+$.50

glucosaminidase and cathepsin B, enzymes found in the lysosomal fraction of proximal tubular cells, and lysozyme (muramidase), a phagocytic enzyme that is reabsorbed into proximal tubular cells after glomerular filtration, are also considered sensitive indicators of injury to this portion of the nephron.

2.2.1 *Alanine aminopeptidase*

Determination of alanine aminopeptidase (AAP) (EC 3.4.11.2) activity in urine has been shown to be a suitable test in the recognition of certain renal diseases[1] as well as of nephrotoxicant exposure. Jung and Scholz[2] have described a spectrophotometric assay in which the activity of urinary AAP is measured after gel filtration of the urine to remove potentially interfering substances. Enzyme activity measurements may be optimized by use of a kinetic processor.[2] Initially, urine samples for AAP analysis are centrifuged to remove debris, and 3 ml of the supernatant is passed through a column of Sephadex G-50 (fine) at room temperature. The column is washed with 0.154 *M* NaCl, and eluates are collected in 1-ml fractions. AAP activity elutes in the 4th to 10th milliliters. For AAP determinations, two solutions are used. Solution A is 59 m*M* TRIS-HCl buffer, pH 7.8, and Solution B is 26 m*M* alanine-4-nitroanilide hydrochloride in the same TRIS-HCl buffer. Mix 1 ml of Solution A and 0.2 ml urine Sephadex eluate, allow to equilibrate at 37°C for 15 min, and start the reaction by adding 0.1 ml Solution B. AAP activity is measured at 410 nm and 37°C in cuvettes with 10 mm light path by monitoring the increase in absorbance resulting from release of 4-nitroaniline catalyzed by AAP in 2 min. Enzyme activity is linear for at least 25 min. Urine samples should be analyzed not later than 4 h after collection to prevent proteolytic deactivation of the enzyme. AAP activities in urine samples collected over a 24-h period from healthy men and women were 7.65 and 12.6 U/l, respectively, where 1 U = 1 μmol of substrate turnover per minute.[2]

2.2.2 *Alkaline phosphatase*

Alkaline phosphatase (AP) (EC 3.1.3.1) can be measured in the same gel filtration eluate as described for AAP above.[2–4] For this assay, 0.2 ml of eluate and 0.4 ml of 0.75 *M* buffer–substrate solution consisting of 2-amino-2-methyl-1-propanol-HCl, pH 10.3, and 4.5 m*M* disodium-*p*-nitrophenylphosphate are used. The initial reaction rate is determined by continuous measurement of the formation of *p*-nitrophenol at 405 nm at 37°C, as described for AAP.

2.2.3 *γ-Glutamyltranspeptidase*

γ-Glutamyltranspeptidase (GGT) (EC 2.3.2.2) is a renal tubular brush border enzyme typically found in low concentrations in normal human urine and in much higher levels in the case of proximal tubular injury. GGT activity is typically measured following gel filtration of the urine sample to remove potentially interfering substances, as described above for alanine aminopeptidase. The assay is based on the broad specificity of GGP toward γ-glutamyl compounds. The most widely used substrate is γ-glutamyl-*p*-nitroanilide, which is incubated with GGP and an acceptor such a glycylglycine. The *p*-nitroaniline released is readily determined from the increase in absorbance at 410 nm.[5]

For the assay, 0.2 ml of 1 m*M* (final concentration) L-γ-glutamyl-*p*-nitroanilide, 0.2 ml 20 m*M* (final concentration) glycylglycine and 0.6 ml 0.1 *M* TRIS-HCl buffer, pH 8.0, are placed in a spectrophotometer cuvette (1-cm light path). The volume of the buffer should be adjusted to allow for that of the enzyme solution added, the final volume of the reaction mixture being 1.0 ml. The solution is heated to 37°C in a spectrophotometer equipped with a thermostatted cuvette holder, and the reaction is initiated by adding a suitable amount of the enzyme solution. The rate of release of *p*-nitroaniline is then recorded at

410 nm (the ε for *p*-nitroaniline is 8800 $M^{-1}cm^{-1}$). GGT activity is expressed as μmol *p*-nitroaniline formed per minute (units), and the specific activity expressed as units per liter.

Diagnostic kits for both colorimetric and kinetic determination of GGT are commercially available, e.g., Sigma No. 545 and 418.

2.2.4 N-*Acetyl-β-*D*-glucosaminidase*

N-acetyl-β-D-glucosaminidase (NAG) (EC 3.2.1.30) is a lysosomal enzyme present in kidney tubule cells. Having a molecular weight of 130 to 140 Kd, NAG is not normally filtered at the glomerulus. Therefore, its presence in the urine is indicative of renal tubular cell injury. NAG has been shown to be a sensitive indicator of renal injury due to a variety of drugs and environmental toxicants.[6–8] A variety of methods have been developed for measuring NAG in urine.[6] Several are described here.

Leaback and Walker[9] have described a fluorometric procedure for measuring urinary NAG levels using the fluorogenic methylumbelliferyl-*N*-acetyl-β-glucosaminide (e.g., Sigma No. M 2133) as substrate. Initially, calibration curves are constructed with 4-methylumbelliferone (MUBF), the product of the enzyme reaction, in 0.15 *M* glycine buffer, pH 10.3. Leaback and Walker described linearity over the MUBF concentration ranges of 0.01 to 0.45 μg/ml and 0.0025 to 0.01 μg/ml. For the NAG assay, a single voided fresh urine sample is diluted 1:3 with ddH_2O, and 50 μl is added to 950 μl of a 0.2 m*M* methylumbelliferyl-*N*-acetyl-β-glucosaminide solution and incubated at 37°C for 30 min. Hydrolysis is stopped by adding 3 ml 0.25 *M* sodium glycinate buffer (pH 10.7), and the 4-methylumbelliferone released is measured by fluorescence at 450 nm after excitation at 365 nm. This method is fairly rapid and inexpensive, but lacks the sensitivity that may be required for monitoring preclinical or subtoxic injury to the kidney resulting from low level exposure to specific nephrotoxicants.

Horak et al.[10] introduced a practical and reliable spectrophotometric NAG assay that improves on the Leaback and Walker method by first removing inhibitors of NAG, which are normally found in the urine, prior to the enzyme assay. In this procedure, 10 ml of fresh urine is centrifuged at 900 × g for 10 min to remove debris, and 1 ml is filtered through a Sephadex G-25 column that has been previously washed with 10 ml 0.15 *M* aqueous NaCl. The urine is washed through the column with an additional 0.5 ml NaCl, and the eluate is discarded after the column is completely drained. The NAG-containing fraction is then eluted from the column into a collecting tube by washing with 2 ml NaCl.

To measure NAG activity, four spectrophotometric cuvettes (1-cm light path) are labeled RB (reagent blank), S (standard), U (urine), and UB (urine blank), and into the respective cuvette following solutions are pipetted: cuvette RB: 0.5 ml 0.15 *M* NaCl; cuvette S: 0.5 ml *p*-nitrophenol solution (100 μmol/l in 0.15 *M* NaCl); cuvettes U and UB: 0.5 ml of urine NAG eluate. All four cuvettes are equilibrated in a water bath at 37°C. Then 0.5 ml of NAG substrate solution (10 m*M* *p*-nitrophenyl-*N*-acetyl-β-D-glucosaminide [Sigma] in 0.1 *M* citrate buffer, pH 4.4) is added to RG, S, and U cuvettes, and samples are then incubated for exactly 15 min at 37°C. AMP buffer (0.75 *M* 2-amino-2-methyl-1-propanol hydrochloride, pH 10.25), 0.5 ml, is pipetted into all cuvettes, and at the same time 0.5 ml NAG–substrate solution is added to cuvette UB. The absorbance of all cuvettes is then measured at 405 nm. NAG activity is computed using the following formula:

$$\text{NAG Activity } (\mu\text{mol/min/l, U/l}) = \frac{\text{Abs}[\text{U-UB}] \times 100 \ \ \mu\text{mol/l} \times 2 \text{ (dilution factor)}}{\text{Abs}[\text{S-RB}] \times 15 \text{ (incubation time)}} \quad (1)$$

$$= \frac{\text{Abs}[\text{U-UB}]}{\text{Abs}[\text{S-RB}]} \times 13.3$$

Measurements of NAG activity in urine specimens of healthy adults derived from this method ranged from 3.3 to 4.1 U/l. NAG activity in spot urine specimens is expressed as units per gram creatinine. Reported values for NAG activities in spot urine samples from healthy adults range from 1.0 to 4.6 U/g creatinine.[10]

Goren et al.[7] have described an adaptation of the manual procedure of Horak et al.,[10] described above, for automated determinations of urinary NAG, using a Micro-KDA analyzer (American Monitor Corp., Indianapolis, IN). The procedure is as follows: 75 µl of urinary NAG Sephadex G-25 eluate is added to 1.4 ml of a solution containing 2.9 m*M* *p*-nitrophenyl-*N*-acetyl-β-D-glucosaminide (PNP) in 0.1 *M* citrate buffer, pH 4.5. After incubation for 25 min at 37°C, 0.3 ml of 1.5 *M* 2-amino-2-methyl-1-propanol hydrochloride is added to stop the reaction and to develop the color. The absorbance of PNP at 410 nm over that of a sample blank is compared with the absorbance of a 2 m*M* *p*-nitrophenol standard (equivalent to the reaction product liberated by 80 U/l of NAG) to obtain NAG activity.*

2.2.5 *Cathepsin B*

Cathepsin B (EC 3.4.4.9) is a lysosomal protein hydrolase that functions to digest proteins that are reabsorbed into proximal tubule cells from the tubular fluid following glomerular filtration. Under normal physiological conditions, small amounts of cathepsin B can be found in the urine, and, as in the case of NAG, levels increase after tubular cell damage.

The assay of cathepsin B is accomplished by a colorimetric procedure based on the detection of 2-naphthylamine, which is released following enzymatic proteolysis of the peptidyl substrate, benzyloxycarbonyl-arginyl-arginyl-2-naphthylamide (Z-Arg-Arg-NNap).[11] The color is formed by coupling 2-naphthylamine with the diazonium salt, Fast Garnet. A thiol (cysteine) is required to activate the enzyme. This would normally destroy the diazonium salt; however, a mercurial compound (Mersalyl–Brij) is introduced to prevent this as well as to terminate the enzymatic reaction. The following reagents are required for the assay:

The buffer/activator, consisting of 88 m*M* KH_2PO_4–12 m*M* Na_2HPO_4–1.33 m*M* disodium EDTA, and pH 6.9, freshly made 2.7m*M* cysteine by addition of the free base.

The substrate stock solution, consisting of Z-Arg-Arg-NNap (available from a number of commercial suppliers), dissolved in water at 20 m*M* and stored at –20°C.

The color reagent, Mersalyl–Brij solution, prepared as follows: first dissolve 2.43 g of mersalyl acid {2-[3-(hydroxymercuri)-2-methoxypropyl]carbamoyl phenoxyacetic acid} (Sigma) in 60 ml of 0.5 *M* NaOH, then add 0.3 g of disodium EDTA and bring up to 450 ml with distilled water. After the EDTA is dissolved, the pH is adjusted to 4.5 by slow addition of 1 *M* HCl with stirring. The volume is then brought up 500 ml with water, and 500 ml of 4% (w/v) Brij 35 (polyoxyethylene lauryl ether) (Sigma) in water is added.

The diazonium salt, Fast Garnet, prepared fresh by diazotization of the base. To prepare the base stock solution, 225 mg of 4-amino-2,3-dimethylazobenzene (U.S. Biochemical Corp.) is crushed to a powder and dissolved in 50 ml ethanol. Thirty milliliters of 1 *M* HCl is added with stirring and the mixture is diluted to 100 ml with water. One milliliter of base stock solution is placed in a test tube standing in a beaker of ice and water, and 0.1 ml of 0.2 *M* $NaNO_2$ is added, mixed, and allowed to stand for at least 5 min. The mixture is then diluted to 100 ml with Mersalyl–Brij reagent. The complete color reagent is stable at 4°C in the dark for 1 day.

* Since metals and other nephrotoxicants, as well as preservatives which might be used to prevent bacterial growth, may directly inhibit urinary NAG activity, it is essential to ascertain the effects of such agents on NAG activity per se prior to the analysis of urinary NAG levels as a measure of tubular injury.

The naphthylamine standard (20 m*M*), made by dissolving 35.9 mg 2-naphthylamine HCl in 10 ml ethanol. If protected from light, this stock solution can be stored at 4°C for up to one month. The working-strength standard is then made by diluting 1 ml of the stock solution to 100 ml with water. This solution should be used on the same day and should also be protected from bright light.

The assay procedure is as follows. To 0.5 ml of the sample containing 10 to 100 ng cathepsin B, diluted as necessary with 0.1% Brij 35, add 1.5 ml of the buffer/activator. Preincubate for 5 min at 40°C, then add 50 µl of substrate stock and mix to start the reaction. After precisely 10 min, add 2 ml of coupling reagent and mix. Allow 10 min for color to develop, then read the absorbance at 520 nm (A_{520}). The color is stable at room temperature. Blanks are prepared by adding the enzyme after the color reagent. Duplicate reagent blanks and standards, prepared by replacing the enzyme with 0.5 ml of 2-naphthylamine standard, are included in each set of assays.

The ΔA_{520} due to 100 nmol of 2-naphthylamine (0.5 ml of 0.2 m*M* solution) corresponds to 10 milliunits (10×10^{-3} µmol/min). The linearity of the color reaction can be ascertained using a standard curve with 0.1, 0.2, 0.3, and 0.4 ml of standard. The $\Delta\varepsilon_{520}$ of the color reaction is 28×10^3; therefore, the 100 nmol standard should give a Δ value of 0.70.

A variation of this procedure that measures urinary cathepsin B activity by fluorescence spectrometry has recently been reported by Schaefer et al.[12] In this case, the fluorogenic peptide Z-Arg-Arg-AMC is substituted for Z-Arg-Arg-NNap as enzyme substrate, and the fluorescence of the free AMC is determined at 460 nm following excitation at 360 nm.

2.2.6 *Lysozyme*

Lysozyme (1,4-*N*-acetylmuraminidase, EC 3.2.1.17) is a phagocytic enzyme found predominantly in monocytes, macrophages, and other phagocytic tissues. It catalyzes the hydrolysis of the peptidoglycan layer of bacterial cell walls. Having a M_r of 15,000, it is readily filtered by the glomerulus and is reabsorbed by the proximal tubule cells.[13] Lysozyme activity in urine increases after proximal tubular cell damage and can be measured by a turbidimetric assay that relies on the catalytic action of the enzyme on the bacterium *Micrococcus leysodeitikus*.[14] However, only immunologic methods are sufficiently sensitive to assay the enzyme in normal urine.[15]

Brouwer et al.[15] have described a very sensitive, competitive enzyme immunoassay (EIA) in which lysozyme is coupled to horseradish peroxidase (HRP) (Sigma, type VI) by means of the heterobifunctional reagent, *N*-succinimidyl 3-(2-pyridyldithiol) propionate (SPDP) (Pharmacia). A conjugate containing 2 mol HRP per mole of lysozyme is isolated by gel filtration on a 1.5 × 93 cm column of Sephacryl S-200 in phosphate-buffered saline (PBS) and is used as a labeled antigen in a competitive enzyme immunoassay against anti-lysosomal rabbit IgG. The assay can detect as little as 1 µg lysozyme/l.

For the assay, urine is centrifuged for 10 min at 1500 × g to remove debris, and the supernatant is used for the EIA. Anti-lysozyme rabbit IgG, raised in New Zealand white rabbits as described[15] or acquired commercially, is diluted to 10 µg/ml in 0.1 *M* sodium carbonate, pH 9.6. Wells of polyvinylchloride (PVC) microliter plates are filled with 150 µl of IgG solution, incubated for 16 to 20 h at room temperature and washed three times with a washing buffer consisting of PBS, Tween (50 m*M* sodium phosphate, pH 7.4; 0.15 *M* sodium chloride; and 0.05% Tween 20). Diluted samples of standards (500 µl) are mixed with 60 µl diluted lysozyme–HRP conjugate. Dilutions are made with PBS containing 1% bovine serum albumin (BSA). One hundred fifty microliters of the sample solutions is added to the wells in duplicate. Wells of the first row of the microtiter plate are set up to contain only PBS containing 1% BSA as blank. Plates are incubated for 2 h at 37°C and washed three times with the washing buffer. One hundred sixty microliters of chromogen solution consisting of 40 mg *o*-phenylenediamine in 100 ml 24 mmol citric acid and 51 m*M* disodium hydrogen phosphate (to which 40 µl 30% hydrogen peroxide is added just before use) is then added, and the reaction is allowed to proceed for 15 min in the dark at room temperature. The reaction is stopped by adding 40 µl of 2.5 *M* sulfuric acid, and the absorbance is measured at 492 nm against the wells of the first row of the plate (blanks). The lysozyme reference interval for human urine is 1.7 to 123 µg/l. Immunoreactive lysozyme is stable in urine at 37°C between pH 3 and 8 for 24 h. Several variations of the EIA for lysosome with HRP-labeled antibodies have been recently described.[13]

2.2.7 Lactate dehydrogenase

Lactate dehydrogenase (EC 1.1.27) (LDH) is a cytoplasmic enzyme that catalyzes the interconversion of pyruvate and lactate. The enzyme is found in many cell types including those which compose the renal cortex and medulla. The presence of LDH activity in the urine has been interpreted as a general measure of injury to the kidney and/or the urogenital tract.

The classical procedure for determination of LDH activity is based on the NADH-dependent reduction of pyruvate to lactate,[16] according to the following reaction:

$$\text{pyruvate} + \text{NADH} + \text{H}^+ \rightarrow \text{L-lactate} + \text{NAD}^+$$

During the reduction of pyruvate, an equimolar amount of NADH is oxidized to NAD^+, resulting in a decrease in absorbance at 340nm. The rate of decrease in absorbance is proportional to LDH activity in the sample.

In preparation for the LDH assay, fresh urine samples are centrifuged at 3000 × g for 10 min and dialyzed against ice-cold distilled water for 3.5 h. Enzyme activity is then measured as follows: 1 ml of dialyzed urine is mixed with 67 m*M* sodium phosphate buffer, pH 7.4, to bring the volume to 2.8 ml. One-tenth milliliter of NADH solution (2.5 mg/ml) is then added, and the mixture is allowed to stand at 30°C for 20 min. The enzyme reaction is started by adding 42 m*M* sodium pyruvate, and the mixture is immediately transferred to a 1-cm silica cuvette in a recording spectrophotometer. The rate of oxidation of NADH is measured by following the decrease in absorbance at 340 nm. Enzyme activity is calculated as nanomoles of NADH oxidized per minute per milligram protein. LDH activity in urine of normal rats has been reported to be on the order of 12 nmoles/min/mg protein.[16] Reagents for the determination of LDH activity by manual and automated procedures are available from Sigma (Procedure No. DG1340-UV).

2.3 Low molecular weight proteins

Studies of humans with renal tubular injury have led to identification and purification of a number of low molecular weight (M_r) urinary proteins (<30,000 Da) including β_2-microglobulin (β_2-mic), α_1-microglobulin (α_1-mic), and retinol-binding protein (RBP, also called α_2-microglobulin). These low M_r proteins share the property of being readily filtered by the glomerulus and almost completely reabsorbed and catabolized by proximal tubular epithelial cells. While largely undetectable in normal urine, these proteins tend to increase in concentration in proportion to tubular damage caused by disease or nephrotoxicant damage. Assays for determining the levels of these proteins in urine are now based largely on immunologic techniques including enzyme-linked immunosorbant assays (ELISA), latex particle immunoagglutination (LIA), and single radial immunodiffusion (SRI). Kits employing these techniques are commercially available.

2.3.1 β_2-Microglobulin

β_2-Microglobulin (β_2-mic) is a low molecular weight protein (M_r = 11,800) that is synthesized in essentially all nucleated cells and is present on their membranes as a component of the class I histocompatibility antigens. Very little β_2-mic is found in the urine of healthy subjects, but levels can increase substantially following renal tubular damage caused by disease or exposure to toxic chemicals. The sensitivity of urinary β_2-mic as an indicator of proximal tubular injury results from the fact that reabsorption of β_2-mic by proximal tubular cells is nearly complete (>99.9%) under normal conditions. Therefore, any increase above normal levels is indicative of proximal tubular cell damage. Numerous methods for the measurement of β_2-mic in urine are available. Determination by single radial immunodiffusion has been described,[17,18] but this method is not sufficiently sensitive for detection of β_2-mic in normal urine without a preliminary concentration step. Radioimmunoassay procedures for measuring β_2-mic have also been developed.[17,18] These techniques are substantially more sensitive, but are time-consuming and require the use of radioisotopes. The latex immunoassay described below has both high sensitivity and precision and is relatively more easily performed than other procedures.

Bernard et al.[19] have described a highly sensitive method for determination of urinary β_2-mic based on the direct agglutination by β_2-mic of latex particles on which an antibody against β_2-mic is adsorbed. The assay consists of incubating urine samples with latex particles on which an anti-β_2-mic antibody has been adsorbed and quantifying the residual unagglutinated particles with an optical particle counter.

For the assay, human urine β_2-mic is obtained from commercial suppliers (e.g., Sigma No. M 4890), and rabbit immunoglobulins against it are either purified from rabbit serum[18] or obtained commercially. Glycine-buffered saline (GBS) is used throughout as the assay buffer and is prepared by a making tenfold dilution of a stock buffer containing 1 *M* glycine, 1.7 *M* NaCl and 76 m*M* NaN_3, adjusted to pH 9.0 with 10 *M* NaOH. To prepare latex particles with β_2-mic antibodies, 5 µl (78.5 µg) of rabbit anti-β_2-mic immunoglobulins are diluted in 0.4 ml GBS, and 50 µl of latex suspension (polystyrene latex particles, 0.79 µm diameter, ESTAPOR K as a 10% suspension, Rhone–Poulenc) is then added with continuous agitation. After a 1-h incubation at room temperature the latex particles are precipitated by centrifugation at 25,000 × g for 10 min, washed twice with several 1-ml portions of GBS, and finally redispersed into 1 ml GBS. To prepare samples and standards, 10- to 20-fold dilutions of urine samples and of purified β_2-mic solutions are made in GBS containing 1 g/l bovine serum albumin (BSA) (e.g., Sigma No. A 2153) adjusted to pH 9.0.

To assay urinary β_2-mic content, pipet in duplicate 20 µl of β_2-mic standard solution or 20 µl of diluted urine samples into glass tubes. In each series of measurements, include at regular intervals tubes containing 20 µl GBS containing BSA only as zero standards. Immediately before incubation, stabilize the latex particles coated with the antibody as follows: resuspend the latex particles from the stock preparation by gentle shaking, then transfer an adequate volume into a plastic tube (i.d. ~1 cm). Vortex for 1 to 2 min to break up any latex aggregates that may have formed during storage. Immediately dilute the latex tenfold with freshly prepared GBS containing 10 g/l BSA, pH 10.0 (which has been previously filtered twice on a 0.45-µm Millipore filter). Then add 50 µl of the stabilized latex to each test tube. Mix the contents of each tube and incubate for 15 to 30 min at 37°C in a shaking water bath (70 to 80 cycles/min). Terminate the incubation by adding 5 ml of GBS containing 1 ml/l Tween 20. (The latter solution should also be filtered on a 0.45-µm Millipore filter before use). Finally, stopper the tubes and invert them three to four times to ensure homogenization of the latex suspension before measuring.

Measurements of β_2-mic are made either by counting the remaining unagglutinated latex particles or by turbidimetry. Unagglutinated particles can be counted using an automated particle counter. The number of unagglutinated latex particles is expressed as a percentage of the total number of free particles obtained with the zero standard. At a tenfold particle dilution, 85% free latex particles corresponded to 1.0 μg/l β_2-mic, whereas 20% free latex particles corresponded to ~90 μg/l β_2-mic, in a nearly linear relationship.[19] At a 20-fold particle dilution, 90% free latex particles corresponded to 1.0 μg/l β_2-mic, whereas 30% free latex particles corresponded to ~90 μg/l β_2-mic.[19] Bernard and Lauwerys[20] have described a continuous flow system for automation of the latex immunoassay by particle counting for β_2-mic and other urinary proteins.

In making β_2-mic measurements by turbidimetry, the absorbance of the latex suspension is read in 2-cm cuvettes at 360 nm (the absorbance maximum) using a conventional spectrophotometer. The agglutination is expressed as the difference between the absorbance of the zero standard and that of the latex incubated with β_2-mic.

A principal concern with regard to measuring urinary levels of β_2-mic is its instability in acid urine; i,e, when the pH of urine is < 5.5, β_2-mic degrades in a time- and temperature-dependent manner.[21] Therefore, rapid neutralization of the urine immediately following collection or, alternatively, consumption of sodium bicarbonate by the subject prior to urine collection is required. Neutralization of the urine can be accomplished by adding 1 ml of 0.4 *M* phosphate buffer, pH 7.6, per 10 ml urine sample and storing at –18°C, if necessary, until β_2-mic analysis can be accomplished. Because of its instability in acid urine, proteins which are more resistant to proteolytic degradation, such as α_1-microglobulin or retinol-binding protein (α_2-microglobulin) (described below), are now preferred to β_2-mic as markers of renal proximal tubular cell injury.

2.3.2 α_1-Microglobulin

α_1-Microglobulin (α_1-mic, also called protein HC) is a glycosylated protein, probably of hepatic origin and with an estimated M_r between 26,000 and 30,000. It occurs in serum both free and bound to several high M_r proteins such as IgA and albumin. Unbound α_1-mic is freely filtered at the glomerulus, but the efficiency of its uptake by renal proximal tubular cells is not yet established. Concentrations of α_1-mic in normal urine are sufficient to permit its accurate determination by single radial diffusion, and kits for this analysis that include the appropriate antisera and standards are available from commercial suppliers. Urinary α_1-mic is stable over the pH range of 4 to 10 and for up to 11 days when stored at 4°C,[22] supporting its utility as a marker of proximal tubular damage and dysfunction.[22,23]

α_1-Mic is most often measured using a single radial immunodiffusion technique initially described by Mancini et al.[24] The single-diffusion reaction is performed by incorporating one of the reactants, the α_1-mic antibody (obtained commercially), into an agar gel at a uniform concentration, while the other reactant, the (urine sample containing the) α_1-mic, is introduced into a circular well, from which it is allowed to diffuse radially into the gel to react with the antibody. The agar gel is prepared as follows: to 100 ml of 0.1 *M* barbiturate buffer, pH 8.6 (made by dissolving 9 g of sodium diethylbarbiturate, 65 ml of 0.1 *N* HCl, and 0.5 g sodium azide in distilled water and adjusting the volume to 1 l), is added 3 g of Special Agar–Noble (Difco) (or other commercially available source). This suspension is placed in a boiling water bath and stirred until the agar is completely dissolved. To prepare the agar–antibody mixture, the required amount of 3% agar solution is cooled to 60°C (or solidified agar gel is melted in a boiling water bath, then cooled to 60°). A suitable dilution of the antibody in barbiturate buffer is brought to 55°, after which equal volumes of both solutions are mixed (thoroughly but avoiding bubbling), using a pipette preheated to 60° in the water bath. After mixing, the antibody–agar mixture is poured without delay into the gel mold (described below), using the same preheated pipette.

A gel mold is used in order to obtain antibody–agar layers of strictly uniform thickness. The base plate supporting the gel typically consists of a glass plate 1 mm thick and measuring on the order 10×7 cm. Frames and siliconized cover plates for accommodating the base plate and which form a compartment into which the gel is introduced, similar to those used for constructing DNA sequencing gels, are available from numerous commercial sources. The gel compartment is filled by holding the frame in a slightly slanting position while the tip of the heated pipette containing the antibody–agar mixture is applied to the lower corner of the compartment. Filling the mold in this way prevents the inclusion of air bubbles. After solidification (10 to 15 min), the frame is disassembled, and circular wells are punched out in the gel using a needle of 2 mm bore. The small cylinders of gel cut out by the needle are removed by suction. Each of the wells receives 2 μl of gel-filtered urine, which is delivered using a micropipette. The plate is now kept in a strictly horizontal position in a moist box until the antigen solutions (urine) have been soaked up by the gel (10 to 30 min). To prevent drying, the antibody–agar plates may be stored under a 2-cm-thick layer of mineral oil. It has been found practical, although not essential, to incubate the oil-covered plates at 37°C.

The ring-shaped precipitates that form around the antigen wells grow in size over a several day period, after which no further increase in dimensions is observed. Final measurements are made when the precipitates are assumed to have reached their final size. After removing the oil by a short rinse in petroleum ether, the silhouettes of the precipitates are projected onto film and the size determined by densitometry. Actual concentrations are determined by comparisons with readings obtained using α_1-mic standards. α_1-Mic concentrations in urine of healthy male volunteers was 0.8 to 5 mg/l.[23]

2.3.3 *Retinol-binding protein*

Retinol-binding protein (RBP), also called α_2-microglobulin, is a low molecular weight plasma protein (M_r = 21,200) that is synthesized in liver and transports vitamin A in its alcoholic form, retinol, from liver to epithelial tissues. Most of RBP in plasma forms a high molecular weight complex with thyroxin-binding prealbumin, which prevents its filtration by the glomerulus.[25] However, after delivering retinol to target tissues, RBP loses its affinity for prealbumin and is freely filtered by the glomerulus. RBP, like β_2-microglobulin, is reabsorbed with an efficiency of >99.9% by proximal tubular cells, and under normal conditions very little RBP is found in the urine (~100 μg/24 h).[26]

Renal tubular insults that compromise low M_r protein reabsorption, e.g., chronic cadmium poisoning, result in considerably increased excretion of RBP in the urine. Several types of immunoassays based on enzyme-linked immunosorbance (ELISA), latex particle agglutination, or single radial immunodiffusion have been described for the measurement of urinary RBP.[25,27-29]

Biagini et al.[29] described an ELISA assay, useful for both urine and serum RBP assessments. Antirat RBP antibodies to RBP are obtained either by treatment of New Zealand white rabbits as described[29] or from commercial sources. Aliquots of the purified antibody are then coupled with biotin for the ELISA assay. For RBP assessments, 96 flat-bottomed wells in disposable PVC microtitration plates are coated with 10 mg/ml of purified antibody in 50 m*M* carbonate/bicarbonate buffer, pH 9.6. Following incubation at 4°C overnight, plates are washed three times with 10 m*M* phosphate buffered saline (PBS), pH 7.2, containing 0.1% bovine serum albumin (BSA). Two hundred microliters of urine sample (diluted 1:10) [or of serum (diluted 1:5000)] or of serial twofold dilutions of purified RBP in 0.1% PBS-BSA is added to each well. Plates are then incubated overnight at 4°C. After washing three times, 200 μl of biotin-conjugated antirat RBP antibodies diluted 800 times is added. Plates are washed again three times and 200 μl of avidin-conjugated alkaline phosphatase (ICN) diluted 2000 times is added. Excess avidin-conjugated alkaline phosphatase is removed by washing plates three times, and enzyme activity is measured by adding *p*-nitrophenylphosphate substrate in diethanolamine buffer (1 g/l, pH 9.8). Following incubation for 30 min at room temperature, absorbance is measured at 405 nm. The detection limit for this assay is reported to be 0.5 μg/l and the working range between 0.8 and 50 μg/l. Urine collections from 20 normal male rats gave mean excretion rates from 310 to 491 ng/24 h, whereas rates from female rats were substantially lower, 65 to 74 ng/24 h.[29]

Topping et al.[27] have described an ELISA assay for human RBP. This assay employs purified human urine RBP and rabbit antibody to human RBP acquired from commercial sources. For the assay, flat-bottomed wells in disposable microtitration plates are coated with antibody (500-fold dilution in 50 m*M* carbonate/bicarbonate buffer, pH 9.6). Following incubation at 4°C overnight, plates are washed three times with 10 m*M* phosphate-buffered saline (PBS), pH 7.2, containing 1 ml/l of Tween 20 polyoxyethylene sorbitan monolaurate (washing buffer). Washed plates should either be used immediately or can be stored at 4°C for as long as four weeks without loss of activity. A standard solution of purified urinary RBP (142 mg/l) is diluted in 5 m*M* phosphate buffer, pH 7.5, containing 10 ml/l of Tween 20 (assay buffer), to give solution with RBP concentrations of 10, 25, 50, 100, and 250 μg/l. Five-microliter aliquots of standards or urine plus 95 μl of assay buffer are added to the wells of the antibody-coated plate, and the plate is incubated overnight at 4°C.

Following incubation, the plate is washed four times with 100 ml of washing buffer over a 15-min period, and a 100-μl aliquot of antibody enzyme conjugate, diluted 500-fold in assay buffer, is added to each well. The plate is agitated for 1 h at room temperature, then washed four times over a 15-min period with 100 ml of 79 m*M* phosphate/27 m*M* citrate buffer, pH 6.0, containing 1 ml/l Tween 20 (substrate buffer). One hundred microliters 7.4 m*M* *o*-phenylenediamine and 5.9 m*M* H_2O_2 in substrate buffer is then added to each well, and the plate is further agitated for 15 min at room temperature. The enzyme reaction is stopped by adding 50 μl of 2 m*M* H_2SO_4, and the absorbance is measured at 490 nm. Each standard and urine sample should be tested in duplicate. The RBP concentration in test samples is calculated from a standard curve. The working range of this assay is reported to be in the range of 10 to 250 μg urinary RBP per liter. The detection limit is 5 μg/l.

Bernard et al.[25] have described a latex immunoassay (LIA) of RBP in human biological fluids. This assay is similar to that described above for β_2-microglobulin, wherein the sample is incubated with antibody-coated latex particles, and the resulting agglutination is then quantified by particle counting or turbidimetry. Purified RBP is used to develop rabbit antihuman RBP antibody, which can also be readily obtained commercially. Antibody is then adsorbed to polystyrene latex particles (0.8 μm in diameter, 100 g/l, Estapor K109) by mixing 5 μl of antibody with 50 μl of the 100 g/l latex suspension in 0.4 ml of glycine-buffered saline (GBS), pH 10, made by diluting tenfold a stock solution containing 1 *M* glycine, 1.7 *M* NaCl, and 76 m*M* sodium azide (NaN_3), and adjusting to pH 9.0 (or pH 10.0 for stabilization of antibody-coated particles) with NaOH.

To measure urinary RBP levels, urine samples are diluted 20-fold in GBS-bovine serum albumin buffer (consisting of GBS buffer containing 1 g/l BSA). The RBP assay is performed as described for β_2-microglobulin above except that 50 μl (instead of 20 μl) of RBP samples are pipetted into 5-ml glass test tubes and incubated with 50 μl of stabilized latex for 30 min at 37°C in a shaking water bath. After incubation, the agglutination can be measured automatically by counting the unagglutinated latex particles with an optical cell counter equipped with a double-threshold system that ignores aggregates. Alternatively, agglutination can be quantified by turbidimetry by measuring the decrease in absorbance of the latex suspension in a 2-mm cuvette at 360 nm.[19] The sensitivity of the LIA agglutination curves is greatly affected by the mode of reading; the most sensitive standard curve for RBP is obtained by using a particle counter equipped with an adjustable upper threshold so that only unagglutinated (0.8 μm) particles are counted.[25] Under these conditions, the working range extends from 0.5 to 32 μg/l, and the detection limit is 0.1 μg/l (of 20-fold diluted urine). Quantifying the agglutination by measuring the decrease in absorbance at 360 nm is less sensitive than particle counting, but has about the same precision.

Urinary RBP can also be assayed by single radial immunodiffusion as described above for α_1-mic.[24] Kits for this assay are available from commercial suppliers.

Several recent review articles have summarized current knowledge regarding the mechanisms of proteinuria and the use of urinary enzymes and proteins as indicators of nephrotoxicity.[30,31] The normal ranges of concentrations of some diagnostic proteins commonly found in human urine are presented in Table 1.

Table 1 Normal Urine Concentrations of Some Common Proteins That are Diagnostic of Renal Toxicity and Disease

Protein	Urine concentration	Ref.
β_2-Microglobulin	21–142 μg/g creatinine	30
	<150–200 μg/l	23
α_1-Microglobulin	4.2 ± 6 mg/g creatinine	30
	0.8–5.0 mg/l	23
Retinol-binding protein	30–130 μg/g creatinine	30
	<250–300 μg/l	23
Tamm-Horsfall glycoprotein	5.1–25.5 mg/g creatinine	30
	22–66 mg/24 h	37

2.4 Kidney-specific antigens

A number of kidney-derived tubular proteins can be measured in the urine on the basis of their immunoreactivity. Under these circumstances, such proteins are referred to as kidney-specific antigens. Examples of renal proteins that have been immunochemically measured in urine are adenosine deaminase-binding protein,[32] glutathione-S-transferases α and π,[33] and carbonic anhydrase,[34] as well as a number of other tubular antigens of currently unknown function.[35,36] Some renal antigens are highly specific for renal tissue, among the best known examples of which is Tamm-Horsfall glycoprotein, which is synthesized exclusively by the thick ascending limb of the loop of Henle and the distal convoluted tubule.[37] Kits that utilize specific immunologic procedures comparable with those described above are available from commercial suppliers for determination of these proteins in urine.

2.5 Kidney-derived porphyrins

Porphyrins are formed in all eukaryotic tissue cells as intermediates in the biosynthesis of heme. In the kidney, most heme biosynthetic activity is localized to renal proximal tubular cells. In healthy renal epithelial cells, porphyrins with 8-, 7-, 6-, 5-, and 4-carboxylated side chains are formed and are excreted into the urine in a well-established pattern.[38,39] Insult to proximal tubular cells by heavy metals and other toxicants impairs porphyrin metabolism resulting in altered urinary porphyrin excretion patterns.[39] Such changes in the urinary porphyrin profile may be indicative both of toxicant exposure as well as of toxicant concentrations in tissue cells. Also, because the excretion of porphyrins from tubular epithelial cells into the tubular luminal fluid is enhanced by oxidative stress, changes in urinary porphyrin concentrations can be indicative of toxicant-induced oxidative injury to renal epithelial cells.[39] These observations have stimulated considerable interest in the evaluation of urinary porphyrin excretion patterns as a biomarker of exposure and toxicity associated with a number of drugs and chemicals.[39-41] Woods and colleagues[42-46] have developed an efficient and sensitive HPLC spectrofluorometric procedure for measuring urinary porphyrin concentrations and have applied this assay to the evaluation of heavy metal exposures in both animals and human subjects. This assay is as follows:

Pretreatment of the C-18 preparatory column. Either Bond Elut extraction columns (Analytichem International, Inc., Harbor City, CA) or SEP-PAK^R C-18 cartridges (Waters Associates, Milford, MA) with a 10-ml plastic syringe as reservoir may be employed as preparatory columns. Before sample application, the C-18 preparatory column is conditioned by attaching to a vacuum filtration apparatus and passing 10 ml of methanol through the column followed by 10 ml of 10 m*M* phosphate buffer, pH 3.5.

Collection of urine samples. To avoid photochemical oxidation of porphyrins, urines should be collected in foil-wrapped 125-ml polypropylene flasks containing ~50 mg/10 ml of $NaHCO_3$ (to maintain neutral pH) and ~4 mg/10 ml EDTA (to prevent potential metal complexation of porphyrins). Following collection, total urine volume should either be processed immediately for porphyrin analysis or frozen at –80°C. For off-site collections, urine samples may be frozen or wrapped in cold-pac and shipped by overnight service to the laboratory where analysis will performed.

Urinary porphyrin analysis. The urine specimen is centrifuged at 2000 × g for 5 min to remove excess bicarbonate and insoluble matter. Three to five milliliters of the supernatant is then acidified to pH 2.5 with 6*N* HCl and loaded onto the preparatory column. Flow through the column is initiated by applying a *slight* vacuum, and the sample is allowed to gravity drip through the column until flow ceases. Facilitated flow using other than a very slight vacuum should be avoided, since this process may cause small amounts of porphyrin to pass through the column. The column is then washed with 3 ml of 10 m*M* pH 3.5 phosphate buffer, which is allowed to gravity drip through the column. At this stage, porphyrins are retained at the top of the column, along with some contaminants. The column is then washed sequentially (using a moderate vacuum): first with 7 ml 10 m*M* pH 3.5 phosphate buffer; second with 40 ml of 35% methanol in 10 m*M* pH 3.5 phosphate buffer (to remove major interfering fluorescent contaminants); third with 3 ml of 10 m*M* pH 3.5 phosphate buffer; and finally with 10 ml of 10 m*M* pH 7.5 phosphate buffer to adjust the column pH for elution of porphyrins. The column is then allowed to dry 10 min. To elute the porphyrins, 1 ml of 100% methanol is passed through the column, followed by 2 ml of 80% methanol in 10 m*M* pH 7.5 phosphate buffer. The sample is warmed briefly in a 40 to 60°C water bath and the eluant evaporated off under nitrogen. The residue, containing the porphyrins, is resuspended in 0.5 ml 1*N* HCl and filtered with a 4-mm Millex-HV 0.45-µm membrane (Millipore Corp., Bedford, MA). Separation and quantitation of individual porphyrins in a 50-µl aliquot is achieved by HPLC (250 × 4.6 mm, packed with Econosphere C18 (5 µm) and equipped with a C-18 guard column cartridge (Alltech/Applied Science, Deerfield, IL), employing a methanol/0.05 *M* sodium phosphate buffer (pH 3.5) gradient mobile phase. Reservoir A contains 0.05 *M* phosphate buffer (pH 3.5). Reservoir B contains 100% methanol. The gradient is programmed to provide an initial 50%

methanol (B) concentration at time 0, 65% B at 3 min, 85% B at 8 min, and 99% B at 18 to 22 min. The gradient is returned to 50% B at 28 min, and the column is allowed to reequilibrate at 50% B for 4 min before the program is terminated at 32 min. Porphyrins are detected by their fluorescent emission at 620 nm after excitation at 395 nm. Eluted porphyrins are calibrated against standard curves developed for chromatographic markers (uroporphyrin I, heptaporphyrin I, hexaporphyrin I, pentaporphyrin I, coproporphyrin I, and mesoporphyrin IX) (Porphyrin Products, Inc., Logan, UT). The sensitivity of this procedure is 0.5 pmol porphyrin. The mean concentrations and ranges of porphyrins in healthy adult human urine are presented in Table 2.

Table 2 Normal Human Urinary Porphyrin Concentrations from 24 Hour and Randomly Collected (Spot) Urine Samples

	Urinary porphyrin concentration Means ± SD and (ranges)	
Porphyrin	24-hour samples (nmol/24 h)	Random (spot) samples (g/l)
Uro	6.0 ± 1.8 (3.2–18.5)	5.1 ± 1.0 (1.7–19.9)
Hepta	3.8 ± 1.5 (1.0–7.8)	3.1 ± 0.5 (0.6–5.3)
Hexa	1.0 ± 1.0 (0–3.5)	1.5 ± 1.2 (0–3.7)
Penta	3.3 ± 3.3 (0.4–15.4)	2.3 ± 1.4 (0.1–4.6)
Copro	52.0 ± 11.4 (29.8–92.6)	30.1 ± 17.3 (12–63)

Note: Porphyrin levels as measured in urine samples collected from healthy adult male subjects presenting to this laboratory during the period 1990 to 1992 for research purposes. Values represent the means and standard deviations of 34 individual determinations for 24-h samples and 75 individual determinations for spot samples.

From Woods, J. S. et al., *J. Toxicol. Environ. Health*, 40, 241, 1993. With permission of Taylor & Francis, Inc., Washington, D.C.

2.6 Acknowledgment

Work in the author's laboratory was supported by NIH grant ES04696.

References

1. Mattenheimer, H., Enzymes in renal disease, *Ann. Clin. Lab. Sci.*, 7, 422, 1977.
2. Jung, K. and Scholz, D., An optimized assay of alanine aminopeptidase in urine, *Clin. Chem.*, 26, 1251, 1980.
3. Amador, E., Zimmermann, T.S., and Wacker, W.E.C., Urinary alkaline phosphatase activity. II. An analytical validation of the assay method, *J. Am. Med. Assoc.*, 185, 953, 1963.
4. The Committee on Enzymes of the Scandinavian Society for Clinical Chemistry and Clinical Physiology, Recommended methods for the determination of four enzymes in blood, *Scand. J. Clin. Lab. Invest.*, 33, 291, 1974.
5. Tate, S.S. and Meister, A., γ-Glutamyltranspeptidase from kidney, *Methods Enzymol.*, 113, 400, 1985.
6. Meyer, B.R., Fischbein, A., Rosenman, K., Lerman, Y., and Reidenberg, M.M., Increased urinary enzyme excretion in workers exposed to nephrotoxic chemicals, *Am. J. Med.*, 76, 989, 1984.
7. Goren, M.P., Wright, R.K., and Osborne, S., Two automated procedures for *N*-acetyl-β-D-glucosaminidase determination evaluated for detection of drug-induced tubular nephrotoxicity, *Clin. Chem.*, 32, 2052, 1986.

8. Jung, K., Pergande, M., Graubaum, H.-J., Fels, L.M., Endl, U., and Stolte, H. Urinary proteins and enzymes as early indicators of renal dysfunction in chronic exposure to cadmium, *Clin. Chem.*, 39, 757, 1993.
9. Leaback, D.E. and Walker, D.G., The fluorimetric assay of *N*-acetyl-β-D-glucosaminidase, *Biochem. J.*, 78, 151, 1961.
10. Horak, E., Hopfer, S.M., and Sunderman, F.W., Jr., Spectrophotometric assay for urinary *N*-acetyl-β-D-glucosaminidase activity, *Clin. Chem.*, 27, 1180, 1981.
11. Barrett, A.J. and Kirschke, H., Cathepsin B, cathepsin H and cathepsin L., *Methods Enzymol.*, 80, 535, 1981.
12. Schaefer, L., Gilge, U., Heidland, A., and Schaefer, R.M., Urinary excretion of cathepsin B and cystatins as parameters of tubular damage, *Kidney Int.*, 46(Suppl. 47), S-64, 1994.
13. Porstmann, B., Jung, K., Shhmechta, H., Evers, U., Perfande, M., Porstmann, T., Kramm, H.-J., and Krause, H., Measurement of lysozyme in human body fluids: comparison of various enzyme immunoassay techniques and their diagnostic application, *Clin. Biochem.*, 22, 349, 1989.
14. Terry, J.M., Blainey, J.D., and Swingler, M.C., An automated method for lysozyme assay, *Clin. Chim. Acta.*, 35, 317, 1971.
15. Brouwer, J., van Leeuwen–Herberts, T., and Otting-van de Ruit, M., Determination of lysozyme in serum, urine, cerebrospinal fluid and feces by enzyme immunoassay, *Clin. Chim. Acta*, 142, 21, 1984.
16. Leathwood, P.D., Gilford, M.K., and Plummer, D.T., Enzymes in rat urine. Lactate dehydrogenase, *Enzymologia*, 42, 285, 1972.
17. Peterson, P.A., Evrin, P.-E., and Berggard, I., Differentiation of glomerular, tubular, and normal proteinuria: determination of urinary excretion of β_2-microglobulin, albumin and total protein, *J. Clin. Invest.*, 48, 1189, 1969.
18. Bernier, G.M. and Conrad, M.E., Catabolism of human β_2-microglobulin by the rat kidney, *Am. J. Physiol.*, 217, 1259, 1969.
19. Bernard, A.M., Vyskocil, A., and Lauwerys, R.R., Determination of β_2-microglobulin in human urine and serum by latex immunoassay, *Clin. Chem.*, 27, 832, 1981.
20. Bernard, A.M. and Lauwerys, R.R., Continuous-flow system for automation of latex immunoassay by particle counting, *Clin. Chem.*, 29, 1007, 1983.
21. Evrin, P.E. and Wibell, L., The serum levels and urinary excretion of beta$_2$-microglobulin in apparently healthy subjects, *Scand. J. Clin. Lab. Invest.*, 29, 69, 1972.
22. Yu, H., Yanagisawa, Y., Forbes, M.A., Cooper, E.H., Crockson, R.A., and MacLennan, I.C.M., Alpha-1-microglobulin: an indicator protein for renal tubular function, *J. Clin. Pathol.*, 36, 253, 1983.
23. Donaldson, M.D.C., Chambers, R.E., Woolridge, M.W., and Whicher, J.T., Stability of alfa$_1$-microglobulin, beta$_2$-microglobulin and retinol-binding protein in urine, *Clin. Chim. Acta.*, 179, 73, 1989.
24. Mancini, G., Carbonara, A.O., and Heremans, J.F., Immunochemical quantitation of antigens by single radial immunodiffusion, *Immunochemistry*, 2, 235, 1965.
25. Bernard, A., Moreau, D., and Lauwerys, R., Latex immunoassay of retinol-binding protein, *Clin. Chem.*, 28, 1167, 1982.
26. Peterson, P.A. and Bergaard, I., Isolation and properties of a human retinol-transporting protein, *J. Biol. Chem.*, 10, 25, 1971.
27. Topping, M., Forster, H.W., Dolman, C., Luczynska, C., and Bernard, A., Measurement of urinary retinol-binding protein by enzyme linked immuno-sorbent assay and its application to detection of tubular proteinuria, *Clin. Chem.*, 32, 1863, 1986.
28. Beetham, R., Dawnay, A., London, J., and Cattell, W.R., A radioimmunoassay for retinol-binding protein in serum and urine, *Clin. Chem.*, 31, 1364, 1985.
29. Biagini, C., Alinovi, R., Bergamaschi, E., Mutti, A., Berni, R., and Franchini, I., An immunoassay method for the determination of rat retinol-binding protein in serum and urine, *Contrib. Nephrol.*, 101, 164, 1993.
30. Bernard, A. and Lauwerys R.R., Proteinuria: changes and mechanisms in toxic nephropathies, *Crit. Rev. Toxicol.*, 21, 373, 1991.

31. Jung, K. Urinary enzymes and low molecular weight proteins as markers of tubular dysfunction, *Kidney Int.*, 46(Suppl. 47), S-29, 1994.
32. Thompson, R.E., Piper, D.J., Galberg, C., Chan, T.H., Tolkoff–Rubin, N.E., and Rubin, R.H., Adenosine deaminase binding protein, a new diagnostic marker for kidney disease, *Clin. Chem.*, 31, 679, 1981.
33. Sundberg, A.G.M., Appelkvist, E.L., Backman, L. and Dallner, G., Urinary π-glutathione transferase as an indicator of tubular damage in the human kidney, *Nephron*, 67, 308, 1994.
34. Taniguchi, N., Tanaka, M., Kishihara, C., Ohno, H., Kondo, T., Matsuda, I. Fujino, T., and Harada, M., Determination of carbonic anhydrase C and beta$_2$-microglobulin by radioimmunoassay in urine of heavy metal-exposed subjects and patients with renal tubular acidosis, *Environ. Res.*, 20, 154, 1979.
35. Falkenberg, F.W., Mai, U., Puppe, C., Risse, P., Hermann, G., Kicking, E., Bremer, K., Mondorf, A., and Shapira, Z., Kidney-derived urinary antigens assayed with monoclonal antibodies for the detection of renal damage, *Clin. Chim. Acta*, 160, 171, 1986.
36. Mutti, A., Lucertini, S., Valcavi, P., Neri, T.M., Fornari, M., Alinovi, R., and Franchini, I., Urinary excretion of brush-border antigen revealed by monoclonal antibody: early indicator of toxic nephropathy, *Lancet*, 2, 914, 1985.
37. Thornley, C., Dawney, A., and Cattell, W.R., Human Tamm–Horsfall glycoprotein: urinary and plasma levels in normal subjects and patients with renal disease determined by a fully validated radioimmunoassay, *Clin. Sci.*, 68, 529, 1985.
38. Woods, J.S., Regulation of porphyrin and heme metabolism in the kidney, *Semin. Hematol.*, 25, 336, 1988.
39. Woods, J.S., Porphyrin metabolism as indicator of metal exposure and toxicity, in *Handbook of Experimental Pharmacology, Vol. 115, Toxicology of Metals, Biochemical Aspects*, Goyer, R.A. and Cherian, M.G., Eds., Springer-Verlag, Berlin, 1995, chap. 2.
40. Marks, G.S., Exposure to toxic agents: the heme biosynthetic pathway and hemoproteins as indicator, *Crit. Rev. Toxicol.*, 15, 151, 1985.
41. Maines, M.D., New developments in the regulation of heme metabolism and their implications, *Crit. Rev. Toxicol.*, 12, 241, 1984.
42. Woods, J.S., Bowers, M.A., and Davis, H.A., Urinary porphyrin profiles as biomarkers of trace metal exposure and toxicity: studies on urinary porphyrin excretion patterns in rats during prolonged exposure to methyl mercury, *Toxicol. Appl. Pharmacol.*, 110, 464, 1991.
43. Bowers, M.A., Aicher, L.D., Davis, H.A., and Woods, J.S., Quantitative determination of porphyrins in rat and human urine and evaluation of urinary porphyrin profiles during mercury and lead exposures, *J. Lab. Clin. Med.*, 120, 272, 1992.
44. Woods, J.S., Martin, M.D., Naleway, C.A., and Echeverria, D., Urinary porphyrin profiles as a biomarker of mercury exposure: studies in dentists with occupational exposure to mercury vapor, *J. Toxicol. Environ. Health*, 40, 239, 1993.
45. Echeverria, D., Heyer, N., Martin, M.D., Naleway, C.A., Woods, J.S., and Bittner, A.C., Behavioral effects of low-level exposure to Hg° among dentists, *Neurotoxicol. Teratol.*, 17, 161, 1995.
46. Gonzales–Ramirez, D., Maiorino, R.M., Zuniga–Charles, M., Xu, Z., Hurlbut, K.M., Junco–Munoz, P., Aposhian, M.M., Dart, R.C., Diaz Gama, J.H., Echeverria, D., Woods, J.S., and Aposhian, H.V., Sodium 2,3-dimercaptopropane-1-sulfonate challenge test for mercury in humans. II. Urinary mercury, porphyrins and neurobehavioral changes of dental workers in Monterrey, Mexico, *J. Pharmacol. Exp. Ther.*, 272, 264, 1995.

chapter three

Histopathologic Methods in Renal Toxicology

Niels Marcussen and Jytte Banner Lundemose

3.1 Background ... 36
3.2 Histopathologic methods ... 36
3.2.1 Fixation of tissue ... 36
3.2.2 Light microscopy ... 37
3.2.2.1 Processing of tissue ... 37
3.2.2.2 Stains ... 37
3.2.2.2.1 Hematoxylin and eosin (H&E) ... 37
3.2.2.2.2 Periodic acid–Schiff (PAS) method ... 37
3.2.2.2.3 Masson's trichrome ... 38
3.2.2.2.4 Silver-methenamine method ... 38
3.2.2.3 Semiquantitative estimation ... 39
3.2.3 Electron microscopy ... 40
3.2.3.1 Transmission electron microscopy (TEM) ... 40
3.2.3.2 Scanning electron microscopy (SEM) ... 40
3.2.4 Immunofluorescence microscopy ... 40
3.2.4.1 Direct immunofluorescence technique ... 42
3.2.4.2 Indirect immunofluorescence technique ... 42
3.2.5 Enzyme and immunohistochemistry ... 43
3.2.6 Stereological and morphometric methods ... 44
3.2.6.1 Unbiased stereological methods ... 44
3.2.6.1.1 Volume fractions and total volumes of structures ... 45
3.2.6.1.2 Volume of single structures ... 46
3.2.6.1.3 Length and surface areas of structures ... 47
3.2.6.1.4 Numbers ... 49
3.2.6.1.5 Counting of glomeruli with the fractionator principle ... 49
3.2.6.2 Morphometric methods relying on assumptions ("biased methods") ... 51
3.2.6.3 Computerized methods of reconstruction of nephrons ... 52
3.2.7 Confocal microscopy ... 52
3.3 Comments on techniques related to specific renal structures ... 52
3.3.1 Glomerular lesions ... 52
3.3.2 Tubular lesions ... 53

0-8493-3341-5/96/$0.00+$.50

3.3.3 Interstitial lesions 53
3.3.4 Vascular lesions 54
3.4 Artifacts 54
3.4.1 Variability in the measurement of structures 55
References 55

3.1 Background

Histologic methods are often used in the investigation of renal toxicology. This may either be in research or in the routine diagnostic use of renal biopsies. In renal biopsies, the histologic investigation is typically done in cases of acute renal failure that in some cases is due to toxic injury to the kidney. Furthermore, toxic injuries may lead to chronic nephropathy that may be diagnosed and investigated by histopathology.

Histopathologic methods of investigating the kidney has expanded during the years. Oliver combined ordinary histology with microdissection and showed that the nephrons in chronic renal failure comprise a very heterogeneous population.[1] The microdissection technique, however, is difficult, and only a limited number of nephrons can be studied. Histopathologic methods, on the other hand, allow examination of many more nephrons. Micropuncture has also been combined with histologic examination allowing for detailed investigations of single nephrons.[2]

The immunofluorescence technique has added to the understanding of immunoreactions in the kidney. Transmission electron microscopy used in a systematic way, or combined with semiquantitative and quantitative methods, has permitted a detailed and precise description of the ultrastructural changes in toxic nephropathies.[3] The quantitative methods, that is, morphometry and stereology, are valuable tools for the investigator. These methods can be used on fresh tissue, frozen tissue, and paraffin or plastic slices or at the ultrastructural level. More and more unbiased stereological methods are being added to the list of available techniques each year. This chapter deals with the many aspects of the histopathologic examination of the kidney that are at hand to the investigator.

3.2 Histopathologic methods

3.2.1 Fixation of tissue

It is a histological maxim that good histology demands good fixation. If fixation is delayed or imperfect, little can be done subsequently to improve the appearance of the section.

The extent of this chapter does not allow a detailed description of the various methods of fixation; instead, the reader is urged to get further information in many of the books on histologic techniques.[4-6] Some fixation methods are commented on briefly.

Formaldehyde forms the basis of most fixatives, and neutral or buffered formol saline is the most popular fixative for various types of specimens. However, it is usually considered a slow fixative. A renal biopsy is very small, and rapid penetration and fixation of the tissue can be obtained with this solution; this is not always the case with other materials. Many other fixatives have been recommended for fixation of renal biopsies, such as Helly's fluid. Corrosive formol (formol-sublimate, 4% formaldehyde in a saturated aqueous solution of mercuric chloride) has been proved very satisfactory as a general routine fixative, particularly suitable for renal biopsies,[7] because it is rapid; only 30 to 45 min are required for renal biopsies. If it is left longer in this fixative, the biopsied tissue will become hard and brittle, making it difficult to cut into thin sections. Excellent histologic detail is achieved and the mercury potentiates many special stains, e.g., PAS and the trichrome method, but unfortunately it appears to interfere somewhat with the methenamine-silver method.

Glutaraldehyde is the preferred fixative for electron microscopy (see Section 3.2.3.1). Perfusion fixation is the technique whereby tissues or organs are fixed by infusion of the fixative in the vessels that are situated in these tissues or organs.[8] This procedure may be used in the experimental animal or in excised kidneys. Often a vasodilator is infused first to ensure dilatation of the vessels. Another method for fast fixation is the so-called dip fixation whereby a fixative is applied on the surface of the kidney. Only a small part of the tissue is then fixed.

3.2.2 *Light microscopy*

3.2.2.1 *Processing of tissue*

When the sample of tissue is small and thin, penetration by alcohol, clearing agents, and wax is rapid; this is especially the case with renal biopsies. Provided that sufficient fixation has occurred, the specimen can be processed overnight on an automated tissue processor set to run for 12 to 14 h, where dehydration occurs through graded alcohols to absolute alcohol. Clearing can be achieved with xylene, toluene, or petroleum. Embedding should be achieved after two changes of melted paraffin wax having a melting point of 56 to 58°C. Although other media are available, paraffin wax remains popular due to the ease with which large numbers of tissue blocks can be processed in relatively short times with minimum supervision. In addition, sectioning and later staining present fewer difficulties than with other media. Paraffin sections can also be obtained rapidly in especially urgent cases by fixation in Carnoy's solution and programming the automated tissue processor to process the tissue in 3 h. It has been proposed that numerous substances can be added to paraffin wax to modify its consistency and frequently its melting point.

Embedding may also take place in plastic. Two groups of resins have been found useful for ultrastructural studies and high-resolution light microscopy; these are epoxy and acrylic resins, like Historesin.

3.2.2.2 *Stains*

3.2.2.2.1 Hematoxylin and eosin (H&E). This is the best known and most widely used staining technique for both normal and pathologic tissue. A well-stained H&E preparation is hard to surpass for the amount of general information it gives, even though it gives rather less information than other stains. It is of value in assessing the cellularity of glomeruli and the degree of necrosis in renal tubules, but is rather ineffective when it comes to examining the glomerular capillary basement membrane. The type of Hematoxylin used is not of any great significance.

3.2.2.2.2 Periodic acid–Schiff (PAS) method. This is an essential staining method that can be used for all renal biopsies in order to obtain a clear impression of glomerular architecture, and in particular of the glomerular basement membrane, especially if a nuclear or counterstain is used. Details for the PAS method are provided below:

1. Bring the section to water; wash for 5 min in running water.
2. Rinse in distilled water.
3. Treat with a 0.5% aqueous solution of periodic acid for 5 min.
4. Wash thoroughly with several changes of distilled water.
5. Treat with Schiff reagent for 15 min.
6. Rinse in three changes of sulfurous acid for 2 min in each rinse.
7. Wash with running water for 3 to 5 min.
8. Stain with hematoxylin and differentiate.

9. Wash in running tap water.
10. Dehydrate, clear, and mount in DPX.

3.2.2.2.3 *Masson's trichrome.* Masson's trichrome is excellent for studying renal architecture with regard to the presence of fibrinoid, the degree of interstitial fibrosis and for detection of basement membrane abnormalities. The procedure is as follows:

1. Bring the sections to water.
2. Stain in Celestin blue iron alum for 5 min.
3. Wash in tap water to remove excess stain.
4. Stain in hematoxylin for 15 min.
5. Wash in tap water, blue for 2 min, and differentiate in 3% acid alcohol for a few seconds.
6. Blue in tap water for 7 to 15 min.
7. Stain in ponceau–acid Fuchsin–orange G for 15 min.
8. Rinse in 0.2% acetified water and differentiate in 5% phosphotungstic acid for 1 to 3 min. Rinse in 0.2% acetified water.
9. Stain in light green for 30 s to 2 min.
10. Rinse in 0.2% acetified water and then in tap water. Dehydrate, clear, and mount.

It is essential to overstain with light green because it cannot be differentiated without spoiling the previous stains.

Ponceau–acid fuchsin–orange G is made up as follows:

ponceau de xylidene	2 g
acid fuchsin	1 g
orange G	2 g

Dissolve in 300 ml of 0.2% acetified water. For use dilute ten times with 0.2% acetified water. A 2% light green solution in 0.2% acetified water is kept as a stock solution, and for use this is diluted 1:10 with 0.2% acetified water.

3.2.2.2.4 *Silver-methenamine method.* This silver stain is useful for evaluation of the glomerular and tubular basement membranes.[9] The reagents needed are

1. 0.5% aqueous periodic acid
2. 0.2% aqueous gold chloride solution
3. 3% aqueous sodium thiosulfate solution
4. Gomori's silver-methenamine solution

Gomori's silver-methenamine solution is made up by taking 100 ml of 3% aqueous methenamine and adding 5 ml of 5% aqueous silver nitrate solution. The resultant mixture is shaken until the white precipitate redissolves. The solution should be stored at 4°C and will keep for six months. To 50 ml of this solution add 6 ml of a 5% aqueous solution of sodium tetraborate. The procedure is as follows:

1. Bring the sections to water and rinse in distilled water.
2. Immerse in periodic acid solution for 15 min.
3. Wash in distilled water.
4. Immerse in silver solution for between 1.5 and 3 h at 50°C in the dark.
5. Wash in distilled water.
6. Immerse in gold chloride for 2 min.

7. Wash in distilled water.
8. Immerse in sodium thiosulfate for 2 min.
9. Wash in running tap water for 5 min.
10. Dehydrate, clear, and mount.

The most satisfactory results with this method are obtained if 1-μm-thick sections are employed. Plastic-embedded, as opposed to paraffin-embedded, material is often best for this purpose, although staining times may have to be considerably prolonged.

Apart from the pictorial or aesthetic value of special staining methods, many are of great diagnostic value in a study of renal disease. Most are directed toward the identification of some substance. The practical methods for carrying out the special staining techniques may be found in the standard texts on practical histopathology such as Lillie.[10]

3.2.2.3 *Semiquantitative estimation*

Semiquantitative methods are often used to investigate the structural changes in various renal conditions. These methods score different parameters at the histologic or electron microscopic level, such as tubular dilatation, disappearance of brush border, and fusion of foot processes, on a scale from 0 to 3+ (Table 1). The investigators may develop their own scoring system and try to make it as reproducible as possible. However, in certain types of renal diseases, schemes for the semiquantitative investigation of renal structures or changes have already been developed and can of course be adopted directly. Use of these standardized scoring schemes makes comparisons with the results of other researchers possible. These standardized schemes, for example, exist in lupus nephritis[11] and renal graft evaluation.[12] The semiquantitative evaluation of interstitial infiltration in renal transplant biopsies is used as an example shown in Table 2.

Table 1 Examples of Parameters That May Be Semiquantitatively Scored

Interstitial inflammation
Tubular dilation
Tubulitis
Disappearance of brush border
Presence of casts
Edema
Mitosis
Regeneration

Table 2 Criteria for Semiquantitative Scoring of Mononuclear Cell Interstitial Infiltration "i" According to the Banff Classification of Kidney Transplant Pathology[12]

i0:	No or trivial interstitial inflammation
i1:	Up to 25% of parenchyma inflamed
i2:	26–50% of parenchyma inflamed
i3:	>50% of parenchyma inflamed

Semiquantitative methods may have certain limitations. Moreover, some data, such as the mean glomerular volume and the distribution of the glomerular volume, can only be evaluated with the use of stereological methods.

In some investigations, semiquantitative scoring may be much easier than it is to obtain morphometric data (Table 3). And in other conditions, it may be possible to show that semiquantitative data are well correlated with the morphometric data. It may then turn out to be simpler to use semiquantitative scoring. Generally, however, morphometric and stereological methods provide the most reproducible results.

Table 3 Histopathological Changes That May Be Difficult to Evaluate Morphometrically

Regeneration of tubules
Tubular vacuolization
Partial brush border loss
Degree of arteritis

3.2.3 *Electron microscopy*

3.2.3.1 *Transmission electron microscopy (TEM)*

For electron microscopy, 1-mm^3 pieces of tissue are immersed in 4% (v/v) aqueous glutaraldehyde buffered with phosphate to pH 7.4 at 4°C. Fixation should take place for periods of between 4 and 12 h. The tissue is then washed with two changes of cold phosphate buffer. Postfixation with cold 1% osmium tetroxide (OsO_4) buffered with phosphate to pH 7.4 for 2 h at 4°C is followed by dehydration in graded ethanol and embedding in araldite epoxy resin. Sections are cut on an ultramicrotome. Thick sections (1 μm) are prepared with glass knives, placed on glass microscope slides, and stained with toluidine blue. Thin sections (60 to 900 nm) are prepared with diamond knives, mounted on copper or nickel grids, and stained with uranyl acetate and lead nitrate or citrate. Silver-stained thin sections may be prepared by the method of Movat.[13] The thin sections are examined by standard transmission electron microscopy.

3.2.3.2 *Scanning electron microscopy (SEM)*

SEM provides significant information regarding the three-dimensional architecture of cells and tissues. Recently, ultrahigh resolution has been developed by the use of a field emission source and an in-lens system.[14] This method has been used to examine the ultrastructure of glomerular and tubular basement membranes.

3.2.4 *Immunofluorescence microscopy*

Immunofluorescence and immunoperoxidase techniques are used to study renal disease, to establish a diagnosis, and to determine pathogenesis.[15] Immunofluorescence is a method for the topographical detection of antigens in cells and tissues and for the demonstration of microorganisms by means of antibodies that are labeled with fluorochromes. Fluorochromes are dyes, the most important being rhodamine derivates and fluorescein isothiocyanate (FITC). In the immunogold staining method, colloidal gold is coupled to antibodies. Some substances have the inherent property of emitting fluorescent light when excited with shortwave radiation. This is called autofluorescence.

Immunofluorescence is best done on fresh frozen tissue, but may in some cases also be done on paraffin-embedded tissue. Refrigerated tissue is usually satisfactory for the detection of immunoglobulins, fibrinogen/fibrin, and albumin. In all cases, tissues should be kept frozen until they are examined. Recurrent freezing and thawing should be avoided.

There are two immunofluorescence methods in use: (1) the *direct* method, in which the tissue is treated with specifically labeled antibodies, like antihuman immunoglobulin conjugated to FITC (Figure 1); and (2) the *indirect* method, in which the tissue is treated first with, for example, an unconjugated antihuman immunoglobulin raised in rabbit or pig and next treated with a fluorescein-conjugated antirabbit or antipig serum (Figure 2). The indirect method may also be used to demonstrate antibodies directed against cells.

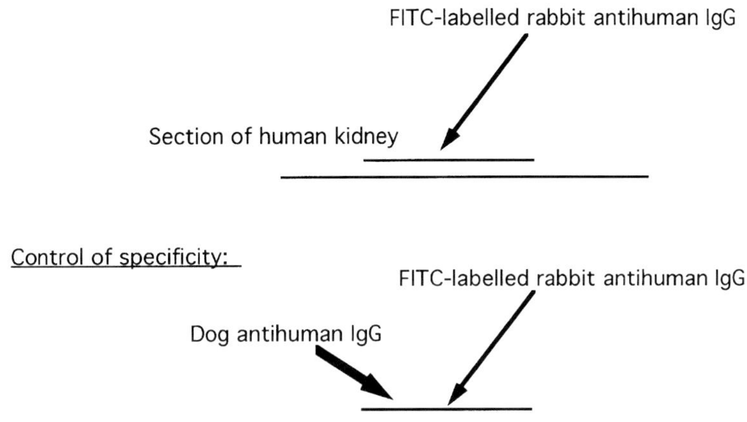

Figure 1 Direct immunofluorescence technique.

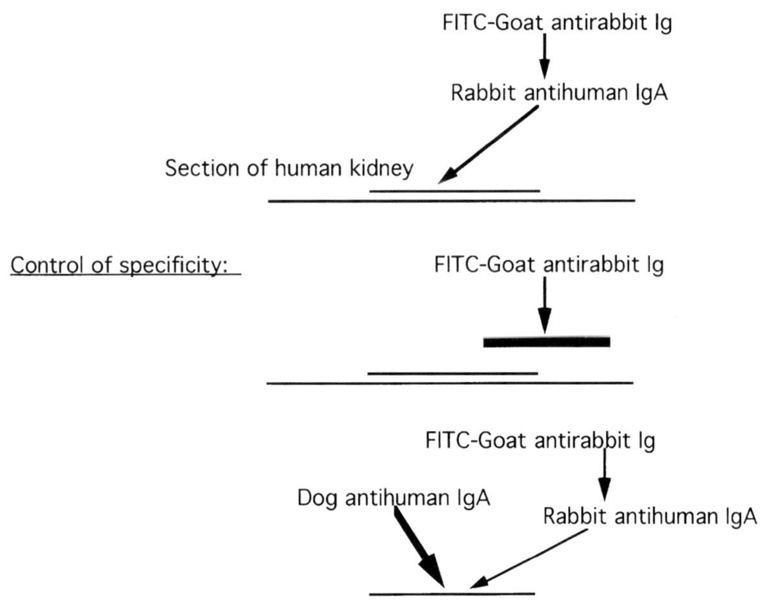

Figure 2 Indirect immunofluorescence technique.

The direct method is shorter than the indirect, which on the other hand is a little more sensitive. The sections produced by either method are examined in a fluorescence microscope with the appropriate filters, so that light of less than 495 nm is available to excite FITC. This will emit light at 525 nm for observation. As fluorescence fades both with exposure to light and with storage, it is necessary to record positive results on fast photographic film.

The processing of the tissue is as follows. Frozen renal tissue is removed from storage and placed on chucks without delay. Needle biopsies can be mounted on a supporting material, e.g., tissue such as liver or artificial material. Both specimen and chuck are refrozen and 7-μm sections cut on a cryostat, air-dried for approximately 5 min on alcohol-cleaned glass slides, and transferred to a moist chamber for the rest of the method. Insufficient or excessive air-drying may cause the sections to float. Sufficient sections are required for the staining with the specifically labeled antibody, and a further one for detection of autofluorescence plus one for immunologic specificity.

Confirmation of the specificity of the antisera is necessary, and the methods used are the Ouchterlony immunodiffusion and immunoelectrophoretic methods.[16] Another technique that can be used for confirmation of specificity is the defined antigen substrate system (DASS), in which purified antigen is coupled to agarose beads and mixed with the antisera.[17-20]

3.2.4.1 *Direct immunofluorescence technique*

1. Wash sections three times, 10 min each, in phosphate-buffered saline (PBS), pH 7.3, to remove unbound plasma protein within vessels and tubules.
2. Drain off excess buffer.
3. Apply antisera labeled with fluorescein isothiocyanate (FITC) diluted in 0.9% saline for 30 min at room temperature (e.g., FITC–rabbit antihuman IgG).
4. Wash sections three times with PBS, pH 7.3, for 10 min, to remove unfixed antiserum.
5. Drain off excess buffer.
6. Mount in 90% glycerol, in PBS, pH 7.3. Blot off excess glycerol.
7. Store overnight in the dark at 4°C.

The specificity must always be controlled and tested in parallel with each antigen, which is applied to an adjacent section. The specificity is obtained with the use of antiserum after absorption with purified antigen. This, however, is expensive, and in many cases purified antigen is not available. "Blocking" reactions are therefore widely used for demonstration of immunologic specificity. In these, the reaction with rabbit antihuman IgG, for example, is inhibited by the prior application of another serum directed against IgG. If this is applied in excess amounts, it will bind to all the antigenic sites on the human IgG and therefore block binding of the second antiserum.[21]

A further modification allows these two steps to be combined as a single step, in which rabbit antihuman IgG/FITC serum is mixed with excess amounts of blocking antibody, and the remainder of the method is performed as before. The result of these controls should be a significant diminution or, preferably, abolition of all positive reactions. If this does not occur, the reaction is not proved to be specific.

3.2.4.2 *Indirect immunofluorescence technique*

1. As in the direct method.
2. As in the direct method.
3. Treat with primary antiserum against human plasma proteins, e.g., rabbit antihuman IgA, diluted in 0.9% saline for 30 min at room temperature.
4. Wash in PBS, pH 7.3, three times, 10 min each, to remove unbound antiserum.
5. Drain off excess buffer.
6. Treat for 30 min with FITC-labeled antisera directed against animal immunoglobulin (e.g., FITC–goat antirabbit Ig).
7. Wash three times, 10 min each, with PBS, pH 7.3, to remove excess unreacted antiserum.
8. Drain off excess buffer.

9. Mount in 90% glycerol in phosphate-buffered saline, pH 7.3. Blot to remove excess glycerol.
10. Store overnight in the dark, 4°C.

There are three possible methods to control specificity. The simplest is one where the application of primary antiserum is omitted. This will ensure that the second antiserum, labeled with FITC, is not binding to the tissue nonspecifically. This is the method most frequently used, although it is not entirely satisfactory. The best method, as described previously, is to use a primary antiserum that has been absorbed with purified antigen. However, this is rarely practicable. Blocking techniques are therefore employed in which prior application of antibody to human IgA (dog antihuman IgA) will fix to the available antigenic sites and prevent binding of subsequently applied antiserum (rabbit antihuman IgA). The second labeled antiserum (goat antirabbit immunoglobulin/FITC) will not fix to the bound dog immunoglobulin, and a significant diminution of specific reaction should occur.

3.2.5 *Enzyme and immunohistochemistry*

Enzyme histochemistry allows one to identify and localize the presence of specific, often tubular, enzymes in tissue sections. It is well known that there is a difference in the distribution of certain enzymes in various segments of the nephron.[22,23] Using enzyme histochemistry to localize different tubular enzymes, it has been possible to define different tubular segments and to show, for example, whether hypotrophy or hypertrophy of these specific segments has taken place.[24] These relatively simple staining methods have provided useful information regarding pathogenic mechanisms.

Enzyme-histochemical methods are preferably used on experimental tissues because they require that the tissue is very rapidly frozen. The method can be summarized shortly as follows. Immediately after removal, the kidney is cut into 2-mm-thick slices. These slices are frozen unfixed in isopentane at –70°C, and 8-μm cryostat sections are collected on coverslips and air-dried. They are incubated at appropriate temperature, often 37°C, for the specific enzyme at various incubation times in order to make the differences between groups as distinctive as possible. After incubation, the tissue is postfixed in formalin (Figure 3).

Immunoperoxidase technique for frozen sections is similar to that described for immunofluorescence, and the enzyme most often used is horseradish peroxidase. Antisera should be checked by immunodiffusion and immunoelectrophoresis and with positive control material. Both direct and indirect immunoperoxidase methods can be used. A further technique involves an unlabeled immunoglobulin bridge that links the primary antiserum to a mixture of soluble complexes of horseradish peroxidase and the antibody to peroxidase (peroxidase–antiperoxidase complexes). The reaction product is a brown polymer produced by the action of oxygen on diaminobenzidine. Free oxygen is released by the reaction of peroxidase with hydrogen peroxide.

The advantages of immunoperoxidase compared to immunofluorescence is that the peroxidase method is a permanent preparation, the localization of immunologic reagents to the kidney is accurate (without subsequent diffusion), and the sections can be examined using light microscopy. H&E counter-stain provides good contrast and better localization than is obtainable with immunofluorescence.

It is possible to demonstrate immunoglobulins in formalin-fixed, paraffin-wax-embedded tissue as well. This can be done using trypsin or microwave treatment prior to the immunofluorescence or immunoperoxidase techniques. Both methods give similar results.[25] Each method, however, has its own disadvantages.[26]

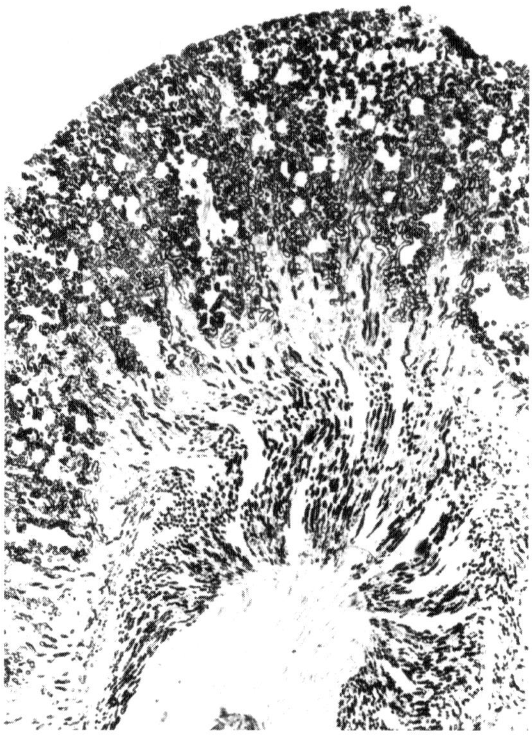

Figure 3 Enzyme histochemical staining for succinate dehydrogenase (SDH) in the kidneys of rats treated with cisplatin for two weeks. Decreased staining is seen in some of the S3 segments of the proximal tubules, indicating the beginning of injury to these segments.

Immunohistologic staining may be used in the identification of intracellular filaments, specific lymphocytic antigens, cytokines, and so on. Immunohistologic staining of tubular cells has been employed most commonly for tumor diagnosis, but is also useful in other renal disorders where the stains can be used to identify tubular segments and localize the target of injury.[27-30] The reader should consult the many review papers and books on immunohistologic methods.

3.2.6 Stereological and morphometric methods

3.2.6.1 Unbiased stereological methods

The use of unbiased stereological and morphometric methods enables the investigator to obtain reliable quantitative data on structure by studying histologic sections or electron micrographs.[31-35] The unbiased quantitative data may be compared with other stereological data or with functional parameters. Using these methods Østerby showed that the peripheral basement membrane in glomeruli increased with the duration of diabetes mellitus.[36] In lithium nephropathy in rats, the renal function was correlated with the volume of proximal tubules.[37] The development of new stereological methods has been very fast in recent years, and it is not possible to give a complete description of these techniques. Instead, this section provides some simple but very useful stereological techniques. For further reading the reader should look into some recent excellent reviews on the subject.[31-34]

The new stereological methods provide unbiased estimates and do not rely upon assumptions regarding the structures under investigation. In contrast, older morphometric methods are based on assumptions, as in, for example, some methods for the estimation of glomerular size where the size distribution and shape of the glomeruli are assumed known.

3.2.6.1.1 Volume fractions and total volumes of structures. In the kidney it is very simple to estimate in an unbiased way the volume fraction of different structures. Volume fraction means the portion of the reference volume (i.e., kidney) that is taken up by a specific structure (i.e., proximal tubules). The volume fraction is also called the relative volume. When the reference volume is known, the absolute volume of the specific structure can be calculated by multiplying the volume fraction by the reference volume.

As an example, the estimation of volume fractions of proximal tubules and interstitial tissue in a rat kidney will be used. After fixation of the kidney (either immersion fixation or perfusion fixation), an effective way of sampling tissue for stereological investigation is to cut it into parallel slices by the use of parallel razor blades mounted on a holder (See Figure 7 in Gundersen et al.[31]). This sampling schema may also be used for many other stereological purposes. All the slices, or every second slice, are/is then embedded in paraffin, and a 3-μm section of each is cut on a microtome. The sections are placed in a microscope where the image is transferred to a TV screen or simply projected onto a table with a mirror. A grid with points is placed on the TV screen or on the table (Figure 4). The sections are then examined in a systematic way so that a few areas from each slide are investigated (Figure 5). In each area, the number of points hitting the proximal tubules and the interstitium is counted (Figure 6). All the counts from each area investigated are added together, and the volume fractions of proximal tubules and interstitium in the kidney can be calculated. The weight of the kidney multiplied by the relative volumes will then provide the absolute volume of proximal tubules and interstitium.

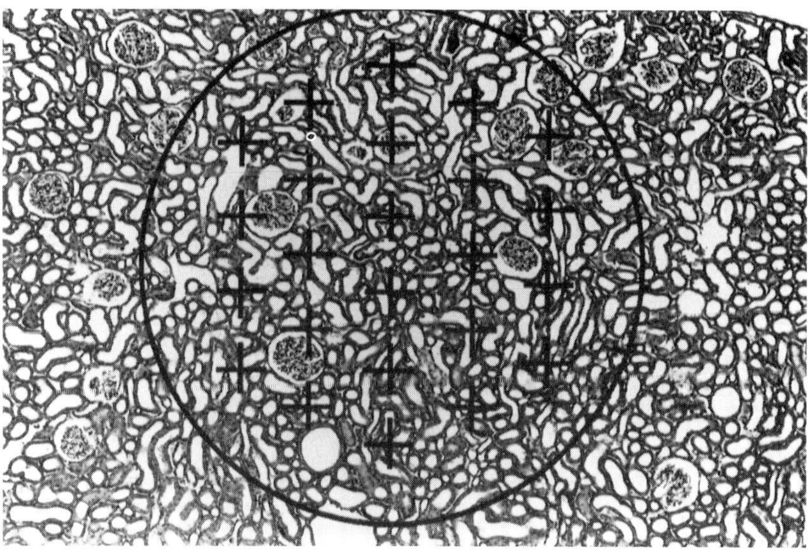

Figure 4 A grid with points with a known distance is placed on the table and the image is projected onto the grid for morphometry.

In the normal human kidney and the normal rat kidney the volume fraction of proximal tubules is about 60%[38,39] and 50 to 60%.[40,41] Measurements of the relative interstitial volume have been more disparate, showing mean values in the normal human kidney ranging from 9 to 30%.[38,39,42-45] These differences are probably due to different fixation and definition of interstitium, although the selection criteria for normal kidneys also has a major impact. The interstitium may be defined with or without intertubular capillaries. The adventitia of major vessels may also be excluded.

Ultrastructural morphometric investigation may be performed on electron micrographs. A point grid is then placed over the pictures and the points counted hitting the

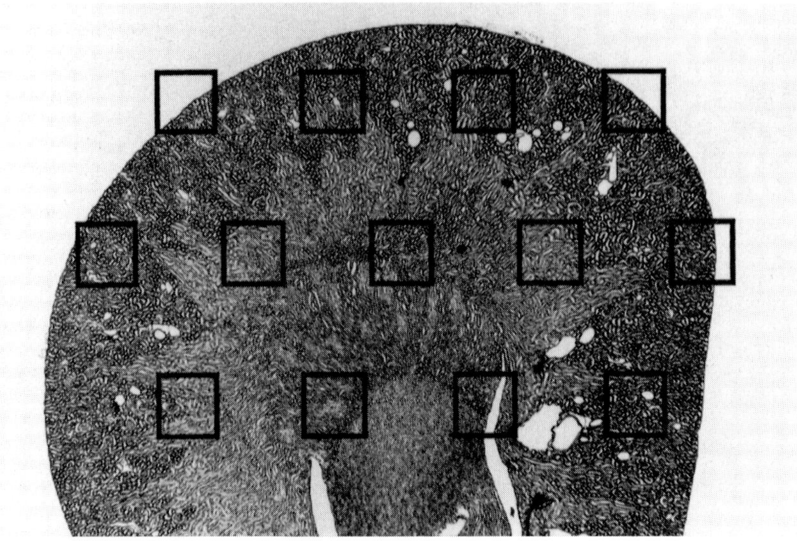

Figure 5 Systematic sampling of cortical tissue for point counting.

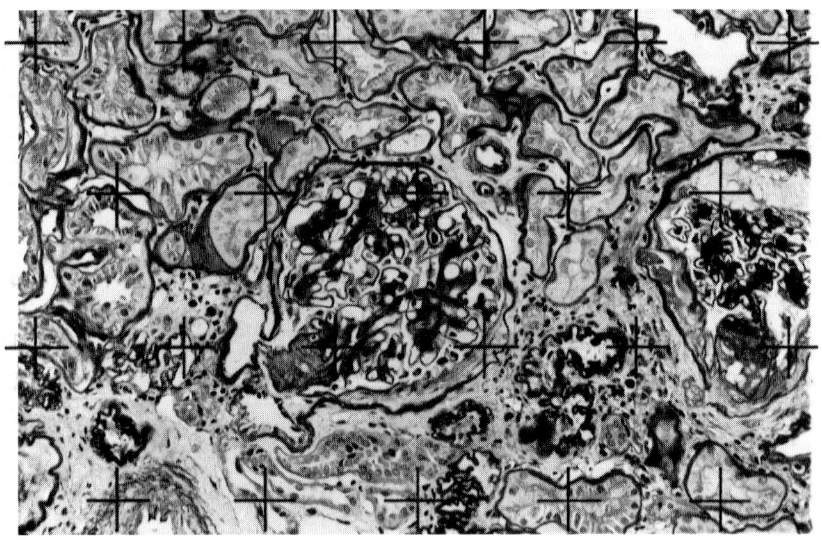

Figure 6 The number of points hitting the different components of the cortex, i.e., proximal tubules, glomerular tuft, interstitium, etc., is counted for the estimation of volume fractions.

structures of interest. For example, in the glomeruli, volume fractions of mesangium, basement membrane, and epithelial cells may be counted, and in the tubules, the relative volume of mitochondria might be of interest. Again, if the reference volume is known, absolute volumes may be calculated.

3.2.6.1.2 Volume of single structures. The individual volume of structures in the kidney may be estimated, and from these values the mean volume can be calculated. It might be of interest to estimate the mean volume of proximal tubular cells or the mean volume of glomeruli.

However, to estimate in an unbiased fashion the number and volume of particles, it is necessary to use the so-called disector.[46] The disector is a stereological sampling device in which randomly selected section pairs are used to count and sample particles (Figure 7). Another mathematical principle, the Cavalieri principle, can then be used to estimate the volume of the correctly sampled particle. If particles are sampled when they are present in a section, their chance of being sampled is proportional to their height, whereas disector-sampled particles have an equal chance of being sampled.

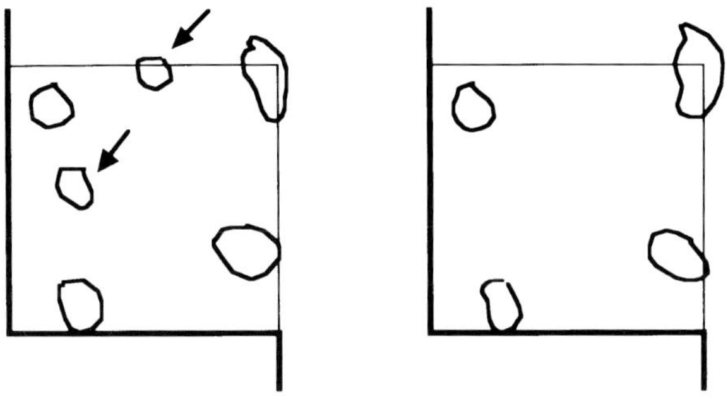

Figure 7 Disector sampling of particles. The particles present in the reference field (left) are counted when they are not present in the look-up field (right).

When the disector principle is used, the samples of renal tissue under investigation are cut into serial sections of a known thickness. The total height of the serial sections must be larger than the height of the highest glomerulus. The first and the second sections are then put into projection microscopes where the images are projected onto a table next to each other. Glomeruli not present in the first section, but present in the second, are sampled. Glomeruli may be sampled in a similar way in the second and third section and so forth. The sampled glomeruli are followed in the subsequent sections, and in each section, or every second section, the area of the glomerular tuft is estimated by point counting. A point grid is randomly placed over the glomerular tuft, and the number of points hitting the tuft is counted. Because the magnification is known, the area associated with each point is known, and the total area of the tuft can be calculated by multiplying the number of points hitting with the point area. The Cavalieri principle is used to estimate the volume of each sampled glomerulus (v_{glom}):

$$v_{glom} = \Sigma a_{glom} \times t_{section} \tag{1}$$

where a_{glom} is the area of the tuft on each section and $t_{section}$ is the thickness of the section. From the volume of each disector-sampled glomerulus the mean glomerular volume is calculated.

The importance of correct sampling of glomeruli for the estimation of their volume has been demonstrated by Marcussen et al.,[47] illustrating that different sampling methods lead to different results. The same principles may be used to estimate volume of other structures, such as cell volumes.

3.2.6.1.3 Length and surface areas of structures. In many instances in renal toxicology it is of major importance to know the length of structures. That could, for example, be the length of proximal tubules in the cortex or the length of capillaries in glomeruli. The estimation of length is simple, and as an example the estimation of the total length of proximal tubules in rat kidney is demonstrated. As described earlier, the kidney is cut into parallel slices, and a number of these are selected and cut into thin sections that are histologically stained. A number of areas are systematically sampled in the sections, and over each area is placed an unbiased counting frame (Figure 8). The number of proximal tubular profiles (Q(PT)) within each counting frame is counted (Figure 9). The area of the counting frame a_{frame} is known because the magnification is known, and the length of the proximal tubules can be calculated from the equation

$$L(PT) = 2 \times \frac{\Sigma Q(PT)}{\Sigma a_{frame}} \times V(kidney) \quad (2)$$

where V(kidney) is the volume of the kidney.

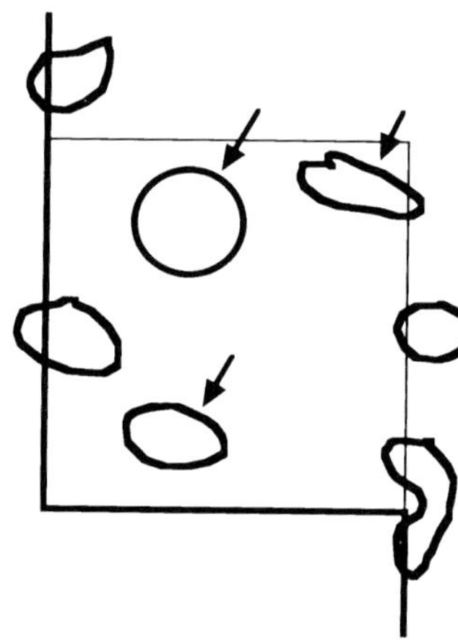

Figure 8 Unbiased counting frame. Particles within the frame and not intersected by the fully drawn forbidden lines are sampled (arrows).

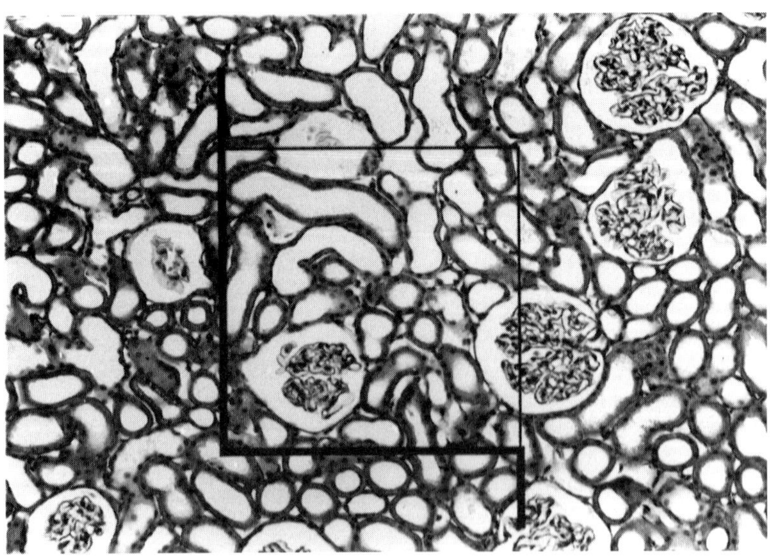

Figure 9 The number of proximal tubular profiles within the unbiased counted frame is counted for the estimation of proximal tubular length.

The surface area of the proximal tubular basement membranes in the kidney may simply be estimated by counting intersection points between the boundary of the tubules and test lines (Figure 10). The surface area of the proximal tubules (S(PT)) is estimated from:

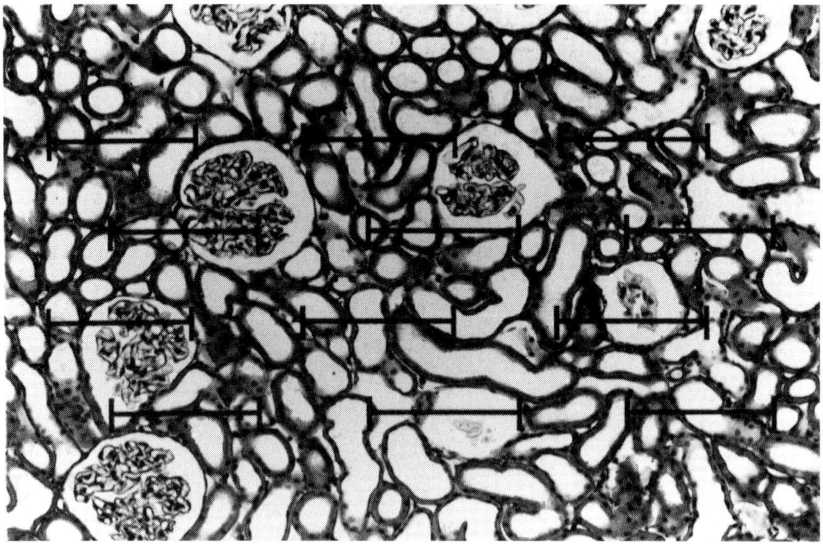

Figure 10 The number of intersections between the proximal tubule boundary and the test lines is counted. In this way the surface area of the proximal tubules may be estimated provided the volume of the reference (cortical) area is known.

$$S(PT) = 2 \times I_L(PT/kidney) \times V(kidney)$$
$$= 2 \times l/p \times \frac{\Sigma I(PT)}{\Sigma P(kidney)} \times V(kidney) \quad (3)$$

where l/p is the test line length per test point, ΣI(PT) is the total number of intersections between the test lines and the proximal tubule basement membrane, ΣP(kidney) is the total number of points hitting the kidney, and V(kidney) is the volume of the kidney.

3.2.6.1.4 Numbers. The total number of structures can also be assessed unbiasedly. For example, the total number of glomeruli in the kidney, or the total number of capillaries in the glomeruli, has been estimated.[48] For the estimation of the total number of structures (i.e., glomeruli) in the kidney, the fractionator design should be used.[49] The main principle is that a certain and known fraction of the kidney is unbiasedly sampled and in that fraction the number of glomeruli is estimated. The glomeruli are counted in the disector to ensure that all glomeruli have an equal chance of being sampled. The number of glomeruli in that fraction is then multiplied with the sampling fraction to provide an estimate of the glomerular number in the whole kidney (for further detail see below). The number of glomeruli has been estimated in humans and rats to be about 600,000[49] and 30,000,[40] respectively. However, the variation in different species is also quite large.[49]

3.2.6.1.5 Counting of glomeruli with the fractionator principle. A human kidney is split in half before fixation in formaldehyde. After fixation, the kidney is weighed. The kidney is then cut into slabs of which a certain fraction is sampled. The medulla is excised from the samples. The slabs are cut into bars and a fraction of them is sampled. These are cut into small blocks of which a fraction is taken. In this way a known fraction (1/140) of the whole kidney is sampled systematically. The sampled tissue pieces are embedded in paraffin in two to four capsules and cut exhaustively by serial sectioning at 25 µm. Every tenth of these sections, and the following section, is sampled and stained with PAS. The sampling fraction for light microscopy f_n is then 140 × 10 = 1400. The counting should be carried out in a darkened room using two projection light microscopes placed so that the fields of vision are projected side by side onto a table. A test system is applied to the fields of vision (see Figure 1 in Marcussen[50]). The magnification is calibrated to about 150× to

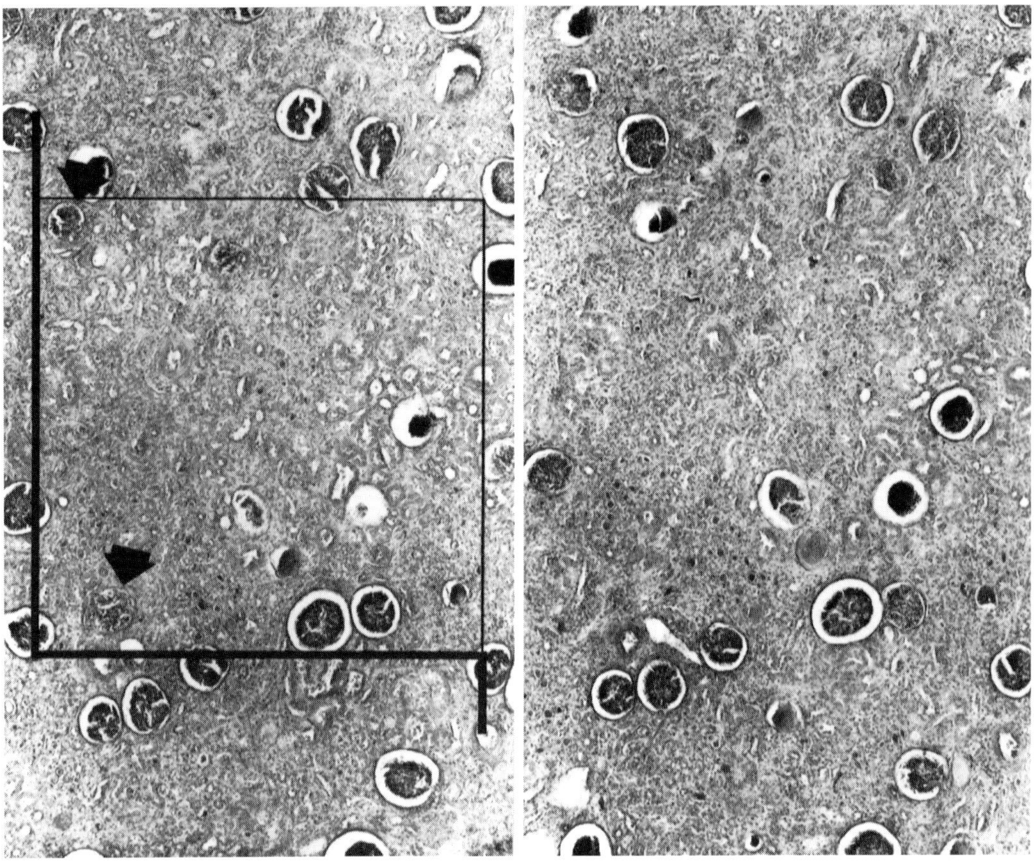

Figure 11 Disector sampling of glomeruli in kidney from patient with renal artery stenosis. The glomeruli present in the left reference field are counted when they are not present in the look-up field (right).

200× by projecting a stage micrometer grid onto the table. A slide with a sampled section is placed in the first microscope and a slide with the following section in the second microscope. The stage of the first microscope is moved by motors in predetermined, equidistant steps in two orthogonal directions. The step size can be controlled using the X–Y axes of the Vernier scales on the stage. In this way, the fraction of a section covered by the test system is well defined. If the grid area is 59,900 mm^2 and the projected magnification is 158×, then the real area of the section covered by the grid is $59{,}900/158^2 = 2.40\ mm^2$. The motor is adjusted to step x and y mm along the length of the microslide. The fraction of the sectional area that is covered by the grid moved in steps is $f_a = 2.40/(x \cdot y)$. The disector is used to count glomeruli. A glomerulus is counted if it appears in a sample frame (in the reference section), but is not present in the corresponding look-up section (Figure 11). In order to optimize the sampling efficiency, both sections are used in two steps as reference and look-up sections. The number of counted glomeruli, Q^-, is then twice what could have been estimated if counting was done in only one direction. Glomeruli are excluded for counting if they are too close to either artificially cut edges or surfaces, where glomerular identity is ambiguous or glomeruli may be lost.[49] The fraction of tissue used for counting is estimated by counting the number of points hitting the tissue, P_s, as well as the number of points hitting the tissue used for counting, P_f. The general formula of estimation of particle number using the fractionator is

$$N = 1/f_n \times 1/f_a \times P_s/P_f \times 1/2 \times \Sigma Q^- \tag{4}$$

where f_n = 1400 and P_s, P_f, and f_a are as defined previously. The factor one half is used because glomeruli are counted in both directions in the microscopic design.

3.2.6.2 *Morphometric methods relying on assumptions ("biased methods")*

Large numbers of methods have been developed that are based upon assumptions regarding the structures under investigation. These assumptions can, for example, pertain to the shape of certain structures or their size distribution. The major problem with morphometric methods based on assumptions is that it is not known whether the assumptions are correct. For example, the size distribution of glomeruli may be different in a group of rats exposed to a nephrotoxic agent compared with a control group. This could be seen if some glomeruli in the toxic group underwent hypertrophy as a response to the toxic agent whereas other glomeruli underwent atrophy. This change may give rise to wrong results, and significant changes could be found that do not exist in reality. However, some of the methods may be useful, especially when it is necessary to estimate the volume of individual renal structures, particularly the glomerular volume. One biased method that may be helpful, and which is also applicable on biopsies, is the method by Weibel and Gomez.[35,51]

Estimation of glomerular volume by the method of Weibel and Gomez is probably the most widely used for estimation of glomerular volume. The following equation is used to estimate mean glomerular volume (v(glom)):

$$\bar{v}(\text{glom}) = \bar{a}(\text{glom})^{3/2} \cdot \beta \cdot k \tag{5}$$

where a(glom) is the mean cross-sectional area of glomeruli in a section, β is a shape coefficient, and k is a size distribution coefficient. The cross-sectional areas of glomeruli are normally estimated on one or more sections so that about 50 to 100 glomerular profiles are measured by point counting or by more automated means. If point counting is used, a grid is randomly placed over each glomerulus and the number of points hitting the glomerular tuft is counted. When the magnification is known, the area associated with each point, a_{point}, is known and then the area of the glomerular tuft, a(glom), is calculated by multiplying a_{point} by the number of points hitting. In a biopsy, it may be necessary to measure glomeruli in more than one section to get enough glomeruli. In these cases, it is preferable that the sections are 50 to 100 μm apart to avoid counting on the same glomerular profiles. When the necessary numbers of glomerular areas have been estimated, the mean glomerular area is calculated and put into the equation. β and k are normally assumed to be 1.38 and 1.1, respectively. The equation is then:

$$\bar{v}(\text{glom}) = \bar{a}(\text{glom})^{3/2} \times 1.38 \times 1.1 \tag{6}$$

Many other biased methods exist for the estimation of structures in the kidney and other organs. However, they do not provide any major advantage over the unbiased stereological methods that have been described previously. Unbiased stereological methods for estimation of total volume, length, and surfaces are so easy and simple that the unbiased methods should be used.

3.2.6.3 *Computerized methods of reconstruction of nephrons*

Reconstruction of nephrons can be important to determine the localization of the nephrotoxic injury or the areas of the nephron that undergo compensatory hypertrophy in certain situations. Computer-assisted three-dimensional reconstruction of the nephron is, however, a very time consuming investigation. Dørup et al.[52] used computer-assisted reconstruction of cortical distal nephron segments to identify the structurally changed segments after lithium treatment in the rat. The method requires that serial sections be made through the area of the kidney that are going to be investigated. The sections or part of them are then scanned into the computer, which is used to locate the segments and which also can be used to draw a three-dimensional map of the nephron. After reembedding of the segments, electron microscopy may be used to identify and further investigate sections of interest. Using this method, Dørup et al.[52] demonstrated that the tubular dilatation in lithium nephropathy took place in the connecting and initial collecting tubules and in the first part of cortical collecting ducts. They also demonstrated changes in individual cell types.

3.2.7 *Confocal microscopy*

Confocal scanning microscopy represents a microscopic technology that can produce noninvasive, high-resolution images from a thick object by eliminating all the reflected light (or fluorescence) from planes above or below the plane in focus. Therefore, instead of seeing an otherwise confusing picture of many cell layers overlying one another, one eliminates all but a single plane of cells. Tandem scanning confocal microscopy permits the noninvasive microscopic viewing of unstained, living, solid organs in real time. The reader is advised to get further information on this subject in the recent articles by Andrews and Cavanagh.[53,54]

3.3 *Comments on techniques related to specific renal structures*

3.3.1 *Glomerular lesions*

Many types of glomerular lesions may be seen in toxic conditions. Toxic agents may damage primarily selective glomerular components, such as in Adriamycin models of the nephrotic syndrome. Endothelial injury is seen after mitomycin administration. However, most often, the nephrotoxic agents may indirectly, via pathophysiologic changes, cause the development of glomerular injury. The various forms of glomerular injury may include immune complex disease, with deposits in various locations in the glomerulus and endothelial, mesangial, or epithelial cellular damage. These changes may be examined with the "normal procedure" for the evaluation of a renal biopsy. Morphometric methods may be applied to histologic sections for the quantitation of percentage of involved glomeruli, glomerular volume, or percentage of damaged glomeruli. Electron microscopically, the morphometric methods may be used to determine the volume of mesangium,[55] thickness of the capillary basement membrane,[36] or the width of the foot processes.[55,56]

Chronic glomerular injury is characterized by glomerular sclerosis. It might typically be due to direct glomerular injury, a consequence of glomerular hypertrophy in remnant glomeruli, or ischemic damage. The earliest detection of chronic glomerular changes may require electron microscopy, while more pronounced changes can be seen in light microscopy. Special stains like Masson's trichrome may be helpful for demonstration of the sclerotic lesion, and immunohistology can be used to identify the type of collagen that is present in the lesion. Morphometry may help quantitate the amount of involved glomeruli.

3.3.2 *Tubular lesions*

Direct tubular injury may be produced by a number of drugs. Aminoglycoside antibiotics are associated with patchy proximal tubular necrosis.[57] Also, amphotericin B and cisplatin may have a direct nephrotoxic effect on proximal tubules.[40,57-59] The direct effect may be studied by histology or enzyme histochemical methods that allow early detection of enzyme changes in the kidneys.[59] If the direct toxic effects are barely visible, stereological methods may not be of much help. However, the ultrastructural changes, such as thinning of brush border, condensation of nuclear chromatin, and focal areas of necrosis can be seen and detected.[58,60,61] It is possible to apply stereological methods to electron micrographs and, for example, to estimate the surface area of the proximal tubules.

Progressive renal changes may be followed by estimation of the volume and length of proximal tubules. These changes are often accompanied by interstitial fibrosis.[62]

The S_3 segment of the proximal tubule is particularly susceptible to ischemic injury.[63] In ischemic acute tubular necrosis (ATN), the most severe morphological changes have also been found in the S_3 segment of the proximal tubule and in the thick ascending loop of Henle.[64,65] Immunostaining for epithelial membrane antigen (EMA), lectins, and cytokeratins of varying molecular weight may help identify the different parts of the nephron in ischemic conditions.

Tubules showing increased staining for various segment-specific enzymes or antibodies can be regarded as hyperplastic or having increased functional activity.[66-68] In patients with chronic renal failure, clusters of hypertrophied nephrons with increased concentration of tubular and glomerular marker proteins can be seen.

3.3.3 *Interstitial lesions*

The interstitial lesions most often investigated are interstitial fibrosis and interstitial infiltrate. For the examination of interstitial fibrosis, histologic methods for the staining of collagen and interstitial tissue should be applied, such as Masson's trichrome, sirius red, or van Gieson. In addition, morphometric assessment of the amount of interstitial tissue with simple point counting that yields the volume fraction of the interstitial tissue is very fast and reliable and often gives a much better figure than semiquantitative estimation. Often one will find a correlation between the reduction in the tubules and the increase in interstitial tissue (Figure 12).

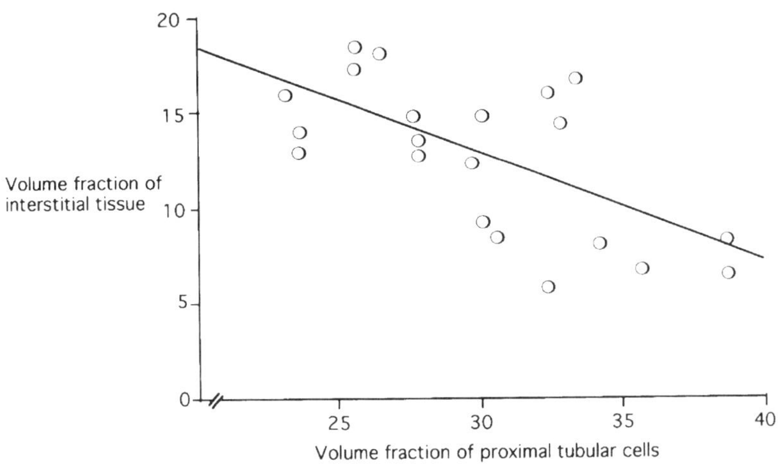

Figure 12 Correlation between the reduction in proximal tubular cells and increase in the amount of interstitial tissue in rats treated with lithium for eight weeks from time of birth.

Interstitial infiltrate consists of inflammatory cells; the amount and type depend on the condition of renal disease. The inflammatory cells may be determined to some extent with the use of normal histologic stains. However, a more precise determination of the type of inflammatory cells may require immunohistologic methods. Exact quantitation of the inflammatory infiltrate based on immunohistologic and morphometric methods may be quite tricky because the immunohistologic staining may be of very different intensity. Morphometrically, one may either estimate the volume fraction of interstitial tissue that is occupied with the specific type of inflammatory cell or one may count the number of inflammatory cells in a certain known area. Both methods may be biased by the varying intensity of the immunohistologic staining, and the method of estimating the number of cells per area is biased by variation in section thickness.

3.3.4 Vascular lesions

Vascular lesions may be present in many toxic renal conditions. Some of them, of course, are secondary to the tubular or glomerular injury or to the accompanying hypertension. Others may be the result of direct vascular injury (cyclosporine) or may give rise to renal vasoconstriction (cyclosporine, nonsteroidal inflammatory drugs in certain patients). Specific histologic stains may help to identify the involved vessels. In biopsies, the sampling error of vessels may be pronounced, and in these cases semiquantitative methods may be as good as morphometric methods. When more renal tissue is available, morphometric methods may be used to estimate the thickness of the vessel wall, the number of capillaries, or the capillary surface area.

3.4 Artifacts

Artifacts may be due to various influences on the tissue. Olsen et al.[69] have described in detail the artifacts that may be present in renal biopsies investigated by electron microscopy. A number of these may also be present in tissue for ordinary light microscopy. They are listed in Table 4. In general, glomeruli are very resistant to the influences of biopsy procedure and fixation.[69] Perfusion fixation dilates the glomerular capillary loops, and the basement membrane may be thinner than in immersion fixed tissue. In contrast to glomeruli, tubular epithelium, and in particular proximal tubular cells, are very vulnerable structures. *In vivo* the proximal tubules are dilated, whereas the lumen of the proximal tubules closes within a few seconds after the blood flow has stopped. The brush border is also very sensitive to delay between fixation and cessation of blood flow to the kidney.

Table 4 Artifacts That May Be Present in Renal Tissue

Mechanical damage to the tissue before fixation
Delay in fixation
Wrong chemical composition of fixation fluid
Changes caused by the processing
Variation in section thickness
Variation in microscopic equipment

These artifacts should be considered when examining renal tissue. It is important to be careful when comparing tissues fixed with one method and tissues fixed with a different method.

3.4.1 Variability in the measurements of structures

Values for the size of structures, such as volume of proximal tubules or mean glomerular volume, may depend on a number of factors. Values reported for glomerular volume in normal rats, for example, vary widely. Some of this variability may reflect differences in the strain, size, sex, and diet of the animals studied. Another source of variability may come from the morphometric method used, as discussed earlier in the section on biased morphometric methods. Additional variability in the measurement of structures may come from differences in the morphological technique. Miller and Meyer[70] showed that the mean glomerular volume obtained in paraffin-embedded tissue was approximately 40% lower than values for the volume obtained in methacrylate-embedded tissue from the same kidneys. Marcussen[40] found that the linear shrinkage in paraffin-embedded rat kidneys was 0.173 ± 0.010 (mean ± SEM) in controls and 0.154 ± 0.013 in a group of cisplatin-treated rats. In contrast, it is known that only an insignificant amount of shrinkage takes place in Epon or methacrylate-embedded tissue.

Sampling variability has to be eliminated as much as possible. One way is to use random sampling whenever possible. This is much easier when one has the entire organ for examination and much more difficult if only a small biopsy is available. Also, whether the lesion is focal or diffuse is important. Diffuse lesions such as in different types of glomerulonephritis may be dealt with in biopsies easier than very focal lesions.

References

1. Oliver, J., *Architecture of the Kidney in Chronic Bright's Disease,* Paul B. Hoeber, New York, 1939.
2. Kramp, R.A., MacDowell, M., Gottschalk, C.W., and Oliver, J.R., A study by microdissection and micropuncture of the structure and the function of the kidneys and the nephrons of rats with chronic renal damage, *Kidney Int.,* 5, 147, 1974.
3. Olsen, S. and Solez, K., Morphological features of acute renal failure, in *Toxicology of the Kidney,* Hook, J.B. and Goldstein, R.S., Eds., Raven Press, New York, 1993, 99.
4. Bancroft, J.D. and Stevens, A., *Theory and Practice of Histological Techniques,* Churchill Livingstone, New York, 1990.
5. Meadows, R., *Renal Histopathology, a Light Microscopy Study of Renal Disease,* Oxford University Press, Oxford, 1973.
6. Dunhill, M.S., *Pathological Basis of Renal Disease,* Balliere Tindall, Oxford, 1976.
7. Lendrum, A.C., On the fixation of postmortem material, *J. Pathol. Bacteriol.,* 52, 132, 1941.
8. Maunsbach, A.B., The influence of different fixatives and fixation methods on the ultrastructure of rat kidney proximal tubule cells. I. Comparison of different perfusion fixation methods and of glutaraldehyde, formaldehyde and osmium tetraoxide fixatives, *J. Ultrastruct. Res.,* 15, 242, 1966.
9. Jones, D.B., Nephrotic glomerulonephritis, *Am. J. Pathol.,* 33, 313, 1957.
10. Lillie, R.D., *Histopathologic Technic and Practical Histochemistry,* McGraw-Hill, New York, 1965, 45 and 174.
11. Balow, J.E., Clinicopathologic correlations in lupus nephritis, *Ann. Intern. Med.,* 91, 596, 1979.
12. Solez, K., Axelsen, R.A., Benediktsson, H., et al., International standardization of criteria for the histologic diagnosis of renal allograft rejection: the Banff working classification of kidney transplant pathology, *Kidney Int.,* 44, 411, 1993.
13. Movat, H.Z., Silver impregnation methods for electron microscopy, *Am. J. Clin. Pathol.,* 53, 528, 1961.
14. Nagatani, T., Saito, S., Sato, M., and Yamada, M., Development of an ultra high resolution scanning electron microscopy by a field emission source and in-lens system, *Scanning Electron Microsc.,* 1, 901, 1987.
15. Larsen, S. and Brun, C., Immune deposits in human glomerulopathy, *Acta Pathol. Microbiol. Scand. Sect. A,* 87, 321, 1979.

16. Ouchterlony, O. and Nilsson, L.Å., Immunodiffusion and immunoelectrophoresis, in *Handbook of Experimental Immunology*, Weir, D.M., Ed., Blackwell Scientific, Oxford, 655, 1973.
17. Capel, P.J.A., The defined antigen substrate spheres (DASS) system and some of its applications, *Ann. N.Y. Acad. Sci.*, 254, 108, 1975.
18. Knapp, W.J., Haaijmann, J.J., Schuit, H.R.E., Radl, J., Van Den Berg, P., Ploem, J.S., and Hijmans, W., Microfluorometric evaluation of conjugate specificity with the antigen substrate spheres (DASS) system, *Ann. N.Y. Acad. Sci.*, 254, 94, 1975.
19. Scales, R.W., Jacobs, N.F., and Skaggs, R., Use of immunoglobulin coupled to agarose beads for examining the specificity of conjugates, *J. Clin. Microbiol.*, 2, 292, 1975.
20. Streefkerk, J.G., Van der Ploeg, M., and Kors, N., Some aspects of immunohistoperoxidase reactions in the agarose bead model system, *Ann. N.Y. Acad. Sci.*, 254, 212, 1975.
21. Goldman, M., *Fluorescent Antibody Methods*, Academic Press, New York, 1968.
22. Harrison, D.J., Kharbanda, R.K., Cunningham, J., et al. Distribution of gluthathione S transferase isoenzymes in human kidney: basis for possible markers of tubular injury, *J. Clin. Pathol.*, 42, 624, 1989.
23. Jacobsen, N.O., The activity of mitochondrial alfa-glycerophosphate dehydrogenase in the rat nephron following triiodo-L-thyrine treatment. A histochemical study, *Histochemistry*, 46, 307, 1976.
24. Jacobsen, N.O., Jørgensen, F., and Thomsen, Å.C., On the localization of some phosphatases in three different segments of the proximal tubules in the rat kidney, *J. Histochem. Cytochem.*, 15, 456, 1967.
25 Davey, F.R. and Busch, G.J., Immunohistochemistry of glomerulonephritis using horseradish peroxidase and fluorescein-labeled antibody: a comparison of two techniques, *Ann. J. Clin. Pathol.*, 53, 531, 1970.
26. Taylor, C.R., Immunoperoxidase technique. Practical and theoretical aspects, *Arch. Pathol. Lab. Med.*, 1021, 113, 1978.
27. Howie, A.J., Gunson, B.K., and Sparke, J., Morphometric correlates of renal excretory function, *J. Pathol.*, 160, 245, 1990.
28. Ivanyi, B. and Olsen, T.S., Immunohistochemical identification of tubular segments in percutaneous renal biopsies, *Histochemistry*, 95, 351, 1991.
29. Marcussen, N., Atubular glomeruli in renal artery stenosis, *Lab. Invest.*, 65, 558, 1991.
30. Scherberich, J.E., Wolf, G., Albers, C., Nowark, A., Stuckhardt, C., and Schoeppe, W., Glomerular and tubular membrane antigens reflecting cellular adaptation in human renal failure, *Kidney Int.*, 36 (Suppl. 27), S38, 1989.
31. Gundersen, H.J.G., Bagger, P., Bendtsen, T.F., et al., The new stereological tools: disector, fractionator, nucleator and point sampled intercepts and their use in pathological research and diagnosis, *Acta Pathol. Microbiol. Immunol. Scand.*, 96, 857, 1988.
32. Gundersen, H.J.G., Bendtsen, T.F., Korbo, L., et al., Some new, simple and efficient stereological methods and their use in pathological research and diagnosis, *Acta Pathol. Microbiol. Immunol. Scand.*, 96, 379, 1988.
33. Braendgaard, H. and Gundersen, H.J.G., The impact of recent stereological advances on quantitative studies of the nervous system, *J. Neurosci. Meth.*, 18, 39, 1986.
34. Gundersen, H.J.G., Stereology of arbitrary particles. A review of unbiased number and size estimators and the presentation of some new ones, in memory of William R. Thompson, *J. Microsc.*, 143, 3, 1986.
35. Weibel, E.R., *Stereological Methods. Practical Methods for Biological Morphometry*, Vol. 1, Academic Press, New York, 1979.
36. Østerby, R., Morphometric studies of the peripheral glomerular basement membrane in early juvenile diabetes. I. Development of initial basement membrane thickening, *Diabetologia*, 8, 84, 1972.
37. Ottosen, P.D., Sigh, B., Kristensen, J., Olsen, S., and Christensen, S., Lithium induced interstitial nephropathy associated with chronic renal failure. Reversibility and correlation between functional and structural changes, *Acta Pathol. Microbiol. Immunol. Scand. Sect. A*, 92, 447, 1984.
38. Marcussen, N. and Olsen, T.S., Atubular glomeruli in patients with chronic pyelonephritis, *Lab. Invest.*, 62, 467, 1990.

39. Møller, J.C. and Skriver, E., Quantitative ultrastructure of human proximal tubules and cortical interstitium in chronic renal disease (hydronephrosis), *Virchows Arch. A*, 406, 389, 1985.
40. Marcussen, N., Atubular glomeruli in cisplatin-induced chronic interstitial nephropathy. An experimental stereological investigation, *Acta Pathol. Microbiol. Immunol. Scand.*, 98, 1087, 1990.
41. Pfaller, W., *Structure Function Correlation on Rat Kidney. Quantitative Correlation of Structure and Function in the Normal and Injured Rat Kidney*, Springer–Verlag, Berlin, 1982.
42. Bohle, A., Bader, R., Grund, K.E., Mackensen, S., and Neunhoeffer, J., Serum creatinine concentration and renal interstitial volume. Analysis of correlations in endocapillary (acute) glomerulonephritis and in moderately severe mesangioproliferative glomerulonephritis, *Virchows Arch. A*, 375, 87, 1977.
43. Dunnill, M.S. and Halley, W., Some observations on the quantitative anatomy of the kidney, *J. Pathol.*, 110, 113, 1973.
44. Hestbech, J., Hansen, H.E., Amdisen, A., and Olsen, S., Chronic renal lesions following long-term treatment with lithium, *Kidney Int.*, 12, 205, 1977.
45. Kappel, B. and Olsen, S., Cortical interstitial tissue and sclerosed glomeruli in the normal human kidney, related to age and sex. A quantitative study, *Virchows Arch. A*, 387, 271, 1980.
46. Sterio, D.C., The unbiased estimation of number and sizes of arbitrary particles using the disector, *J. Microsc.*, 134, 127, 1984.
47. Marcussen, N., Ottosen, P.D., Christensen, S., and Olsen, T.S., Atubular glomeruli in lithium-induced chronic nephropathy in rats, *Lab. Invest.*, 61, 295, 1989.
48. Nyengaard, J.R. and Marcussen, N., The number of glomerular capillaries estimated by an unbiased and efficient stereological method, *J. Microsc.*, 171, 27, 1993.
49. Nyengaard, J.R. and Bendtsen, T.F., The practical use of the fractionator in glomerular counting, *Acta Stereol.*, 8, 275, 1989.
50. Marcussen, N., Atubular glomeruli in renal artery stenosis, *Lab. Invest.*, 65, 558, 1991.
51. Weibel, E.R. and Gomez, D.M., A principle for counting tissue structures on random sections, *J. Appl. Physiol.* 17, 343, 1962.
52. Dørup, J., Ottosen, P.D., et al. Lithium-induced structural changes in the cortical distal nephron. Localized by computer-assisted three-dimensional reconstruction, *J. Ultrastruct. Mol. Struct. Res.*, 100, 212, 1988.
53. Andrews, P.M., The histopathology of kidney uriniferous tubules as revealed by noninvasive confocal vital microscopy, *Scanning*, 16, 174, 1994.
54. Cavanagh, H.D., Petroll, W.M., and Jester, J.V., The application of confocal microscopy to the study of living system, *Neurosci. Biobehav. Rev.*, 17, 483, 1993.
55. Marcussen, N., Ottosen, P.D., and Christensen, S., Ultrastructural quantitation of atubular and hypertrophic glomeruli in rats with lithium-induced chronic nephropathy, *Virchows Arch. A*, 417, 513, 1990.
56. Seefeldt, T., Bohman, S.-O., Gundersen, H.J.G., Maunsbach, A.B., Petersen, V.B., and Olsen, S., Quantitative relationship between glomerular foot process width and proteinuria in glomerulonephritis, *Lab. Invest.*, 44, 541, 1981.
57. Bennett, W.M. and Porter, G.A., Overview of clinical nephrotoxicity, in *Toxicology of the Kidney*, Hook, J.B. and Goldstein, R.S., Eds., Raven Press, New York, 1993, 63.
58. Dobyan, D.C., Levi, J., Jacobs, C., Kosek, J., and Weiner, M.W., Mechanism of cis-platinum nephrotoxicity. II. Morphologic observations, *J. Pharmacol. Exp. Ther.*, 213, 551, 1980.
59. Marcussen, N. and Jacobsen, N.O., The progression of cisplatin-induced tubulointerstitial nephropathy in rats, *Acta Pathol. Microbiol. Immunol. Scand.*, 100, 256, 1992.
60. Chopra, S., Kaufman, J.S., Jones, T.W., Hong, W.K., Gehr, M.K., Hamburger, R.J., Flamenbaum, W., Trump, B.F., and Chase, D.H., Cis-diamminedichlorplatinum-induced acute renal failure in the rat, *Kidney Int.*, 21, 54, 1982.
61. Jones, T.W., Chopra, S., Kaufman, J.S., Flamenbaum, W., and Trump, B.F., Cis-Diamminedichloroplatinum (II)-induced acute renal failure in the rat. Correlation of structural and functional alterations, *Lab. Invest.*, 52, 363, 1985.
62. Dobyan, D.C., Long-term consequences of cis-platinum-induced renal injury: a structural and functional study, *Anat. Rec.*, 212, 239, 1985.

63. Venkatachalam, M.A., Bernard, D.B., Donohue, J.F., and Levinsky, N.G., Ischemic damage and repair in the rat proximal tubule: differences among the S1, S2 and S3 segments, *Kidney Int.*, 14, 31, 1978.
64. Brezis, M., Rosen, S., Silva, P., and Epstein, F.H., Transport activity modifies thick ascending limb damage in the isolated perfused kidney, *Kidney Int.*, 25, 65, 1984.
65. Olsen, T.S. and Hansen, H.E., Ultrastructure of medullary tubules in ischemic acute tubular necrosis and acute interstitial nephritis in man, *Acta Pathol. Microbiol. Immunol. Scand.*, 98, 1139, 1990.
66. Gröne, H.-J., Weber, K., Gröne, E., Helmchen, U., and Osborn, M., Coexpression of keratin and vimentin in damaged and regenerating tubular epithelia of the kidney, Am. J. Pathol., 129, 1, 1987.
67. Jacobsen, N.O., Olesen, O.V., Thomsen, K., Ottosen, P.D., and Olsen, S., Early changes in renal distal convoluted tubules and collecting ducts of lithium-treated rats, Lab. Invest., 46, 298, 1982.
68. Jacobsen, N.O., Ottosen, P.D., and Christensen, S., Early renal changes in lithium-treated normal and vasopressin-deficient rats, *Acta Pathol. Microbiol. Immunol. Scand. Suppl.*, 4, 56, 1988.
69. Olsen, T.S., Racusen, L.C., and Solez, K., Ultrastructural investigation of renal biopsies: a discussion of artifacts and special methodology, *J. Electron Microsc. Tech.*, 9, 283, 1988.
70. Miller, P.L. and Meyer, T.W., Effects of tissue preparation on glomerular volume and capillary structure in the rat, *Lab. Invest.*, 63, 862, 1990.

chapter four

The Isolated Perfused Kidney*

Gary L. Diamond

4.1 Introduction 59
4.2 Advantages of the isolated perfused kidney preparation over other *in vitro* preparations 60
4.3 Limitations of the isolated perfused kidney preparation 61
4.4 Basic methods for isolation and perfusion of the kidney 62
4.4.1 Isolation of the kidney 62
4.4.1.1 Laparotomy 62
4.4.1.2 Ureteral cannulation 63
4.4.1.3 Cannulation of the vasculature 63
4.4.2 Perfusion apparatus 65
4.4.3 Perfusate 66
4.4.3.1 Substrates 66
4.4.3.2 Colloid 67
4.4.3.3 Oxygen carriers 67
4.5 New developments in methodology 68
4.5.1 Isolated perfused rat kidney-liver preparation 68
4.5.2 Nuclear magnetic resonance (NMR) spectroscopy measurements of renal tissue metabolism 68
4.5.3 Continuous microscopy of renal microvasculature during perfusion 68
4.5.4 Perfusion of remnant kidneys 69
4.5.5 Moment analysis of single-pass transit times 69
4.5.6 Isolated perfused amphibian kidney 69
4.6 Applications of the isolated perfused kidney for evaluating nephrotoxic chemicals 71
References 71

4.1 Introduction

The history of the use of isolated perfused kidney preparations for studying nephrotoxicology extends to at least 1876, when Bunge and Schmiedeberg reported the synthesis of hippurate from glycine and benzoic acid in the isolated perfused dog kidney.[1] Since this early report, the technique has been applied to a variety of problems in renal physiology, biochemistry, and toxicology. Perfusions described in the early literature were limited to relatively short duration; perfusate flow and glomerular filtration rates became severely

* In memory of Dr. Julius J. Cohen.

0-8493-3341-5/96/$0.00+$.50

depressed or ceased entirely within 60 to 80 min.[2,3] Modern improvements on these techniques have extended perfusion time to several hours.[4] Several refinements of the perfusion apparatus and media have contributed to the improved function of the isolated kidney, including the use of in-line filters and dialyzers and perfusion media containing purified natural colloids such as bovine serum albumin,[5-7] selected metabolic substrates,[8-11] and red blood cells or other synthetic oxygen binding chemicals.[12-22]

The basic isolated perfused kidney preparation consists of the whole kidney isolated from the systemic vasculature, and usually removed from the animal, and perfused through the renal artery with a synthetic plasma- or blood-like medium. Perfusate is delivered into the renal vasculature with a variable speed pump that can be adjusted to achieve a constant mean arterial pressure. Oxygenation of the perfusate is achieved with an in-line gas exchange system. Urine is collected through a cannula placed in the ureter.

Several variations of this basic technique have been developed to suit specific experimental designs. These include the placement of various in-line monitoring devices for perfusate temperature, pH, and oxygen content. The perfusate leaving the renal vein can be either recirculated to the renal artery or collected in a reservoir to achieve a single-pass perfusion. The single-pass technique ensures a constant arterial perfusate composition, since it is not modified by renal metabolism or excretion. However, it also consumes large quantities of perfusate and can be very expensive if the perfusate contains physiologic colloids such as serum albumin.

Perfusion methods for various mammalian species including the dog,[13] rabbit,[23,24] guinea pig,[25] pig,[20,26,27] and toad[28,29] have been reported. However, most of the recent literature has focused on the isolated perfused rat kidney preparation. This reflects, to some extent, the size of the rat in relation to its cost and availability as a research animal. Isolation of the kidney for perfusion requires an extensive surgical procedure that can be readily performed on rats; it is much more difficult to accomplish with smaller mammals.

The isolated perfused kidney preparation is useful for probing certain problems in nephrotoxicology; however, as is true for all experimental techniques, it also has certain limitations. These are summarized briefly in the following sections.

4.2 *Advantages of the isolated perfused kidney preparation over other* in vitro *preparations*

The isolated perfused kidney is the least destructive of the kidney macrostructure of the numerous *in vitro* approaches currently available for studying the kidney; therefore, it is particularly well-suited for studies requiring intact renal morphology. It is the only *in vitro* preparation in which glomerular filtration and tubular functions are retained. Thus, it is particularly useful for studying effects of chemicals on glomerular function and renal blood flow and related effects on tubular transport function. The preparation has been used extensively to examine the mechanism of ischemic and hypoxic injury.[11,12,16,17,30-42] Although the renal nerves are severed in the isolation procedure, the sectioned nerves and vasculature can be electrically or chemically stimulated to examine humoral and neuronal control of the vasculature and tubular function, and the effects of chemicals on this control.[43-52] The isolated perfused kidney is uniquely suited for studies of the relationship between the control of the renal vasculature and renal metabolism.[11,16,33-36]

Control over almost all aspects of the composition of the perfusate is possible with the isolated perfused kidney. Controllable components include the concentrations of dissolved and gaseous metabolic substrates and electrolytes, colloids, oxygen carriers, xenobiotics and metabolites, and binding ligands in the perfusate. This control facilitates establishing reproducible exposures to any specific toxicants or mixtures that are being studied. Since the kidney is isolated, it is also possible to achieve higher concentrations of toxic chemicals in the perfusate and kidney than might be achieved or tolerated *in vivo*. An example of this is the use of colloid-free perfusates to rapidly establish high levels of cadmium in the kidney.[53] The colloid osmotic pressure of the perfusate can be increased sufficiently to effectively stop filtration in order to isolate and study peritubular transport and metabolism.[54-57]

Isolation of the kidney from the *in vivo* circulation greatly facilitates the identification of renal metabolites of xenobiotics.[58-63]

4.3 Limitations of the isolated perfused kidney preparation

Perfusion flow rate, glomerular filtration rate, and tubular function decline progressively over several hours in most isolated perfused kidney preparations. Therefore, the preparation can be useful for examining directly the toxic effects of *in vitro* exposures to chemicals that result from relatively short duration exposures and to effects with very short latencies. For the study of the effects of more chronic exposures or effects that have longer latencies, animals must be exposed to the chemical and their kidneys isolated at various times after exposure.

The isolated perfused kidney exhibits several functional abnormalities that must be considered when designing or evaluating toxicologic studies. These abnormalities include relatively high perfusion flow rates and low filtration fractions in the initial stages of perfusion, loss of concentrating ability, and glomerular proteinuria.[4,11,64] The inability of the isolated rat kidney to concentrate the urine appreciably above the perfusate may be related to the high perfusion flow rate and structural abnormalities of the thick ascending limb of the loop of Henle, discussed below.

The filtration fraction of the isolated perfused rat kidney (and kidneys of other species) is lower than *in vivo* by a factor of 5 to 10 at *in vivo* GFR (approximately 1 ml $\cdot$ min^{-1} $\cdot$ g wet wt^{-1}) and arterial perfusion pressure (approximately 100 mmHg). Addition of erythrocytes to the perfusate decreases perfusion flow rate and increases filtration fraction.[18] The mechanisms for the low filtration fraction and the increase in filtration fraction induced by erythrocytes in the isolated *in situ* perfused rat kidney have been studied with micropuncture techniques. At similar perfusion pressures and superficial nephron glomerular filtration rates, single nephron plasma flow was higher by a factor of ten, and single nephron filtration fraction was lower by a factor of ten in cell-free perfused kidneys than in erythrocyte-perfused kidneys. Glomerular hydrostatic pressure, transcapillary hydrostatic pressure, and afferent arteriolar protein concentration were similar in cell-free and erythrocyte-perfused kidneys; the glomerular ultrafiltration coefficient was higher by a factor of two in the erythrocyte perfused kidneys, but within the *in vivo* range.[65] These observations suggest that the lower filtration fraction in cell-free perfusions results primarily from a higher perfusion flow rate and lower glomerular ultrafiltration coefficient rather than changes in Starling forces.

Isolated rat kidneys perfused with a substrate-supplemented perfusate containing bovine serum albumin (BSA) excrete relatively large amounts of albumin.[64] This albuminuria is at least in part of glomerular origin; the sieving coefficient of albumin, determined by micropuncture of the early proximal tubule of superficial nephrons, is higher than the *in vivo* sieving coefficient by a factor of ten.[64] Morphological studies of isolated cell-free perfused rat kidneys have shown that, within minutes of perfusion at a pressure of 105 mmHg, glomerular capillaries expand and the surface area of the glomerular basement membrane increases. Podocyte processes stretch to accommodate the expanded endothelium, maintaining the apparent structural integrity of the filtration barrier intact.[66,67] Glomerular proteinuria observed in the isolated perfused kidney may result from changes in the composition or charge of the glomerular basement membrane; inclusion of oxygen radical scavengers in the perfusate decreases proteinuria and decreases the loss of heparin sulfate-derived sulfur from the glomerulus.[68]

Certain structural anomalies have been observed in the tubules of isolated perfused kidneys. These include cellular necrosis of the medullary thick ascending limb of the loop of Henle (mTAL) and terminal segments of the proximal tubule.[15,69] The lesion in the proximal tubule is particularly significant to toxicological studies since this region is highly sensitive to chemical injury resulting from *in vivo* exposures. The structural lesions appear to be related to regional hypoxia in the outer medulla and can be partially or completely prevented by increasing the oxygen-carrying capacity of the perfusate or decreasing metabolic work.[12,15,16,17,33,34] Conversely, the mTAL lesions can be exacerbated by increasing metabolic work or decreasing oxygen delivery.[35,36] The sensitivity of the isolated perfused kidney to changes in regional oxygen delivery and oxygen demand should be considered in any evaluations of toxic chemicals made in these preparations.

Evaluation of the effects of chemicals on function of specific regions of the nephron is not easily accomplished with the perfused whole kidney. For example, distinguishing transport lesions in the proximal tubule from those in the distal tubule can be approached with clearance techniques or moment analysis of single-pass transit times; however, these techniques are less definitive than direct evaluations of isolated tubular segments. With considerably greater technical effort, micropuncture techniques can be applied to the perfused rat kidney to evaluate proximal and distal reabsorptive function.[8,64]

Setup and maintenance of a perfusion laboratory is labor-intensive and requires trained and experienced personnel to ensure quality control. Each animal must be surgically prepared prior to the perfusion and yields only one perfused kidney. This limits the rate at which multiple variables, such as various chemical mixtures, can be examined.

4.4 Basic methods for isolation and perfusion of the kidney

4.4.1 Isolation of the kidney

Functional vitality of the perfused kidney requires a proficient and consistent isolation procedure that minimizes surgical stress to the animal, renal ischemia, and structural damage to the kidney. A general procedure for isolation and perfusion of the rat kidney is described here. Numerous modifications of this procedure have been described that may be more or less advantageous, depending on the objectives and surgical skills of the investigator. The best way to learn to isolate kidneys for perfusion is to be tutored by someone who has experience with a given technique. After mastering one technique, modifications can be implemented to suit the objectives.

4.4.1.1 Laparotomy

The donor rat is anesthetized with an intraperitoneal injection of a thiobarbiturate to achieve anesthesia for at least 30 to 60 min. The rat is secured on its back on a heating pad to maintain normal body temperature during surgery; the extensive laparotomy required to isolate the ureter and kidney is a substantial thermal challenge to the rat. Body temperature can be monitored during surgery with a rectal probe, and the heating pad adjusted accordingly.

After anesthesia is achieved, the femoral vein is exposed through an incision made in the hind limb; this allows subsequent intravenous injections of mannitol, heparin, and more anesthetic if needed. An intravenous injection of isotonic mannitol (e.g., 100 mg dissolved in 0.5 ml isotonic sodium chloride) is given to achieve osmotic diuresis. This facilitates isolation and cannulation of the ureter and may also provide some protection from ischemic injury of the kidney during the isolation procedure.[68,70]

A midline incision is made from the sternum to the pelvis and the abdominal cavity is exposed with clamps. The mesentery is resected to expose the inner dorsal surface of the abdominal cavity, right kidney area, and right ureter (from the perspective of the surgeon, the right kidney and ureter will be on the left side of the rat). The resected mesentery can be covered with gauze moistened with warm aqueous isotonic sodium chloride.

4.4.1.2 *Ureteral cannulation*

The ureter must be cannulated if urine is to be collected from the isolated kidney. Cannulation of the right ureter is achieved with a 3- to 5-cm length of polyethylene or polypropylene tubing (Clay Adams, PE-50). Cannulas narrower than PE-50 may provide high enough resistance to decrease glomerular filtration and urine flow rates.[7] Insertion of the cannula into the ureter is made easier if the tip is tapered and beveled. Although tubing smaller than PE-50 can be used without tapering, it will increase resistance to flow. A 0.5- to 1.0-cm taper at the end of a length of PE-50 tubing can be achieved by inserting a wire halfway into a 10-cm length of PE tubing, grasping either end of the tubing with hemostats or pliers, and pulling the wireless end of the tubing until it breaks. The resulting tapered end can be beveled with a razor. The taper should be no more than needed to achieve cannulation to avoid unnecessary resistance to flow. The beveled end of the cannula should be viewed through a magnifying glass to ensure that it is perfectly smooth and free of burrs. Several cannulas should be prepared and inspected prior to initiating surgery.

The right ureter, 1 to 2 cm below the kidney, lies on the inner dorsal surface of the abdominal cavity, to the left (from the perspective of the surgeon) of the descending vena cava and dorsal aorta; it can be identified by its pale yellow color and peristaltic contractions. The latter will be particularly evident during a mannitol-induced diuresis. Three loose ligatures are placed under the ureter approximately 1 to 2 cm below the kidney. Care should be taken at this point to avoid contacting the ureter or applying tension to it as this may precipitate muscle spasms that may disrupt urine flow. A 1.5× to 3× magnifying binoculars and a good light source (e.g., fiber-optic) will make it easier to visualize the ureteral incision and insertion of the cannula. The more posterior (rostral) ligature can be tightened just prior to the ureteral incision to expand the ureter slightly; this will create a bigger target for the incision and better visualization of the incision (e.g., expulsion of urine). A small nick is made across the ureter with an iris scissors, approximately one third of the diameter of the ureter, midway between the two ligatures. The tapered end of the cannula is inserted into the ureter, and the cannula is advanced up to, but not into, the renal pelvis and is tied securely to the ureter with the remaining two ligatures. The ligatures should be cut free of the surrounding tissue.

Urine should begin flowing immediately from the end of the cannula; if not, the cannula and ureter should be inspected for kinks, plugs, or leaks. Recannulation of a plugged ureter is difficult but can be attempted. The left ureter can be inspected to determine if the anuria is unilateral or bilateral; bilateral anuria would be indicative of cardiovascular stress. If leakage or blockage does explain the anuria, another dose of isotonic mannitol can be administered to stimulate urine formation. If flow is not initiated promptly, it is probably best to abort the preparation or risk anuria after perfusion is initiated.

4.4.1.3 *Cannulation of the vasculature*

Arterial perfusate is delivered to the isolated kidney through a cannula inserted into the renal artery. Venous perfusate can be allowed to drain from the posterior inferior vena cava or into a cannula placed in the inferior vena cava. The latter arrangement allows the venous perfusate to be directed to an oxygen electrode cell or other type of flow cell or sampling port.

A renal arterial cannula can be made from an 18- or 19-gauge stainless steel hypodermic needle; however, more elaborate designs have been described.[5,7,9] The end of the needle should be ground and polished to achieve a smooth bevel; the bevel should be inspected under a magnifying glass to ensure that it has no burrs. A 19- or 18-gauge cannula may produce significant resistance to flow at perfusion flow rates achieved in the isolated perfused rat kidney. Therefore, it is advisable to measure and record the pressure–flow relationship of the cannula prior to each use. Hydrostatic pressure resulting from cannula resistance can be subtracted from arterial pressure measured during perfusion to estimate the actual arterial pressure that is translated to the renal artery.

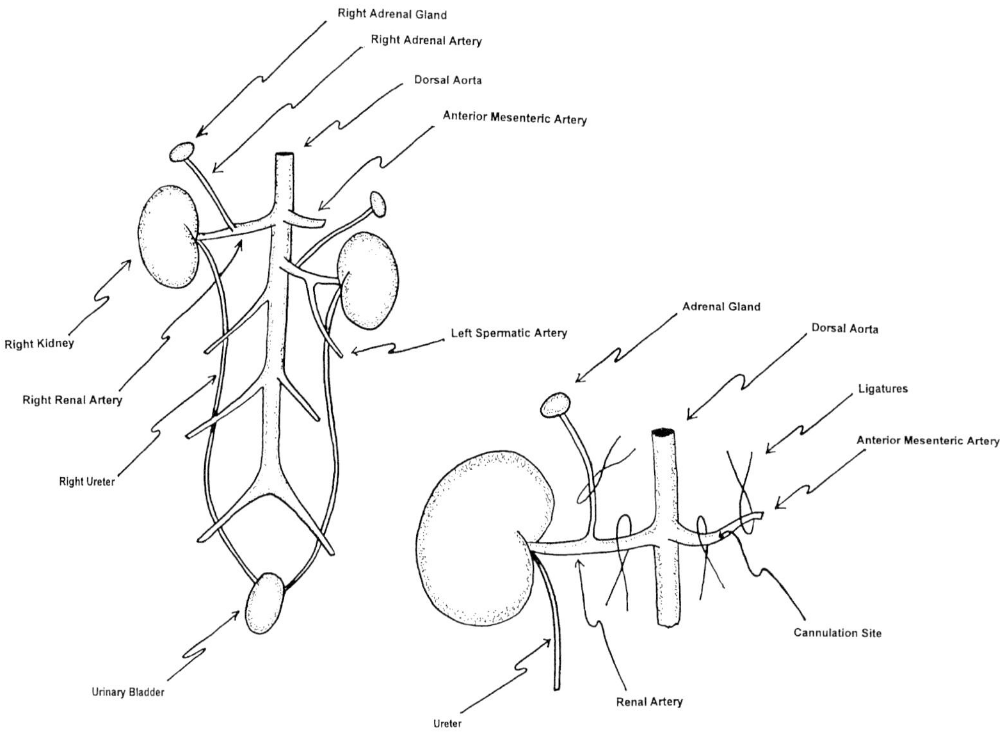

Figure 1 Schematic drawing of the surgical field for cannulation of the renal artery showing the major anatomical landmarks and placement of ligatures.

The renal artery should be cannulated with no disruption of oxygen delivery to the kidney. To achieve this end, the renal artery can be cannulated from the anterior mesenteric artery, which usually originates from the dorsal aorta directly opposite the right renal artery (Figure 1). An alternative approach is to insert the cannula into the dorsal aorta, caudal to the renal arteries, and advance the cannula into the right renal artery. However, this requires that the dorsal aorta be occluded caudal to the kidneys prior to perfusion, which may produce transient changes in renal blood flow and perfusion pressure. The dorsal aorta approach also requires that the cannula be turned approximately 90° while in the dorsal aorta in order to cannulate the right renal artery; this can be difficult to accomplish, although it can be made somewhat easier with a bent cannula.

The surgical preparation for the mesenteric arterial approach to the cannulation of the renal artery requires isolation and placement of loose ligatures under the anterior mesenteric artery, renal artery, and right adrenal artery (Figure 1). The adrenal artery is tied prior to cannulation of the renal artery to prevent the possibility of leakage of perfusate through the adrenal artery after the kidney is excised from the body. Some investigators excise the adrenal gland prior to cannulating the renal artery. After all loose ligatures are in place, sodium heparin (20 to 40 IU) should be administered intravenously to prevent blood clots from forming during the cannulation procedure. A second dose of mannitol also may be given at this time. The arterial cannula, connected to the perfusion apparatus and filled with oxygenated perfusate, is inserted into the anterior mesenteric artery; perfusion is initiated and the cannula is then advanced through the dorsal aorta and into the right renal artery where it is secured with ligatures. The cannulation procedure is more easily accomplished with aid from an assistant who can secure the ligatures while the surgeon holds the cannula in the renal artery.

Certain anatomical variations can increase the difficulty of achieving good cannulations. A common variation is displacement of the right renal artery along the dorsal aorta, anterior or posterior from the origination of the anterior mesenteric artery. Multiple right renal arteries originating from the dorsal aorta also occur.

After cannulation of the renal artery, the right kidney and ureter, with cannula intact, can be excised from the body and transferred into the perfusion chamber. Alternatively, the kidney can be perfused *in situ*.

4.4.2 *Perfusion apparatus*

The perfusion apparatus consists of a thermostatically regulated chamber, a platform on which to place the kidney and collect urine and venous perfusate, reservoirs for the perfusate, a filtration system for the perfusate, an oxygenation system, calibrated pumps for delivering perfusate, and various metering devices to assess perfusion pressure, temperature, pH, or other variables to be monitored. A typical design is illustrated in Figure 2.

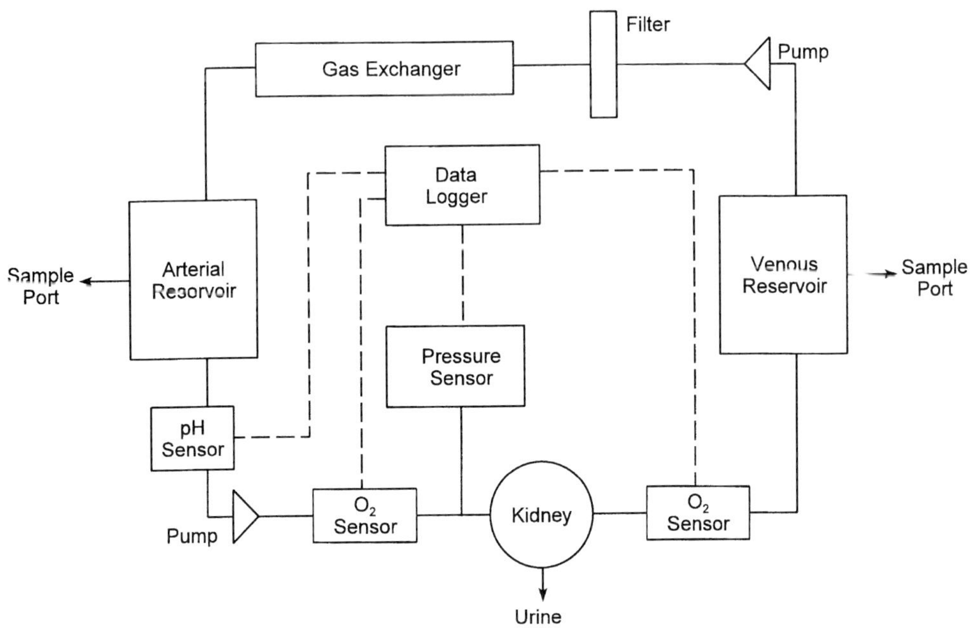

Figure 2 Typical perfusion circuit for the isolated perfused kidney.

Arterial perfusate can be delivered to the kidney using calibrated variable speed peristaltic pumps to achieve a desired arterial pressure. Pulsations in pressure can be damped by installing a pulsation chamber on the arterial side of the pump.[7] Modifications in pulsation pressure may affect certain functions of the isolated kidney, including renin release.[71] Arterial perfusate should be passed through a 10- to 15-μm filter to remove any debris that might have entered the perfusate during isolation of the kidney or that might be released from the preparation during perfusion; this is particularly important if the venous perfusate is recirculated to the kidney.

Oxygenation of a protein-free perfusate can be achieved by bubbling an oxygen gas mixture directly into the arterial perfusate reservoir through a fine bubble diffuser. The diffusion bubbler will produce extensive foaming if the perfusate contains even small amounts of protein. This can be avoided by oxygenating the perfusate through a semi-permeable membrane. A simple oxygenator consists of 25 ft of Silastic tubing placed in a glass jar that is continuously purged with the gas mixture.

Perfusate pH can be monitored continuously by placing a pH electrode in the flow of the perfusate. It is particularly important to monitor pH if the perfusate is recirculated, because renal excretion and metabolism can result in the loss or addition of bicarbonate during the perfusion.

Colloid osmotic pressure of the perfusate may need to be monitored if a small volume of perfusate is recirculated (e.g., 200 ml) and urine volumes are high. Sustained excretion of low-protein urine can result in a rise in colloid osmotic pressure, which can decrease glomerular filtration rate.[7,72] A rise in colloid osmotic pressure can be prevented by infusion of protein-free perfusate.

4.4.3 *Perfusate*

Function of the isolated perfused kidney is highly dependent on the composition of the perfusate. A given perfusate can be expected to achieve a certain functional profile that can be characterized in several dimensions: levels of various functions supported (e.g., mean glomerular filtration rate), change in the levels of function with perfusion time (i.e., functional stability), interkidney variability. The functional profile of a given perfusate will define the types of studies that can be supported by that preparation. The investigator can leverage this attribute in order to design a preparation that supports those dimensions of the functional profile that achieves the objectives of the research. It is incumbent on the investigator to report information about the functional profile of his or her preparation, as this provides the only basis for comparing results across laboratories.

The basic perfusate used by many investigators is a Krebs–Ringer–bicarbonate (KRB) solution equilibrated with a mixture of 95% carbon dioxide and 5% oxygen (95%/5% CO_2/O_2) gas and to which may be added substrates for energy metabolism and synthesis, protein or nonprotein colloid to provide a desired colloid osmotic pressure, and oxygen carriers to increase the oxygen carrying capacity of the perfusate.

4.4.3.1 *Substrates*

Transport and synthesis in the isolated kidney are dependent on the availability of energy from substrate catabolism, primarily oxidative catabolism. Isolated rat kidneys perfused under extreme hypoxic conditions (e.g., KRB equilibrated with 95% N_2/5% CO_2) will sustain low rates of sodium transport and low fractional reabsorption of sodium if provided substrates for anaerobic metabolism.[73] Kidneys perfused with oxygenated substrate-free KRB sustain low rates of sodium transport and fractional reabsorption of sodium by oxidizing endogenous fatty acids.[74] Higher rates of transport are achieved with oxygenated perfusates supplemented with substrates for the glycolytic pathway or precursors and substrates for the tricarboxylic acid cycle.[9,74-77] However, higher rates of transport and related oxygen demand also may exacerbate hypoxic injury to the outer medullary tubular epithelium; this is thought to result when transport-driven oxygen demand exceeds oxygen delivery.[17]

The isolated rat kidney utilizes amino acids. Net utilization of alanine, aspartate, glycine, and proline occurs in rat kidneys perfused with a substrate-supplemented KRB perfusate.[78] Addition of a full complement of amino acids to a substrate-supplemented perfusate reduces the severity of hypoxic lesions that otherwise occur in the mTAL.[10] The mechanism for this protective effect was thought to be support of renal synthesis of glutathione, because protection is afforded by the addition of glutathione and/or amino acids that support synthesis of glutathione (glycine, glutamate, and cysteine).[10] However, glycine or alanine also have been shown to prevent or lessen the severity of this lesion and to reduce enzyme release from the perfused kidney.[40,79] Glycine and alanine also lessen the severity of severe mTAL injury that occurs when kidneys are perfused with a hypoxic substrate-supplemented perfusate; glutamate and cysteine, alone or in combination do not protect against this injury.[40] Thus, the protective effect of glycine and alanine may involve mechanisms other than, or in addition to, support of glutathione synthesis.[42] These observations have prompted many investigators to include glycine and alanine as part of a standard substrate mixture for perfusion of rat kidneys.

A recent development has been the elucidation of the importance of nitric oxide and its metabolic precursor, arginine, in regulating regional vascular resistance in the isolated perfused kidney.[49,80-87] The inhibitor of nitric oxide formation from L-arginine, L-NG-monomethylarginine, increases the severity of mTAL injury that otherwise occurs in isolated rat kidneys perfused with a substrate-supplemented perfusate; this effect can be prevented by the addition of L-arginine to the perfusate.[80] Thus, the inclusion or exclusion of L-arginine to the perfusate should be considered in light of these observations.

Additional data on the function of kidneys perfused with various amino acid mixtures are available.[7,10,11,78,88-91]

4.4.3.2 *Colloid*

Rat kidneys perfused with bovine serum albumin (BSA) and energy substrates in the perfusate have higher perfusion flow rates, lower glomerular filtration rates, and higher fractional reabsorption of sodium than kidneys perfused with BSA-free perfusates of similar nonprotein composition.[7,53] Increasing the concentration of BSA in substrate-supplemented and substrate-free perfusates increases perfusion flow rate, decreases glomerular filtration rate, and increases fractional reabsorption of sodium.[7,72] Glomerular filtration rate remains stable for longer perfusion times if BSA is included in a substrate-supplemented perfusate.[7]

Bovine serum albumin should be dialyzed and defatted prior to use in perfusions, particularly if control of substrates is an objective.[92] Continuous dialysis of the perfusate during perfusion has been reported to improve stability of glomerular filtration rate in some preparations.[7]

Nonprotein colloids are an alternative to albumin when having albumin in the perfusate conflicts with a given experimental objective. The synthetic polymer polyvinylpyrrolidone (PVP) has been used as a replacement for albumin in the isolated perfused rat kidney.[61,93] Glomerular filtration rate and fractional reabsorption of sodium in kidneys perfused with a KRB-PVP substrate supplemented perfusate were lower than in kidneys perfused with a KRB-BSA perfusate of similar colloid osmotic pressure and composition.[94]

4.4.3.3 *Oxygen carriers*

The inclusion of erythrocytes in the perfusate has been shown to increase perfusion flow rate and filtration fraction, reduce or prevent cellular necrosis in outer medullary segments of the proximal tubule and mTAL, and decrease glomerular proteinuria that otherwise occurs in isolated rat kidneys perfused with a KRB–albumin substrate-supplemented perfusate.[15,65,95] Including erythrocytes in the perfusate introduces a second tissue into the perfusion preparation; the transport and metabolic characteristics of the erythrocyte preparation should be considered in the design of a perfusion approach to explore a given research problem.

Cell-free oxygen carriers can be explored if introducing erythrocytes into the perfusate conflicts with experimental objectives. Stroma-free hemoglobin has been used in isolated perfused rat kidney preparations as an oxygen carrier in KRB perfusates.[96] These kidneys excrete large amounts of hemoglobin, and it is likely that the high filtered load of hemoglobin would have some metabolic consequences; this has not been rigorously explored. Rat kidneys perfused with a mixture of stroma-free erythrocytes and a synthetic oxygen carrier, Fluosol-DA (an emulsion of perfluorodecalin and perfluorotrypropylamine), in a KRB perfusate excreted less hemoglobin than kidneys perfused with either stroma-free hemoglobin or Fluosol-DA in a similar KRB perfusate.[22] Other synthetic oxygen carriers that have been used in isolated kidney preparations include hemoglobin derivatives,[21,97] emulsified FC43,[20,97] and pluronic F108 (methyl oxirane polymer).[19]

4.5 New developments in methodology

The isolated perfused kidney preparation continues to evolve as an important model for studying renal metabolism and physiology. Several recent advances in methodology have great potential for further expanding the utility of this preparation in the study of mechanisms of nephrotoxicity.

4.5.1 Isolated perfused rat kidney-liver preparation

An isolated perfused rat kidney-liver preparation has been recently reported in which the kidney and liver are perfused in parallel with a recirculated perfusate; the venous perfusate from both organs is delivered to a common reservoir.[98] The preparation has been used to explore interorgan activation and clearance of steroid hormones.[99-103] One outcome of these studies was the demonstration of kaliuresis induced from hepatic metabolites of aldosterone.[102] Thus, the preparation could be used to study the nephrotoxicity of chemicals that might be activated to nephrotoxicants or proximate nephrotoxicants in the liver.

4.5.2 Nuclear magnetic resonance (NMR) spectroscopy measurements of renal tissue metabolism

A recent and important advancement of the study of the energy metabolism of the kidney is the application of NMR spectroscopy to the isolated perfused kidney. The technique provides real-time measurements of tissue adenosine mono-, di-, and triphosphate (AMP, ADP, ATP) in whole kidney during perfusion. A standard perfusion technique has been described with certain enhancements to accommodate the NMR spectroscopy and analysis.[25,104] The cannulated rat or guinea pig kidney is suspended in a 16-mm (outer diameter, O.D.) NMR tube that is inserted into the bore of a 20-mm-O.D. vertical magnet of a Varian XL 200 NMR spectrometer. Two percent $^{2}H_2O$ is added to the perfusate to quantify water present in the NMR window. Chloride space measurements are obtained on the same kidney by tuning the NMR to the ^{35}Cl-NMR frequency; this, together with the ^{2}H-NMR spectrum, allows the estimation of total tissue water volume (i.e., $^{2}H_2O$ space) and intracellular water volume (i.e., $^{2}H_2O$ space minus ^{35}Cl space) and, thereby, tissue adenine nucleotide concentrations.

4.5.3 Continuous microscopy of renal microvasculature during perfusion

Direct visualization of the glomerular microvasculature has been achieved in isolated perfused hydronephrotic rat kidneys.[105] This technique allows continuous measurements of afferent and efferent arteriolar constriction and dilation during perfusion and can be used to assess the vasoactive properties of chemicals. Unilateral hydronephrosis is induced in the rat by surgical isolation and ligation of the right ureter. Ureteral ligation results in progressive renal tubular atrophy which allows the microvasculature of surface cortical glomeruli to be visualized directly under a microscope.[106] Eight to ten weeks after ureteral ligation, the right kidney is isolated and perfused using a modified recirculating perfusion technique.[105] The cannulated kidney is placed on the stage of an inverted microscope; the stage is heated and has a viewing port on the bottom surface. The image from the microscope is captured with a video camera and can be digitalized for analysis and measurements of microvessel diameter.

4.5.4 Perfusion of remnant kidneys

Isolated perfused remnant kidney preparations recently have been developed for exploring physiological and biochemical adaptations that occur in the remnant kidney following unilateral or 80% nephrectomy.[78,107-109] Toxicological ramifications of adaptations to partial loss of functional renal mass are currently a subject of considerable interest. Partial nephrectomy induces compensatory growth in the remnant kidney; associated with this are changes in the severity of toxicity and disposition of metals,[110-113] glutathione metabolism,[114,115] and metallothionein metabolism.[116-117] The isolated perfused kidney preparation offers a relatively unexplored approach to studying the metabolic bases for these changes.

4.5.5 Moment analysis of single-pass transit times

Single-pass perfusion of the isolated kidney allows continuous collection of both urine and venous perfusate, which in turn allows precise measurements of arterial–urine and arterial–venous transit times of chemicals injected into the arterial perfusate. Transepithelial transit times and epithelial cell residence times for injected transport substrates can be estimated by comparing the transit time of the substrate with the transit times of plasma and extracellular space markers injected simultaneously with the transport substrate. The computational method used is known as moment analysis.[118] This type of multiple indicator dilution experiment is not novel, nor is its use in the study of nephrotoxicity in the whole animal; however, its recent application to the isolated perfused rat kidney provides an additional tool for research on the effects of toxicants on tubular transport in whole kidney.[119] The approach has been used to explore the time course of impaired tubular secretion of organic ions that is induced by uranyl nitrate[120] and to study mechanisms of renal tubular transport of aminoglycoside antibiotics,[121] epidermal growth factor,[122] and neutral and charged colloids.[123]

4.5.6 Isolated perfused amphibian kidney

The amphibian kidney has a double blood supply; an arterial supply delivers blood to the glomerulus and subsequently to the peritubular capillaries; a portal supply delivers blood directly to the peritubular capillaries. Isolation and perfusion of the portal circulation of the African clawed toad (*Xenopus laevis*) has been reported.[28] This preparation can be used to study tubular uptake and release of chemicals introduced directly into the peritubular vascular space without glomerular filtration. Although glomerular filtration is prevented by ligation of the renal arterial supply, urine formation can be induced by infusing *p*-aminohippurate into the portal circulation. Presumably, under these conditions, urine formation is driven by hydrostatic pressure in the tubule induced by the osmotic pressure of *p*-aminohippurate secreted into the tubule lumen. The preparation has been used to study peritubular uptake of amino acids in the kidney[28,29] and has great potential for exploring renal tubular metabolism and transport of nephrotoxicants.

Table 1 Examples of Toxicologic Applications of the Isolated Perfused Kidney

Chemical	Species	Type of study	Ref.
Aminoglycosides	Rat	Effects on function	124
Bacitracin	Rat	Metabolism, effects on vascular resistance	125
Cadmium	Rat	Uptake, excretory clearance, and effects of *in vitro* exposure on function	53
Cefonicid	Rat	Excretory clearance	126
Cimetidine	Rat	Excretory clearance	127
Cisplatin	Rat	Uptake and effects on function	128,129
Cyclosporin A	Rat	Effects on function	130–133
Cytochalasin D	Rat	Effects of microtubule disruption on function and structure	134
Dimercaptopropane sulfonate	Rat	Excretory transport and metabolism	61,135
Dimethylsulfoxide	Rabbit	Effects on excretion of gamma-glutamyl transpeptidase	23
Dipeptides	Rat	Metabolism	62
Enalapril	Rat	Metabolic and excretory clearance	136
Endotoxin	Rat	Effects on function	137
5-Dimethylsulfamoyl-6,7-dichloro-2,3-dihydrobenzofuran-2-carboxylic acid (DBCA)	Rat	Excretory clearance	138
Gamma-L-glutamyl-L-dopa	Rat	Metabolic activation and vascular effects	54
Ibuprofen	Rat	Excretory and metabolic clearance	139
Loop diuretics	Rat	Diuretic mechanisms of furosemide and ethacrynic acid	140
Menadione	Rat	Metabolism and effect of glutathione conjugate on function and structure	141
Mercuric chloride	Rat	Effects on vascular resistance, relation to adenosine production; excretion	61,135,142
Methotrexate	Rat	Excretory clearance	143
1-Naphthol	Rat	Metabolism and excretory clearance	63
Nonsteroidal anti-inflammatory agents	Rat	Effects on function, uptake, metabolism, and excretory clearance	19,58–60, 144,145
Opiates	Rat	Effects on function; excretory clearance of morphine and glucuronide and sulfate conjugates	146,147
Polycations	Rat	Effects of exposure on function	148
Puromycin aminonucleoside	Rat	Mechanism of disruption of renal handling of sodium	149
Shockwave	Pig	Shockwave-induced renal lesions	26,27
Sodium fluoride	Rat	Effect on structure and function	150
Tobramycin	Rat	Mechanisms of tubular uptake examined; moment analysis of single-pass transit times	121
Triamterene	Rat	Excretory clearance	151
Trichloroethene	Rabbit	Effect of S-cysteine conjugate on function	152
Uranium	Dog, rat	Effects on function; moment analysis of single-pass transit times of organic ions	13,120
Water-soluble contrast agents	Rat	Effects on function and structure	153–156

4.6 Applications of the isolated perfused kidney for evaluating nephrotoxic chemicals

The isolated perfused rat kidney has been used in two principal ways in toxicological research: (1) to examine the effects of nephrotoxic chemicals on renal function and structure and (2) to examine the renal metabolism, binding, and excretion of xenobiotics. Specific examples are listed in Table 1.

References

1. Smith, H. W., *The Kidney*, Oxford University Press, New York, 1951, 153–543.
2. Weiss, C., Passow, H., and Rothstein, A., Autoregulation of flow in isolated rat kidney in the absence of red cells, *Am. J. Physiol.*, 196, 1115, 1959.
3. Bauman, Arthur W., Clarkson, T. W., and Miles, E. M., Functional evaluation of isolated perfused rat kidney, *J. Appl. Physiol.*, 18, 1239, 1963.
4. Maack, T., Physiological evaluation of the isolated perfused rat kidney, *Am. J. Physiol.*, 238, F71, 1980.
5. Little, J. R. and Cohen, J. J., Effect of albumin concentration on function of the isolated perfused kidney, *Am. J. Physiol.*, 226, 512, 1974.
6. Cohen, J. J., Kook, Y. J., and Little, J. R., Substrate-limited function and metabolism of the isolated perfused rat kidney: effects of lactate and glucose, *J. Physiol. London*, 266, 103, 1976.
7. Schurek, H. and Alt, J. A., Effect of albumin on the function of perfused rat kidney, *Am. J. Physiol.*, 240, F569, 1981.
8. De Mello, G. and Maack, T., Nephron function of the isolated perfused rat kidney, *Am. J. Physiol.*, 231, 1699, 1976.
9. Cohen, J. J., Merkens, L. S., and Peterson, O. W., Relation of Na^+ reabsorption to utilization of O_2 and lactate in the perfused rat kidney, *Am. J. Physiol.*, 238, F415, 1980.
10. Epstein, F. H., Brosnan, J. T., Tange, J. D., and Ross, B. D., Improved function with amino acids in the isolated perfused kidney, *Am. J. Physiol.*, 243, F284, 1982.
11. Brezis, M., Silva, P., and Epstein, F. H., Amino acids induce renal vasodilatation in isolated perfused kidney: coupling to oxidative metabolism, *Am. J. Physiol.*, 247, H999, 1984.
12. Franke, H., Barlow, C. H., and Chance, B., Oxygen delivery in perfused rat kidney: NADH fluorescence and renal functional state, *Am. J. Physiol.*, 231, 1082, 1976.
13. Nizet, A., Influence of uranyl nitrate upon tubular reabsorption and glomerular filtration in blood perfused isolated dog kidneys, *Eur. J. Physiol.*, 391, 296, 1981.
14. Swanson, J. W., Besarab, A., Pomerantz, P. H., and DeGuzman, A., Effect of erythrocytes and globulin on renal functions of the isolated rat kidney, *Am. J. Physiol.*, 241, F139, 1981.
15. Schurek, H. and Kriz, W., Morphologic and functional evidence for oxygen deficiency in the isolated perfused rat kidney, *Lab. Invest.*, 53, 145, 1985.
16. Brezis, M., Rosen, S., Silva, P., and Epstein, F. H., Selective vulnerability of the medullary thick ascending limb to anoxia in the isolated perfused rat kidney, *J. Clin. Invest.*, 73, 182, 1984.
17. Brezis, M., Rosen, S., Stoff, J. S., Spokes, K., Silva, P., and Epstein, F. H., Inhibition of prostaglandin synthesis in rat kidney perfused with and without erythrocytes: implication for analgesic nephropathy, *Miner. Electrolyte Metab.*, 12, 326, 1986.
18. Lieberthal, W., Vasilevsky, M. L., Valeri, C. R., and Levinski, N. G., Interactions between ADH and prostaglandins in isolated erythrocyte-perfused rat kidney, *Am. J. Physiol.*, 21, F331, 1987.
19. Cox, P. G., Moons, W. M., Russel, F. G., and van Ginneken, C. A., Renal disposition and effects of naproxen and its l-enantiomer in the isolated perfused rat kidney, *J. Pharmacol. Exp. Ther.*, 255, 491, 1990.
20. Moore, K. P., Taylor, G. W., Gove, C., Wood, J., Tan, K. C., Eason, J., and Williams, R., Synthesis and metabolism of cysteinyl leukotrienes by the isolated pig kidney, *Kidney Int.*, 41, 1543, 1992.
21. Nishi, K., Ueda, S., and Nishi, R., Effects of pyrdoxalated hemoglobin polyoxethylene conjugate (PHP) on renal circulation in isolated perfused rat kidney, *Biomed. Artif. Cells Immob. Biotech.*, 20, 751, 1992.

22. Millis, R. M., Barber, J. D., Anderson, W. A., Dehkordi, O., Toussaint, R. M., and Ertugrul, L., Acute beneficial effect of Fluosol-DA on urinary excretion of stroma-free hemoglobin in the isolated rat kidney, *Renal Failure*, 16, 325, 1994.
23. Pillion, D. J., Teske, A. H., and Leibach, F. H., γ-Glutamyl transpeptidase in the urine from an isolated rabbit kidney perfused with and without DMSO, *Biochem. Pharmacol.*, 25, 913, 1976.
24. Li, T., Croce, K., and Winquist, R. J., Vasoconstrictor and vasodilator effects of serotonin in the isolated rabbit kidney, *J. Pharmacol. Exp. Ther.*, 263, 928, 1992.
25. Barac-Nieto, M., Dowd, T. L., Gupta, R. K., and Spitzer, A., Changes in NMR-visible kidney cell phosphate with age and diet relationship to phosphate transport, *Am. J. Physiol.*, 261, F153, 1991.
26. Back, W., Kohrmann, K. U., Bensemann, J., Rassweiler, J., and Alken, P., Histomorphologic and ultrastructural findings of shockwave-induced lesions in the isolated perfused kidney of the pig, *J. Endourol.*, 8, 257, 1994.
27. Kohrmann, K. U., Back, W., Bensemann, J., Florian. J., Weber, A., Kahmann, F., Rassweiler, J., and Alken, P., The isolated perfused kidney of the pig: new model to evaluate shock wave-induced lesions, *J. Endourol.*, 8, 105, 1994.
28. Gekle, M. and Silbernagl, S., Basolateral uptake and tubular metabolism of L-citrulline in the isolated-perfused non-filtering kidney of the African clawed toad (Xenopus laevis), *Pflügers Arch.*, 419, 492, 1991.
29. Gekle, M. and Silbernagl, S., On leaking into the lumen, amino acids cross the tubule cells. Secretion of L-citrulline in the isolated-perfused non-filtering kidney of the African clawed toad (Xenopus laevis), *Pflügers Arch.*, 419, 499, 1991.
30. Linas, S. L., Whittenburg, D., and Repine, J. E., O_2 metabolites cause reperfusion injury after short but not prolonged renal ischemia, *Am. J. Physiol.*, 253, F685, 1987.
31. Linas, S. L., Shanley, P. F., White, C. W., Parker, N. P., and Repine, J. E., O_2 metabolite-mediated injury in perfused kidneys is reflected by consumption of DMTU and glutathione, *Am. J. Physiol.*, 253, F692, 1987.
32. Gamelin, L. M. and Zager, R. A., Evidence against oxidant injury as a critical mediator of postischemic acute renal failure, *Am. J. Physiol.*, 255, F450, 1988.
33. Brezis, M., Rosen, S., Spokes, K., Silva, P., and Epstein, F. H., Transport dependent anoxic cell injury in the isolated perfused rat kidney, *Am. J. Pathol.*, 116, 327, 1984.
34. Brezis, M., Rosen, S., Silva, P., and Epstein, F. H., Transport activity modifies thick ascending limb damage in the isolated perfused kidney, *Kidney Int.*, 25, 65, 1984.
35. Brezis, M., Rosen, S., Spokes, K., Silva, P., and Epstein, F. H., Polyene toxicity in renal medulla: injury mediated by transport activity, *Science*, 224, 66, 1984.
36. Brezis, M., Rosen, S., Spokes, K., Silva, P., and Epstein, F. H., Substrates induce hypoxic injury to medullary thick ascending limbs of isolated rat kidneys, *Am. J. Physiol.*, 251, F710, 1984.
37. Brezis, M., Greenfeld, Z., Shina, A., and Rosen, S., Angiotensin II augments medullary hypoxia and predisposes to acute renal failure, *Eur. J. Clin. Invest.*, 20, 199, 1990.
38. Epstein, F. H., Rosen, S., Galicka-Piskorska, G., Spokes, K., Brezis, M., and Silva, P., Relation of adenosine to medullary injury in the perfused rat kidney, *Miner. Electrolyte Metab.*, 16, 185, 1990.
39. Silva, P., Rosen, S., Spokes, K., Taylor, M., and Epstein, F. H., Influence of endogenous prostaglandins on mTAL injury, *J. Am. Soc. Nephrol.*, 1, 808, 1990.
40. Silva, P., Rosen, S., Spokes, K., and Epstein, F. H., Effect of glycine on medullary thick ascending limb injury in perfused kidneys, *Kidney Int.*, 39, 653, 1991.
41. Shanley, P. F. and Johnson, G. C., Calcium and acidosis in renal hypoxia, *Lab. Invest.*, 65, 298, 1991.
42. Heyman, S., Spokes, K., Rosen, S., and Epstein, F. H., Mechanism of glycine protection in hypoxic injury: analogies with glycine receptor, *Kidney Int.*, 42, 41, 1992.
43. Marre, M., Misumi, J., Raemsch, K., Cormol, P., and Menard, J., Diuretic and natriuretic effects of nifedipine on isolated perfused rat kidneys, *J. Pharmacol. Exp. Ther.*, 223, 263, 1982.
44. Mejia, G., Challoner–Hue, L., and Steele, T. H., Calcium in neural control of renal circulation, *Am. J. Physiol.*, 247, F739, 1984.

45. Logan, A. G. and Chatzilias, A., The role of calcium in the control of renin release from the isolated rat kidney, *J. Physiol. Pharmacol.*, 58, 60, 1980.
46. Cooper, C. L. and Malik, K. U., Mechanism of action of vasopressin on prostaglandin synthesis and vascular function in the isolated rat kidney: effect of calcium antagonists and calmodulin inhibitors, *Am. J. Pharmacol.*, 229, 139, 1984.
47. Steele, T. H. and Challoner–Hue, L., Renal interactions between norepinephrine and calcium antagonists, *Kidney Int.*, 26, 719, 1984.
48. Gerkens, J. F., Reproducible vasodilatation by platelet-activating factor in blood- and Krebs-perfused rat kidneys is albumin-dependent, *Eur. J. Pharmacol.*, 177, 119, 1990.
49. Reid, J. J. and Rand, M. J., Renal vasoconstriction is modulated by nitric oxide, *Clin. Exp. Pharmacol. Physiol.*, 19, 376, 1992.
50. Schwartz, D. D. and Malik, K. U., Characterization of prejunctional alpha-2 adrenergic receptors involved in modulation of adrenergic transmitter release in the isolated perfused rat kidney, *J. Pharmacol. Exp. Ther.*, 261, 1050, 1992.
51. Oellerich, W. F. and Malik, K. U., Neuropeptide Y modulates the vascular response to periarterial nerve stimulation primarily by a postjunctional action in the isolated perfused rat kidney, *J. Pharmacol. Exp. Ther.*, 266, 1321, 1993.
52. Sehic, E., Ruan, Y., and Malik, K. U. Attenuation by alpha,beta-methylenadenosine-5′-triphosphate of periarterial nerve stimulation-induced renal vasoconstriction is not due to desensitization of purinergic receptors, *J. Pharmacol. Exp. Ther.*, 271, 983, 1994.
53. Diamond, G. L., Cohen, J. J., and Weinstein, S. L., Renal handling of cadmium in perfused rat kidney and effects on renal function and tissue composition, *Am. J. Physiol.*, 251, F784, 1986.
54. Barthelmebs, M., Caillette, A., Ehrhardt, J. D., Velly, J., and Imbs, J. L., Metabolism and vascular effects of gamma-L-glutamyl-L-dopa on the isolated rat kidney, *Kidney Int.*, 37, 1414, 1990.
55. Helwig, J. J., Musso, M. J., Judes, C., and Nickols, G. A., Parathyroid hormone and calcium: interactions in the control of renin secretion in the isolated, nonfiltering rat kidney, *Endocrinology*, 129, 1233, 1991.
56. Gillatt, D. J., Shulkes, A., Read, D. M., and Hardy, K. J., Metabolism of neurotensin by isolated perfused rat kidney, *Am. J. Physiol.*, 258, E930, 1990.
57. Saussine, C., Massfelder, T., Parnin, F., Judes, C., Simeoni, U., and Helwig, J. J., Renin stimulating properties of parathyroid hormone-related peptide in the isolated perfused rat kidney, *Kidney Int.*, 44, 764, 1993.
58. Bekersky, I., Fishman, L., Kaplan, S. A., and Colburn, W. A., Renal clearance of salicylic acid and salicyluric acid in the rat and in the isolated perfused rat kidney, *J. Pharmacol. Exp. Ther.*, 212, 309, 1980.
59. Bekersky, I., Colburn, W. A., Fishman, L., and Kaplan, S. A., Metabolism of salicylic acid in the isolated perfused rat kidney, *Drug Metab. Dispos.*, 8, 319, 1980.
60. Newton, J. F., Yoshimoto, M., Bernstein, J., Rush, G. F., and Hook., J. B. 1983. Acetaminophen nephrotoxicity in the rat. I. Strain difference in nephrotoxicity and metabolism, *Toxicol. Appl. Pharmacol.*, 69, 291, 1983.
61. Klotzbach, J. M. and Diamond, G. L., Complexing activity and excretion of 2,3-dimercaptopropane sulfonate in rat kidney, *Am. J. Physiol.*, 254, F871, 1988.
62. Fonteles, M. C., Oliveira, J. V., and Carvalho, K. M., Metabolism of dipeptides by isolated and perfused nonfiltering kidneys, *Braz. J. Med. Biol. Res.*, 23, 785, 1990.
63. Redegeld, F. A., Hofman, G. A., Koster, A. S., and Noordhoek, J., Flow-dependent extraction of 1-naphthol by the rat isolated perfused kidney, *Naunyn Schmiedebergs Arch. Pharmakol.*, 343, 330, 1991.
64. Stolte, H., Schurek, H. J., and Alt, J. M., Gomerular albumin filtration: a comparison of micropuncture studies in the isolated perfused rat kidney with in vivo experimental consitions, *Kidney Int.*, 16, 377, 1979.
65. Gabbai, F. B., Peterson, O. W., Khang, S., Wilson, C. B., and Blantz, R. C., Glomerular hemodynamics in cell-free and erythrocyte-perfused isolated rat kidney, *Am. J. Physiol.*, 267, F423, 1994.
66. Sakai, T., Lemley, K. V., Hackenthal, E., Nagata, M., Nobiling, R., and Kriz, W., Changes in glomerular structure following acute mesangial failure in the isolated perfused kidney, *Kidney Int.*, 41, 522, 1992.

67. Kriz, W., Hackenthal, E., Nobiling, R., Sakai, T., Elger M., and Hahnel, B., A role for podocytes to counteract capillary wall distension, *Kidney Int.*, 45, 369, 1994.
68. Tay, M., Comper, W. D., Vassiliou, P., Glasgow, E. F., Baker, M. S., and Pratt, L., The inhibitory action of oxygen radical scavengers on proteinuria and glomerular heparan sulfate loss in the isolated perfused kidney, *Biochem Int.*, 20, 767, 1990.
69. Alcorn, D., Emslie, K. R., Ross, B. D., Ryan, G. B., and Tange, J. D., Selective distal nephron damage during isolated kidney perfusion, *Kidney Int.*, 19, 638, 1981.
70. Lieberthal, W., Sheridan, A. M., and Valeri, C. R., Protective effect of atrial natriuretic factor and mannitol following renal ischemia, *Am. J. Physiol.*, 258, F1266, 1990.
71. Nobiling, R., Munter, K., Buhrle, C. P., and Hackenthal, E., Influence of pulsatile perfusion upon renin release from the isolated perfused rat kidney, *Pflügers Arch.*, 415, 713, 1990.
72. Zamlauski–Tucker, M. and Cohen, J. J., Effect of substrate-free albumin on perfused rat kidney function, *Renal Physiol.*, 10, 352, 1988.
73. Gronow, G. H. and Cohen, J. J., Substrate support for renal functions during hypoxia in the perfused rat kidney, *Am. J. Physiol.*, 247, F618, 1984.
74. Fonteles, M. C., Cohen, J. J., Black, A. J., and Wertheim, S. J., Support of kidney function by long-chain fatty acids derived from renal tissue, *Am. J. Physiol.*, 244, F235, 1983.
75. Cohen, J. J. and Black, A. J., Substrate-selective maintenance of tissue K+ in perfused rat kidney, *Am. J. Physiol.*, 242, F360, 1982.
76. Anaizi, N. H., Cohen, J. J., Black, A. J., and Wertheim, S. J., Renal tissue citrate: independence from citrate utilization, reabsorption, and pH, *Am. J. Physiol.*, 251, F547, 1986.
77. Anaizi, N. H. and Cohen, J. J., Kinetics of glucose decarboxylation in the substrate-limited isolated perfused kidney, *Renal Physiol. Biochem.*, 14, 81, 1991.
78. Perez, G., Epstein, M., Reitberg, B., Horton, C., and Loutzenhiser, R., Uptake and release of amino acids by normal and remnant kidneys: studies in the isolated perfused kidney, *Am. J. Clin. Nutr.*, 33, 1373, 1980.
79. Baines, A. D., Shaikh, N., and Ho, P., Mechanisms of perfused kidney cytoprotection by alanine and glycine, *Am. J. Physiol.*, 259, F80, 1990.
80. Brezis, M., Heyman, S. N., Dinour, D., Epstein, F. H., and Rosen, S., Role of nitric oxide in renal medullary oxygenation. Studies in isolated and intact rat kidneys, *J. Clin. Invest.*, 88, 390, 1991.
81. Cachofeiro, V. and Nasjletti, A., Increased vascular responsiveness to bradykinin in kidneys of spontaneously hypertensive rats. Effect of *N*-omega-nitro-L-arginine, *Hypertension*, 18, 683, 1991.
82. Gardes, J., Poux, J. M., Gonzalez, M. F., Alhenc-Gelas, F., and Menard, J., Decreased renin release and constant kallikrein secretion after injection of L-NAME in isolated perfused rat kidney, *Life Sci.*, 50, 987, 1992.
83. Radermacher, J., Klanke, B., Schurak, H. J., Stolte, H. F., and Frolich, J. C., Importance of NO/EDRF for glomerular and tubular function: studies in the isolated perfused rat kidney, *Kidney Int.*, 41, 1549 1992.
84. Kikuchi, K., Nagano, T., Hayakawa, H., Hirata, Y., and Hirobe, M., Detection of nitric oxide production from a perfused organ by a luminol-H2O2 system, *Anal. Chem.*, 65, 1794, 1993.
85. Zhang, B. L. and Sassard, J., Eicosanoid-dependence of responses of pre- but not postglomerular vessels to noradrenaline in rat isolated kidneys, *Br. J. Pharmacol.*, 110, 235, 1993.
86. Simeoni, U., Massfelder, T., Saussine, C., Judes, C., Geisert, J., and Helwig, J. J., Involvement of nitric oxide in the vasodilatory response to parathyroid hormone-related peptide in the isolated rabbit kidney, *Clin. Sci.* 86, 245, 1994.
87. Vargas, F., Sabio, J. M., and Luna, J. D., Contribution of endothelium derived relaxing factors to acetylcholine induced vasodilatation in the rat kidney, *Cardiovasc. Res.*, 28, 1373, 1994.
88. Terao, N., Suzuki, M., Asano, Y., and Hosoda, S., Enhanced reabsorption of bicarbonate and phosphorus by the addition of amino acids in the isolated perfused kidney, *Kidney Int.*, 27, 951, 1985.
89. el Sayed, A. A., Haylor, J., and el Nahas, A. M., Differential effects of amino acids on the isolated perfused rat kidney, *Clin. Sci.*, 79, 381, 1990.
90. el Sayed, A. A., Haylor, J., and el Nahas, A. M., Mediators of the direct effects of amino acids on the rat kidney, *Clin. Sci.*, 81, 429, 1991.

91. el Sayed, A. A., Haylor, J., and el Nahas, A. M., Involvement of renal autacoids in the direct effects of mixed amino acids on the kidney, *Miner. Electrolyte Metab.*, 18, 117, 1992.
92. Chen, R. F., Removal of fatty acids from serum albumin by charcoal treatment, *J. Biol. Chem.*, 242, 173, 1967.
93. Bullivant, M., Volume changes in cells of the outer medulla during perfusion of the rat kidney, *J. Physiol.*, 280, 125, 1978.
94. Klotzbach, J. M., Studies on the Mechanism of Action of 2,3-Dimercaptopropane Sulfonate (DMPS): A Mercurial Complexing Agent, Ph.D. Dissertation, University of Rochester, Rochester, NY, 1987.
95. Pagel, H. and Stolte, H., On the glomerular mechanism of the renal protein excretion. Studies in the isolated perfused rat kidney, *Renal Physiol. Biochem.*, 15, 249, 1992.
96. Millis, R. M., Barber, J. D., Anderson, W. A., Toussaint, R. M., Baker, F. W., and Hackley, B. E., Jr., Amelioration of nephrotoxicity associated with synthetic oxygen transport media, *J. Natl. Med. Assoc.*, 84, 773, 1992.
97. Franke, H. and Weiss, C., The O_2 supply of the isolated cell-free perfused rat kidney, *Adv. Exp. Med. Biol.*, 75, 425, 1976.
98. Daugaard, H., Egfjord, M., and Olgaard, K., Isolated perfused rat kidney and liver combined: a new experimental model, *Eur. J. Physiol.*, 401, 220, 1987.
99. Daugaard, H., Egfjord, M., and Olgaard, K., Influence of calcium on the metabolism of intact parathyroid hormone by isolated perfused rat kidney and liver, *Endocrinology*, 126, 1813, 1990.
100. Daugaard, H., Egfjord, M., and Olgaard, K., Metabolism of parathyroid hormone in isolated perfused rat kidney and liver combined, *Kidney Int.*, 38, 55, 1990.
101. Daugaard, H., Egfjord, M., Lewin, E., and Olgaard, K., Metabolism of *N*-terminal and C-terminal parathyroid hormone fragments by isolated perfused rat kidney and liver, *Endocrinology*, 134, 1373, 1994.
102. Egfjord, M., Daugaard, H., and Olgaard, K., Aldosterone metabolism in combined isolated perfused rat liver and kidney, *Am. J. Physiol.*, 260, F536, 1991.
103. Egfjord, M., Daugaard, H., and Olgaard, K., Influence of glucocorticoid on the metabolism of aldosterone in the isolated perfused rat liver and kidney, *Steroids*, 57, 335, 1992.
104. Barac–Nieto, M., Gupta, R. K., and Spitzer, A., NMR studies of phosphate metabolism in the isolated perfused kidney of developing rats, *Pediatr. Nephrol.*, 4, 392, 1990.
105. Loutzenhiser, R., Epstein, M., Hayashi, K., and Horton, C., Direct visualization of effects of endothelin on the renal microvasculature, *Am. J. Physiol.*, 258, F61, 1990.
106. Steinhausen, M., Snoel, H., Parekh, N., Baker, R., and Johnson, P. C., Hydronephrosis: a new method to visualize vas afferens, efferens and glomerular network, *Kidney Int.*, 23, 794, 1983.
107. Shohat, J., Erman, A., Boner, G., and Rosenfeld, J., Mechanisms of the early and late response of the kidney to contralateral nephrectomy, *Renal Physiol. Biochem.*, 14, 103, 1991.
108. Price, D. A., Okolicany, J., and Maack, T., Renal receptors and effects of atrial natriuretic factor in compensatory renal hypertrophy, *Kidney Int.*, 42, 75, 1992.
109. Harris, D. C., Tay, C., Egan, M. A., and Stewart, A., Altered metabolism in the ex vivo remnant kidney. I. Effects of time, substrate and perfusion pressure, *Nephron*, 54, 410, 1993.
110. Zalups, R. K. and Diamond, G. L., Mercuric chloride-induced nephrotoxicity in the rat following unilateral nephrectomy and compensatory renal growth, *Virchows Arch. B*, 53, 336, 1987.
111. Zalups, R. K., Klotzbach, J. M., and Diamond, G. L., Enhanced accumulation of injected inorganic mercury in renal outer medulla after unilateral nephrectomy, *Toxicol. Appl. Pharmacol.*, 89, 226, 1987.
112. Zalups, R. K., Gelein, R. M., Morrow, P. E., and Diamond, G. L., Nephrotoxicity of uranyl fluoride in uninephrectomized and sham-operated rats, *Toxicol. Appl. Pharmacol.*, 94, 11, 1988.
113. Zalups, R. K., Gelain, R. M., and Cherian, M. G., Shifts in the dose-effect relationship for the nephropathy induced by cadmium-metallothionein in rats after a reduction of renal mass, *J. Pharmacol. Exp. Ther.*, 262, 1256, 1992.
114. Zalups, R. K. and Veltman, J. C., Renal glutathione homeostasis in compensatory renal growth, *Life Sci.*, 42, 2171, 1988.
115. Zalups, R. K. and Lash, L. H., Effects of uninephrectomy and mercuric chloride on renal glutathione homeostasis, *J. Pharmacol. Exp. Ther.*, 254, 962, 1990.

116. Zalups, R. K. and Cherian, G., Renal metallothionein metabolism after a reduction of renal mass. I. Effect of unilateral nephrectomy and compensatory renal growth on basal metal-induced renal metallothionein metabolism, *Toxicology*, 71, 83, 1992.
117. Zalups, R. K. and Cherian, G., Renal metallothionein metabolism after a reduction of renal mass. II. Effect of zinc pretreatment on the renal toxicity and intrarenal accumulation of inorganic mercury, *Toxicology*, 71, 103, 1992.
118. Kamiya, A., Tanigawara, Y., Saito, Y., Hayashi, Y., Aiba, T., Inui, K., and Hori, R., Moment analysis of drug disposition in kidney. II. Urine pH-dependent tubular secretion of tetraethylammonium in the isolated perfused rat kidney, *J. Pharm. Sci.*, 79, 692, 1990.
119. Foulkes, E. C., Effects of heavy metals on renal aspartate transport and the nature of solute movement in kidney cortex slices, *Biochim. Biophys. Acta*, 241, 815, 1971.
120. Tanigawara, Y., Saito, Y., Aiba, T., Ohoka, K., Kamiya, A., and Hori, R., Moment analysis of drug disposition in kidney. III. Transport of *p*-aminohippurate and tetraethylammonium in the perfused kidney isolated from uranyl nitrate-induced acute renal failure rats, *J. Pharm. Sci.*, 79, 249, 1990.
121. Aiba, T., Itoga, Y., Shimizu, H., Tanigawara, Y., and Hori, R., Renal handling of tobramycin in the isolated perfused rat kidney, *J. Pharm. Sci.*, 83, 723, 1994.
122. Kim, D. C., Sugiyama, Y., Sawada, Y., and Hanano, M., Renal tubular handling of *p*-aminohippurate and epidermal growth factor (EGF) in filtering and nonfiltering perfused rat kidneys, *Pharm. Res.*, 9, 271, 1992.
123. Mihara, K., Mori, M., Hojo, T., Takakura, Y., Sezaki, H., and Hashida, M., Disposition characteristics of model macromolecules in the perfused rat kidney, *Biol. Pharm. Bull.*, 16, 158, 1993.
124. Cojocel, C., Dociu, N., Maita, K., Sleight, S. D., and Hook, J. B., Effects of aminoglycosides on glomerular permeability, tubular reabsorption, and intracellular catabolism of the cationic low-molecular-weight protein lysozyme, *Toxicol. Appl. Pharmacol.*, 68, 96, 1983.
125. Drapeau, G., Petitclerc, E., Toulouse, A., and Marceau, F., Dissociation of the antimicrobial activity of bacitracin USP from its renovascular effects, *Antimicrob. Agents Chemother.*, 36, 955, 1992.
126. Rodriguez, C. A. and Smith, D. E., Influence of the unbound concentration of cefonicid on its renal elimination in isolated perfused rat kidneys, *Antimicrob. Agents Chemother.*, 35, 2395, 1991.
127. Boom, S. P., Moons, M. M., and Russel, F. G., Renal tubular transport of cimetidine in the isolated perfused kidney of the rat, *Drug Metab. Dispos.*, 22, 148, 1994.
128. Sumpio, B. E., Chaudry, I. H., and Baue, A. E., Reduction of the drug-induced nephrotoxicity by ATP-MgCl2. I. Effects on the cis-diamminedichloroplatinum-treated isolated perfused kidney, *J. Surg. Res.*, 38, 429, 1985.
129. Miura, K., Goldstein, R. S., Pasino, D. A., and Hook, J. B., Cisplatin nephrotoxicity: role of filtration and tubular transport of cisplatin in isolated perfused kidney, *Toxicology*, 44, 147, 1987.
130. Mehring, N., Neumann, K. H., Rahn, K. H., and Zidek, W., Mechanisms of cyclosporin A-induced vasoconstriction in the isolated perfused rat kidney, *Nephron*, 60, 477, 1992.
131. Roby, K. A. and Shaw, L. M., Effects of cyclosporine and its metabolites in the isolated perfused rat kidney, *J. Am. Soc. Nephrol.*, 4, 168, 1993.
132. Besarab, A., Jarrell, B. E., Hirsch, S., Carabasi, R. A., Cressman, M. D., and Green, P., Use of isolated perfused kidney model to assess the acute pharmacologic effects of cyclosporine and its vehicle, Cremophor EL, *Transplantation*, 44, 195, 1987.
133. Luke, D. R., Kassiske, B. L., Matzke, G. E, Awni, W. M., and Weane, W. F., Effects of cyclosporine on the isolated perfused rat kidney, *Transplantation*, 43, 795, 1987.
134. Kellerman, P. S., Clark, R. A, Hoilien, C. A., Linas, S. L., and Molitoris, B. A., Role of microfilaments in maintenance of proximal tubule structural and functional integrity, *Am. J. Physiol.*, 259, F279, 1990.
135. Diamond, G. L., Klotzbach, J. M., and Stewart, J. R., Compexing activity of 2,3-dimercapto-1-propanesulfonate and its disulfide auto-oxidation product in rat kidney, *J. Pharmacol. Exp. Ther.*, 246, 270, 1988.
136. de Lannoy, I. A., Hirayama, H., and Pang, K. S., A physiological model for renal drug metabolism: enalapril esterolysis to enalaprilat in the isolated perfused rat kidney, *J. Pharmacokinet. Biopharm.*, 18, 561, 1990.

137. Cohen, J. J., Black, A. J., and Wertheim, S. J., Direct effects of endotoxin on the function of the isolated perfused rat kidney, *Kidney Int.*, 37, 1219, 1990.
138. Higaki, K., Kadono, K., Goto. S., and Nakano, M., Stereoselective renal tubular secretion of an organic anion in the isolated perfused rat kidney, *J. Pharmacol. Exp. Ther.*, 270, 329, 1994.
139. Ahn, H. Y., Jamali, F., Cox, S. R., Kittayanond, D., and Smith, D. E., Stereoselective disposition of ibuprofen enantiomers in the isolated perfused rat kidney, *Pharm. Res.*, 8, 1520, 1991.
140. Bowman, R. H., Dolgin, J., and Coulson, R., Furosemide, ethacrynic acid and iodoacetate on function and metabolism in perfused rat kidney, *Am. J. Physiol.*, 224, 416, 1973.
141. Redegeld, F. A., Hofman, G. A., van de Loo, P. G., Koster, A. S., and Noordhoek, J., Nephrotoxicity of the glutathione conjugate of menadione (2-methyl-1,4-naphthoquinone) in the isolated perfused rat kidney. Role of metabolism by gamma-glutamyltranspeptidase and probenecid-sensitive transport, *J. Pharmacol. Exp. Ther.*, 256, 665, 1991.
142. Rossi, N., Ellis, V., Kontry, T., Gunther, S., Churchill, P., and Bidani, A., The role of adenosine in HgCl2-induced acute renal failure in rats, *Am. J. Physiol.*, 258, F1554, 1990.
143. Statkevich, P., Fournier, D. J., and Sweeney, K. R., Characterization of methotrexate elimination and interaction with indomethacin and flurbiprofen in the isolated perfused rat kidney, *J. Pharmacol. Exp. Ther.*, 265, 1118, 1993.
144. Cox, P. G., Moons, W. M., Russel, F. G., and van Ginneken, C. A., Renal handling and effects of salicylic acid in the isolated perfused rat kidney, *Pharmacol. Toxicol.*, 68, 322, 1991.
145. Cox, P. G., Moons, M. M., Russel, F. G., and van Ginneken, C. A., Indomethacin: renal handling and effects in the isolated perfused rat kidney, *Pharmacology*, 42, 287, 1991.
146. Ellis, A. G. and Adam, W. R., Effects of opiates on sodium excretion in the isolated perfused rat kidney, *Clin. Exp. Pharmacol. Physiol.*, 18, 835, 1991.
147. Van Crugten, J. T., Sallustio, B. C., Nation, R. L., and Somogyi, A. A., Renal tubular transport of morphine, morphine-6-glucuronide, and morphine-3-glucuronide in the isolated perfused rat kidney, *Drug Metab. Dispos.*, 19, 1087, 1991.
148. Firth, J. D., Effect of polycations on the function of the isolated perfused rat kidney, *Clin. Sci.*, 79, 591, 1990.
149. Firth, J. D. and Ledingham, J. G., Effect of natriuretic agents, vasoactive agents and of the inhibition of metabolism on sodium handling in the isolated perfused kidney of the nephrotic rat, *Clin. Sci.*, 79, 559, 1990.
150. Willinger, C. C., Moschen, I., Kulmer, S., and Pfaller, W., The effect of sodium fluoride at prophylactic and toxic doses on renal structure and function in the isolated perfused rat kidney, *Toxicology*, 95, 55, 1995.
151. Muirhead, M. R. and Somogyi, A. A., Effect of H2 antagonists on the differential secretion of triamterene and its sulfate conjugate metabolite by the isolated perfused rat kidney, *Drug Metab. Dispos.*, 19, 312, 1991.
152. Hassall, C. D., Gandolfi, A. J., and Brendel, K., Correlation of the *in vivo* and *in vitro* renal toxicity of S-(1,2-dichlorovinyl)-L-cysteine., *Drug Chem. Toxicol.*, 6, 507, 1983.
153. el Sayed, A. A., Haylor, J. L., el Nahas, A. M., Salzano, S., and Morcos, S. K., Haemodynamic effects of water-soluble contrast media on the isolated perfused rat kidney, *Br. J. Radiol.*, 64, 435, 1991.
154. Haylor, J. L., el Sayed, A. A., el Nahas, A. M., and Morcos, S. K., The effect of sodium iothalamate on the vascular resistance of the isolated perfused rat kidney, *Br. J. Radiol.*, 64, 50, 1991.
155. Brown, P., Haylor, J., Morcos, S. K., Cope, G. H., and el Nahas, A. M., Effect of diatrizoate on the function of the isolated perfused rat kidney, *Br. J. Radiol.*, 65, 1011, 1992.
156. Brown, P. W., Haylor, J. L., Morcos, S. K., and el Nahas, A. M., The functional effects of gadolinium-DTPA on the isolated perfused rat kidney, *Eur. J. Radiol.*, 16, 85, 1993.

chapter five

Micropuncture and Microperfusion Techniques

Carla R. Ramsey and Franklyn G. Knox

5.1 Introduction 79
5.2 Background and history 80
5.3 Preparation 81
  5.3.1 Animals and surgical preparation 81
  5.3.2 Identification of nephron segments 82
  5.3.3 Equipment 83
    5.3.3.1 Microscope 84
    5.3.3.2 Micromanipulators 84
    5.3.3.3 Micropipettes 84
5.4 Procedures 85
  5.4.1 Micropuncture 85
    5.4.1.1 Measurement of single nephron glomerular filtration rate 86
    5.4.1.2 Evaluation of tubular transport 86
    5.4.1.3 Advantages and disadvantages 87
  5.4.2 Microperfusion 88
    5.4.2.1 Microperfusion of proximal tubules 89
    5.4.2.2 Microperfusion of the loop of Henle 90
    5.4.2.3 Microperfusion of distal tubules 90
    5.4.2.4 Advantages and limitations 90
5.5 Microdissection and measurement of tubular segments 91
5.6 Microanalytic techniques 91
References 93

5.1 *Introduction*

The nephron is highly complex and heterogeneous from a morphological, biochemical, and physiologic point of view.[1] Additionally, there is a strong correlation between the morphological and functional attributes of each nephron segment and the potential development of nephrotoxicity.[2] *In vivo* microperfusion and micropuncture are two valuable techniques that are used to study the function of individual nephron segments in the intact kidney and the effects of drugs or nephrotoxins on tubular function.[3-11]

0-8493-3341-5/96/$0.00+$.50

These techniques can directly determine the tubular handling of drugs and nephrotoxicants. For example, recent *in vivo* micropuncture studies have been used to determine the ultrafilterability and tubular handling of various inorganic metal ions such as cadmium and aluminum.[3,4] Micropuncture techniques have also been used to characterize the organic anion transporter and organic cation transporter.[5-8] Micropuncture was used to determine the active tubular secretion of *p*-aminohippurate (PAH) by the organic anion transporter and also demonstrated that *N*-methylnicotinamide (NMN) was secreted into the proximal tubule by the organic cation transporter.

Microperfusion and micropuncture are also used to determine the specific effects that a particular drug or nephrotoxicant may have on tubular function. For example, micropuncture studies have determined the effect of the acute administration of cisplatin on glomerular filtration and segmental tubular transport.[9] Likewise, a recent study by Kidwell et al. utilized *in vivo* micropuncture to determine that gentamicin had no significant effect on single nephron glomerular filtration rate or proximal reabsorption but significantly decreased transport by the loop of Henle.[10]

The application of the micropuncture and microperfusion techniques have provided considerable information concerning the physiology and toxicology of the kidney. Micropuncture is the method of choice to determine the *in vivo* concentration profile and composition of luminal fluid along the nephron. Microperfusion is a valuable technique in the study of renal toxicology since specific drugs or substances of interest may be applied directly to the tubule in the luminal perfusate to determine their effect on tubular function.

5.2 Background and history

The micropuncture technique for collecting tubular luminal fluid from individual nephron segments originated in the early 1920s when Joseph Wearn and Alfred Richards first analyzed fluid from Bowman's space of the *in vivo* frog kidney.[12] This initial description of the micropuncture technique has been described as "one of the most important single contributions to renal physiology".[13] A series of studies during the next two decades then delineated the properties of glomerular filtrate and tubule fluid in amphibian kidneys. In 1941 the first application of micropuncture to the mammalian kidney was published by Walker and Oliver.[14] In collaboration with Phyllis Bott, who was instrumental in developing microanalytic techniques for the nanoliter volume of tubular fluid collected during micropuncture, Walker and colleagues collected the first data describing the function of individual mammalian nephron segments.[15]

Important variations and modifications of the micropuncture technique were also developed during that period that are still valued for studying the function of individual nephron segments. In 1937, Richards and Walker first described stationary microperfusion of the proximal tubule in the *Necturus* kidney.[16] Stationary microperfusion was further modified, and in 1961, Gertz and Ullrich introduced the shrinking droplet technique for determination of isotonic fluid reabsorption.[17] In contrast to stationary microperfusion, continuous microperfusion was developed by Sonnenberg and Deetjen in 1964.[18] Subsequently, microinjection techniques and microperfusion of peritubular capillaries have been developed and employed in the study of renal function.[19] It is the aim of this chapter to detail the advantages, application, and limitations of *in vivo* micropuncture and microperfusion techniques to study nephron function and tubular transport. Several comprehensive reviews have dealt with both the history and technical aspects of the micropuncture methodology. Some of these references are listed here and are suggested for additional information.[20-26]

5.3 Preparation

5.3.1 Animals and surgical preparation

As described above, the micropuncture methodology was first applied to the study of the amphibian kidney. The advantages of using kidneys from amphibians such as the frog, *Necturus* (mudpuppy), *Amphiuma* (Congo eel), and *Triturus* (Japanese newt) for micropuncture include the accessibility, large size, and slow reabsorption rate of amphibian tubules. Micropuncture and microperfusion are also performed in a variety of mammalian species, including dogs and small rodents. Although used extensively in *in vitro* studies, *in vivo* micropuncture of the rabbit is relatively uncommon due to instability during anesthesia.[20] The most common experimental animal in use for micropuncture and microperfusion studies is the rat and, therefore, the methodologies in this chapter are described as applied to the rat kidney.

Sprague–Dawley, Wistar, and Munich–Wistar rat strains are extensively used in micropuncture and microperfusion experiments. Munich–Wistar rats are often used in studies of glomerular function because their glomeruli are visible and accessible at the surface of the kidney. Other strains such as the spontaneously hypertensive rat or the Brattleboro rat are also used to study nephron function during specific pathophysiologic conditions. Rats of 200 to 250 grams body weight are usually chosen for micropuncture of superficial cortical nephron segments. Young rats weighing less than 150 grams are chosen for micropuncture of collecting ducts, loops of Henle, or vasa recta because the papilla protrudes into the ureter and is accessible at this stage of development.

Animals are anesthetized with a long-acting anesthetic such as Inactin (thiobutabarbital, 5-sec-butyl-5-ethyl-2-thiobarbituric acid; 100 to 120 mg/kg body weight, injected intraperitoneally) or a mixture of ketamine (Ketaset; 50 mg/kg body weight) and Inactin (30 to 40 mg/kg body weight).[20] Rats are placed on a thermostatically controlled table to maintain body temperature at 36 to 38°C.[27] A tracheostomy is then performed using a small segment of PE-240 (O.D. = 0.095″, I.D. = 0.066″; Clay Adams, Parsippany, NJ) tubing that is short enough to minimize deadspace. Catheters (PE-50, O.D. = 0.038″, I.D. = 0.023″) are then inserted into the carotid or femoral artery for blood sampling and measurement of blood pressure. Catheters (PE-50) are also inserted into the jugular veins for infusions. A 3 to 6% inulin* solution in isotonic saline is initiated in micropuncture experiments for the later determination of tubular-fluid-to-plasma-inulin concentration and single nephron filtration rate. Rats often also receive an additional saline or albumin infusion intravenously to replace surgical losses and maintain an adequate blood volume and urine flow for optimal collections. Last, one or both ureters are catheterized for urine collection. A PE-50 catheter is recommended for the ureter because it provides much less resistance, and subsequent obstructions are less likely than with a PE-10 (O.D. = 0.024″, I.D. = 0.011″) catheter, particularly with high urine flow rates.[28] A catheter with an inner diameter that is too small will impede urine flow, trap particles, and lead to renal obstruction.

Micropuncture or microperfusion are most often performed on the left kidney because of its accessibility and longer vascular pedicle when compared to the right kidney. The left kidney is isolated via a flank incision made at the left subcostal margin. The kidney is then carefully separated from the surrounding tissue and placed in a clear Lucite kidney holder or cup to immobilize and support it during microperfusion.[29] The abdominal cavity is filled with a light mineral oil to cover the kidney and also to prevent heat and fluid losses.

The kidney is carefully dissected free from the surrounding fat and connective tissue with fine, rounded forceps. It is often helpful to leave a very small fringe of connective tissue attached to the kidney that can be used to hold and maneuver the kidney into the

* Or an appropriate solution of another extracellular marker such as iothalamate.

kidney holder. Care must be taken not to damage the surrounding blood vessels or the adrenal gland. When the kidney is thoroughly dissected and attached only at the pedicle, it is carefully placed in an appropriately sized kidney holder. A thin layer of cotton soaked in mineral oil should line the bottom and sides of the kidney holder. Care should be taken to avoid stretching the pedicle and causing subsequent vasoconstriction of the renal artery while placing the kidney in the holder. Obstruction of the ureter or renal vein by bands of connective tissue should also be avoided. The renal capsule of the rat is transparent and is left intact for micropuncture or microperfusion. However, in the dog the renal capsule is thicker and opaque and a portion of the capsule must be removed to visualize the tubules.

Following surgery and isolation of the kidney, blood pressure should be stable and should be within the level of autoregulation, above 90 mmHg. The surface of the kidney should appear healthy, with a smooth surface and reddish color. An obstruction of the ureter or vein will result in a tense, poorly functioning kidney, often with transparent-looking areas. A constriction of the renal artery will produce a soft kidney with patchy distribution of blood flow and the appearance of a pitted surface. Urine flow should usually be between 1 and 10 μl/min under control conditions in the rat.

5.3.2 *Identification of nephron segments*

Once the kidney is isolated in a kidney holder, the superficial nephron segments can be visualized with a stereomicroscope. The majority of the tubules visible on the surface of the kidney are convolutions of the proximal tubule. Superficial glomeruli are also visible on the surface of the kidney in the Munich–Wistar strain of rat. Peritubular capillaries appear as thin red lines between and around the tubules. A few distal tubular segments are also visible on the surface of the rat kidney and under control conditions are often distinguished from proximal tubules by their thinner walls and smaller lumina. In the dog and rat approximately 60% of the length of the proximal tubule is accessible to micropuncture. Figure 1 shows a microscopic view of the latest accessible convolution of a proximal tubule that had been injected with latex (see Section 5.5).[30,31] This tubule was subsequently dissected free and straightened, as shown in Figure 2. The point shown by the arrow corresponds to the point on the surface marked by the arrow in Figure 1.

Most of the nephron segments on the surface of the kidney are proximal tubules, and with experience, these segments can be visually distinguished from distal segments of nephron. However, a reliable method to positively identify proximal and distal segments on the surface of the kidney is the use of dyes such as lissamine green. The use of lissamine green dye to identify surface tubules was first developed in 1963 by Steinhausen.[32] When a small bolus of lissamine green dye (25 to 50 μl of a 10% solution) is infused intravenously, the distinct timed appearance of the dye within surface structures of the kidney allows identification of specific tubular segments.

Shortly after the bolus infusion, the surface of the kidney appears green and the dye first appears in the capillaries near the surface of the kidney. As the dye is filtered at the glomerulus, it appears along the nephron. Within about 10 s the dye will reach the last loops of the proximal tubule in the rat. The dye then disappears from the surface as it enters the loops of Henle. Then, the dye reappears on the surface of the kidney about 20 s after its initial appearance in the capillaries as it enters segments of the distal tubule. The dye then reaches the late distal segments approximately 35 s after it first enters the renal vasculature. By using this technique, nephron segments can be identified and particular segments can be drawn on a map of the surface of the kidney in the field of view for relocation of these segments at a later time. It is important to note that the intravenous infusion of lissamine green should be kept at a minimum because large doses of lissamine

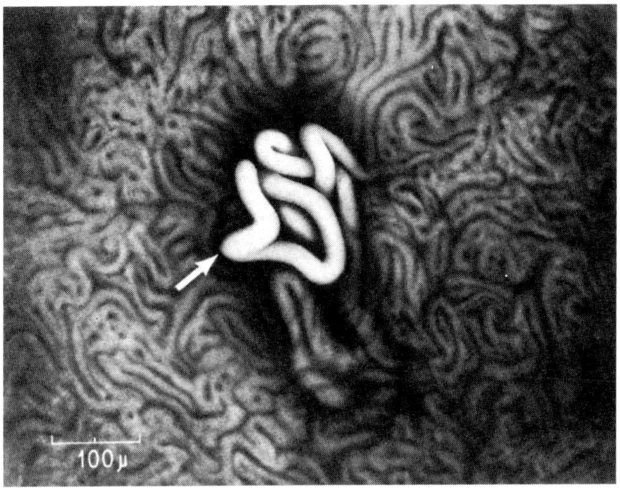

Figure 1 Photomicrograph of the latest accessible surface convolution (arrow) of a proximal tubule that was injected with latex in a dog kidney. (From Knox, F. G. and Marchand, G. R., in *Methods in Pharmacology*, Vol. 4A, Martinez-Maldonado, M., Ed., Plenum Press, New York, 1976, 76. With permission.)

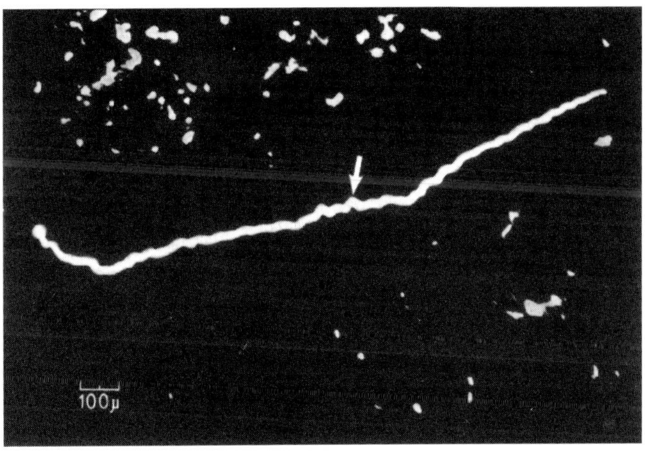

Figure 2 Photomicrograph of the entire proximal convoluted tubule shown in Figure 1. The arrow indicates the point along this nephron segment that corresponds to the latest accessible surface convolution. (From Knox, F. G. and Marchand, G. R., in *Methods in Pharmacology*, Vol. 4A, Martinez-Maldonado, M., Ed., Plenum Press, New York, 1976, 77. With permission.)

green have been shown to be natriuretic and to increase single nephron glomerular filtration rate.[33-35] However, these effects were rapidly reversible and several repeated injections of small doses of lissamine green, as used for micropuncture, failed to result in sustained renal effects. Nevertheless, micropuncture or microperfusion should be performed only after the dye has completely disappeared from the kidney. Preferably, lissamine green should be infused at least one half hour prior to micropuncture or microperfusion.

5.3.3 Equipment

The experimental setup and tools necessary for micropuncture and microperfusion are shown in Figure 3.

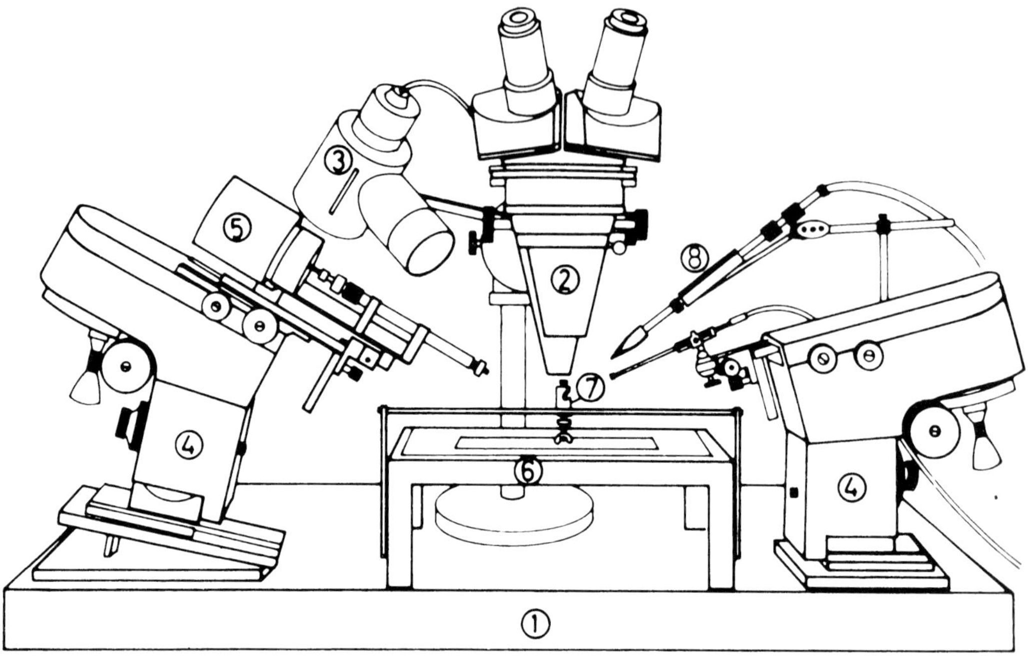

Figure 3 Experimental setup for micropuncture in the rat. (1) Stone plate; (2) microscope; (3) light source; (4) micromanipulators; (5) microperfusion pump; (6) thermostatically heated table; (7) kidney holder; (8) heated oil dropper. (From Lang, F., Greger R., Lechene, C., and Knox, F. G., in *Methods in Pharmacology,* Vol. 4B, Martinez-Maldonado, M., Ed., Plenum Press, New York, 1978, 77. With permission.)

5.3.3.1 Microscope

Micropuncture and microperfusion are performed under a stereo dissecting microscope. The essential features of this microscope include: a magnification range up to 200×, preferably with a zoom optic system for changing magnification, and a working distance of 3 to 4 cm for the manipulation of micropipettes between the surface of the kidney and the objective. This microscope is then mounted in a stand that allows adjustment of the microscope in three dimensions. A cool light source, such as fiber-optic light, is used to illuminate the kidney under the microscope to avoid producing intense heat on the kidney surface. An oil dropper is used to continuously drip oil heated to 37°C from a supply tube wrapped with a heating coil onto the surface of the kidney.

5.3.3.2 Micromanipulators

Since micropuncture and microperfusion involve impalement of individual nephron segments with the tip of a glass micropipette, accurate controlled movement of the pipette over micrometer distances is necessary. This is accomplished by placing the pipette in a micromanipulator that smoothly and precisely maneuvers the pipette in all dimensions across the surface of the kidney. The most commonly used have been the Lietz and De Fonbrune micromanipulators.

5.3.3.3 Micropipettes

The micropipettes are made from borosilicate (Pyrex, Kymex) glass capillary tubes with an outer diameter of approximately 1 mm. The pointed tip of the pipette is produced by mechanical pipette pullers that heat the middle of the capillary tube, by an electric coil, until the capillary tube melts and is pulled apart by a mobile magnet. Vertical or horizontal pipette pullers are available, and the size and shape of the pipette tip can be regulated by adjusting the heat and magnetic pull delivered to the glass. The pipette must then be beveled and sharpened with the use of a rotating grinding stone.[36]

Micropipettes of the appropriate shape and size are crucial for a successful micropuncture or microperfusion experiment. The pipette is sharpened, under a low-power stereoscope, by using a micromanipulator to lower the tip of the pipette at about a 30° angle onto a rotating grinding stone. After sharpening, the tip of the pipette is rinsed with distilled water and acetone. The size and shape of the micropipette is then determined under a compound microscope with a micrometer. Pipettes should have smooth edges and an appropriate outer diameter. For micropuncture of proximal tubules, pipettes having tips with an outer diameter of 10 μm are used, while for distal tubules pipettes with tips of 8 μm are used; pipettes having tips with an outer diameter of 12 μm are used to inject latex into the tubule (see below).

5.4 Procedures

5.4.1 Micropuncture

Collection of tubular luminal fluid during micropuncture is accomplished by advancing the tip of a micropipette into the lumen of the specific tubule to be studied. A timed complete collection of the ultrafiltrate or tubular fluid that flows into the pipette is then obtained.

Micropipettes that are to be used for the collection of tubular fluid are first filled at the tip with a 2% solution of castor oil stained with Sudan black B. Micropipettes are easily filled by inserting a 30-gauge needle attached to a syringe into the pipette and injecting an oil column approximately 2 to 3 mm in length into the pipette tip. This pipette is then attached to a length of tubing connected to a glass syringe with a stopcock and mounted in a micromanipulator. To precisely puncture the tubule, the micropipette is lowered onto the kidney at an angle of 10 to 40 degrees to the surface of the kidney. Puncture is easiest if the pipette is oriented with the long axis of the tubule. The opening of the beveled tip should be facing upward, and the pointed, sharpened side of the pipette tip should be touching the surface of the tubule. With the micromanipulator, the pipette is then lowered and the tip is advanced into the center of the tubular lumen. The tip of the pipette should be located in the center of the tubule without deforming the tubule. It is also important not to produce a fistula to other nephrons by "overshooting" the tubular lumen and then adjusting the tip position.

Once the tip of the pipette is placed in the lumen, oil is then injected into the lumen of the tubule by applying pressure to the glass syringe attached to the micropipette. The length of the oil column introduced into the lumen should be equal to 4 or 5 tubular diameters. This column of oil is placed into the lumen of the tubule to act as an oil block to ensure complete collection of the tubular luminal fluid that reaches the pipette. Too small an oil block may allow retrograde collection of tubular fluid from more distal segments to contaminate the micropuncture sample. Too large an oil block may cause an increase in intraluminal pressure.

Immediately after the oil column is in place, the collection of tubular fluid is initiated by gentle negative pressure from the glass syringe. Once fluid has initially entered the pipette, collection should occur spontaneously and negative pressure should no longer be necessary. During collection, the diameter of the tubule should remain constant and similar to the other tubules, and the oil column should remain in position just downstream adjacent to the pipette tip. For timed collections, the timer is started at the moment the collection is initiated. The use of a footswitch to start and stop the timer is recommended to improve the accuracy of both the initiation and termination of the timed collection. Additionally, small errors in the timing of collection are minimized in longer collection times. Therefore, collection times should be at least 2 min, with most collections being 3 to 6 min. The length of collection time is also dependent on the amount of sample that is needed for the analytical procedures.

At the end of the collection, the tubing connected to the pipette is opened to atmospheric pressure by the stopcock. The pipette is quickly moved from the tubular lumen to the oil covering the kidney. A small amount of oil is aspirated into the tip of the pipette to prevent evaporation of the sample of tubular fluid. Likewise, the pipette is then stored with its tip placed in oil for later analysis.

After control collections of fluid from several tubules, the animal can be subjected to an experimental condition, and a second collection of tubular fluid can be obtained from the same tubules used for the control collections. In this re-collection procedure, the second collection is taken from the same site in the tubule where the first collection was made.[37] Therefore, the second pipette should be placed in the same puncture site in the tubule and should have the same shape and taper as the first and may have a slightly larger tip diameter (1 μm) than the first pipette.

5.4.1.1 *Measurement of single nephron glomerular filtration rate*

The collection time, the volume of the sample of tubular fluid, the concentration of inulin in the collected tubular fluid (TF_{In}), and the concentration of inulin in the plasma (P_{In}) are used to calculate single nephron glomerular filtration rate (SNGFR). The flow rate of the tubular fluid (V_{TF}) is calculated as the volume of the collected sample divided by the time of the collection.

Using these above values, the calculation for SNGFR is analogous to that for whole kidney glomerular filtration rate. The equation used for this calculation is presented below as Equation 1.

$$\text{SNGFR (nl min}^{-1}) = V_{TF}\ (\text{nl min}^{-1}) \times (TF_{in}/P_{in}) \tag{1}$$

When the single nephron filtration rate has been estimated by dividing the whole kidney glomerular filtration rate by an average number of nephrons in the kidney, a value of 30 nl min^{-1} was obtained for the SNGFR. However, this value is based on the assumption that all nephrons are filtering and that the rate of filtration is similar in all glomeruli.[21] Perhaps a more precise estimate of SNGFR for the superficial nephrons of the rat is based on previous measurements during control euvolemic conditions.[38,39] Thus, values considerably above or below these values indicate errors in the micropuncture collection, such as retrograde collection, fistula formation, or blocked flow.

5.4.1.2 *Evaluation of tubular transport*

The ratio of the concentration of inulin in the sample of tubular fluid to the concentration of inulin in the plasma (TF_{in}/P_{in}) is a measure of fractional volume reabsorption by the tubule up to the point of collection. When the ultrafiltrate is first formed at the glomerulus, it has the same concentration of inulin as plasma, and the TF_{in}/P_{in} ratio is equal to one. As fluid, but not inulin, is reabsorbed by the tubule, the concentration of inulin in the tubular fluid increases, and therefore, the TF_{in}/P_{in} also increases.

The net fractional transport of a substance by the nephron up to the point of micropuncture can also be determined. The net reabsorption or secretion of the substance of interest (X) can be determined using the concentrations of inulin and substance X in the sample of tubule fluid and the concentrations of inulin and substance X in a corresponding sample of plasma. The calculation of net reabsorption or net secretion of a substance in individual nephron segments is analogous to the calculation of fractional excretion for the whole kidney. The fraction of filtered substance X remaining at the point of tubule puncture or the fractional delivery of X (FD_X) from the site of micropuncture is calculated as a ratio, which is presented in Equation 2:

$$(TF_X \div P_X) \div (TF_{In} \div P_{In}) \tag{2}$$

where TF_X and TF_{In} represent the concentrations of substance X and inulin in samples of tubular fluid, and P_X and P_{In} represent the concentrations of substance X and inulin in the plasma.

If the above ratio is less than one, then net reabsorption of the substance has occurred along the nephron. If the above ratio is more than one, then there has been net secretion of substance X by the nephron. When the above value is multiplied by 100, the percentage of filtered substance X remaining at the site of puncture is known.

The net transport by specific individual segments of the nephron can also be determined from puncturing successive segments.[40-42] Free-flow micropuncture samples of tubular fluid from successive nephron segments such as the early proximal tubule, the late proximal tubule, and the early and late distal tubule can be used to determine the transport of water and solutes between the glomerulus and the site of micropuncture. Therefore, a comparison of the amount of fluid or solute that is remaining at successive sites of micropuncture can be used to calculate net transport by the segment(s) of the nephron between the two puncture sites. For example, although the loop of Henle is inaccessible to micropuncture, a comparison of transport between the late proximal tubule segment and the early distal tubule can be used to determine transport by the loop of Henle. Likewise, the differences in fractional delivery at early and late distal tubular puncture sites can be used to indicate transport by the distal convoluted tubule.

The function of papillary structures such as the thin limbs of Henle's loop and the collecting duct can also be determined by directly collecting tubular fluid samples from these structures.[43,44] Papillary micropuncture has also been used to determine transport by the deep, juxtamedullary nephrons of the kidney.[45,46] However, micropuncture of papillary structures requires the use of animals in which the papilla can be exposed. The golden hamster is one species in which the papilla protrudes into the ureter and has, therefore, been used widely for these purposes.[23] Likewise, young Wistar rats are also used, because the tip of the papilla in their kidneys protrudes several millimeters into the renal pelvis. In these animals, the papilla is exposed by removing the fat surrounding the papilla. Lateral and perpendicular incisions are then made in the ureter to expose the papilla to allow visualization of the tubules and vessels. When viewed under the microscope, the loops of Henle appear as thin, white loops with very small lumina, while the collecting ducts have larger lumina and are visualized easily. Micropuncture samples are then collected as described above for superficial segments except that micropipettes having a smaller tip diameter (3 to 5 μm) are used to puncture these papillary structures.

5.4.1.3 *Advantages and disadvantages*

Micropuncture has been important in understanding the *in vivo* function of individual segments of the nephron during physiologic and pathophysiologic conditions in the presence and absence of various drugs, toxic substances, and hormones. This technique has been instrumental in determining tubular reabsorption and secretion of various endogenous and exogenous substances. Free-flow *in vivo* micropuncture has the advantage that the tubule is studied in the intact functioning kidney, and a physiologically stable preparation can be studied for several hours. However, micropuncture can, therefore, be done only in certain species, and extrapolation to other species and humans must be made. Moreover, micropuncture requires surgical preparation and is performed in the presence of appropriate anesthesia. While the effect of anesthesia on tubule function must be considered, the effect of anesthetics can be controlled by making paired control and experimental collections in the same anesthetized animal.[20,47,48] Another limitation of the micropuncture technique is that sampling of tubular fluid is usually limited to collections from accessible portions of surface nephrons only. Since internephron heterogeneity is known to exist, results from surface nephrons may or may not be representative of all nephrons.[45,46] The fact that a single segment of the nephron is studied can be advantageous because only small quantities of drugs and reagents are necessary. On the other hand, this also requires meticulous fluid collection and methods of sensitive microanalysis.

The exposure of the nephron to micropuncture may alter its normal function. The first important consideration is placement of the micropipette into the tubule. The major concern in placement of the pipette is the formation of a fistula to adjacent nephron loops. It has been estimated that fistula formation occurs in approximately 10% of all punctures.[49,39] Tubule leaks can be indicated by visualization, excessively fast tubular flow rates or SNGFR and unreasonable values for concentrations of inulin in the tubular fluid. It is important to establish criteria for acceptance of fluid samples and to adhere to them throughout the experiment. Any samples not meeting the predetermined criteria should be rejected.[20]

The placement of an adequate oil block is also a necessary consideration since retrograde contamination of collected tubular fluid can significantly increase the estimate of SNGFR and alter the composition of the collected sample. An oil block of sufficient length that remains in place during the collection is necessary to prevent retrograde contamination.[50] Once the oil block is in place, suction is applied to the pipette to initiate collection. It has been suggested that changes in intratubular pressure during filtrate collection may be transmitted to the glomerulus and affect SNGFR.[51] However, it has been demonstrated that intentional decreases in intratubular pressure during tubular fluid collection has no significant effect on SNGFR.[38] Furthermore, standard collection techniques do not alter intraluminal pressure significantly.

Considerable controversy has centered around the site of puncture and subsequent placement of the oil block for the determination of SNGFR. Insertion of an oil block interrupts the flow of tubular fluid to the macula densa. When placed in the proximal tubule, the oil block ceases downstream flow and could activate the tubuloglomerular feedback mechanism so that the measured SNGFR would not be representative of filtration in the tubule if an oil block were not present.[53,54] However, when proximal collections were compared to distal collections in studies performed in rats, no significant difference in SNGFR or in autoregulatory capability was detected. Single nephron filtration rate was comparable when collections were made in the presence or absence of flow to the macula densa.[55,56] Thus, it was concluded by these investigators that proximal micropuncture is a reliable technique for the measurement of single nephron filtration rate. However, during conditions that increase the rate of flow of tubular fluid above physiologic levels, placement of an oil block that interrupts flow to the macula densa may have significant effects on the autoregulation of SNGFR.[57]

5.4.2 *Microperfusion*

Continuous *in vivo* microperfusion is a useful technique to determine the function of a specific segment of the nephron. The segment of interest is first isolated from the glomerular filtrate between a wax and oil block. This nephron is then perfused with a known specific solution and at a chosen flow rate. Because the tubular segment can be perfused with a solution of known composition, microperfusion is useful for determining the net rate for secretion of substances into the tubular lumen, as well as net reabsorptive rates. In addition to determining the net transport of fluid or solutes by a specific segment of the nephron, *in vivo* microperfusion is also a particularly valuable technique to add specific drugs or hormones to the luminal perfusate and to determine their effect on tubular function. The procedure for microperfusion is shown schematically in Figure 4.

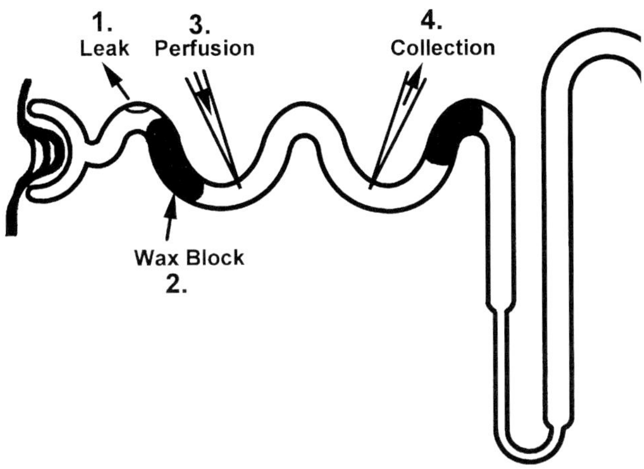

Figure 4 Schematic representation of proximal tubule microperfusion. First a tubule with several surface loops is identified by infusing stained fluid in an early portion of the tubule segment. (1) The pipette is withdrawn and a small hole remains in the tubule to allow the glomerular filtrate to leak from the tubule. (2) A paraffin wax block is inserted into the next loop of the tubule. (3) The tubule is perfused with a pipette attached to a microperfusion pump. (4) The luminal perfusate is collected downstream after the placement of a distal mineral oil block.

5.4.2.1 *Microperfusion of proximal tubules*

To microperfuse proximal tubular segments it is first necessary to identify a proximal tubule that has at least four to five surface loops. A micropipette containing a stained solution is inserted into the first loop of the segment to identify the four to five surface loops. Once the segment of interest has been identified and mapped, the first micropipette is removed leaving a hole to allow the native glomerular filtrate to escape from the tubular lumen. A second micropipette is then placed into the second surface loop for the injection of stained paraffin wax to block the glomerular filtrate. This pipette is then removed, and a third pipette, which is connected to a perfusion pump and contains stained perfusion fluid, is inserted into the third loop to perfuse the tubular segment. Perfusion of the tubular segment is initiated, and the luminal perfusate is then collected downstream in the fourth or fifth surface loop by a fourth micropipette, which contains a 2% Sudan black B in mineral oil solution. The samples of microperfusate are then collected as described above for micropuncture. After the pipette is inserted into the tubular lumen, a column of stained mineral oil is injected into the lumen and the timed collection of perfusate is made. Paired control and experimental collections are often made in the same perfused tubule. It is necessary to reduce leaks during perfusion and collection of the second sample. Therefore, for these samples, the pipettes used for control and experimental collections should be matched for size and shape.

One of the most important steps in the microperfusion technique is the introduction of the wax block into the initial loop of the tubular segment to obstruct the flow of the native glomerular filtrate. Inadequate blockade will allow for contamination of the luminal perfusion fluid with substances that have been filtered. If the animal is receiving a systemic infusion of inulin, microperfusate samples can be analyzed for inulin. Microperfusion samples that contain no inulin indicate that the wax block was effective and did indeed obstruct the flow of the inulin-containing glomerular filtrate. In contrast, if the microperfusate samples do contain inulin, this indicates that the wax block did not completely block the glomerular filtrate and the sample was contaminated with the native glomerular filtrate (which contained inulin).

For most wax blocks, paraffin that has been filtered and stained with Sudan black B is used. The wax is injected into the tubular lumen with the use of a micropipette (10 to 12 μm) that contains the stained wax at the tip. This wax-containing pipette is then placed in a micromanipulator that is attached to a hydraulic microdrive.[58] This microdrive forces the semisolid wax out of the tip of the pipette and into the tubule lumen by hydraulically advancing a wire that is placed in the wax-containing pipette. This advancing wire, which has a diameter that is matched with the pipette inner diameter, displaces the wax and forces it out of the pipette.

The other essential step in *in vivo* microperfusion is the perfusion of the tubular segment with a solution of known composition at a known flow rate. This is accomplished with a micropipette that is filled with the perfusate solution using a syringe fitted with a 30-gauge needle and is then connected to a microperfusion pump. The first motor-driven microperfusion pump was introduced in the 1960s by Sonnenberg and Deetjen.[18] Subsequent modifications of this pump have included the addition of a servo control device to keep the flow speed constant at the set rate.[59] These microperfusion pumps use an electric motor to advance a small piston into a holding device which seals the micropipette and the pump. As the piston is advanced, fluid is forced out of the tip of the pipette, and the flow rate out of the pipette is equal to the volume displacement by the advancing piston.

5.4.2.2 *Microperfusion of the loop of Henle*

Microperfusion of the loop of Henle is similar to that described above for the proximal tubule. However, before microperfusion of the loop of Henle, a pipette filled with a stained solution (FD&C blue or lissamine green) is inserted in the mid or early proximal tubule. The stained solution is then infused into the tubule to identify the remaining portions of the proximal tubule and the corresponding distal segments of that nephron. The perfusion micropipette is placed in the last accessible surface loop of the proximal tubule. The wax block is then placed upstream to the perfusion pipette or in the next upstream loop. The segment is perfused and the subsequent collections are made from the earliest distal segment possible.

5.4.2.3 *Microperfusion of distal tubules*

For microperfusion of the distal tubule, at least two distal convolutions must be accessible on the surface of the kidney. As in microperfusion of the loop of Henle, dyed fluid is first infused into the proximal tubule to identify at least two subsequent distal segments of the same nephron. When a sufficiently long distal tubular segment is found, a perfusion pipette with a tip diameter of 5 to 7 μm, is placed into the upstream loop of the distal tubule. The nephron is then blocked with wax upstream to the perfusion pipette. The block may be placed in the late proximal tubule to avoid damaging or distending the distal segment being perfused.[20] Collections are made from the downstream loop of the distal tubule with a collection pipette having a tip diameter of 8 to 12 μm.

5.4.2.4 *Advantages and limitations*

Continuous microperfusion is used to regulate both the composition and flow rate of the fluid perfusing the nephron segment without altering the systemic circulation or overall renal function. Microperfusion is a valuable technique to determine and discriminate between luminal and peritubular action of a drug or nephrotoxicant in the *in vivo* kidney. The drug or nephrotoxicant can be added to the tubular perfusion solution to study luminal action or to the systemic circulation to determine peritubular effects.

The composition of an artificial tubular perfusate may alter the function of the nephron segment under study. However, variations in the composition of the perfusate can be one method to determine the parameters that regulate tubular transport. Microperfusion also has the advantage of discriminating between net reabsorption or secretion. Therefore, the effect of the drug or nephrotoxin on nephron function, as well as the transport of the drug or nephrotoxin, can be determined during *in vivo* microperfusion.

Microperfusion is subject to many of the same limitations and difficulties that were discussed above for micropuncture. Microperfusion involves the placement of several pipettes in the tubule lumen. Therefore, leaks are the major source of error during these experiments. Increased permeability to various substances may occur in the vicinity of the puncture site.[60] Therefore, the presence of systemic inulin in samples from tubules perfused with inulin-free solutions should be used to test for contamination.

5.5 Microdissection and measurement of tubular segments

Following either micropuncture or microperfusion and subsequent collections, the length of the perfused segment and the exact site of puncture can be determined with the use of latex casts.[30,31] To accomplish this, the segment is repunctured at the collection site with a pipette that contains a brightly colored latex (Microfil) solution. This pipette, which contains the latex solution, should have a tip diameter about 2 μm larger than the micropuncture pipette so that it completely seals the micropuncture opening in the tubule. The latex is injected into the tubule with enough pressure to completely fill the segment. After completion of the experiment, the kidney is removed and partially digested in a 25% NaOH solution for at least 2 h at room temperature. The kidney is then rinsed with distilled water and the latex tubular casts are gently dissected free under water with the use of microdissection tools. The tubular cast is then straightened and measured with an ocular micrometer and planimetry.

5.6 Microanalytic techniques

Both micropuncture and microperfusion produce minute samples (nanoliter volumes) which must be analyzed for concentrations of one or more substances of interest and for exact volume of fluid. Thus, considerable effort has been directed toward developing microanalytic approaches to determine the composition of the tubular fluid or collected perfusate.

The volume of the sample in the collection pipette is measured using a constant-bore, 1-μl glass capillary tube that has been filled with oil.[61,62] Briefly, under a dissecting microscope, the sample of fluid is transferred into the capillary tube by inserting the pipette, which is attached to a glass syringe, into the end of the capillary tube. Slight pressure is then applied to the syringe to expel the sample into the capillary tube and split the column of oil. The volume of the sample is calculated by measuring the length of the sample column with an ocular micrometer and multiplying it by the calibration factor for the constant-bore capillary tube.

The techniques that have been useful to determine the composition of micropuncture or microperfusion samples include radioactive tracers, spectrophotometry, fluorophotometry, helium glow photometry, HPLC, or microprobe analysis.[63] Concentrations of substances in collected samples are also often determined using microadaptations of macrochemical methods. Since the method of microanalysis is particularly dependent on the specific experimental design, volume of sample, and substances of interest, the following section is a brief description of some of the techniques that have been most commonly used to analyze micropuncture or microperfusion samples.

Inulin is perhaps the most often measured component of collected samples. If labeled inulin was used during the experiment, the radioactivity of ^{14}C- or ^{3}H-labeled inulin can be measured to determine the concentration of inulin in the collected samples. Otherwise, inulin is measured chemically.[64,65] This method was developed by Vurek and Pegram and utilizes the hydrolysis of inulin to fructose.[65] Fructose reacts with the reagent dimedone to form a fluorescing compound. The fluorescence is then detected with a fluorometer fitted with a cuvette adapter for the sample capillary tube.

Fluorometry is also used to determine the concentrations of protein, urea, and ammonia in samples of tubular fluid or perfusate.[66-69] Additionally, another common method used to determine the concentration of protein in collected samples is a colorimetric assay that was modified from the original protein macroassay described by Lowry.[70,71] A second assay available for urea also uses colorimetry to detect a product derived from urea in the diacetyl monoxime reaction.[72,73] Phosphate concentrations in the collected samples are generally determined colorimetrically with a method first developed by Chen et al. and later adapted by Greger et al. for use with an ultramicrocuvette to measure optical density in a spectrophotometer.[42,74]

Chloride, in subnanoliter volume of fluid, and other halide anions are commonly measured with electrometric titration as developed by Ramsay et al.[75] Bicarbonate and carbon dioxide in micropuncture or perfusate samples can be determined with several different techniques; however, one of the most common uses the method of calorimetry.[76-80] First, all bicarbonate is converted to carbon dioxide, which then reacts with solid lithium hydroxide. A thermistor then measures the temperature at the reaction site and the integral of the temperature vs. time is proportional to the concentration of carbon dioxide in the sample. Para-aminohippurate (PAH) has been measured using the radioactivity of radiolabeled ^{3}PAH, colorimetrically as developed by Deetjen and Sonnenberg or with reversed-phase HPLC using a C-18 column and UV detection.[5,81]

Most metal cations and biologically relevant elements can be analyzed using atomic absorption spectrometry.[63] With this method the element is atomized in an electrically heated graphite cuvette. Thus samples are analyzed without any dilution or adding of reagents. Very minute quantities (subnanoliter) of sample are required for analysis and picomole levels of detection are possible for many elements. With atomic absorption spectrometry, more than one element can be determined in a small fraction of the sample, which leaves most of the sample for other assays requiring a much larger sample volume.

One of the most sensitive, powerful, and versatile methods for determining picomole concentrations of most elements is the X-ray microspectrometric method, electron microprobe analysis.[20,63,82,83] Electron microprobe analysis can analyze practically any element of the periodic table above the low atomic number for carbon-6. The volume of sample needed for analysis is extremely small (femtoliters) and the method is highly sensitive. Often, 1×10^{-16} g of an element is easily quantifiable. This method is also nondestructive, so the same sample can be reanalyzed. However, this method requires expensive equipment and considerable technical support; therefore, it is not as commonly used as some of the above mentioned techniques.

Micropuncture and microperfusion require careful animal preparation, meticulous collection of fluid samples, and precise ultramicroanalysis. Future applications of micropuncture and microperfusion may require the development of novel analytic techniques. Throughout decades of use, micropuncture and microperfusion have been invaluable tools to study the function of individual nephron segments and the tubular effects of drugs and nephrotoxins. With the continual evolution of microanalytic techniques, micropuncture and microperfusion techniques will undoubtedly continue to contribute to the study and understanding of renal transport.

References

1. Trump, B. F., Berezesky, I. K., Lipsky, M. M., and Jones, T. W., Heterogeneity of the nephron: significance to nephrotoxicity, in *Renal Heterogeneity and Target Cell Toxicity*, Bach, P. H. and Lock E. A., Eds., John Wiley & Sons, Chichester, 1985, 31.
2. Walker, R. J. and Duggin, G. G., Cellular mechanisms of drug nephrotoxicity, in *The Kidney: Physiology and Pathophysiology*, Vol. 3, Seldin, D. W. and Giebisch, G., Eds., Raven Press, New York, 1992, chap. 106.
3. Felley-Bosco, E. and Diezi, J., Fate of cadmium in rat renal tubules: a micropuncture study, *Toxicol. Appl. Pharmacol.*, 98, 243, 1989.
4. Burnatowska-Hledin, M. A., Mayor, G. H., and Lau, K., Renal handling of aluminum in the rat: a clearance and micropuncture study, *Am. J. Physiol.*, 249, F192, 1985.
5. Deetjen, P. and Sonnenberg, H., Der tubulare Transport von *p*-aminohippursaeure. Mikroperfusionsversuche am Einzelnephron der Rattenniere *in Situ*, *Pflügers Arch.*, 285, 35, 1965.
6. Cortney, M. A., Mylle, M., Lassiter, W. E., and Gottschalk, C. W., Renal tubular transport of water, solute, and PAH in rats loaded with isotonic saline, *Am. J. Physiol.*, 209, 1199, 1965.
7. Haeberle, D., Influence of glomerular filtration rate on the rate of para-aminohippurate secretion by the rat kidneys: micropuncture and clearance studies, *Kidney Int.*, 7, 385, 1975.
8. Ross, C. R., Diezi–Chomety, F., and Roche–Ramel, F., Renal excretion of N_1-methylnicotinamide in the rat, *Am. J. Physiol.*, 228, 1641, 1975.
9. Daugaard, G., Cisplatin nephrotoxicity: experimental and clinical studies, *Dan. Med. Bull.*, 37, 1, 1990.
10. Kidwell, D. T., McKeown, J. W., Grider, J. S., McCombs, G. B., Ott, C. E., and Jackson, B. A., Acute effects of gentamicin on thick ascending limb function in the rat, *Eur. J. Pharmacol.*, 270, 97, 1994.
11. Lacchini, M. L. S., Lopes, A. G., Malnic, G., and Giebisch, G., Cisplatinum-induced lesion of proximal tubule acidification in the rat, *Renal Physiol. Biochem.*, 15, 106, 1992.
12. Wearn, J. T. and Richards, A. N., Observations on the composition of glomerular urine, with particular reference to the problem of reabsorption in the renal tubules, *Am. J. Physiol.*, 71, 209, 1924.
13. Gottschalk, C. W., The application of micropuncture techniques to analysis of renal function: a personal view, *Am. J. Kidney Dis.*, 16, 536, 1990.
14. Walker, A. M. and Oliver, J., Methods for the collection of fluid from single glomeruli and tubules of the mammalian kidney, *Am. J. Physiol.*, 134, 562, 1941.
15. Walker, A. M., Bott, P. A., Oliver, J., and McDowell, M. C., The collection and analysis of fluid from single nephrons of the mammalian kidney, *Am. J. Physiol.*, 134, 580, 1941.
16. Richards, A. N. and Walker, A. M., Methods of collecting fluid from known regions of the renal tubules of amphibia and of perfusing the lumen of a single tubule, *Am. J. Physiol.*, 118, 111, 1937.
17. Gertz, K. H. and Ullrich, K. J., Methode zur Analyse des Stofftransportes am einzelnen Tubulus der intakten Rattenniere, *Pflügers Arch.*, 274, 61, 1961.
18. Sonnenberg, H. and Deetjen, P., Methode zur Durchströmung einzelner Nephronabschnitte, *Pflügers Arch.*, 278, 669, 1964.
19. Lechene, C. and Morel, F., Microinjections de sodium et d'inuline marques dans les capillaires du rein de Hamster. I. Permeabilié au sodium des segments tubulaires corticaux, *Nephron*, 2, 207, 1965.
20. Velazquez, H. and Wright, F. S., Renal micropuncture techniques, in *Handbook of Physiology*, Vol. 1, Windhager, E. E., Ed., Oxford University Press, New York, 1992, chap. 6.
21. Gottschalk, C. W. and Lassiter, W. E., Micropuncture methodology, in *Handbook of Physiology*, Orloff, J. and Berliner, R. W., Eds., American Physiological Society, Washington, D.C., 1973, chap 6.
22. Lang, F., Greger, R., Lechene, C., and Knox, F. G., Micropuncture techniques, in *Methods in Pharmacology*, Vol. 4B, Martinez–Maldonado, M., Ed., Plenum Press, New York, 1978, chap. 4.
23. Knox, F. G. and Marchand, G. R., Study of renal action of diuretics by micropuncture techniques, in *Methods in Pharmacology*, Vol. 4A, Martinez–Maldonado, M., Ed., Plenum Press, New York, 1976, chap. 3.

24. Quamme, G. A. and Dirks, J. H., Micropuncture techniques, *Kidney Int.*, 30, 152, 1986.
25. Gottschalk, C. W., Renal tubular function: lessons from micropuncture, *Harvey Lect.*, 58, 124, 1962–63.
26. Windhager, E. E., *Micropuncture Techniques and Nephron Function*, Butterworth and Co. Ltd., Cambridge, England, 1968.
27. Oberg, P. A., Persson, E., Pettersson, H., and Stalbecker, S., DC temperature-regulating device for anesthetized experimental animal, *J. Appl. Physiol.*, 39, 680, 1975.
28. Cortell, S., Davidman, M., Gennari, F. J., and Schwartz, W. B., Catheter size as a determinant of outflow resistance and intrarenal pressure, *Am. J. Physiol.*, 223, 910, 1972.
29. Andreucci, V. E., Surgery in the rat, in *Manual of Renal Micropuncture*, Andreucci, V. E., Ed., Idelson, Naples, Italy, 1978, chap. 4.
30. Cortell, S., Silicone rubber for renal tubular injection, *Am. J. Appl. Physiol.*, 26, 158, 1969.
31. Tisher, C. C. and Clapp, J. R., Intraluminal latex injection: an aid to the histological identification of renal tubules, *Kidney Int.*, 2, 54, 1972.
32. Steinhausen, M., Ein Methode zur Differenzierung proximaler und distaler Tubuli der Nierenrinde von Ratten *in vivo* und ihre Anwendung zur Bestimmung tubularer Stromungsgeschwindigkeiten, *Arch. Ges. Physiol.*, 277, 23, 1963.
33. Roch–Ramel, F. and Jotterand, N., Natriuretic effect of lissamine green, *Experientia*, 26, 683, 1970.
34. Heller, J., The influence of lissamine green on tubular reabsorption of electrolytes and water in rats, *Arch. Ges. Physiol.*, 323, 27, 1971.
35. Lynch, R. E., Schneider, E. G., Strandhoy, J. W., Willis, L. R., and Knox, F. G., Effect of lissamine green dye on renal sodium reabsorption in the dog, *J. Appl. Physiol.*, 35, 169, 1973.
36. Vurek, G. G., Bennett, C. M., Jamison, R. L., and Troy, J. L., An air-driven micropipette sharpener, *J. Appl. Physiol.*, 22, 191, 1967.
37. Dirks, J. H., Cirksena, W. J., and Berliner, R. W., The effect of saline infusion on sodium reabsorption in the proximal tubule of the dog, *J. Clin. Invest.*, 44, 1160, 1965.
38. Brenner, B. M. and Daugharty, T. M., The measurement of glomerular filtration rate in single nephrons of the rat kidney, *Yale J. Biol. Med.*, 45, 200, 1972.
39. Andreucci, V. E., Herrara–Acosta, J., Rector, F. C., and Seldin, D. W., Measurement of single-nephron glomerular filtration rate by micropuncture: analysis of error, *Am. J. Physiol.*, 221, 1551, 1971.
40. Haas, J. A., Berndt, T. J., Haramati, A., and Knox, F. G., Nephron sites of action of nicotinamide on phosphate reabsorption, *Am. J. Physiol.*, 246, F27, 1984.
41. Berndt, T. J. and Knox, F. G., Nephron site of resistance to phosphaturic effect of PTH during respiratory alkalosis, *Am. J. Physiol.*, 249, F919, 1985.
42. Greger, R., Lang, F., Marchand, G., and Knox, F. G., Site of renal phosphate reabsorption, *Pflügers Arch.*, 369, 111, 1977.
43. Gottschalk, C. W., Lassiter, W. E., Mylle, M., Ullrich, K. J., Schmidt–Nielsen, B., O'Dell, R., and Pehling, G., Micropuncture study of composition of loop of Henle fluid in desert rodents, *Am. J. Physiol.*, 204, 532, 1963.
44. Sakai, F., Jamison, R. L., and Berliner, R. W., A method for exposing the rat renal medulla *in vivo*: micropuncture of the collecting duct, *Am. J. Physiol.*, 209, 663, 1965.
45. Haas, J. A., Granger, J. P., and Knox, F. G., Effect of renal perfusion pressure on sodium reabsorption from proximal tubules of superficial and deep nephrons, *Am. J. Physiol.*, 250, F425, 1986.
46. Jamison, R. L., Micropuncture study of superficial and juxtamedullary nephrons in the rat, *Am. J. Physiol.*, 218, 46, 1970.
47. Dev, B., Häberle, D., Schnermann, J., and Wunderlich, P., Effect of barbiturates on GFR and fluid reabsorption along proximal convoluted tubules and loops of Henle in rats, *Pflügers Arch.*, 344, 21, 1973.
48. Elmer, M., Eskildsen, P. C., Kristens, L. O., and Leyssac, P. P., A comparison of renal function in rats anesthetized with inactin and sodium amytal, *Acta Physiol. Scand.*, 86, 41, 1972.
49. Andreucci, V. E. and Rector, F. C., Some artifacts in measuring single-nephron glomerular filtration rate, *Yale J. Bio. Med.*, 45, 217, 1972.

50. Brenner, B. M., Keimowitz, R. I., Wright, F. S., and Berliner, R. W., An inhibition effect of furosemide on sodium reabsorption by the proximal tubule of the rat nephron, *J. Clin. Invest.*, 48, 290, 1969.
51. Schnermann, J., Horster, M., and Levine, D. Z., The influence of sampling techniques on the micropuncture determination of GFR and reabsorptive characteristics of single rat proximal tubules, *Pflügers Arch.*, 309, 48, 1969.
52. Davidman, M., Lalone, R. C., Alexander, E. A., and Levinsky, N. G., Some micropuncture techniques in the rat, *Am. J. Physiol.*, 221, 1110, 1971.
53. Schnermann, J., Wright, F. S., Davis, J. M., Stackelberg, W. V., and Grill, G., Regulation of superficial nephron filtration rate by tubulo-glomerular feedback, *Pflügers Arch.*, 318, 147, 1970.
54. Navar, L. G., Burke, T. J., Robinson, R. R., and Clapp, J. R., Distal tubular feedback on the autoregulation of single nephron glomerular filtration rate, *J. Clin. Invest.*, 53, 516, 1974.
55. Maddox, D. A., Troy, J. L., and Brenner, B. M., Autoregulation of filtration rate in the absence of macula densa-glomerulus feedback, *Am. J. Physiol.*, 227, 123, 1974.
56. Knox, F. G., Ott, C. E., Cuche, J. L., Gasser, J., and Haas, J., Autoregulation of single nephron filtration rate in the presence and absence of flow to the macula densa, *Circ. Res.*, 34, 836, 1974.
57. Schnermann, J., Persson, E. G., and Agerup, B., Tubuloglomerular feedback. Nonlinear relation between glomerular hydrostatic pressure and loop of Henle perfusion rate, *J. Clin. Invest.*, 52, 862, 1973.
58. Gutsche, H. U., Müller–Suur, R., Hegel, U., Hierholzer, K., Lüderitz, S., A new method for intratubular blockade in micropuncture experiments, *Pflügers Arch.*, 354, 197, 1975.
59. Deetjen, P. and Silbernagl, S., Some new developments in continuous microperfusion technique, *Yale J. Biol. Med.*, 45, 301, 1973.
60. Morel, F. and Murayama, Y., Simultaneous measurements of unidirectional and net sodium fluxes in microperfused rat proximal tubules, *Pflügers Arch.*, 320, 1, 1970.
61. Andreucci, V. E., Volume measurement of microsamples, in *Manual of Renal Micropuncture*, Andreucci, V. E., Ed., Idelson, Naples, Italy, 1978, chap. 16.
62. Spinelli, F., Pehling, G., and Witz, H., A simplified method of determining the volume of renal tubular fluid samples, *Nephron*, 10, 271, 1973.
63. Greger, R., Lang, F., Knox, F. G., and Lechene, C., Analysis of tubule fluid, in *Methods in Pharmacology*, Vol. 4B, Martinez–Maldonado, M., Ed., Plenum Press, New York, 1978, chap. 5.
64. Conger, J. D., Rhoads, H. N., Christie, S. N., and Bruke, T. J., A modification of the fluorescence method for micro-inulin determinations, *Kidney Int.*, 8, 334, 1975.
65. Vurek, C. G. and Pegram, S. E., Fluorometric method for the determination of nanogram quantities of inulin, *Anal. Biochem.*, 10, 409, 1966.
66. Viets, J. W., Deen, W. N., Troy, J. L., and Brenner, B. M., Determination of serum protein concentration in nanoliter blood samples using flourescamine or o-phthaldehyde, *Anal. Biochem.*, 88, 513, 1978.
67. Roch–Ramel, F., An enzymic and fluorophotometric method for estimating urea concentrations in nanoliter specimens, *Anal. Biochem.*, 21, 372, 1967.
68. Roman, R. J., Bonventre, J. V., and Lechene, C. P., Fluorometric assay for urea in urine, plasma, and tubular fluid, *Anal. Biochem.*, 98, 136, 1979.
69. Good, D. W. and Vurek, G. G., Picomole quantitation of ammonium ions by flow-through fluorometry, *Anal. Biochem.*, 130, 199, 1983.
70. Lowry, O. H., Rosebrough, N. J., Farr, A. L., and Randall, R. J., Protein measurement with the folin-phenol reagent, *J. Biol. Chem.*, 193, 265, 1951.
71. Brenner, B. M., Falchuk, K. H., Keimowitz, R. I., and Berliner, R. W., The relationship between peritubular capillary protein concentration and fluid reabsorption by the renal proximal tubule, *J. Clin. Invest.*, 48, 1519, 1969.
72. Vurek, G. G. and Knepper, M. A., A colorimeter for measurement of picomole quantities of urea, *Kidney Int.*, 21, 656, 1982.
73. Marsh, D. J., Frasier, C., and Decter, J., Measurement of urea concentrations in nanoliter specimens of renal tubular fluid and capillary blood, *Anal. Biochem.*, 11, 73, 1965.
74. Chen, P., Toribara, T., and Warner, H., Microdetermination of phosphorus, *Anal. Chem.*, 28, 1756, 1956.

75. Ramsay, J. A., Brown, R. H. J., and Croghan, P. C., Electrometric titration of chloride in small volumes, *J. Exp. Biol.*, 32, 822, 1955.
76. Vurek, G. G., Warnock, D. G., and Corsey, R., Measurement of picomole amounts of carbon dioxide by calorimetry, *Anal. Chem.*, 47, 765, 1975.
77. Warnock, D. G. and Burg, M. B., Heterogeneity of CO_2 transport in proximal straight tubules, *Am. Soc. Neph. Abstr.*, 96, 1975.
78. Hevert, F., Microdetermination of carbonate using a strain gauge pressure transducer, *Pflügers Arch.*, 344, 271, 1973.
79. Karlmark, B. and Sohtell, M., The determination of bicarbonate in nanoliter samples, *Anal. Biochem.*, 53, 1, 1973.
80. Maffly, R. H., A conductometric method for measuring micromolar quantities of carbon dioxide, *Anal. Biochem.*, 23, 252, 1968.
81. Astier, A. and Deutsch, A. M., High-performance liquid chromatographic determination of hippuric acid in human urine, *J. Chromatogr.*, 182, 88, 1980.
82. Ingram, M. J. and Hogben, C. A., Electrolyte analysis of biological fluid with the electron microprobe, *Anal. Biochem.*, 18, 54, 1967.
83. Morel, F., Roinel, N., and LeGrimellec, C., Electron probe analysis of tubular fluid composition, *Nephron*, 6, 350, 1969.

chapter six

Microdissection and Microanalysis of Specific Nephron Segments from Mammalian Kidney

Eduardo N. Chini and Thomas P. Dousa

6.1 Summary 97
6.2 Introduction 98
6.3 Microdissection of nephron segments 99
  6.3.1 General considerations 100
    6.3.1.1 Species differences 100
    6.3.1.2 Expressing data 101
  6.3.2 Methods of preparation of tissue and dissection 102
    6.3.2.1 Preparation of rat renal tissue 102
    6.3.2.2 Microdissection 102
  6.3.3 Identification of nephron segments 102
    6.3.3.1 Glomeruli 103
    6.3.3.2 Proximal convoluted tubules (PCT) 103
    6.3.3.3 Proximal straight tubules (PST) 103
    6.3.3.4 Medullary thick ascending limbs (MTAL) 103
    6.3.3.5 Cortical thick ascending limbs (CTAL) 103
    6.3.3.6 Distal convoluted tubules (DCT) 103
    6.3.3.7 Cortical collecting ducts (CCD) 104
    6.3.3.8 Outer medullary collecting ducts (OMCD) 104
    6.3.3.9 Inner medullary collecting ducts (IMCD) 104
6.4 Microdissection combined with molecular biology method 104
6.5 Conclusion 105
6.6 Appendix 105
  6.6.1 Buffers and solutions 105
6.7 Acknowledgments 105
References 106

6.1 Summary

Mammalian kidney is an enormously complex organ in terms of structural diversity, metabolism, function, and hormonal regulation. Mammalian nephrons consist of at least 14 distinct segments (Figure 1),[1] some with very specifically localized functions. The precise

0-8493-3341-5/96/$0.00+$.50

determination of biochemical and physiological processes within specific nephron segments is one of the major goals of modern renal physiology and pathophysiology. Although a number of other methods for separation of specific tubule segments have been developed and used, localization of a specific property within the nephron by measuring the function in question in microdissected segments is considered the most rigorous standard for identifying specific intranephron localization of a biochemical process.

6.2 *Introduction*

Due to the complex nature and heterogeneity of the kidney (Figure 1),[1] the precise localization of biochemical processes within nephron segments is a necessary approach to the study of renal function and pathophysiology. For example, the lack of a biochemical characteristic in extracts or homogenates of renal tissue may be due to the great diversity of cell populations in this organ. In some notable cases, one specific nephron segment or cell population is the exclusive site of localization for an enzyme or transporter. Of particular interest is the site of action of hormones and therapeutic drugs, which may be confined to one particular segment of the kidney.

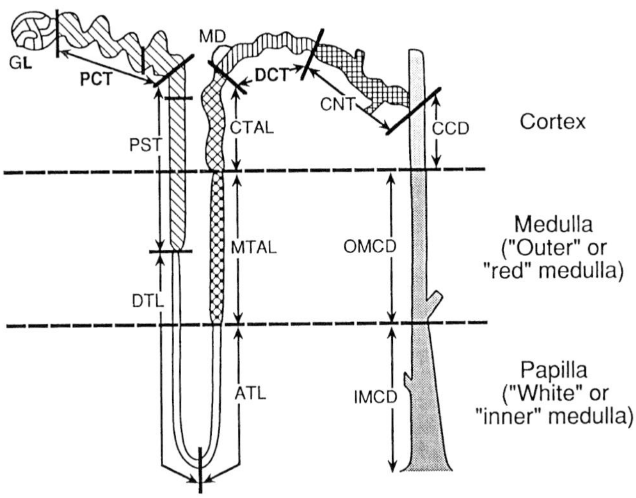

Figure 1 Microanatomic subdivision of mammaliam nephron. Diagram of the structural organization of the mammalian kidney demonstrating the relations between various segments of the nephron and the microscopic zones of the kidney. GL, glomeruli; PCT, proximal convoluted tubule; PST, proximal straight tubule; DTL, descending thin limb; ATL, ascending thin limb; MTAL, medullary thick ascending limb; CTAL, cortical thick ascending limb; MD, macula densa; DCT, distal convoluted tubule; CNT, connecting tubule; CCD, cortical collecting duct; OMCD, outer medullary collecting duct; IMCD, inner medullary collecting duct. (Adapted from Kriz, W. and Bankir, L., *Am. J. Physiol.*, 254, F1, 1988.)

The precise determination of physiological processes in a specific nephron segment is of extreme importance. Several techniques have been used to determine the phenotypical heterogeneity of the nephron, including microperfusion, immunohistochemistry, and microdissection, which are the "gold standard" procedures for the study of isolated nephron segments. In addition, procedures were developed for isolation of homogenous populations of single nephron segments such as glomeruli, proximal convoluted tubules, and others. Primary cultures of specific renal epithelial cells are also valuable tools for the study of renal function and dysfunction, especially for the understanding of the cell biology within particular nephron segments.

Studies of microdissected segments have led to a broad number of unexpected and sometimes surprising findings. For example, Morel and associates found, in kidneys of rabbits, that the adenylate cyclase sensitive to vasopressin (AVP) is not only present in the collecting ducts (where it was expected to be found), but also in the thick ascending limb of Henle's loop (MTAL).[2-3] Although AVP-sensitive adenylate cyclase in MTAL is considered nonessential for elaboration of concentrated urine, it forced a reevaluation and reinterpretation of results of previous enzyme studies of AVP in preparations from the whole medulla. A strain of mice with nephrogenic diabetes insipidus (NDI mice) was also studied using microdissection techniques. Findings indicated that increased activity of one of the cAMP phosphodiesterases (PDE) isozymes — not a defect in AVP receptors — precludes AVP-stimulated cAMP accumulation and antidiuretic response and is the basis for this disease.[4-6] Recently, studies on microdissected tubules using the RT-PCR technique demonstrated the localization of mRNA encoding numerous nephron components, for example, an unusual distribution of the plasma membrane Ca^{2+}-ATPase isoform type III,[7] which is otherwise found only in some excitable tissues. The cognate mRNA for this isoform III was found exclusively in the descending thin limb (DTL) of rat kidney.[7] In short, the microdissection technique is a powerful tool for the study of renal pathophysiology and toxicology and should be employed when use of other techniques fails to solve the problem in question. The major limitation of microdissection is the limited amount of sample that can be collected and analyzed.

In this chapter we discuss some salient aspects of kidney microdissection for isolation of nephron segments and its application in the biochemical study of kidney.

6.3 Microdissection of nephron segments

The principles of the microdissection technique were developed by Burg et al. for the microperfusion of isolated nephron segments.[8] In 1975, Chabardes et al. adapted with great success the original technique developed by Burg et al. for the analyses of enzymatic activity of adenylate cyclase and ATPases in isolated segments (Figure 2).[9] Since then, several laboratories have been able to perform microdissection and use it as a tool for biochemical analyses of nephron segments.[2-7,9-13] For example, our laboratory applied microdissection techniques to investigate the mode of action of AVP. Of particular interest was the use of microdissection combined with measurement of cAMP phosphodiesterase activity (PDE).[4-6] We applied this technique to the study of a strain of mice with hereditary nephrogenic diabetes insipidus (NDI) and demonstrated that increased PDE activity in the collecting duct system, particularly in the inner medullary collecting duct, leads to a functional resistance to AVP in this segment and consequent increase in urinary volume.[4-6]

However, as pointed out by Moriyama et al., microdissection combined with determination of enzymatic activity is of limited use in distinguishing between very similar enzymatic and transporter protein activities.[14] Recently, an elegant technique for the detection of specific mRNAs in single nephron segments was developed by the group of Garcia-Perez in Dr. Knepper's laboratory at the National Institutes of Health.[14] This technique combines nephron microdissection with reverse transcription (RT) of mRNA, followed by polymerase chain reaction (PCR) for amplification of a target cDNA (Figures 2 and 3). Recently the RT-PCR procedure in combination with microdissection has been applied to study nephron localization of many specific mRNAs, e.g., aldolase reductase, plasma membrane Ca^{2+}-ATPase, ANF receptor, and others.[7,14-17]

Next, we discuss some important details pertaining to the microdissection of nephron segments and its applications. In addition, we provide some technical comments about the use of microdissection for RT-PCR.

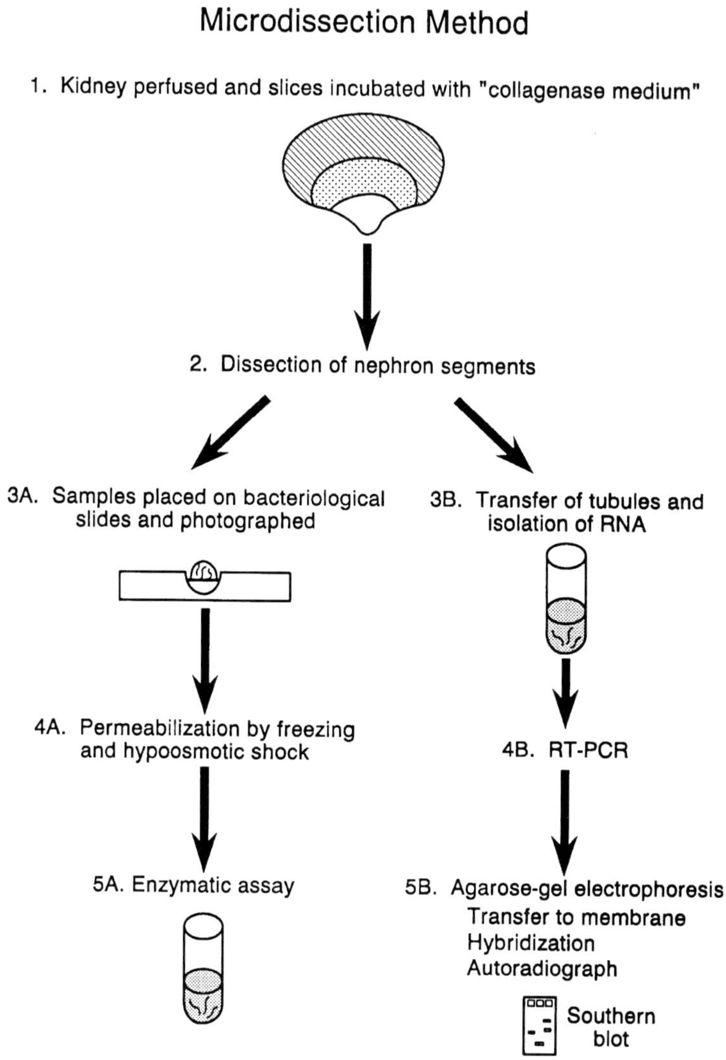

Figure 2 Scheme of procedure outlining experiments with use of microdissection methodology. Study of enzymatic activity or mRNA distribution in nephron segments. (1) Kidney is prepared as described by Morel et al.[2] (2) Nephron segments are dissected out under stereomicroscope (magnification 30×). Samples can be processed for enzymatic analysis (Dousa et al.[5]); or the nephron segments may be used for determination of specific mRNAs by combination of isolation of RNA, RT-PCR, and Southern blot. (Adapted from Dousa, T. P., Jackson, B. A., and Edwards, R. M., in *Antidiuretic Hormone*, Yoshida, S., Share, L., and Yagi, K., Eds., Japan Scientific Press, Tokyo, 1979, 193.)

6.3.1 General considerations

6.3.1.1 Species differences

Microdissection of nephron segments can be applied to a number of species of experimental animals as well as to human kidney. When approaching selection of a model for study, several items should be kept in mind. Technically, virtually all parts of the nephron from rabbit kidney can be well identified and isolated; divisions of the distal nephron are especially accessible for dissection. It is advisable for investigators learning microdissection technique to conduct several training microdissections in rabbit kidney. However,

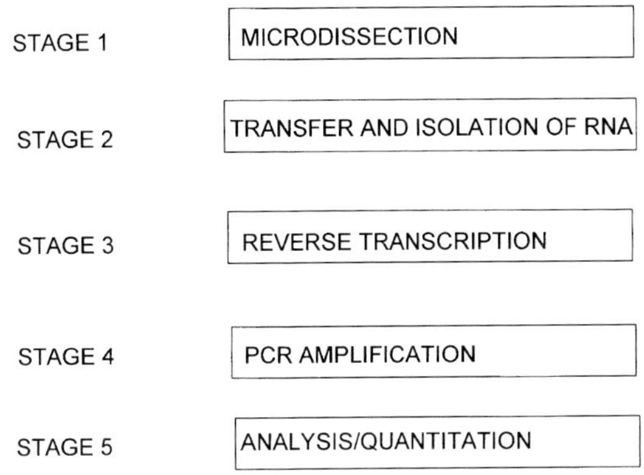

Figure 3 Steps in axial localization of specific mRNAs along the nephron. Stages are described in text.

information on pathophysiology in rabbit kidney is rather limited. Mouse kidney is also relatively easy for dissection studies.

Despite the fact that rat kidney is considered one of the more difficult for dissection primarily due to the presence of a well-developed connective tissue, the rat kidney is one of the most studied since it is almost a universal model for the study of renal function. Dissection of human kidney is feasible,[18] although not easy, and can employ uninvolved regions of kidneys removed from patients with renal cell carcinoma. Segments of kidney are then perfused from the lobar artery, and regions of the kidney are dissected as described for animal kidneys. Alternatively, cadaveric kidneys rejected for transplantation have been employed. In this case, a whole kidney can be perfused, but the organ usually had been on perfusion apparatus for numerous hours when it was rejected. Few microdissections have been performed on dog kidney.[19] The majority of studies in the literature have been conducted on rat and rabbit kidneys. When a method is set up for any given species, it is imperative to follow in detail the method described in the original study.

6.3.1.2 Expressing data

The enzyme activity, generated metabolite, or content of mRNA evaluated in microdissected nephron segments should be related to an appropriate reference point. The most common and easiest point for comparison is the total length of the tubules in the sample (or number of glomeruli in the sample). This may be sufficient information if only one type of nephron segment is studied, since the length of the tubule is proportional to its protein content. However, in comparing different nephron segments, protein content may differ severalfold when the same lengths of tubules are used. In our opinion, the use of protein content of the microdissected tubules as a reference point is a more appropriate method. The protein content in the studied segment is determined, based on a large number of samples, and is expressed in nanograms per millimeter of length; then tubular lengths are multiplied by typical segment protein content in an established standard.

When large quantitative differences are encountered or when the presence or absence of the studied phenomenon in a given nephron segment is the objective of the study, expression of the results with length as a reference may be permissible. However, expression of parameters per protein is especially important in cases in which the enzyme activity from tubular segments in control animals is compared with that in animals with an experimentally induced renal disorder. How the pathologic state influences the typical protein/length content of the nephron segment in each study should be determined. The mentioned considerations are of primary importance prior to embarking on a new project.

6.3.2 Methods of preparation of tissue and dissection

Since the rat kidney is most frequently used for microdissection studies, we outline some methodologic features applied to microdissection of nephron segments from the rat kidney.

6.3.2.1 Preparation of rat renal tissue

Briefly, the rat is anesthetized with an injection (i.p.) of pentobarbital sodium (90 mg/kg body wt) prior to insertion of a polyethylene catheter (PE-90) into the abdominal aorta, inferior to the renal artery bifurcation. The aorta is then clamped above the bifurcation of the renal arteries and below the site of the cannulation. The renal vein is cut and the kidneys are perfused *in situ* with 20 ml of cold Hank's saline solution until both are completely blanched.[20-22] After perfusion with Hank's solution, kidneys are perfused with 20 ml of prewarmed (37°C) collagenase medium (as described previously).[2] Following perfusion, the kidneys are quickly removed and sliced (0.5 to 1.0 mm) with a razor blade along the corticomedullary axis. The slices are then incubated in a collagenase medium (see Appendix below) at 35–37°C for 35 to 60 min, depending on the segment to be dissected (to dissect IMCD extensive digestion of the tissue is desirable), with constant aeration (aeration provides oxygen for the tissue and constant mixing of the solution). After incubation, the tissue is rinsed with a microdissection solution that is identical to the collagenase medium except that it does not contain collagenase or hyaluronidase, and the concentration of $CaCl_2$ is lower (see Appendix).

6.3.2.2 Microdissection

Microdissection is performed in a glass petri dish, with ice-cold microdissection solution, as described previously.[2,4-7,9-15] Tubular segments are dissected under a stereomicroscope (magnification 30×) using the criteria outlined below. The dissection can be performed with either a sharpened stainless steel needle, or sharp forceps (Dumont Medical No. 5 is a good choice). The illumination of the petri dish should come from underneath and run horizontally. After dissection, the tubules are transferred to another petri dish for cleaning of the segments and measurement of their lengths. Transfer of tubules is possible using a 20-ml pipette, with an albumin-saturated tip, to avoid the sticking of the tubule to the plastic. As previously discussed, microdissection of rat renal cortex is difficult due to the well-developed connective tissue matrix. When we perform dissection of the renal cortex from the rat in our laboratory,[15] the key step in the preparation of the tissue is collagenase digestion. Several concentrations of collagenase and varying times of incubation should be used in preliminary experiments for determination of ideal conditions. Overdigestion of the tissue may lead to complete disintegration of the tubular structure. Insufficient digestion can be attributed frequently to the collagenase activity itself; therefore purchasing or reserving a brand and lot of collagenase from a specific supplier that has been proved successful, is recommended to prevent complications arising from enzymatic variations.

6.3.3 Identification of nephron segments

Identification of microdissected nephron segments is the next key step in good microdissection technique. Extensive training is the only way to become confident in identification of the major segments of the nephron. Several criteria have been described previously for the identification of nephron segments during microdissection,[2,8-13] some of which are outlined below for the rat kidney. However, similar criteria can be used for dissection of nephron segments from other mammalian kidneys. In addition to dissection of nephron segments, microdissection of renal microvessels can also be performed, as first described by Edwards and colleagues.[23-26]

6.3.3.1 Glomeruli

Glomeruli are one of the easiest renal structures to be dissected. In well-prepared tissues this structure will pull out of the surrounding tissue by simple manipulation of the cortex. The glomeruli can be identified by their ovoid or spherical shape.

6.3.3.2 Proximal convoluted tubules (PCT)

Proximal convoluted tubules are identified under the stereomicroscope as tortuous tubules with a large diameter when compared with other segments. In addition, they have a "milky" appearance. The definitive criterion for identification of the proximal convoluted tubules is their attachment to a renal corpuscle. This feature is always desired. It is important to note the significant variation in the length and diameter of these segments. This variation is due to the differences between the superficial and the juxtamedullary types of proximal convoluted tubules.

6.3.3.3 Proximal straight tubules (PST)

Proximal straight tubules are continuations of the proximal convoluted tubule. They are found in the medullary rays of the cortex and in the outer medullary portion of the kidney, and their appearance closely resembles that of proximal convoluted tubules. The most valuable criterion for identification of the proximal straight tubule is its attachment to a descending thin limb of Henle's loop (DTL), a thin segment of the nephron that is almost transparent under a stereomicroscope and that extends from the outer medulla deep into the inner medulla. Conversely, the major criterion for the identification of the descending thin limb of Henle's loop is its attachment to the terminal portion of the proximal straight tubule.

6.3.3.4 Medullary thick ascending limbs (MTAL)

Medullary thick ascending limbs are located in the outer medulla. They are continuous extensions of the ascending thin limbs of Henle's loop (ATL) in the inner medulla and extend into the cortex as cortical thick ascending limbs (CTAL). The major criteria for identification of the medullary thick ascending limb are (1) its localization in the outer medulla; (2) the smooth appearance of the tubule, which contains two outer dense borders with a transparent inner line; and (3) its attachment to the ascending thin limb of Henle's loop. The diameter of the medullary thick ascending limbs is intermediate between that of the thin limbs of Henle's loop and that of the outer medullary collecting ducts (OMCD).

6.3.3.5 Cortical thick ascending limbs (CTAL)

Cortical thick ascending limbs are almost identical to medullary thick ascending limbs. However, they tend to be somewhat smaller in diameter; they are localized in the cortex; and they are attached to the macula densa region of the distal tubule. All these differences are used as criteria for distinguishing cortical thick ascending limbs from medullary thick ascending limbs.

6.3.3.6 Distal convoluted tubules (DCT)

Distal convoluted tubules are the most difficult of all segments of the nephron to dissect from the rat kidney. On the other hand, dissection of the distal convoluted tubule from the kidneys of rabbits and mice is relatively easy. The distal convoluted tubule is a very short, V-shaped structure (noted to be convoluted as the name suggests) present in the cortex between the macula densa and the first branch within the collecting duct system. In the kidneys of rabbits and mice, a continuous dissection from the cortical thick ascending limb to the cortical collecting duct is possible. Also, several distal convoluted tubules feeding into one cortical collecting duct can be dissected from the kidneys of rabbits and mice.

6.3.3.7 *Cortical collecting ducts (CCD)*

Cortical collecting ducts represent the initial segment of the collecting system. They are localized in the cortex and can be identified as branching tubules having a granular appearance due to the presence of two different cell types.

6.3.3.8 *Outer medullary collecting ducts (OMCD)*

Outer medullary collecting ducts are long segments that span the entire depth of the outer medulla and are continuous with the inner medullary collecting duct. In the outer medulla, outer medullary collecting ducts can be easily identified under the stereomicroscope by their granular appearance. The external border of the tubule has been described as "fuzzy" (although we think that this description may not be appropriate). When compared with the other tubular segments present on the outer medulla (medullary thick ascending limbs and descending thin limbs), the outer medullary collecting duct can be distinguished by its larger diameter. Of particular interest is the fact that during microdissection of the outer medulla, when the tissue is pulled longitudinally from the medulla, this segment is more resistant and will appear as a long tubule between the cortex and the medulla. During the process of separating the outer medulla on the longitudinal axis, both medullary thick ascending limbs and descending thin limbs can be broken. However, in our hands, the outer medullary collecting ducts appear to be more resistant, and very long segments can be separated and dissected free.

6.3.3.9 *Inner medullary collecting ducts (IMCD)*

Extensive branching occurs in the inner medullary collecting ducts. They appear to be very similar to the outer medullary collecting ducts. In our experience the inner medullary collecting ducts can be dissected free from papillary connective tissue only after extensive digestion with collagenase.

6.4 *Microdissection combined with molecular biology method*

Recently, a method for determination of mRNA in nephron segments was described. In this method, a combination of microdissection, isolation of RNA, and RT-PCR has proved valuable for the study of renal tubular and cellular biochemistry. We previously developed a modification of this method in our laboratory.[7] Some specific points when performing microdissection for RT-PCR are described below (Figure 3).

To obtain good preparations of RNA from microdissected tubules, it is necessary to minimize the activity of RNase during the entire procedure.[27-28] For this purpose a number of precautions should be taken. (1) Disposable gloves should be used during the manipulation of all material. (2) All solutions and glassware should be sterile for molecular biology. In our laboratory we treat all the glassware with 0.1% diethyl pirocarbonate (DEPC), followed by baking. (3) Forceps and pipette tips are autoclaved prior to the experiment. (4) All solutions are obtained sterile or prepared with DEPC-treated water and autoclaved. (5) Of particular importance for the microdissection step is the inclusion of 5 to 10 m*M* vanadyl ribonuclease complex (VRC, Life Technologies) and RNase-free albumin in the microdissection solution to minimize RNA hydrolysis. After microdissection, the tubules are rinsed in a VRC-free solution and transferred to a tube containing 1 U/ml of human placental RNase inhibitor (Boehringer Mannheim, Indianapolis, IN) and frozen quickly in liquid nitrogen.

The RT-PCR is performed using standard techniques after isolation of the mRNA using affinity chromatography with oligo(dT)sepharose using, e.g., the Micro Fast Track kit (Invitrogen, San Diego, CA).[27]

RT-PCR can determine the presence and relative levels of specific mRNAs in single nephrons. However, it is difficult to accurately quantify mRNA levels with this technique. Another inherent limitation of the RT-PCR is that it gives no information about the relative abundance of protein encoded by mRNA in different nephron segments. Thus, although it can document differences in the amount of message between nephron segments, this technique does not determine if this translates into different amounts of protein. Recently, protein content within tubular segments has been determined using a combination of microdissection and Western blot analysis.[29]

The only renal structure that can be isolated pure, well-preserved, and in relatively large quantities is the glomerulus. One example is the isolation of glomeruli by differential sieving.[20] We have recently used isolated glomeruli to study the role of PDE isozymes in the control of superoxide production.[20] Even microdissection cannot avoid the fact that glomeruli consist of at least three distinct cell-type populations and these should be analyzed further, for example, by the study of primary, cultured, specific cell populations.[30-31]

6.5 Conclusion

Because of the heterogeneity of renal tissue, microdissection of specific nephron segments is a valuable and sometimes indispensable tool for the study of renal function or dysfunction. In microdissected segments, virtually any parameter can be measured provided a given analytic method can be scaled down. Microdissection is a time-demanding technique and is limited by the small amount of tubules that can be isolated. Thus, it should be used judiciously when very specific questions are investigated, since it represents a considerable investment of time and effort.

6.6 Appendix

6.6.1 Buffers and solutions

The solutions described here are in current use in our laboratory.

Collagenase solution. In millimolar: 137 NaCl, 5 KCl, 0.8 $MgCl_2$, 0.33 NaH_2PO_4, 0.44 KH_2PO_4, 1 $MgCl_2$, 10 tris(hydroxymethyl)aminomethane (TRIS) hydrochloride, 1 $CaCl_2$, 0.15 to 0.2% collagenase (type I, Sigma), 0.1 to 0.2% hyaluronidase (Sigma), pH 7.4. This solution is used for both perfusion of the kidney and collagenase digestion of the kidney.

Microdissection solution. The composition of this medium is identical to the collagenase medium except that it does not contain collagenase or hyaluronidase and the $CaCl_2$ concentration is 0.25 m*M*. In the case of dissection, for the RT-PCR technique 5 to 10 m*M* of vanadyl ribonuclease complex (VRC, Life Technologies) and 0.1% bovine serum albumin (BSA, RNase-free, Promega) are added.

Washing solution. Identical to the microdissection solution except for the absence of VRC and BSA, even when microdissection is carried out for RT-PCR (see Morel et al.[2]).

6.7 Acknowledgments

This work was supported by NIH grants DK-30597 and DK-16105 and by Mayo Foundation. E. N. Chini is a recipient of a National Kidney Foundation Research Fellowship. We would like to thank Dr. J. P. Grande and C. C. S. Chini for discussion of the manuscript.

References

1. Kriz, W. and Bankir, L., A standard nomenclature for structures of the kidney, *Am. J. Physiol.*, 254, F1, 1988.
2. Morel, M., Chabardes, D., and Imbert-Teboul, M., Methodology for enzymatic studies of isolated tubular segments: adenylate cyclase, in *Methods in Pharmacology*, Vol. 4B, Martinez-Maldonado, M., Ed., Plenum Press, New York, 1976, 297.
3. Morel, F., Sites of hormone action in the mammalian nephron, *Am. J. Physiol.*, 240, F159, 1981.
4. Jackson, B.A., Edwards, R.W., Valtin, H., and Dousa T.P., Cellular action of vasopressin in medullary tubules of mice with hereditary nephrogenic diabetes insipidus, *J. Clin. Invest.*, 66, 110, 1980.
5. Dousa, T.P., Jackson, B.A, and Edwards, R.M., Cellular action of vasopressine in medullary collecting tubules and in ascending limbs of Henle's loop, in *Antidiuretic Hormone*, Yoshida, S., Share, L., and Yagi, K., Eds., Japan Scientific Press, Tokyo, 1979, 193.
6. Dousa, T.P., Cyclic-3′,5′-nucleotide phosphodiesterase in the cyclic adenosine monophosphate (cAMP)-mediated action of vasopressine, *Semin. Nephrol.*, 14, 333, 1994.
7. Caride, A.J., Chini, E.N., Dousa,T.P., and Penniston J.T., Unique localization of mRNA encoding plasma membrane Ca^{2+} pump isoform 3 in rat thin descending loop of Henle, *Am. J. Physiol.*, 1995 (in press).
8. Burg, M., Grantham, J., Abramow, W., and Orloff, J., Preparation and study of fragments of single rabbit nephrons, *Am. J. Physiol.*, 210, 1293, 1966.
9. Chabardes, D., Imber, M., Clique, A., Montegut, M., and Morel, F., PTH-sensitive adenyl cyclase activity in different segments of rabbit nephron, *Pflügers Arch.*, 354, 329, 1975.
10. Schmidt, U. and Hoster, M., Sodium-potassium-activated adenosine triphosphatease: methodology for quantification in microdissected renal tubule segments from freeze-dried and fresh tissue, in *Methods in Pharmacology*, Vol. 4B, Martinez-Maldonado, M., Ed., Plenum Press, New York, 1976, 259.
11. Chabardes, D., Imber-Teboul, M., Mountegut, M., Clique, A., and Morel, F., Catecholamine-sensitive adenylate cyclase activity in different segments of rabbit nephron, *Pflügers Arch.*, 361, 9, 1975.
12. Imber, M., Chabardes, D., Montegut, M., Clique, A., and Morel, F., Adenylate cyclase activity along the rabbit nephron as measured in single isolated segments, *Pflügers Arch.*, 354, 213, 1975.
13. Imbert, M., Chagardes, D., Monyegut, M., Clique, A., and Morel, F., Vasopressin-dependent adenylate cyclase in single segments of rabbit kidney tubule, *Pflugers Arch.*, 357, 173, 1975.
14. Moriyama, T., Murphy, H.R., Martin, B.M., and Garcia-Perez, A., Detection of specific mRNAs in single nephron segments by use of the polymerase chain reaction, *Am. J. Physiol.*, 258, F1470, 1990.
15. Magocsi, M., Yamaki, M., Penniston, J.T., and Dousa, T.P., Localization of mRNAs coding for isozymes of plasma membrane Ca^{2+}-ATPase pump in rat kidney, *Am. J. Physiol.*, 263, F7, 1992.
16. Terada, Y., Moriyama, T., Martin, B.M., Knepper, M.A., and Garcia-Perez, A., RT-PCR microlocalization of mRNA for guanilyl cyclase-coupled ANF receptor in rat kidney, *Am. J. Physiol.*, 258, F1080, 1991.
17. Custer, M., Meier, F., Schlatter, E., Greger, R., Garcia-Perez, A., Biber, J., and Murer, H., Localization of NaPi-1, a Na-Pi cotransporter, in rabbit kidney proximal tubules, *Pflügers Arch.*, 424, 203, 1993.
18. Schmid, H., Mall, A., and Bockhorn, H., Altered distribution pattern of Na+-K+-ATPase and succinate dehydrogenase activities along the nephron in human acute post-transplant renal failure, *J. Clin. Chem. Clin. Biochem.*, 23, 27, 1985.
19. Takaori, K., Iwao, H., Ikemoto, F., and Yamamoto, K., Specific distribution of renin binding protein in rat and dog kidney, *Clin. Exp. Hypert.*, 4, 2097, 1982.
20. Chini, C.C.S., Chini, E.N., Williams, J.M., and Dousa, T.P., Formation of reactive oxygen metabolites in glomeruli is suppressed by inhibition of cAMP phosphodiesterase isozyme type IV, *Kidney Int.*, 46, 28, 1994.
21. Shah, S.V., Northrup, T.E., Hui, Y.S.F., and Dousa, T.P., Action of serotonin (5-hydroxytryptamine) on cyclic nucleotides in glomeruli of rat renal cortex, *Kidney Int.*, 15, 463, 1979.

22. Abboud, H.E., Ou, S.L., Velosa, J.A., Shah, S.V., and Dousa, T.P., Dynamics of renal histamine in normal rat kidney and in nephrosis induced by aminonucleoside of puromycin, *J. Clin. Invest.*, 69, 327, 1982.
23. Edwards, R.M., Segmental effect of norepinephrine and angiotensin II on isolated renal microvessels, *Am. J. Physiol.*, 244, F526, 1983.
24. Edwards, R.M., Direct assessment of glomerular arteriole reactivity, *NIPS*, 3, 216, 1988.
25. Edwards, R.M., Trizna, W., and Kinter, L.B., Renal microvascular effect of vasopressin and vasopressin antagonists, *Am. J. Physiol.*, 256, F-274, 1989.
26. Edwards, R.M., Trizna, W., and Ohlstein, E.H., Renal microvascular effect of endothelin, *Am. J. Physiol.*, 259, F-217, 1990.
27. PCR Technology, Principles and Applications for DNA Amplification, Erlich, H.A., Ed., Stockton Press, New York, 1989, 7.2.
28. Sambrook, J., Fritsh, E.F., and Maniatis, T., in *Molecular Cloning*, Cold Spring Harbor Laboratory Press, Cold Spring Harbor, NY, 1989.
29. McDonough, A.A., Magyar, C., and Komatsu, Y., Expression of Na+-K+-ATPase a- and b-subunits along rat nephron: isoform specific and response to hypokalemia, *Am. J. Physiol.*, 267, C901, 1994.
30. Matousovic, K., Grande, J.P., Chini, C.C.S., Chini, E.N., and Dousa, T.P., Inhibitors of cyclic nucleotide phosphodiesterase isozymes type-III and type-IV suppress mitogenesis of rat mesangial cells, *J. Clin. Invest.*, 96, 401, 1995.
31. Grande, J.P., Jones, M.L., Swenson, C.L., Killen, P.D., and Warren, J.S., Lipopolysaccharide induced monocyte chemoattractant protein production by rat mesangial cells, *J. Lab. Clin. Med.*, 124, 112, 1994.

chapter seven

Preparation and Use of Precision-Cut Renal Cortical Slices in Renal Toxicology

A. Jay Gandolfi, Klaus Brendel, and Quintus Fernanado

7.1 Introduction....110
7.2 Slicers and slicing....110
7.2.1 Slicers....110
7.2.2 Species used for renal slice preparation....110
7.2.3 Renal tissue coring....112
7.2.4 Renal slicing....112
7.2.5 Slice thickness....113
7.2.6 Slice storage and loading....113
7.3 Renal slice incubation systems....113
7.3.1 Dynamic organ culture....113
7.3.2 Submersion culture....113
7.3.3 Orbital suspension incubations....113
7.3.4 Incubation media....115
7.4 Viability and toxicology assays....115
7.4.1 Preincubation....115
7.4.2 Normalization....115
7.4.3 K^+ content in slices....115
7.4.4 Intracellular enzyme leakage....116
7.4.5 Cellular ATP....116
7.4.6 Respiration....116
7.4.7 Biosynthesis....116
7.4.8 Transport function....116
7.4.9 Microscopic evaluation....117
7.4.10 Length of viability....117
7.5 Metallic toxicant accumulation....117
7.5.1 Uptake and toxicity of metals....117
7.5.2 Proton induced X-ray emission (PIXE)....118
7.5.3 Application of PIXE....118
7.6 Toxicant studies with precision-cut renal slices....119
7.6.1 Halogenated hydrocarbons and glutathione/cysteine conjugates....119
7.6.2 Antibiotics....119

0-8493-3341-5/96/$0.00+$.50

7.6.3 Antineoplastic agents 120
7.6.4 Other chemicals 120
7.7 Conclusions and future studies 120
7.8 Acknowledgments 121
References 121

7.1 Introduction

Renal slices have provided a useful tool to study renal physiology and biochemistry and the effect of toxicants in these areas.[1] Historically, organic ion transport and renin release, which are functions of paramount importance to the kidney, have been extensively examined using the slice system.[2] Although renal slices have been used to study biochemical, physiological, and toxicological responses in the kidney, these studies have been hampered by the lack of a system that can produce slices of reproducible dimensions and response.[3,4] The development of a system to produce positional precision-cut renal slices as well as the development of incubation systems to maintain their viability in culture has overcome some of these limitations.[5] This chapter focuses on the preparation and incubation of positional, precision-cut renal slices as well as methods for assessing their viability and intoxication.

7.2 Slicers and slicing

7.2.1 Slicers

There are currently two mechanical slicers in use for the preparation of precision-cut renal slices. The first slicer developed for precision-cut tissue studies was the Krumdieck slicer,[6] which has undergone several modifications (Figure 1). Its current version is described in recent studies.[7,8] The slicer can be filled with oxygenated physiological solution to preserve the physiological activity of tissue during preparation. The slicer operates on the principle that a core of tissue (tissue coring will be described later) is fed into an oscillating blade that is drawn across the core to make a slice. The slice is then swept away into a collection device. The slice thickness can be adjusted, with optimum thickness around 250 μm. The diameter of the core is preset by the coring device, with diameters ranging from 4 to 8 mm.

Recently another mechanical slicer has been developed that works on the same principle as the Krumdieck slicer except it is simpler in design (Brendel–Vitron) (Figure 2). The Brendel–Vitron slicer is possibly more rugged and "user friendly."[9] Its major difference from the Krumdieck slicer is that the core of tissue is manually drawn across a rotating blade. As with the Krumdieck slicer, the slice is swept into a collection device such that sequential slices can be collected.

7.2.2 Species used for renal slice preparation

Precision-cut renal slices have been prepared from various species, including rabbit,[10] rat,[11] mouse, dog, and humans.[12] When renal slices are prepared from smaller species (rat, mouse), the kidney is trimmed rather than cored to fit into the tissue holder in the mechanical slicer.[11] In this case when slices are prepared, the slice reflects the complete cross section of the kidney (cortex, outer and inner medulla, and pelvis). For larger species, the kidney can be cored, allowing for precision-cut slices to be prepared from different sections of the kidney.[7,13] Rabbits (1.5 to 2.3 kg) are recommended for these studies since they are the largest laboratory animals with unipapillary kidneys in which detailed anatomical studies have been conducted.[14]

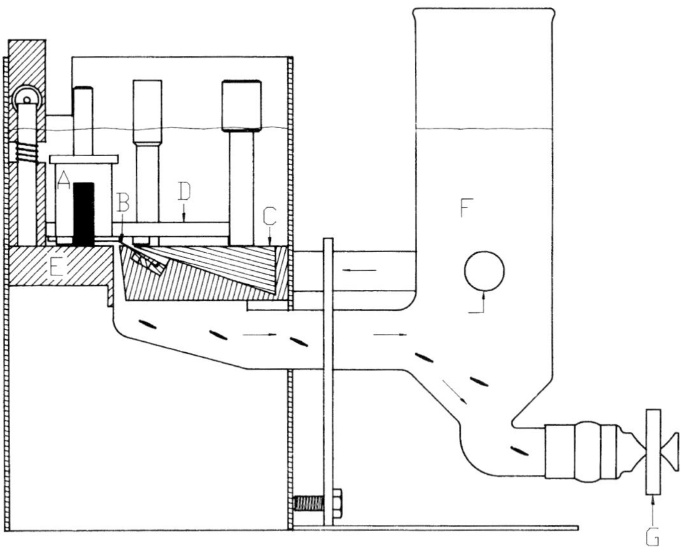

Figure 1 A schematic representation of the Krumdieck/Alabama Research & Development tissue slicer. Slices are produced by the movement of the tissue core (A) across the leading edge of an oscillating microtome blade (B), which is protected by a wedge (C). The tissue is fully submerged in buffers and is supported in a stainless steel insert held in a mechanically driven pivot arm (D). Only the portion of the tissue being cut off is exposed. Slice thickness is determined by the amount of weight over the tissue core and the height of the slicing stage (E), which is controlled by a micrometer-type horizontal screw. Buffer is continually circulated and oxygenated by an internal centrifugal pump. The slices are deposited in a glass trap (F) using the buffer flow and are then retrieved by the opening of a simple pinch clamp (G), which allows slices to flow out with a small amount of buffer. The autoclavable, stainless steel Krumdieck tissue slicer is fully automated and can be used with precooled buffer or with buffer cooled by an external refrigeration unit connected to the reservoir. (Courtesy of Alabama Research and Development Corporation, Munford, AL.)

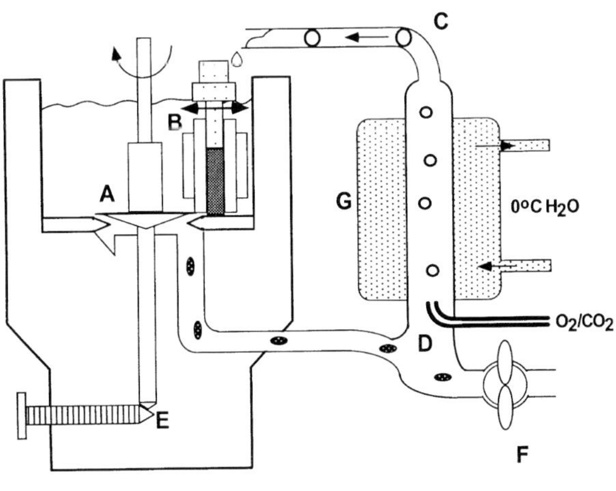

Figure 2 Brendel–Vitron slice diagram. Slices are produced by a rotating circular blade (A) that is motor driven. The tissue contained in the cutting arm (B) is moved across the blade by the operator. Slicing buffer is returned to the slicing chamber (C) by a gas elevator pump from the slice collection vessel (D). Slice thickness is controlled by weight over the tissue core and by a cone/countercone micrometer adjustment (E). Slices are retrieved by release of a valve in the collection vessel (F) and buffer is cooled during the procedure by an ice water circulation system (G). (Courtesy of Vitron, Inc., Tucson, AZ.)

7.2.3 Renal tissue coring

After kidneys have been removed from the animal (usually rabbit), they are decapsulated in preparation for slicing.[13] Kidneys need not be perfused to remove blood components. The slicing and incubation processes flush most of the blood components from the slices. Cylindrical cores (up to seven per kidney for the rabbit), are cut along the cortical–papillary axis by pushing the kidneys against a rotating (300 rpm) piece of thin-walled sharpened stainless steel tubing (Figure 3). Coring can also be performed by hand with a sharpened core bore, but the resulting cores are less satisfactory. Cores of 4 to 10 mm have been used, with the 6- to 8-mm size used most routinely. By taking the cores from the cortex through the papilla the renal tubular anatomy is aligned for positional slicing.[15]

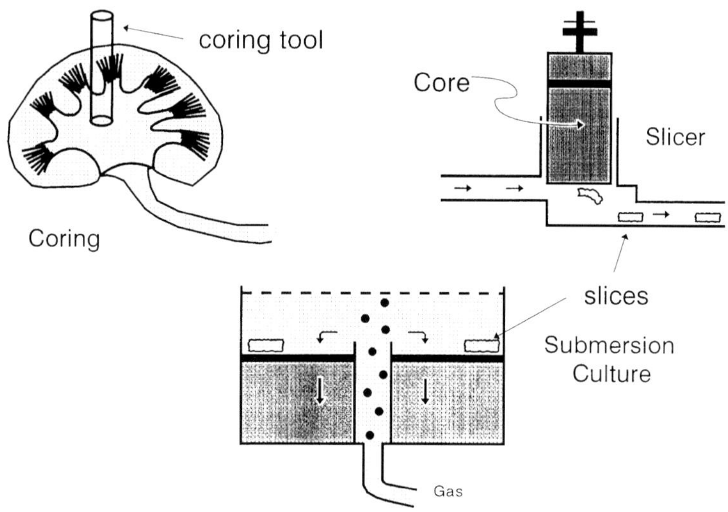

Figure 3 Steps in renal slice preparation. (Adapted from Gandolfi, A. J. and Brendel, K., *Toxicol. In Vitro*, 4, 337, 1990. With permission of Elsevier Science Ltd., U.K.)

7.2.4 Renal slicing

Renal cores are placed into the tissue holder of one of the mechanical slicers (Krumdieck or Brendel–Vitron), which holds these cores in a rigid position submerged in the oxygenated, physiological buffer.[13] Although various physiological buffers or minimal salts buffers can be used, the most common solution utilized is ice-cold Dulbecco's Modified Eagle's: Ham's Nutrient Mix F12 (DME/F12) in a 1:1 mixture.[7,15] In both slicers, a weighted piston is placed above the core to maintain a constant pressure for advancement of the core while slicing. The tissue core is drawn either manually or mechanically (depending on slicer) across the blade, and the slices swept away into a collection chamber by the circulating medium. Since the slices are cut at right angles to the tubular axis of the kidney, the resulting slices consist of an array of short tubular segments. The slice thickness can be set between 100 and 500 µm. Two hundred and fifty to 350 µm has been found to be optimal to allow exchange of gases, nutrients, and wastes. Thinner slices are too friable, while thicker slices restrict the exchange of nutrients and gases.

Slices can be made from all sections of the core, but typically the first slice is discarded and the next six to eight slices used for studies since they contain all the cell types of the cortex.[15] Different slices from the core can be used to specifically examine various components of the nephron from the cortex to the medulla.[7]

7.2.5 Slice thickness

One of the primary reasons for the success of precision-cut tissue slices is the reproducibility of the thickness of the slices prepared by the mechanical slicers (Krumdieck or Brendel–Vitron). Variations in thickness between slices is usually 10% or less. Further, the thickness of slices is consistent throughout the slice; that was not the case with hand-held slices such as the Stadie–Riggs slices. Slice thickness must be maintained between 250 and 350 μm to allow optimum exchange of nutrients, wastes, gases as well as exposure to toxicants.

Slice thickness can be measured by a variety of methods. A fresh slice can be wet mounted on a cover slip with the slice positioned by the edge. A dissecting microscope equipped with a calibrated ocular micrometer can then be used to measure the slice thickness.[15] Another method is to embed the slices and then section them on end. The thickness of the slices can then be determined with a calibrated ocular microscope.

Recently two other approaches have been taken. Since the slice diameter is preset by the coring tool and the slice wet weight can be obtained easily, it is fairly straightforward to calculate mathematically the thickness of the slice once the density of the tissue has been established. Even simpler is the placing of the slice between two cover slips that have been previously calibrated with an electronic micrometer. The cover slips with the slice between them are then remeasured and the slice thickness obtained.

7.2.6 Slice storage and loading

Precision-cut slices are fragile and must be handled with care. After preparation, slices can be stored for a short period in ice-cold medium that is oxygenated.[10] Slices are usually moved by a ladle or by allowing them to wrap around a glass rod. When the slice is lifted with fine tweezers, care must be taken to not puncture it or allow it to rip due to its own weight.

7.3 Renal slice incubation systems

There are several methods for incubating precision-cut renal slices. The choice of the incubation technique depends on the length of incubation, the type of chemical under investigation (volatility, solubility), the reactivity of the chemical with incubation components, and the subsequent assays to be performed. Dynamic organ culture, aerated submersion culture, and orbital suspension cultures are three incubation techniques that have been utilized successfully for the incubation of renal slices. The incubation systems have several features in common in that they deliver nutrients and oxygenated medium to both surfaces of the slice while limiting mechanical injury to the slices.[7]

7.3.1 Dynamic organ culture

Dynamic organ culture was developed by Smith et al.[16] and incorporates the concepts of roller bottle culture with Trowell culture[17] techniques (Figure 4). In this incubation system, the slices are mounted on stainless steel titanium or Teflon mesh cylinders (260 μm core size), which are then circumscribed with either stainless steel titanium or Teflon wheels or cradels and inserted into glass scintillation vials containing 1.6 to 1.7 ml of culture medium. This volume of medium wets but does not submerge the slice. The vials are gassed (usually 95:5 O_2/CO_2), capped, and placed on a 37°C vial rotator[18] set at approximately 3 rpm. This allows the slice to rotate into and out of the culture medium, thus allowing for aeration and nutrient/waste exchange. This closed incubation system has been used when volatile and hazardous substances are being examined. In addition, this system is useful when only small amounts of test chemical are available since it requires less medium than some of the other incubation systems.[19] Problems, though, may be encountered due to surface tension effects, which may cause the brush border membrane to slough off from the proximal tubular epithelial cells.

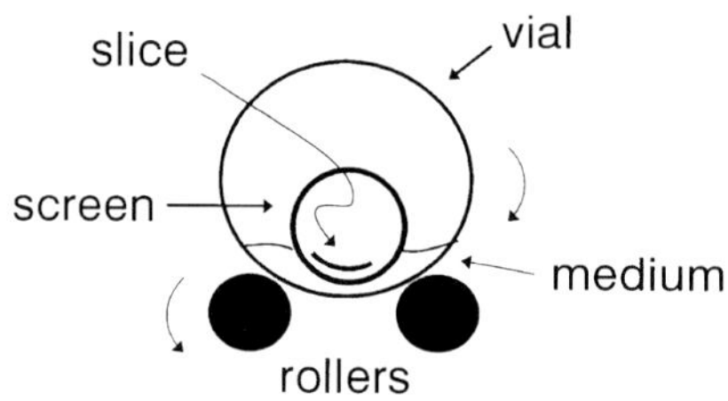

Figure 4 Dynamic organ culture diagram.

7.3.2 *Submersion culture*

Submersion culture, also called bubble culture, was developed as a gentle system to support slices on a porous membrane submerged beneath a constantly circulating aerated medium.[13] The culture incubation system has been described previously and basically consists of an incubation vessel containing Teflon cups (Figure 5).[15] Slices are placed on stainless steel screens located near the base of the cup such that the slices are submerged in the medium. A needle is placed through the base of the vessel extending into a central tube to serve as a gas port. When this system is lightly aerated, a gentle circulation of the medium occurs that ensures constant gas concentrations, maintains pH throughout the experiment, and "holds" the slices in place submerged on the screens. The system is very gentle, thus causing virtually no mechanical stress to the slices. It has its limitations because it is an open system and thus is usually restricted to chemicals with minimal vapor pressure (ions, metals). In addition, protein cannot be added to the medium because it will cause excessive foaming.

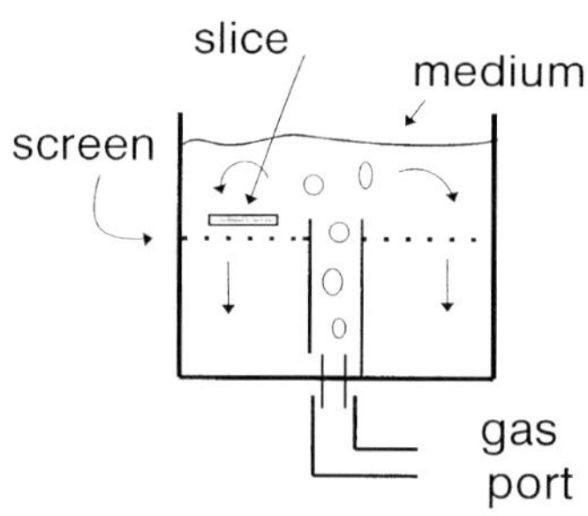

Figure 5 Submersion culture diagram.

7.3.3 *Orbital suspension incubations*

Twenty-four-well tissue culture plates were previously used for incubation of precision-cut liver slices.[20] This was considered a dynamic version of Trowell culture[17] since the slices were placed in individual baskets and barely submerged in 1 ml of medium present in each well. The culture plates were placed in a gyratory shaker to allow mixing of medium and exchange of gases. Recently this system was modified for incubations with renal slices.[7,21] Either 12- or 24-well plates are used, with one slice incubated in each well containing 1 ml of medium. The slices are maintained in suspension by placing the plates on an orbital shaking plate that is then housed in a 37°C air/CO_2 incubator. As with the bubble culture, this system utilizes low volumes of culture medium and is easy to set up. However, there has been some controversy about how well this incubation system maintains slice viability.[22]

7.3.4 *Incubation media*

A serum-free mixture of Dulbecco's Modified Eagle's and Ham's Nutrient Mix F-12 (1:1) was the initial medium used for preparing and incubating precision-cut renal slices.[13] A serum-free mixture was used to avoid foaming, and phenol red was omitted since it interfered with organic ion transport studies. The medium was gassed with 95/5% O_2/CO_2 for 15 min at room temperature and the pH then adjusted to 7.4. With few exceptions, this has remained the medium of choice for all precision-cut renal slice studies. For incubations using the roller culture system, a Krebs–HEPES buffer has been utilized[20] while a Waymouth's culture medium has been utilized for some human kidney slice studies[12] and for cold- and cryopreserved tissue slice studies.[23] Antibiotics are usually not used with the medium to eliminate any of the effects produced by these compounds in renal cells (toxicity or alterations in transport).

7.4 *Viability and toxicology assays*

A variety of assays have been applied to assess that the renal slices in culture maintain their viability and unique renal functions.

7.4.1 *Preincubation*

It normally takes the slices 1 h to adjust to their incubation conditions. During the preincubation, cellular debris (cut cells, blood components, etc.) are released into the medium. Since the slices are cut from the tissue cores submerged in ice-cold medium, the slices must readjust to 37°C incubation temperatures. During the preincubation, many viability indicators are changing. Thus, it is imperative to acclimate the slices before beginning viability and toxicity investigations.

7.4.2 *Normalization*

For many *in vitro* cellular systems, assays are normalized to cell number. For the precision-cut tissue slices, this would be impractical, so other methods of normalization have been used. The easiest method is slice weight, which is performed by removing the slice after incubation, blotting it dry on a paper towel, and weighing it.[12] However, if the slices should become edematous during incubation or should they dehydrate, the normalization can be inaccurate. Many assays are based on protein content, but this may not be optimal since renal cells may lose protein (sloughing of brush border) during incubation.[15] Thus, the standard method we have used for normalizing assays is by slice DNA content.[8,10,13] The DNA content of each slice is measured using a fluorometric technique.[24] Basically a cell homogenizer is used to homogenize each slice in 0.5 ml distilled water. A 0.1-ml aliquot is processed and reacted with diaminobenzoic (DABA) acid to produce a DABA–DNA conjugate which is fluorescent. Sensitivity of the assay is 0 to 50 μg DNA.

7.4.3 *K^+ content in slices*

In a variety of *in vitro* systems, it has been found that the K^+ content of the tissue slice is a good reflection of the Na^+, K^+-ATPase activity and membrane integrity, and losses in K^+ content are an early sensitive sign of intoxication.[8] Slices are removed from the incubation system, blotted, and placed in 0.5 ml of distilled water. A cell sonicator is then used to homogenize each slice, and a 0.1-ml aliquot is removed for DNA analysis.[24] The remaining sample is precipitated with trichloroacetic acid (3% final concentration), centrifuged, and the supernatant measured for intercellular K^+ content by flame photometry.[25] The slice K^+ content (nanomoles) is normalized per microgram of slice DNA.

7.4.4 *Intracellular enzyme leakage*

A number of intracellular proteins have been used as indicators of leaky membranes or total disruption of the renal cell.[26] In fact, selected proteins have been suggested as markers for specific cells within the nephron.[27] The intracellular enzyme concentrations and the leakage of enzymes are measured, and the results expressed as a percent of total activity which has leaked out. Loss of slice lactic dehydrogenase is used to profile a variety of organic nephrotoxicants in rabbit renal slices.[10] Wolfgang et al.[28] examined the leakage of multiple enzymes following exposure of precision-cut renal cortical slices to dichlorovinyl cysteine and other toxicants. These included lactic dehydrogenase, γ-glutamyl transpeptidase, and alkaline phosphatase. The enzyme leakage was normalized per microgram slice DNA or reported as percent decrease as described above.

7.4.5 *Cellular ATP*

ATP content reflects the energy status of the cells of the slice. Coupled with slice K^+ content (ATPase activity) and respiration, it provides information on the status of the viability of the cells in the slice. Slice ATP has been quantified by the luciferin–luciferase assay.[29] For these analyses, slices are removed after incubation and blotted on tissue paper. Slices are placed in 0.5% trichloroacetic acid, sonicated, and centrifuged to separate the supernatant fraction for ATP analysis.[19] The remaining pellet is used to measure slice DNA content by the fluorometric technique.[24]

7.4.6 *Respiration*

For selected toxicants, respiration has been observed to be an early indicator of toxicity to slices.[28] O_2 consumption is monitored by a Clark-type electrode attached to a chart recorder. After incubation, slices are removed and placed individually in a closed chamber with Krebs–HEPES buffer at 37°C and stirred with a magnetic stirrer such that the stirrer does not touch the slice.[19] Oxygen consumption is monitored for 5 min, and the slices are then removed and used to determine DNA content for normalization.

7.4.7 *Biosynthesis*

Biosynthesis requires uptake of precursors, cellular energy, and proper functioning of cellular organelles. Alterations in biosynthesis, such as of proteins, has been observed at times to be an even more sensitive indicator of tissue slice viability.[30] Protein synthesis is measured by ^{3}H-leucine incorporation.[12] Slices are incubated in the presence of ^{3}H-leucine and then homogenized in 1 ml of 1 *N* NaOH. Following the addition of 1.5 *N* acetic acid, the samples are centrifuged and washed twice, and the pellets dissolved in 0.5 ml of 0.5 *N* NaOH. The incorporation of ^{3}H-leucine is determined and normalized to slice protein content.

7.4.8 *Transport function*

Functional assessments are important indicators of the unique properties of the kidney. Since transport of a variety of organic and inorganic cations and anions is a key function of the cortex of the kidney, it is most often evaluated.[1] Although the lumens of the nephron segments in slices seem to close after 60 to 90 min of incubation, it has been demonstrated that glucose uptake (which is luminal) occurs for up to 6 h of incubation and is inhibitable by phlorhizin.[15] Thus uptake processes by luminal or basolateral routes appear possible.

Typically uptake is evaluated on slices removed from one of the incubation systems. Uptake of radiolabeled organic anion (*p*-aminohippuric acid) or organic cation (tetraethyl ammonium [TEA]) is measured by placing the slice in a scintillation vial containing the transport substrate and allowing it to incubate in the dynamic roller culture system.[19] Slices are allowed to take up the transport substrate for 40 min. The slices are then removed and blotted. The radioactive substrate content in the slice and medium are determined. ^3H_2O is also present in the medium to normalize the volumes. Accumulation ratios are expressed as slice (^{14}C substrate/^3H_2O) to medium (^{14}C substrate/^3H_2O) ratio.

7.4.9 Microscopic examination

One of the most attractive features of using tissue slices is the ability to evaluate cell specific injury by microscopic techniques.[5,31] Both light and electron microscopic evaluations have been used.[25,28,29] For renal slices, site-specific lesions have been observed with a wide variety of nephrotoxicants.[10,19] Chronologically coupling biochemical and functional alterations with microscopic changes allows for a fuller examination of the mechanism of toxicity. Samples for histology are fixed in phosphate buffered 4% formaldehyde/1% glutaldehyde solution.[28] Slices are then dehydrated with increasing concentrations of ethyl alcohol and embedded in methacrylate plastic. Sections (1.5 to 2.0 μm) are cut and stained with 1% toluidine blue. For electron microscopy examination, slices are fixed flat in Karnovsky's solution for 4 h and subsequently transferred to 7.5% sucrose overnight. Thick sections are prepared, regions are selected, and grids are prepared. Final sections are stained with lead citrate and uranyl acetate.

7.4.10 Length of viability

Precision-cut renal slices have routinely been maintained for 24 h of incubation using good laboratory technique (nonsterile). Incubations can be extended to 48 to 72 h with sterile technique and exchanging media every 24 h. Longer term incubations, though, will produce artifacts in the microscopic analysis due to the impressions by the slice lying on the support screens of the submersion culture and general realignment of cells. Antibiotics are typically not added to the medium to avoid the potential renal toxicity seen with these compounds.

7.5 Metallic toxicant accumulation

Most heavy metals are potent nephrotoxicants.[32] Precision-cut rabbit renal cortical slices have been used to examine the site-specific nephrotoxicity of metals,[25] mechanisms of nephrotoxic injury,[33] toxicity of metal mixtures,[34] and toxicity of metal conjugates.[35]

7.5.1 Uptake and toxicity of metals

The rank order of metals in rabbit renal cortical slices has been established as $HgCl_2 \gg K_2Cr_2O_7 > CdCl_2 > NaAsO_2$.[34] These metals produce a site-specific injury which reflects that seen *in vivo*.[25] $HgCl_2$ produced an initial injury to the S_3 segment of the proximal tubule while $K_2Cr_2O_7$ produced an injury in the S_1 to S_2 segments of the proximal tubule. Since the entire kidney slice is exposed to the nephrotoxicant, the susceptibility must be unique to the targeted cell population. Studies indicate that uptake of the toxicant by specific target cells may be the key event in the initial expression of the injury.[33]

The uptake (and localization) of metallic nephrotoxicants has been previously performed on studies with cisplatin, in which the platinum content on the slice was measured by atomic absorption analysis;[29] with $HgCl_2$, in which the Hg was detected microscopically by silver amplification of Hg-selenide complexes[33] or as monitored in its radioactive form;[36] and with $K_2Cr_2O_7$, in which the localization was attempted with electron probe X-ray analysis.

Due to the multiple metals under study we required an analytical technique that did not require radiolabeled metals, was nondestructive, and could measure multiple metals simultaneously. Thus, we employed proton-induced X-ray analysis for our studies.

7.5.2 Proton induced X-ray emission (PIXE)

Proton-induced X-ray emission is a powerful multielement analysis technique with high sensitivity. The PIXE technique involves bombarding a sample with protons, which eject inner shell electrons of the elements in the sample. The emission of X-rays whose energies are characteristic of the elements present in the sample can be quantified using a liquid-nitrogen-cooled solid-state Si (Li) detector and a multichannel analyzer. The PIXE analysis provides information on concentrations of elements above atomic number 11 and is the only analytical technique that can determine 20 to 30 elements non-destructively in a single, small sample, with detection limits of 1 to 5 ppm. The PIXE technique has been used successfully for the elemental analysis of renal slices following incubation with metallic toxicants.[37] To utilize this technique, after incubation, renal slices are blotted dry and placed on 3.5-μm Mylar film stretched across X-ray fluorescence sample cups (diameter = 3.2 cm, open ended). Another piece of film is placed on top to create a sandwich (Figure 6). Two holes are punched in the sandwich to allow air to escape and the sample to dry. Samples are placed in the freezer immediately after preparation until the day before analysis, at which point they are placed in a desiccator and allowed to thaw and dry. The dried samples are analyzed by PIXE. The slice in the sample holder is placed into a ten-sample chamber. The proton beam strikes the target and generates the X-rays that are detected by the Si (Li) detector. Sample beam size is kept at 4 mm × 4 mm, which covers 60% of the area of the slice surface. Values are reported as nanograms of element per square centimeter and can be converted to parts per million by dividing by the areal/density of the sample (grams per square centimeter) since the sample is treated as a thin target.[37]

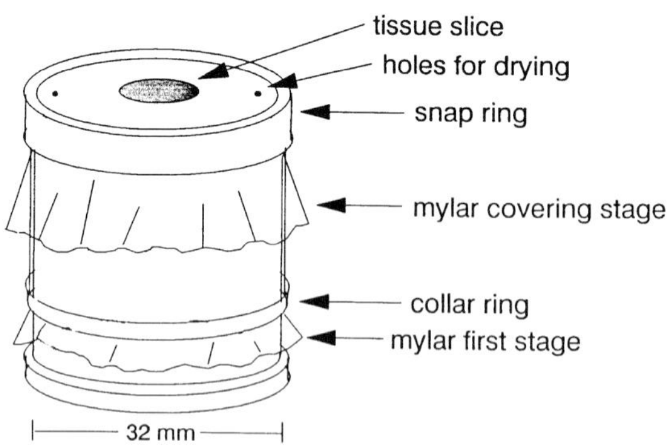

Figure 6 PIXE sample holder diagram.

7.5.3 Application of PIXE

Using PIXE analysis, it was demonstrated that there is a correlation between the potency of the metal toxicant and the amount of metal accumulated.[34] This system also proved valuable to demonstrate the interactive effects of multiple metals on uptake and subsequent toxicity. Since PIXE can readily quantify multiple elements, pairs of metallic toxicants can be incubated and the accumulation of the various metals determined in the renal slice simultaneously. Our initial studies indicate that incubation of pairs of metals with renal slices do not produce synergistic toxicity and only in rare cases is the toxicity additive. Most of the time infra-additive toxicity is observed, which is related to the ability of one metal to inhibit the uptake of a second metal.[34]

The mechanism of renal uptake of nephrotoxic heavy metal species, such as $HgCl_2$ and $NaAsO_2$, is not clear. The metals are known to react with endogenous sulfhydryls, such as glutathione, so metal–glutathione conjugates may be delivered to the kidney. To study this possibility, the toxicity and uptake of metals, metal glutathione conjugates, and metal/glutathione co-incubations have been examined.[35] Synthetic Hg–glutathione conjugate was found to be less cytotoxic than $HgCl_2$ whereas As–glutathione conjugate exhibited a 2-h delay in producing cytotoxicity compared to $NaAsO_2$ itself. This delay in toxicity, however, was not correlated to changes in uptake. In fact, As and Hg accumulations determined by PIXE analysis were almost identical for the metal salts and metal glutathione conjugates. However, exogenous glutathione decreased $HgCl_2$ cytotoxicity, which correlated with a decrease in Hg accumulation in the slice. While exogenous glutathione had limited, if any, protective effect against the cytotoxicity of $NaAsO_2$, a decrease in arsenate accumulation was not observed. It appears that Hg–glutathione and arsenic–glutathione conjugates can be cytotoxic and are not totally responsible for the accumulation of these metals in renal cortical slices.[35]

7.6 *Toxicant studies with precision-cut renal slices*

Besides the metallic toxicants mentioned in Section 7.5, numerous other toxicants have now been studied with precision-cut renal slices.

7.6.1 *Halogenated hydrocarbons and glutathione/cysteine conjugates*

Several halogenated hydrocarbons form glutathione, cysteine, or mercapturic acid conjugates that are subsequently biotransformed in the kidney to potent specific nephrotoxicants.[8] Using dichlorovinylcysteine as a model toxicant, it was demonstrated that renal slices could specifically accumulate, biotransform, and bioactivate dichlorovinylcysteine.[28,38,39] It was demonstrated that the accumulation of DCVC was critical for toxicity to occur and that once the DCVC was taken up in the renal cortical slices it was rapidly biotransformed. Light microscopic examination provided a sequence of histopathological changes from an initial S_3 lesion between 4 to 8 h to a lesion encompassing all the proximal tubular elements by 12 h.[28] Electron microscopy demonstrated not only the specificity of DCVC toxicity, but also illustrated mitochondrial damage and loss of brush borders. *N*-acetyl dichlorovinylcysteine was less toxic in renal slices than DCVC. However, both compounds produced damage to the S_3 segment of the proximal tubule similar to that found *in vivo*.[39] Subsequent studies have demonstrated that accumulation of cysteine conjugates may involve multiple transport mechanisms to the different segments of the nephron.

7.6.2 *Antibiotics*

The nephrotoxicity of cephaloridine and gentamicin has been examined in rabbit renal cortical slices.[10] Cephaloridine produced a concentration-dependent decrease in intracellular K^+ content. However, the decreases were not dramatic. Some decreases were noted as early as 4 h, while in many instances it took almost 24 h of incubation before decreases were noted. Cephaloridine also produced decreases in slice lactic dehydrogenase content and inhibited both PAH (organic anion) and TEA (organic cation) sliced media accumulations.

For gentamicin, only the highest concentrations studied caused alterations in intracellular K^+ content and this required 24 h of incubation.[10] Histopathological investigation demonstrated minimal damage to S_3 segments and thick ascending limbs of Henle's loop following 12 and 24 h of incubation. However an S_3 lesion was noted by 24 h of incubation following exposure to high concentrations of gentamicin along with injury to the ascending thick segments. This pattern of injury is unique to *in vitro* exposure and may be due to alternative delivery mechanisms not utilized *in vivo*.

7.6.3 *Antineoplastic agents*

Cisplatin is a potent antineoplastic agent, whose major limiting side effect is nephrotoxicity. The S_3 segment of the proximal tubule appears to be the major site of injury, but the exact mechanism of cisplatin nephrotoxicity has not been fully elucidated. Phelps et al.[29] utilized precision-cut rabbit renal slices to study the effect of four platinum coordination complexes. The complexes were ranked for nephrotoxic potential based on intracellular K^+ and ATP content. The ranking was found to be quite similar to clinical reports. Furthermore, platinum uptake was comparable to *in vivo* levels in the concentration range for producing cisplatin toxicity and was similar to or lower than peak blood levels in cancer patients. However, the lesion produced in the rabbit renal cortical slices was in the S_1 and S_2 segments of the nephron segments. This is different from that observed in animal studies and may be related to a susceptibility of these segments to hypoxia caused by the incubation technique.[15]

7.6.4 *Other chemicals*

In an attempt to examine the importance of transport in producing toxicity, a number of studies have been undertaken looking at various organic anions and organic cations. McGuinness et al.[40] found that the toxicity of the antineoplastic agent celiptium was related to its accumulation by the organic cation pathway. Further studies demonstrated that the quaternary amine structure was needed for these chemical structures to be nephrotoxic. To further understand the key features needed for accumulation of organic cations in the kidney, a series of aromatic quaternary amines was examined for their toxicity to renal slices.[19] It was discovered that differences in toxicity could not be completely explained by slight structural variations. Thus, a single model organic cation, 1-benzylquinolinium (BQ) was used to assess organic cations in rabbit renal cortical slices. Histopathological evaluation revealed that BQ produced site-specific injury in the S_3 region of the proximal tubule. Biochemical assays revealed dose- and time-dependent decreases in BQ-exposed slices over a 12-h incubation. Cation transport export was decreased by BQ at subtoxic doses within 12 h, while organic anion transport was unaffected. This is the first demonstration of the importance of organic cation transport in the nephrotoxicity of these aromatic quaternary amine compounds.

7.7 *Conclusions and future studies*

Positional precision-cut renal cortical slices (and precision-cut slices from other sections of the kidney) have proven to be a valid *in vitro* system for examining the nephrotoxicity of a wide variety of chemicals. The renal slices maintain their viability over 24 h of incubation and are capable of retaining many of the functions unique to the kidney. Accumulation of toxicants in target cells has been shown to be critical for the demonstration of site-specific injury. Future studies will need to focus on the specific cells that are injured to demonstrate that they are specifically accumulating, bioactivating (if necessary), and becoming intoxicated as a result of the presence of the chemical being studied.

7.8 Acknowledgments

The authors wish to acknowledge the following individuals whose research efforts formed the basis of this chapter: C. Ruegg, G. Wolfgang, H. Sheevers, T. Lowe, J. Leavitt, L. McIntyre, D. Ashbaugh, R. Keith, J. Phelps, C. Burton, S. Hasal, Q. Chen, R. Fisher, S. Connors, I. Setiarahardjo. The development of this technique and the research studies were sponsored by NIH (ES 05790, P42 ES04940, DK 41006) and Johns Hopkins Center for Alternatives to Animal Testing.

References

1. Rose, R. C., Bianchi, J., and Schuette, S. A., Effective use of renal cortical slices in transport and metabolic studies, *Biochem. Biophys. Acta*, 821, 431, 1985.
2. Smith, M. A., Hewitt, W. R., and Hook, J. B., *In vitro* methods in renal toxicology, in *In Vitro Methods in Toxicology*, Atterwill, C. K. and Steele, C. E., Eds., Cambridge University Press, New York, 1987, 13.
3. Bach, P. H. and Lock, E. A., The use of renal tissue slices, perfusion and infusion techniques to assess nephrotoxicity related changes, in *Nephrotoxicity: Assessment and Pathogenesis*, Bach, P. H., Bonner, F. W., Bridges, J. W., and Lock, E. A., Eds., John Wiley & Sons, New York, 1982, 128.
4. Smith, J. H., The use of renal cortical slices from the Fisher 344 rat as an *in vitro* model to evaluate nephrotoxicity, *Toxicol. Appl. Pharmacol.*, 11, 132, 1988.
5. Brendel, K., Gandolfi, A. J., Krumdieck, C. L, and Smith P. F., Organ slices revisited, *Trends Pharmacol. Sci.*, 8, 11, 1987.
6. Krumdieck, C. L., Santos, J. E. D., and Ho, K. J., A new instrument for the rapid preparation of tissue slices, *Anal. Biochem.*, 104, 118, 1980.
7. Ruegg, C. E., Preparation of precision-cut renal slices and renal proximal tubular fragments for evaluating segment-specific nephrotoxicity, *J. Pharmacol. Toxicol. Methods*, 31, 125, 1994.
8. McGuinness, S. G., Gandolfi, A. J., and Brendel, K., Use of renal slices and renal tubule suspensions for *in vitro* toxicity studies, *In Vitro Toxicol.*, 6, 1, 1993.
9. Parrish, A. R., Gandolfi, A. J., and Brendel, K., Precision-cut tissue slices: applications in pharmacology and toxicology, *Life Sci.*, 57, 1887, 1995.
10. Wolfgang, G. H. I., Gandolfi, A. J., and Brendel, K., Evaluation of organic nephrotoxins in rabbit renal cortical slices, *Toxicol. In Vitro*, 3, 341, 1989.
11. Ziegler, T. L., Winter, S. M., Sell, R., Gandolfi, A. J., and Sipes, I. G., Metabolism of acrylic acid in Sprague–Dawley rat liver and kidney slices, *Toxicologist*, 13, 138, 1993.
12. Fisher, R. L., Sanuik, J. T., Gandolfi, A. J., and Brendel, K., Toxicity of cisplatin and mercuric chloride in human kidney cortical slices, *Hum. Exp. Toxicol.*, 13, 517, 1994.
13. Ruegg, C. E., Gandolfi, A. J., and Brendel, K., Preparation and incubation of precision-cut, positional renal slices, *Pharmacol. Methods*, 17, 111, 1987.
14. Kaissling, B. and Kriz, W., Structural analysis of the rabbit kidney, *Adv. Anat. Embryol. Cell Biol.*, 56, 1, 1979.
15. Ruegg, C. E., Wolfgang, G. H. I., Gandolfi, A. J., Brendel, K., and Krumdieck, C. L., Preparation and utilization of positional renal slices for *in vitro* nephrotoxicity studies, in *In Vitro Models in Toxicology*, McQueen, C. A., Ed., Telford Press, Caldwell, NJ, 1989.
16. Smith, P. F., Gandolfi, A. J., Krumdieck, C. L., Putnam, C. W., Zukowski, C. F., Davis, W. M., and Brendel, K., Dynamic organ culture of precision liver slices for *in vitro* toxicology, *Life Sci.*, 36, 1367, 1985.
17. Trowell, D. A., The culture of mature organs in a synthetic medium, *Exp. Cell Res.*, 16, 118, 1959.
18. Smith, P. F., Fisher, R., McKee, R., Gandolfi, A. J., Krumdieck, C. L., and Brendel, K., Precision-cut liver slices: a new *in vitro* tool in toxicology, in *In Vitro Models in Toxicology*, McQueen, C.A., Ed., Telford Press, Caldwell, NJ, 1989, 93.
19. Sheevers, H. V., Brendel, K., Wright, S. H., Nagle, R. B., and Gandolfi, A. J., Nephrotoxicity and uptake of 1-benzyl quinolinium in precision-cut rabbit renal cortical slices, *Toxicol. In Vitro*, 8, 1243, 1994.
20. Connors, S., Rankin, D. R., Gandolfi, A. J., Krumdieck, C. L., Koep, L. J., and Brendel, K., Cocaine hepatotoxicity in cultured liver slices: a species comparison, *Toxicology*, 61, 171, 1990.

21. Silber, P. M., Greenwalt, T. M., and Ruegg, C. E., Tissue slices as an *in vitro* model for studying heart, liver, and kidney toxicity, in *Animal Testing Alternatives*, Salem, H., Ed., Marcel Dekker, New York, 1995, 83.
22. Fisher, R. L., Shaughnessy, R. P., Jenkins, P. L., Austin, M. L., Roth, G. L, Gandolfi, A. J., and Brendel, K., Dynamic organ culture is superior to multiwell plate culturing systems for maintaining liver slice viability, *Toxicologist*, 15, 108, 1995.
23. Fisher, R. L., Hasal, S. J., Sanuik, J. T., Scott, K. S., Gandolfi, A. J., and Brendel, K., Cold- and cryo-preservation of human liver and kidney slices, *Cryobiology*, 30, 250, 1993.
24. Kissane, J. M. and Robbins, E., The fluorometric measurement of deoxyribonucleic acid in animal tissues with special reference to the central nervous system, *J. Biol. Chem.*, 233, 184, 1958.
25. Ruegg, C. E., Gandolfi, A. J., Brendel, K., and Nagle, R. B., Differential patterns of injury to the proximal tubule of renal cortical slices following *in vitro* exposure to mercuric chloride, potassium dichromate, or anoxic conditions, *Toxicol. Appl. Pharmacol.*, 90, 261, 1987.
26. Ross, B. D. and Guder, W. G., Heterogeneity and compartmentation in the kidney, in *Metabolic Compartmentation*, Sies, H., Ed., Academic Press, London, 1982, 363.
27. Stonard, M., Proteins, enzymes and cells in urine as indicators of the site of renal damage, in *Nephrotoxicity in the Experimental and Clinical Situation, Part 2*, Bach, P. H. and Lock, E. A., Eds., Martinus Nijhoff Publishers, Dordrecht, The Netherlands, 1987, 563.
28. Wolfgang, G., Gandolfi, A. J., Nagle, R., Brendel, K., and Stevens, J., Assessment of S-(1,2-Dichlorovinyl)-L-cysteine induced toxic events in rabbit renal cortical slices, biochemical and histological evaluation of uptake, covalent binding, and toxicity, *Chem. Biol. Interact.*, 75, 153, 1990.
29. Phelps, J. S., Gandolfi, A. J., Dohr, R., and Brendel, K., Cisplatin nephrotoxicity: *in vitro* studies with precision cut renal cortical slices, *Toxicol. Appl. Pharmacol.*, 90, 501, 1987.
30. Ghantous, H. N., Fernando, J. L., Keith, R. L., Gandolfi, A. J., and Brendel, K., Effects of halothane and other volatile anaesthetics on protein synthesis and secretion in guinea pig liver slices, *Br. J. Anaesth.*, 68, 172, 1992.
31. Smith, P. F., Fisher, R., Shubat, P. J., Gandolfi, A. J., Krumdieck, C. L., and Brendel, K., In vitro cytotoxicity of allyl alcohol and bromobenzene in a novel organ culture system, *Toxicol. Appl. Pharmacol.*, 87, 509, 1987.
32. Conner, E. A. and Fowler, B. A., Mechanisms of metal-induced nephrotoxicity, in *Toxicology of the Kidney*, Hook, J. B. and Goldstein, R. G., Eds., Raven Press, New York, 1993, 437.
33. Ruegg, C. E., Gandolfi, A. J., and Brendel, K., Regioselective acute tubular necrosis in renal cortical slices following $HgCl_2$ and $K_2Cr_2O_7$: localization and transport studies, in *Nephrotoxicity: Extrapolation from In Vitro to In Vivo Animals to Man, Proc. 3rd Int. Symp. Nephrotoxicity*, Guildford, England, 1987, 107.
34. Keith, R. L, McGuinness, S. J., Gandolfi, A. J., Lowe, T. P., Chen, Q., and Fernando, Q., Interaction of metals during their uptake and accumulation in rabbit renal cortical slices, *Environ. Health Perspect.*, 103, 77, 1995.
35. Burton, C. A., Hatlelid, K., Divine, K., Carter, D. E., Fernando, Q., Brendel, K., and Gandolfi, A. J., Glutathione effects on toxicity and uptake of $HgCl_2$ and $NaAsO_2$ in rabbit renal cortical slices, *Environ. Health Perspect.*, 103, 81, 1995.
36. Hasal, S. J., Aposhian, H. V., Gandolfi, A. J., and Brendel K., Human and rabbit renal cortical slices as a model to evaluate heavy metal chelators, in *Mountain West Society of Toxicology*, Inhalation Toxicology Research Institute, Kirkland Air Force Base, Albuquerque, NM, September, 1994.
37. Lowe, T., Fernando, Q., Keith, R., and Gandolfi, A. J., Elemental analysis of renal slices by proton induced X-ray emission, *Environ. Health Perspect.*, 101, 302, 1993.
38. Wolfgang, G. H. I., Gandolfi, A. J., Stevens, J. L., and Brendel, K., *In vitro* and *in vivo* nephrotoxicity of the L and D isomers of S-(1,2-dichlorovinyl)-cysteine, *Toxicology*, 58, 33, 1989.
39. Wolfgang, G. H. I., Gandolfi, A. J., Stevens, J. L., and Brendel, K., *N*-acetyl S-(1,2-dichlorovinyl)-L-cysteine produces a similar toxicity to S-(1,2-dichlorovinyl)-L-cysteine in rabbit renal slices: differential transport and metabolism, *Toxicol. Appl. Pharmacol.*, 101, 205, 1989.
40. McGuinness, S. J., Rankin, D. R., Bezruvczyk, P., Brendel, K., and Gandolfi, A. J., Nephrotoxicity and transport of celiptium in rabbit renal proximal tubule suspensions, *In Vitro Toxicol.*, 8, 169, 1995.

chapter eight

In Vitro *Perfusion of Isolated Nephron Segments: A Method for Renal Toxicology*

Rudolfs K. Zalups and Delon W. Barfuss

8.1 Introduction 124
8.2 Historical development 124
8.3 Application to renal toxicology 124
8.4 Technical aspects and procedures 129
8.4.1 Harvesting of renal tissue 129
8.4.2 Dissection and identification of segments of the nephron 129
8.4.2.1. S1 segments of the proximal tubule 130
8.4.2.2 S2 segments of the proximal tubule 130
8.4.2.3 S3 segments of the proximal tubule 131
8.4.2.4 Cortical collecting ducts and ascending thick limbs of Henle's loop 131
8.4.2.5 Outer medullary collecting ducts and ascending thick limbs of Henle's loop 131
8.4.3 Transferring a dissected tubular segment to the perfusion chamber 132
8.4.4 Attaching a dissected tubular segment to the holding and collection pipettes 132
8.4.5 Composition of perfusing and bathing solutions 133
8.4.6 Collecting samples 134
8.4.7 Perfusion of tubular segments immersed in mineral oil 135
8.4.8 Harvesting a perfused tubular segment at the end of an experiment 135
8.4.9 Analysis of samples 137
8.4.10 Volume markers 138
8.4.11 Calculations 138
8.4.11.1 Lumen-to-bath flux 138
8.4.11.2 Bath-to-lumen flux 139
8.4.11.3 Cellular concentration of solute 139
8.4.11.4 Leak 140
8.4.12 Perfusion chamber 142
8.5 Crafting pipettes used for perfusing segments of the nephron 142
8.5.1 Holding pipette 143
8.5.2 Collection pipette 145
8.5.3 Perfusion pipette 145

0-8493-3341-5/96/$0.00+$.50

8.5.4 Constant volume pipette 145
8.5.5 Cleaning pipettes 145
8.5.6 Pipette holders 146
References 146

8.1 Introduction

The techniques of isolating and perfusing individual segments of the nephron (and collecting duct) *in vitro* have been used widely in the fields of physiology and medicine to evaluate the characteristics of transport of numerous plasma solutes along the nephron *in vivo*. Until recently, however, these techniques had apparently never been applied to the field of renal toxicology to study the transport and toxicity of nephrotoxicants along the nephron. We feel that these techniques hold much promise for investigators to gain a better understanding of the mechanisms involved in the renal transport, metabolism, and toxicity of various nephrotoxicants. Therefore, one of the major aims of this chapter is to reintroduce the isolated perfused tubule technique to investigators in the renal sciences, with a specific slant toward renal toxicology. We provide in this chapter an overview and a description of the various methods needed to carry out experiments intended to evaluate the transport, metabolism, and toxicity of nephrotoxicants in isolated perfused segments of the nephron and collecting duct.

8.2 Historical development

In the mid-1960s, the isolated perfused renal tubule technique (for studying transport and metabolism of plasma solutes along individual segments of the nephron) was developed at the National Institutes of Health under the direction of Maurice Burg.[1] After initially working out the mechanics for perfusing, Burg and colleagues discovered that the dissected tubular segments they obtained contained holes in them. The holes were found to be caused by collagenase digestion, which was used as an aid in the dissection of individual segments of the nephron. After several months of futile attempts at trying to obtain suitable specimens for perfusing, Jared J. Grantham (who was one of investigators in the group) attempted dissecting segments of the nephron from the rabbit without the aid of collagenase. His attempts proved to be successful, which made it possible for Maurice Burg to perform the first isolated perfused tubule experiment. During the initial experiments, however, Burg and colleagues found that the collection pipettes they had forged did not seal tightly around the perfused tubular segments, which allowed bathing fluid to leak into their collected samples of luminal fluid. Jared Graham solved this problem by constricting the opening of the collection pipette and coating the tip of the pipette with a thin layer of a cured elastomer (Dow Corning Sylgard 184). Since its original development, the isolated perfused tubule technique has been used extensively by numerous groups of investigators around the world.

8.3 Application to renal toxicology

Beginning in the early 1990s, we were the first investigators to begin studying and characterizing the toxicity, transport, accumulation, and metabolism of heavy metals along isolated segments of the nephron using the isolated perfused tubule technique.[2-6] One of our first studies involved examining the toxicity and transport of radiolabeled inorganic mercury ($^{203}Hg^{++}$) along isolated S1, S2, and S3 segments of the proximal tubule of the rabbit.[2] We subsequently studied the transport and toxicity of radiolabeled inorganic mercury when it was bound to compounds containing free sulfhydryl groups.[3] We have also studied the toxicity, transport, accumulation, and metabolism of cadmium,[4] cadmium–metallothionein,[5] and methylmercury[6] along isolated perfused segments of the proximal tubule.

A low power and a higher power photographic view of some of the more important components and equipment used to carry out experiments with isolated perfused tubules are presented in Figures 1 (low power view) and 2 (higher power view). In addition, Figures 3 and 4 depict a typical setup and configuration we have used to study mechanisms of transport, metabolism, and toxicity of nephrotoxic substances along isolated segments of the nephron (and collecting duct). As shown in these two figures, an individual segment of the nephron (usually 0.5 to 2.0 mm in length) is attached (at opposite ends) to a holding pipette and a collection pipette made of glass, while fluid (of any desired composition) is perfused through the lumen via the perfusion pipette, which is present inside the center of the holding pipette.

Lumen-to-bath transepithelial transport (absorption) of a toxicant can be studied by placing the toxicant in the perfusing solution (perfusate) and simultaneously measuring its rate of disappearance from the luminal compartment while measuring its rate of appearance in the bathing solution. These simultaneous measurements have proved helpful in understanding how particular segments of the nephron handle filtered plasma solutes. For example, some substances disappear from the lumen at the same rate they appear in the bathing solution, indicating very little interaction or binding with cellular components. On the other hand, some substances disappear from the luminal fluid at a much faster rate than they appear in the bathing solution. And in some instances, there are substances that disappear from the luminal fluid, but do not appear in the bathing solution. In these latter two cases, the substances being studied are being retained by some mechanism(s) in the epithelial cells of the segment being studied. This retention can be explained by any combination of the following: (1) the substances are binding to some cellular ligand(s), (2) the substances are being metabolically converted to some nonreadily transported form, and/or (3) the substances are incapable of exiting the epithelial cells across the basolateral membrane. These same insights can also be applied in experiments where the bath-to-lumen transepithelial flux (secretion) of a substance is being studied. In this particular application, the rate of bath-to-lumen transepithelial flux of a substance can be determined by measuring the rate at which the substance appears in the luminal fluid.

In both lumen-to-bath and bath-to-lumen flux studies, the intracellular concentration of a substance being studied can also be determined from the perfused segment. This information, along with bidirectional rates of flux, can be used to gain insight into the characteristics and mechanisms of transport of a particular solute across the luminal and basolateral membranes.

As stated above, a substance can be metabolized during the process of absorption or secretion by the different epithelial cells present along the nephron and collecting duct. Combining various analytical techniques with the isolated perfused tubule technique, one can determine if, and to what extent, a particular toxicant or solute is metabolized as it is translocated across the epithelium of a specific tubular segment.

In addition to evaluating the transport and metabolism of a substance, the cytotoxicity of that substance can also be evaluated simultaneously in specific segments of the nephron and collecting duct using the isolated perfused tubule technique. Cytotoxicity in isolated perfused tubular segments can be evaluated mainly by two methods. The first method is by microscopic visualization, characterization, and recording and then subsequent quantitation of pathological changes occurring along tubular segments perfused with, or exposed to, a specific toxicant. Some of the toxic or pathological effects that can be observed microscopically in the renal epithelial cells of a perfused tubular segment include cellular

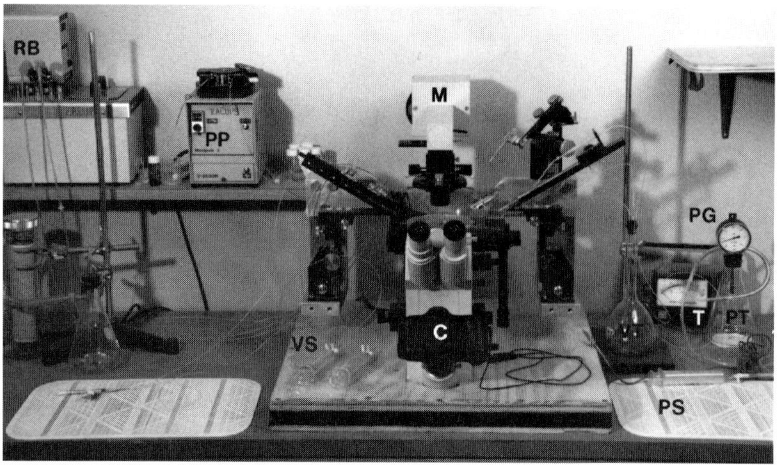

Figure 1 A photograph of a typical setup used in the perfusion and study of isolated segments of the nephron or collecting duct. In the center of the field is an inverted biological microscope (M) equipped with phase-contrast (or Normarski or Hoffman) optics and other components needed to carry out isolated perfused tubule experiments. An aluminum support system for micromanipulators is attached to the mechanical stage of the microscope. In the center of the stage is a thin cylindrical plate of Plexiglas. In the center of this cylindrical Plexiglas is the chamber in which isolated segments of the nephron and collecting duct are perfused. Also attached to the microscope is a camera (C) that is used for photomicrography. An X,Y, and Z micromanipulator is attached on the base portion of both left and right sides of the aluminum support bar. Just to the left of the base of the microscope, two vacuum syringes (VS) can be seen. These syringes are used to aid in mounting an isolated tubular segment in the holding and collection pipettes and to help draw up collected fluid. On the right side of the photograph, a pressure syringe (PS) and a pressure trap (PT) can be seen just below the platform for the microscope. The pressure syringe is used to generate positive air pressure in the pressure trap, which is used as a reservoir for pressure needed to drive the perfusate out of the perfusion pipette into and through the isolated tubular segment. The pressure trap is equipped with a pressure gauge (PG) to monitor the perfusion pressure. To the back and left of the pressure trap is a telethermometer (T), which is used to monitor the temperature of the bathing fluid in the perfusion chamber via a temperature probe. In front, and to the left of, the telethermometer is a volumetric flask, which serves as a vacuum trap (VT). Polyethylene tubing goes into the vacuum trap from a vacuum system and reservoir (part of which is seen in the lower portion of the left side of the photograph). The vacuum trap is connected to a pipette mounted on a micromanipulator set on the top of the aluminum support bar. This pipette is used to maintain a constant volume of bathing fluid in the perfusion chamber and to collect samples of the bath. On the left side of the photograph, a thermoregulated recirculating bath (RB) and peristaltic pump (PP) can be seen. The recirculating bath is used to heat the perfusion chamber and bathing fluid to the desired temperature, and the peristaltic pump is used to deliver the bathing solution into the perfusion chamber via a piece of polyethylene tubing.

swelling, formation of intracellular vacuoles, shedding of the brush border (from proximal tubular epithelial cells), bleb-formation, and necrosis. Visualization and confirmation of cellular necrosis is best accomplished when the perfusing solution contains a vital dye (such as FD&C green No. 3, mol wt = 809 Da) that is excluded from the cytoplasm of healthy, viable epithelial cells. The second way is by evaluating the effect(s) of a toxicant on the tubular transport (or lack of transport) of well-characterized substances (such as certain volume makers, sugars, amino acids, etc.). For instance, when renal tubular epithelial cells have become significantly injured after being exposed to a toxicant, their intercellular junctions become leaky, which allows small molecules to pass through them. Measurement of tubular leak of volume markers (such as ^{3}H-L-glucose, which is not

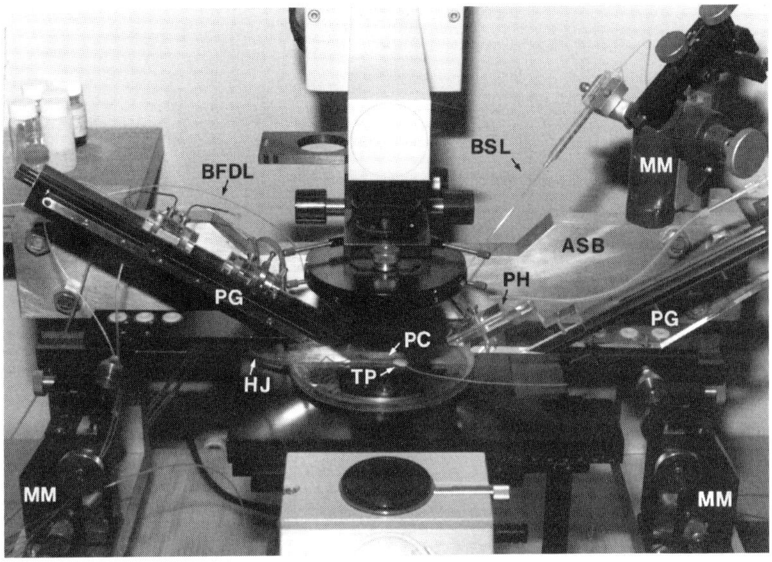

Figure 2 This photograph shows a higher power view of the apparatus surrounding the perfusion (bathing) chamber (PC). One can see that the micromanipulators (MM) mounted on the left and right platforms of the aluminum support bar (ASB) have pipette guides (PG) mounted on them. Pipette holders (PH), which are used to move and secure in place the pipettes used to perfuse a tubular segment, are mounted on the guides. The pipette guide and holders on the left side of the stage are used to hold and move the holding and perfusion pipettes, while the pipette guide and holder on the right side of the stage are used to hold and move the collection and constant volume pipettes. A temperature probe (TP) can be seen at the side of the perfusion chamber. The bathing fluid delivery line (BFDL) coming from the peristaltic pump and the bath siphon line (BSL) going to the vacuum trap can also be seen. Generally the bathing fluid delivery line is wrapped around the copper heating jacket (HJ) used to heat the perfusion chamber. This helps to efficiently heat the bathing fluid. Also seen in the photograph is the micromanipulator (MM) to support the bath siphon line, which is used to maintain a constant volume of fluid in the perfusion chamber and to collect samples of bathing fluid for analysis.

transported by renal epithelial cells) is an effective means of evaluating the level of epithelial integrity of an intoxicated perfused segment of the nephron. Moreover, if a toxicant affects oxidative metabolism significantly, then sodium-dependent transport (either luminal or basolateral) of numerous plasma solutes (such as L-amino acids and D-glucose) would be affected greatly. The magnitude of this effect can be determined in each of the specific segments of the nephron and collecting duct.

Toxic effects can be specific for a particular transport process, or they can be general, affecting many cellular processes. With the isolated perfused tubule technique, one can determine whether a toxic substance influences a single transport system or multiple transport processes.

There are several unique features of the isolated perfused tubule technique. One is that an intact tubular epithelium (including the tubular basal lamina), in which the *in vivo* orientation and polarity of the epithelial cells are maintained can be studied. This is in contrast to some other *in vitro* renal systems, in which bipolar orientation is lost and some dedifferentiation of the tubular epithelial cells occurs. Another unique feature is that the investigator has complete control over the luminal and basolateral environment surrounding the perfused tubular segment. The physical condition and composition of both the perfusing and bathing solutions can be very carefully controlled and manipulated. For example, ionic and osmotic composition; presence or absence of toxicants; presence or

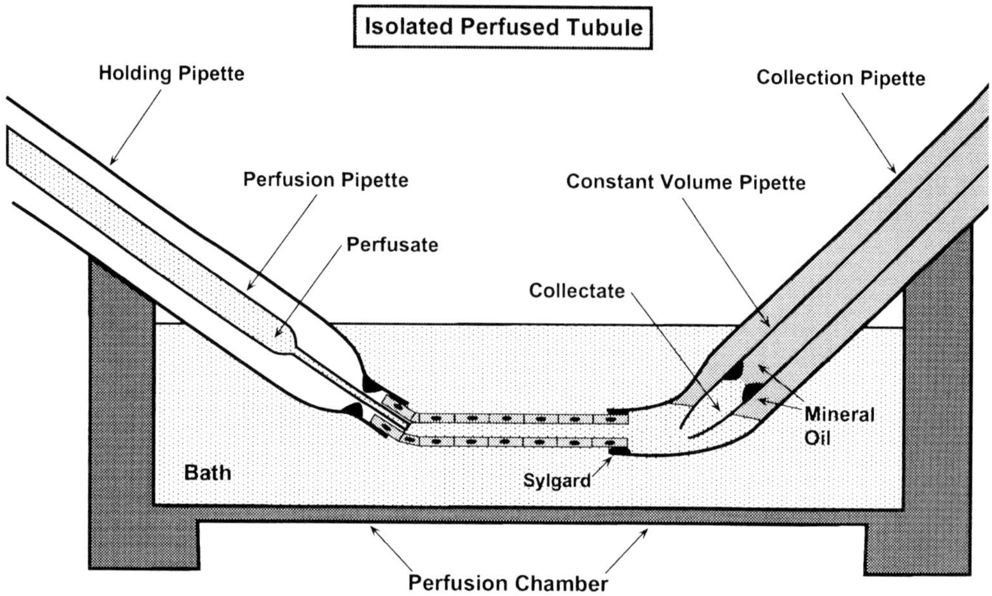

Figure 3 A schematic diagram illustrating the important features of the isolated perfused tubule technique. As can be seen, a segment of the nephron or collecting duct is attached to, and suspended between, a holding pipette (on the left) and a collection pipette (on the right) while it is immersed in a bathing solution (which is normally exchanged at a chosen rate) present in the perfusion chamber. The base of the perfusion (or bathing) chamber is made from a coverslip for a microscope slide and is generally positioned over the objective lens of an inverted biological microscope. This allows one to visualize all aspects of a perfused tubular segment during an experiment. After a tubular segment is first suspended between the holding and collection pipettes, a perfusion pipette is guided down inside the center of the holding pipette until the tip of the perfusion pipette is in the lumen of the tubular segment. Once the perfusion pipette is in place, fluid that was preloaded in the pipette is perfused into the lumen of the tubule. Fluid and solutes that are not reabsorbed, or that are secreted into the lumen, are collected at the opposite end of the perfused segment by the collection pipette. The fluid that enters the tip of the collection pipette can then be collected by a constant volume (volumetric) pipette, which is placed down the center of the collection pipette through a layer of mineral oil used to prevent evaporation of collected samples. This pipette is usually designed to hold 20 to 50 nl. Samples of collectate, perfusate, and bathing solution are generally analyzed for content of a specific solute being studied. With the isolated perfused tubule technique, one can measure both lumen-to-bath and bath-to-lumen transport of solutes, including nephrotoxicants.

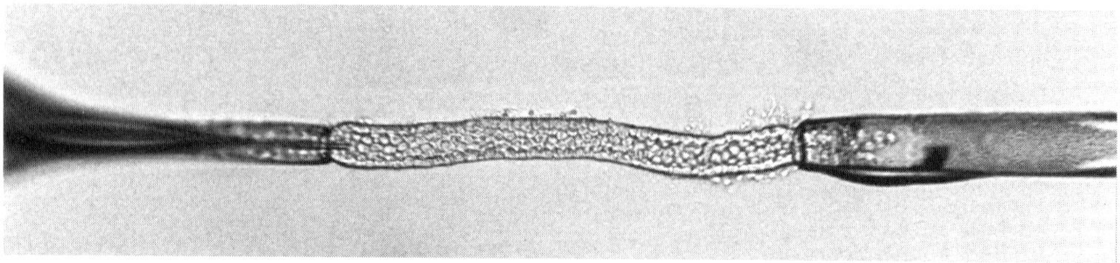

Figure 4 Photomicrograph of an S2 segment of a proximal tubule from the kidney of a rabbit being perfused through the lumen with a simple electrolyte solution. On the left side of this photomicrograph, the S2 segment is being held in place by the holding pipette. The perfusion pipette can be seen within the center of the holding pipette and projecting into the lumen of the S2 segment. On the right side, the perfused S2 segment is being held in place by the collection pipette. The volumetric pipette cannot be seen in this view.

absence of amino acids, proteins, hormones, and/or other plasma solutes; temperature; transepithelial hydrostatic pressure; and other factors can all be controlled. This capability gives this technique a great advantage over other *in vivo* and *in vitro* renal systems, in which the tubular environment cannot be very well controlled.

In summary, the isolated perfused tubule technique is one of the most powerful techniques that one can use to study the renal tubular transport, metabolism, and toxicity of nephrotoxic substances.

8.4 Technical aspects and procedures

The isolated perfused tubule technique allows access to segments of the nephron that are otherwise inaccessible for examination with other methods. In the rabbit, virtually every segment of the nephron has been studied using the isolated perfused tubule technique. Other species, such as rats, mice, snakes, salamanders and frogs are also being used, but because of difficulties in tubular dissection, only a few segments can be studied. The discussion in this chapter focuses on dissection and perfusion of segments of the nephron and collecting duct obtained from the kidneys of rabbits.

8.4.1 Harvesting of renal tissue

Prior to obtaining renal tubular segments from a rabbit (the younger the better), the animal should be anesthetized with a combination of ketamine (70 mg/kg) and xylazine (30 mg/kg) administered intramuscularly. After anesthesia is induced, the left and/or right kidney(s) is/are removed through an abdominal incision and is/are quickly cut (with a razor blade) into 1-mm-thick coronal sections, which are placed in a cold (on ice) phosphate/sucrose buffer solution used for the preservation of renal tissue.[7] Each kidney will provide at least eight to ten sections or slices. We have found that these slices can be used for up to 8 h to obtain segments for perfusion if they are kept on ice. One can also perfuse about 60 ml of the cold phosphate/sucrose buffer solution through the renal vasculature *in situ* before harvesting the kidney. In our hands, this more extensive procedure has proved to be unnecessary. The only advantage this protocol provides is that the kidney(s) is/are cleared of blood and the clotting factors found in blood. This aids in preventing the tubular segments from becoming sticky and difficult to dissect and transfer to the perfusion chamber.

8.4.2 Dissection and identification of segments of the nephron

In general, a couple of pairs of very fine tipped forceps and/or dissecting needles are required to dissect individual segments of the nephron and collecting duct. In all instances, care must be taken not to pull or stretch a tubular segment excessively during the process of tubular isolation and dissection. The forceps of choice for dissection are Dumont No. 5. The tips of these forceps should be filed down with very fine sandpaper (5- to 30-μm grain size) to obtain a tapered sharp tip while one is viewing the forceps through a dissecting microscope. To prevent stretching a tubular segment or placing holes in it during the process of dissection, one must pull the tubular segment by its ends with minimal force so that the outside diameter of the tubule does not become smaller. Too much tension on the tubule will disrupt the epithelial cells from one another and the basal lamina. To minimize the tension that is required to separate a prospective tubule from its place among other segments of the nephron, one can strip other tubular segments away until only two to five tubules remain attached in a bundle. Then the prospective tubule can be grabbed by one of its ends and can be gently pulled free. All dissection should be done under a binocular dissecting microscope.

Once a tubular segment has been dissected free, it can be visually inspected for disrupted or damaged areas (which generally appear as opaque, "milky" spots). If the segment passes initial inspection, then the ends of the segment are trimmed. This is usually necessary because the ends have been damaged by the forceps or dissecting needles during dissection. Trimming the ends of the tubular segment is accomplished by using the sharp edges of two 20-gauge hypodermic needles as scissors. One needle is placed across the segment at the location to be cut, with the point of the needle held on the bottom of dissecting dish (petri dish). The second needle is then drawn across the tubule in such a manner that the two sharp edges of the needles slice past each other like the blades of a pair of scissors. This trimming approach prevents crushing the ends of the tubule closed, which would render the tubular segment nonperfusable. After trimming, the tubular segment is ready to be transferred to the perfusion chamber.

Identification of the various segments of the nephron is accomplished primarily by anatomical or zonal location and structural characteristics unique to each segment. The following are characteristics used to identify the three segments of the proximal tubule (S1, S2, and S3), cortical collecting ducts, cortical thick ascending limbs of the loop of Henle, outer medullary segments of the collecting duct, and outer medullary portions of thick ascending limbs of the loop of Henle.

8.4.2.1 *S1 segments of the proximal tubule*

S1 segments of the proximal tubule are dissected from the cortical region of the 1-mm-thick coronal slices of kidney. They are identified by their large outside diameter and very convoluted shape. Occasionally a renal corpuscle is found to be attached to the isolated S1 segment, which serves as positive identification for this segment. To obtain S1 segments, the kidney slices are pulled in half, along the natural cleavage plane, from the tip of the papilla to the capsular surface overlying the outer cortex. The free edges of each of the two cleaved wedge-shaped portions of renal tissue are then probed for ends of S1 segments, which on occasion are found dangling free. Subcapsular, midcortical, or juxtamedullary S1 segments can be selected by noting the region of the cortex from which they are dissected. By gently pulling on the free end of the segment and teasing it free from the surrounding tubular segments, an S1 segment can be obtained. If the segment is found to be sufficiently long enough, one should grab the end of the segment at the point where it is still attached to the surrounding tubules and gently pull it free. Subsequently the free ends of the dissected tubular segment should be trimmed.

8.4.2.2 *S2 segments of the proximal tubule*

S2 segments of the proximal tubule are found in the medullary rays and are identified as tubules that span the entire length of the cortex and have a very straight shape. The S2 segments have a larger diameter than any other segments of the nephron present in the medullary rays. The best approach to dissect and isolate S2 segments of the proximal tubule is to first pull a wedge-shaped strip of renal tissue from a 1-mm-thick coronal slice of the kidney while viewing the slice of tissue through a dissecting microscope. The wedge is pulled apart systematically along its longitudinal axis, from the tip of the papilla to the outer cortex (with fine forceps), which is the natural cleavage plane running parallel to the direction of most straight segments of the nephron. Continuing this process results in the wedge of renal tissue becoming progressively smaller until there is only a small bundle of tubules remaining. During the process of dissection, one must keep in mind, at all times, where the representative zones of the kidney are located in the wedge of tissue. This will aid in identifying specific segments of the nephron. When the wedge of tissue has become small enough, an individual tubular segment can be identified for isolation. All but one or two of the remaining tubules near the prospective S2 tubular segment are stripped away, during which one avoids pulling on the prospective tubule. Then, one end of the prospective tubule is grabbed and gently stripped free from the remaining tubules. The free ends of the dissected S2 segment are then trimmed as described above.

8.4.2.3 S3 segments of the proximal tubule

The S3 segment of the proximal tubule is identified as the last 1 mm of the proximal straight tubule that is attached to the descending thin limb of Henle's loop. The S3 segment can be dissected and isolated in two ways. The easiest method is to look for loose ends of descending thin limbs of Henle's loop, which are common in the region of the inner stripe of the outer medulla. Once a loose end of a descending thin limb is identified, one can grab the thin descending limb and pull it gently toward the corticomedullary junction. The S3 segment that is continuous with the thin limb will usually strip free until it reaches the corticomedullary junction. At this junction, the beginning of the S3 segment can be grabbed with another pair of forceps and pulled free. Once free, the thin descending limb can be trimmed off. If the loose end of a thin descending limb cannot be found, then S3 segments can be isolated from a group of straight-appearing tubules in the region of the corticomedullary junction, which one can grab and pull toward the inner medullary region to free. With a group of tubules isolated, an S3 segment can be identified by its larger outer diameter and dissected free with blunt dissection, as described for the S2 segments.

8.4.2.4 Cortical collecting ducts and ascending thick limbs of Henle's loop

Cortical collecting ducts are dissected from the column of tubules in the medullary rays, which contain proximal straight tubules, thick ascending limbs of Henle's loop, and a few cortical collecting ducts. The approach is to strip away the proximal straight tubules until a cortical collecting duct is visualized (which is usually attached to the side of one or more cortical thick ascending limbs). It can be identified by its smaller diameter and somewhat granular appearance (due to the presence of principal cells and intercalated cells). These segments do not dissect as cleanly as the pars recta (straight) segments of proximal tubules. They usually are perfused with small portions (50 to 100 μm) of thick ascending limbs attached. Removing these portions of thick ascending limbs is generally risky, since this can disrupt the basal lamina of the cortical collecting duct.

Cortical thick ascending limbs of the loop of Henle are also dissected from the medullary rays in the cortex with the same approach that is used to dissect cortical collecting ducts. When the bundle of tubules in a medullary ray is reduced to a few segments, the thick ascending limb can be identified by its small outside diameter and frail appearance. The outer diameter of the cortical thick ascending limbs of the loop of Henle is smaller than the outer diameter of cortical collecting ducts. The frail appearance of these segments comes from the epithelial cells being very flat, or squamous (about 2 μm in thickness). The tubule can be pulled away from the remaining tubules with gentle dissection. Because of its frailty, the thick ascending limb is difficult to dissect free from other segments in the medullary rays.

8.4.2.5 Outer medullary collecting ducts and ascending thick limbs of Henle's loop

Outer medullary collecting ducts and ascending thick limbs of the loop of Henle are obtained from wedges of renal tissue from the inner stripe region of the outer medulla. The tubular segments found in this zone of the kidney are descending thin limbs and ascending thick limbs of the loop of Henle and outer medullary segments of the collecting duct. One can differentiate the ascending thick limbs from the collecting ducts on the basis of two main structural characteristics. The outer medullary segments of the collecting duct tend to be somewhat granular in appearance (because they also contain both principal and intercalated cells), and they are more translucent than the medullary ascending thick limbs. Ascending thick limbs in the inner stripe of the outer medulla also have a slightly smaller outer diameter than that of collecting ducts in this same zone. The ascending thick limbs tend to be more hardy and resilient in appearance than any of the other segments in the inner stripe of the outer medulla.

8.4.3 *Transferring a dissected tubular segment to the perfusion chamber*

Transferring an isolated segment of the nephron or collecting duct to the perfusion chamber can be somewhat difficult to master. It is accomplished with a 1.0-ml plastic syringe attached to the transfer pipette. With one hand, one brings the open end of the transfer pipette very near to, but not touching, the trimmed tubular segment, which is lying free on the bottom of a dissection dish. With the free hand, one draws out the plunger of the 1.0-ml syringe slowly until the tubule, with a little of the dissecting fluid, is sucked 1 to 2 mm into the transfer pipette. If a minimal amount of fluid is drawn into the transfer pipette, the fluid and the tubule will remain stationary in the tip while the transfer pipette is relocated to the perfusion chamber. While one views through the compound microscope to which the perfusion chamber is attached, the tip of the transfer pipette is placed into the bathing solution present in the perfusion chamber. Gently pushing the plunger of the 1-ml syringe will force the fluid with the tubule out of the transfer pipette into the bathing fluid of perfusion chamber. Caution should be taken to avoid pushing too hard or quickly on the plunger or air bubbles will form in the bathing solution and the tubule may be lost. If executed properly, the tubular segment will be seen slowly coming out of the transfer pipette and settling onto the bottom of the perfusion chamber (which consists of a thin microscope coverslip). If the transfer pipette is new and has not been used, there is a strong possibility that a tubular segment will stick to the inside wall of the pipette. This problem can be minimized by repeatedly using the same transfer pipette and not cleaning it too thoroughly after use. It is best if the pipette is cleaned with a quick rinse of distilled water and then dried with acetone and air suction.

8.4.4 *Attaching a dissected tubular segment to the holding and collection pipettes*

Once a dissected tubular segment is transferred to the perfusion chamber and has settled to the bottom, it will probably need to be oriented parallel to the long axis of the chamber to make one of its free ends available to be sucked into the holding pipette. This is best accomplished by nudging the tubule with a glass needle (made from a glass rod having a diameter of 2.0 mm). Once the tubule is in place, the holding pipette is maneuvered with the aid of a micromanipulator (to which it is attached) so that the open end of the pipette is about 25 to 50 μm from the end of the tubule. This places the tip of the holding pipette on, or very close to, the bottom of the perfusion chamber. Caution should be used while moving the pipette around or it can be easily broken by coming in contact with the bottom of the perfusion chamber. When the pipette and tubular segment are in position, gentle suction is manually applied to the holding pipette with a 30- to 50-ml glass syringe attached by polyethylene tubing to the pipette. This suction will pull the closest free end of the tubule into the holding pipette to the alignment constriction of the holding pipette (Figures 3 and 4). Too much suction will pull the tubule completely into the holding pipette, and the tubule will be lost. This can also ruin the holding pipette. Next, the holding pipette, with the tubule attached, is maneuvered by a micromanipulator (Figure 2) off the bottom of the perfusion chamber approximately 1 to 2 mm. The perfusion pipette is then advanced through the alignment constriction of the holding pipette into the lumen of the tubule (Figure 3). Pressure is gently applied to the fluid in the perfusion pipette to force perfusion fluid into the lumen of the tubule. One monitors this process through the microscope by watching the lumen of the tubule progressively open up from the perfusion end to the free end. With the lumen open, the tubular epithelial cells can be inspected more closely for damage. Once it has been determined that the tubular segment is healthy, the perfusion pipette is advanced until its tip is just beyond the opening of the holding pipette.

With the tubule being perfused through the lumen, the collection pipette can be attached. It is brought into place 25 to 50 μm from the remaining free end of the tubular segment. The end of the collection pipette is sealed with 50 to 100 μm of a liquid elastomer that has been placed there to prevent bathing fluid from freely flowing into the collection pipette and sealing the tubule in the collection pipette. As with attaching the holding pipette, manual suction is applied to the collection pipette with a 30- to 50-ml glass syringe. Extreme caution is required when applying this suction or the tubule will be pulled out of the holding pipette and drawn completely into the collection pipette. This suction should be applied with very light pulses. The proper pulse will pull a small volume of bathing solution through the liquid elastomer with the tubule close behind. If performed properly, about 50 to 100 μm of the tubular segment will be pulled into the collection pipette, and the liquid elastomer (Sylgard 184) will flow back to the tip and around the tubule making a tight seal between the bathing solution and the collectate. The maturation of this seal may take 5 to 10 min as the bathing fluid is warmed to 38°C.

If excess bathing fluid is drawn into the collection pipette while one is attaching the tubule, it will need to be removed and the collection pipette cleaned. This is done by placing a cleaning pipette into the collection pipette with its tip at the narrow junction of the collection pipette and sucking the excess bathing fluid into the cleaning pipette. With the cleaning pipette still in place, about 500 μl of water is placed in the collection pipette via the cleaning pipette. This water is sucked out and replaced with about 750 μl of acetone, which is then sucked out of the collection pipette. This cleaning procedure will clean all the aqueous solution out of the collection pipette. If this is not done, samples of perfused fluid are difficult to collect, and they will be contaminated with bathing solution that entered while the tubule was being attached. Subsequently, the cleaning pipette is removed, cleaned, and filled with about 25 μl of light mineral oil by oral suction. Next, this light mineral oil is placed in the collection pipette on top of the sample being collected. This prevents evaporation of water from the sample. This is accomplished with oral pressure forcing the oil out of the cleaning pipette after the tip of the cleaning pipette is placed on, or very near, the surface of the collected fluid.

8.4.5 *Composition of perfusing and bathing solutions*

In many experiments, it is desirable to have the perfusing and bathing solutions be simple electrolyte solutions that can be easily controlled and modified. In many of our studies, we use a perfusing solution that contains the following: 145 m*M* Na^+, 140 m*M* Cl^-, 5 m*M* K^+, 2.5 m*M* Ca^{2+}, 1.2 m*M* Mg^{2+}, 1.2 m*M* SO_4^{2-}, 2 m*M* $HPO_4^{2-}/H_2PO_4^-$, and 1 m*M* D-glucose, with pH adjusted to 7.4. In experiments where the cytotoxicity of a nephrotoxicant is being evaluated, it is useful to have the vital dye FD&C green No. 3 (mol wt = 809 Da) in the perfusate at a concentration of 250 n*M*.

In general, the composition of the bathing solution in our experiments is the same as the composition perfusing solution, except that the bathing solution contains 0.5 m*M* glutamine or glutamate as a substrate for energy metabolism.

When it is desirable to mimic closely the *in vivo* state, isolated segments of the nephron can be perfused with an ultrafiltrate of rabbit plasma, which can be made by filtering samples of rabbit plasma through a 50,000 mol wt cutoff filter. In addition, the perfused tubular segments can be separately or simultaneously bathed in rabbit plasma.

In general, a great deal of control over the fluid environment surrounding a perfused segment of the nephron is afforded an investigator using the isolated perfused tubule technique.

8.4.6 Collecting samples

Samples of luminal fluid exiting from a perfused tubular segment (collectate) and bathing solution are collected for each perfused tubule in order to measure lumen-to-bath (or bath-to-lumen) flux (moles [generally femtomoles] per minute per millimeter) of a solute and a volume marker. This is accomplished by measuring the rate of disappearance of the solute and volume marker from the luminal fluid and the rate of appearance of that solute and volume marker into the bathing solution.

As shown in Figure 3, samples of perfused fluid entering the collection pipette are collected into a constant volume pipette (50 to 100 nl) that is advanced through the layer of oil at the tip of the collection pipette. As the constant volume pipette is advanced through the layer of oil, suction is applied orally or by a syringe to fill the constant volume pipette to its constriction with oil. The collection pipette is then advanced until its tip barely penetrates into the aqueous collectate. The collectate is drawn into the constant volume pipette with suction until the level of the collectate in the collection pipette is lowered to the elbow (30° bend) in the collection pipette. This point in the elbow region of the collection pipette will serve as the end reference point to which all subsequent collectate samples are drawn. The first sample of collectate is discarded as waste, and the constant volume pipette is cleaned by rinsing it three times with water and then dried with acetone and accompanying vacuum. This is the standard cleaning procedure used for all the pipettes when they need cleaning after an experiment. The collection pipette is cleaned between every collected sample. The cleaned constant volume pipette is then placed back into the center of the collection pipette and is advanced toward the collectate in the tip of the collection pipette. Suction needs to be applied on the constant volume pipette as it is passed through the oil, so that by the time the tip of the pipette reaches the collectate it will be filled with light mineral oil. During the time required to clean the constant volume pipette and replace it in position in the collection pipette, 10 to 20 nl of collectate will have accumulated. This is drawn into the constant volume pipette so the level of collectate is lowered to the reference point of the collection pipette. The filling of the constant volume pipette with collectate is monitored through the microscope. If the microscope is a compound microscope, it will require a 1 to 2× objective to visualize the reference point and the constriction of the constant volume pipette simultaneously. Any objective with greater magnification has too narrow of a focal plane and visual field to see both ends of the constant volume pipette chamber simultaneously. The time required to fill the constant volume pipette is used to calculate the volume collection rate (nanoliters per minute).

During a typical lumen-to-bath flux experiment, the bathing solution is routinely collected and analyzed for the appearance of the solute (being studied) and volume marker into the bathing solution. The sampling is accomplished easily, in part because the bathing solution is continuously flowing through the perfusion chamber at a constant rate (generally around 0.3 ml min^{-1}). The bathing fluid is delivered to the perfusion chamber with a peristaltic pump (Figure 1) that forces bathing fluid into one end of the chamber while vacuum aspirates the fluid out of the chamber at the opposite end at the same rate. This keeps the level of the bathing fluid constant and exchanges the complete volume of bathing fluid three times per minute (chamber volume is generally around 0.3 ml). The aspirated bathing solution is collected in 20-ml scintillation vials configured into a vacuum trap. Scintillation vials are changed every 5 min during experiments. Usually, the solute being studied is radiolabeled, and therefore scintillation fluid is generally added directly into the vial containing the collected bathing solution, which is later assayed for the presence of the radiolabel being used.

8.4.7 Perfusion of tubular segments immersed in mineral oil

A unique variation of isolating and perfusing tubules is to perfuse them while they are immersed in mineral oil, as depicted in Figure 5.[8,9] This results in the absorbed fluid (absorbate), which contains reabsorbed solutes, collecting on the contraluminal (capillary) side of the tubular basal lamina. The physical force present at the oil–aqueous interface results in the absorbate collecting in the form of torus-shaped droplets at regular intervals along the perfused tubule. It has been shown that each torus-shaped droplet of absorbate is isolated from the other droplets of absorbate.[10] This isolation prevents solutes in the droplets from diffusing laterally along the tubule. These droplets of absorbate can be collected with a small (1 to 5 nl) constant volume pipette as individual droplets or they can be pushed together with a glass needle and taken up collectively. With these characteristics, the lumen-to-absorbate transport of a toxic substance can be studied in terms of how concentrated a solute or toxicant can become in the basolateral fluid environment adjacently lining a tubular segment. Analysis of each individual droplet of absorbate from a perfused tubule (2 mm or longer) can provide insight to any longitudinal heterogeneity of transport and metabolism of a solute or toxicant.

There are some special maneuvers required to perfuse tubules that are immersed in light mineral oil. Each tubular segment is initially perfused normally in an aqueous bathing solution. A 5-mm layer of light mineral oil is placed on top of the aqueous bathing solution. The bathing solution is then aspirated through an exit port at the bottom of the perfusion chamber. As the aqueous bathing solution is removed, the light mineral oil lowers and surrounds the perfusing tubule and the pipettes. S1 segments of proximal tubules slide into the oil very easily, whereas S2 and S3 segments resist going into the oil. When the layer of oil comes in contact with these segments at the oil–water interface, the S2 and S3 segments prefer to remain with the aqueous bathing solution. To prevent the tubule from being pulled out of the holding and collection pipettes, suction is applied to both the holding and collection pipettes until the oil layer is low enough to cover the tubule. Once the tubular segment is pulled into the oil, it relaxes and perfuses normally, except that higher hydrostatic pressure (10 to 15 mmHg) is usually required to keep the tubule perfusing. This higher perfusion pressure does not appear to increase the luminal hydrostatic pressure, as indicated by the shape of the tubular epithelial cells remaining unchanged. In general, they become flattened in appearance when the transepithelial hydrostatic pressure is much above 20 mmHg. The pressure gradient appears to be at the absorbate–oil interface, which does not change the transepithelial pressure (transmural pressure).

Tubular segments perfused immersed in oil are more viable than tubules perfused in artificial peritubular fluid. Segments of the proximal tubule perfused in a typical aqueous bathing solution lose about 5% of their function per hour. This is usually not a problem, since most experiments are complete within an hour of beginning perfusion. On the other hand, segments of proximal tubules have been perfused immersed in oil for up to 3.5 h with no diminution in the rate of fluid volume absorption. It is speculated that a perfused tubule under oil is surrounded by a fluid environment that more closely approximates the tubular fluid environment found *in vivo*. The fluid that is in direct contact with the basolateral membrane of these perfused tubules generally contains higher concentrations of preferentially absorbed solutes (D-glucose, bicarbonate, amino acids, etc.) than the fluid found around tubules bathed with a standard aqueous bath.

8.4.8 Harvesting a perfused tubular segment at the end of an experiment

In order to calculate the cellular concentration of a toxicant in an isolated perfused segment of the nephron, it is necessary to harvest the perfused tubule at the end of the experiment.

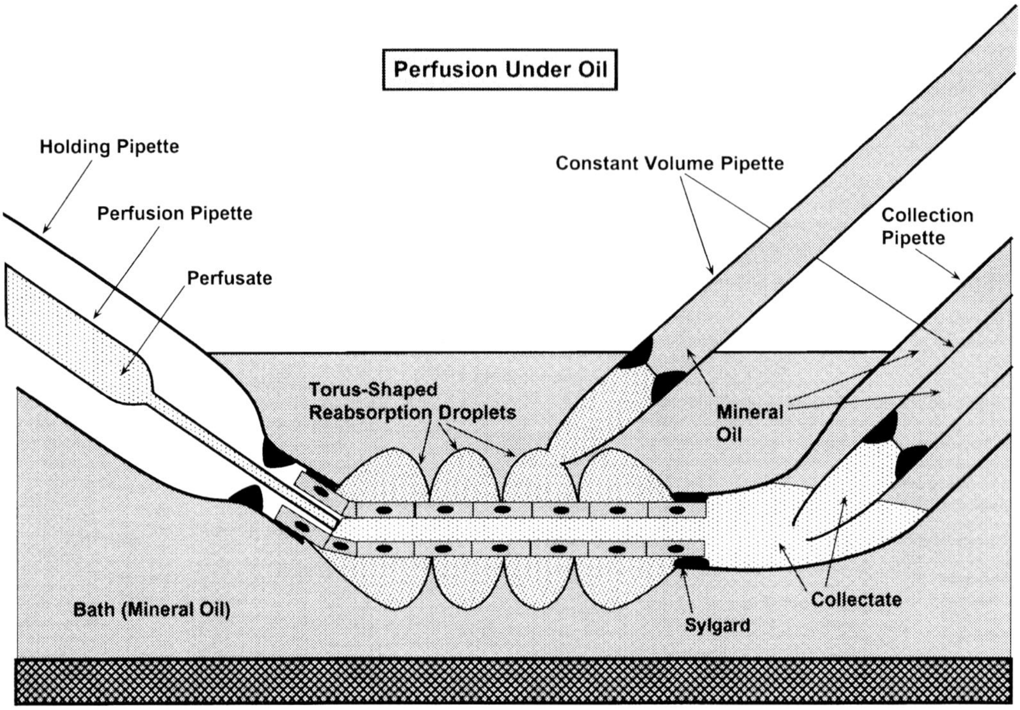

Figure 5 A schematic drawing illustrating a modification of the isolated perfused tubule technique used to evaluate the composition of reabsorbed fluid emanating from the basolateral membrane of an isolated perfused segment of the nephron or collecting duct immersed in mineral oil. In this modification of the isolated perfused tubule technique, an isolated renal tubular segment is first suspended between a holding and a collection pipette in a typical aqueous bathing solution and then is perfused through the lumen with some type of an aqueous perfusate. Once the tubular segment has been suspended between the holding and collection pipettes, the bathing solution is removed from the bathing chamber in a retrograde manner and is replaced with a light-weight mineral oil. When the tubular segment becomes completely surrounded with oil, torus-shaped reabsorption droplets form on the extracellular surface of the basolateral membrane of the epithelial cells lining the perfused tubular segment. These droplets can be taken up in timed collections with a constant volume (volumetric) pipette, and the rate of fluid formation and the concentration of solutes in the fluid can be determined subsequently. This technique may prove to be very useful in evaluating the transport and leak of nephrotoxicants across the basolateral membrane after they have left the luminal fluid. By knowing the composition of the fluid environment bathing the basolateral membrane of a segment of the nephron or collecting duct, much can be gained in understanding the factors and mechanisms involved in the handling of a solute (nephrotoxicant) in that tubular segment.

The tubular segment is harvested while it is being perfused, by grabbing it near the end attached to the holding pipette with a pair of fine forceps (preferably Dumont No. 5). It is then pulled free from the holding, perfusion, and collection pipettes, and removed from the bathing solution, and placed in 10 μl of 3% (w/v) trichloroacetic acid (TCA). This maneuver takes less than 1 s to complete. During this short time interval, very little of a rapidly transported solute will exit the cells of the tubular epithelium. Plastic tissue-typing dishes that have small 10-μl wells are commonly used. With the tip of the forceps holding the tubule in the TCA solution, the tissue-typing dish and the forceps are moved in unison to the stage of a dissecting microscope. While one is viewing the tubular segment, it is shaken free from the forceps. The TCA precipitates all the larger cellular proteins and releases the cytosolic contents. This process occurs within a few seconds after the tubular segment is placed in the TCA solution and can be documented by the appearance of the tubular segment changing to an opaque white color. After a few minutes, the tubular segment is removed from the TCA solution and is placed in a vial of scintillation fluid and analyzed later (by standard isotopic methods) for the content of the solute or toxicant being studied. The presence of the solute or toxicant in this TCA-precipitable fraction of the tubular segment indicates that the solute or toxicant is in some manner associated with the larger proteins of the epithelial cells. The soluble fraction of the tubular segment that is mixed in the TCA solution is added to scintillation fluid and is also assayed for the solute or toxicant. The data obtained from the TCA-soluble and TCA-precipitable fractions and the estimate of cellular volume of water permits one to approximate the cellular concentration of the solute or toxicant being studied. The value for the cellular concentration that is obtained by the method outlined above should be considered as a minimal or low estimate if one assumes that the solute being studied is distributed equally in all cellular compartments. This is probably not the case. Many solutes are confined to restricted regions or compartments within the tubular epithelial cells, and therefore they are at greater concentrations in these compartments than is being calculated on the basis of uniform distribution. Another possible error resulting in the estimation of the cellular concentration of a solute is that some fraction of the radiolabel used to follow and measure a particular solute may no longer be associated with the solute as a result of metabolism. To correct for this potential error, a portion of the TCA-precipitable fraction of the tubular segment must be analyzed by some method to determine the percentage of the radiolabel that remains associated with the original solute being studied.

8.4.9 Analysis of samples

Since samples of fluid obtained from isolated perfused tubules are small (sometimes as little as 20 nl), very sensitive analytical methods must used for determining the concentration of solutes in these samples. In most cases, chemical analysis is incapable of detecting solutes in the amounts that they are present in the collected samples. Since only a few samples can be collected from each perfused tubular segment, the analytical techniques used must be precise and repeatable. For these reasons, compounds labeled with radioisotopes (γ- and/or β-emitters) are most commonly used in isolated perfused tubule experiments, inasmuch as they can be detected accurately in very small quantities (femtomoles).

Coupling the use of radiolabeled compounds with HPLC (high-performance liquid chromatography), when one is analyzing samples from isolated perfused tubules can be helpful in determining the extent to which a substance is metabolized as it is transepithelially transported from lumen to bath or from bath to lumen. In essence, HPLC can be used to separate the original radiolabeled compound from any radiolabeled metabolites. This is accomplished by adding enough nonlabeled compound to the sample so the detection system (UV or fluorescence) on the HPLC can detect when the compound being studied is coming off the HPLC column. This portion of the HPLC effluent can be collected, and the amount of radioactivity can be quantitated with standards and compared to the total amount of radioactivity that was in the whole (all of the effluent) sample. With this procedure, one can determine the percentage of the original radiolabeled compound that remains intact. This approach has proved very effective in the study of adenosine transport.[11] This same approach can also be very helpful when studying the transport and renal metabolism of nephrotoxic compounds.

Mass spectrometry is another very sensitive method that can be applied to isolated perfused tubule experiments to study the transport and metabolism of toxicants. The major shortcomings of using this technique are cost and gaining access to a sensitive mass spectrometer.

8.4.10 Volume markers

The ideal volume marker is a substance that will remain in the compartment to which it is added. Consequently, any change in the concentration of a transportable substance relative to the concentration of the volume marker will indicate the rate the substance is being transported. Without a volume marker, any change in the concentration of a solute could be explained on the basis of the movement of water into or out of the tubular lumen. If the concentration of a solute in a fluid compartment is not compensated for by the change in the concentration of a volume marker in that same compartment, a miscalculation will occur when one computes rates of epithelial transport of a solute being studied. An ideal volume marker for isolated perfused tubules is one that does not adhere to cell membranes, is not transported, does not penetrate tight junctions or cell membranes, and is water soluble.

A volume marker is also required if the integrity of a tubular segment is being monitored. The rate at which the volume marker leaks from the tubular lumen into the bathing solution can be used as an indicator of the rate of nonspecific leak of a tubular segment. If this leak is too great during any one experiment, then it becomes justifiable to disregard the findings from that experiment. The generally accepted normal lumen-to-bath leak of a volume marker is about 1% of the total volume marker being perfused into the lumen via the perfusion pipette. This value may differ depending on the volume marker used. Substances most commonly used as volume markers in isolated perfused tubules are ^{3}H- or ^{14}C-inulin, ^{3}H- or ^{14}C-polyethylene glycol, and ^{3}H- or ^{14}C-L-glucose.

8.4.11 Calculations

8.4.11.1 Lumen-to-bath flux

Transport of a solute (including toxicants) in lumen-to-bath flux experiments is generally evaluated by measuring the rate at which that solute disappears from the luminal fluid (J_D, disappearance flux rate) and the rate at which it appears in the bathing solution (J_A, appearance flux rate). The disappearance flux rate of a solute (J_D, generally femtomoles per minute per millimeter), is measured by Equation 1:

$$J_D = (([Solute]_P \times V_P) - ([Solute]_C \times V_C)) \div L \tag{1}$$

where $[Solute]_P$ and $[Solute]_C$ are the concentrations (femtomoles per nanoliter) of the solute being studied in the perfusate and collectate, respectively. $[Solute]_P$ and $[Solute]_C$ are generally determined from the specific activity (sa, disintegrations per minute per femtomole) of the radioisotope being used for the solute. V_C (nanoliters per minute) is the volume collection rate, which is calculated from the time required to fill the constant volume pipette. V_P is the rate at which fluid is being perfused into the tubular segment (perfusion rate, nanoliters per minute), and is calculated by the following equation:

$$V_P = ([VM]_C \div [VM]_P) \times V_C \tag{2}$$

where $[VM]_C$ and $[VM]_P$ are the concentrations of the volume marker (usually ^{3}H-L-glucose, ^{3}H-inulin, ^{14}C-PEG) in the collectate and perfusate, respectively. When the volume marker is labeled with a traceable radioisotope, the concentration of the volume marker in either the perfusate or collectate is expressed as the amount of disintegrations per minute (dpm) of the radioisotope being used per nanoliter. L (Equation 1) is the length (millimeters) of the perfused tubular segment.

The appearance flux rate (J_A, femtomoles per minute per millimeter) of a solute is determined by Equation 3:

$$J_A = ([Solute]_B \times V_B) \div L \tag{3}$$

where $[Solute]_B$ is the concentration (femtomoles per milliliter) of the solute in the bathing solution, V_B is the rate (milliliters per minute) at which the bathing solution is being collected, and L is the length of the tubular segment being perfused. When a radioisotope is being used to study a particular solute, then J_A can be computed with a modification of Equation 3:

$$J_A = (\text{dpm}_{\text{Solute}} \div (\text{sa}_{\text{Solute}} \times T)) \div L \tag{4}$$

where $\text{dpm}_{\text{Solute}}$ is the amount of disintegrations per minute of the radioisotope being used to study the solute that appears in the bathing solution in T time (minutes), $\text{sa}_{\text{Solute}}$ is the specific activity (disintegrations per minute per femtomole) of the radioisotope used to study the solute, and L is the length (milliliters) of the tubular segment.

8.4.11.2 Bath-to-lumen flux

In bath-to lumen flux experiments one can determine the rate at which a solute appears in the luminal fluid from the bathing fluid. This appearance flux (J_{BL}, femtomoles per minute per millimeter) is calculated by measuring the rate of appearance of the solute in the lumen when it is placed in the bathing solution only. Equation 5 is used for this calculation:

$$J_{BL} = ([Solute]_C \times V_C) \div L \tag{5}$$

where $[Solute]_C$ is the concentration (femtomoles per nanoliter) of the solute in the collectate and V_C is the rate (nanoliters per minute) at which fluid is being collected in the collection pipette. This rate is calculated from the time required to fill the constant volume pipette. L in this equation is the length of the tubular segment.

When a radioisotope is being used to study the bath-to-lumen transport of a solute, then J_{BL} can be calculated with a modified form of Equation 5, which is presented below:

$$J_{BL} = (\text{dpm}_{\text{Solute}} \div (\text{sa}_{\text{Solute}} \times T)) \div L \tag{6}$$

where $\text{dpm}_{\text{Solute}}$ is the amount of disintegrations per minute of the radioisotope used for the solute that appears in the luminal fluid, $\text{sa}_{\text{Solute}}$ is the specific activity (disintegrations per minute per femtomole) of the radioisotope used for the solute, T is the time (minutes) required to collect the sample, and L is the length (millimeters) of the tubular segment. For J_{BL} to represent a unidirectional flux from bath to lumen, the perfusion rate must be rapid enough to prevent the solute from moving back into the bathing solution. A perfusion rate of at least 20 nl per minute per milliliter is usually rapid enough to prevent flux from the lumen to the bathing solution, even if the solute is actively transported.

8.4.11.3 Cellular concentration of solute

In order to calculate the cellular concentration of a solute in a perfused tubular segment, one must determine (estimate) the cellular content of water (H_2O_{Cell}) in that segment. The H_2O_{Cell} in a tubular segment is calculated in picoliters (pl) using Equation 7:

$$H_2O_{Cell} = \pi\,(OR^2 - IR^2) \times L \times 0.7 \tag{7}$$

where OR and IR are the average outer and inner tubular radii (microns), respectively, L is the length of the tubular segment (microns), and 0.7 accounts for the fraction of cellular volume that is water.[12]

Once the cellular volume or content of water has been determined, then one can go on and compute (estimate) the cellular concentration of a solute ($[Solute]_{Cell}$, molar [generally micro- or millimolar]) in a tubular segment that was perfused. Assuming that a radiolabel for the solute is used, the cellular concentration of the solute can be estimated using Equation 8:

$$[Solute]_{Cell} = (\mathrm{dpm}_{Solute} \div \mathrm{sa}_{Solute}) \div H_2O_{Cell} \tag{8}$$

where dpm_{Solute} is the disintegrations per minute of radioisotope being used for the solute that was in the TCA-soluble fraction of the perfused tubular segment, sa_{Solute} is the specific activity (disintegrations per minute per femtomole) of the radioisotope for the solute that is taken from standards, and H_2O_{Cell} is the cellular volume of water. Values for disintegrations per minute of the radioisotope for the solute are corrected for any radioactivity that may remain in the lumen. This fraction can be determined by the amount of volume marker that is extracted with the tubular segment. This correction factor is always very small (about 1% or less).

8.4.11.4 Leak

Since the epithelial cells in various segments of the nephron permit the intercellular (through junctional complexes) passage of certain solutes to varying degrees, it is important to determine, and to factor in, the magnitude of intercellular leak of a solute when computing the rates of transport of a solute in a perfused tubular segment. Ideally this leak should be measured with an isomeric form of the solute that is not actively transported by the epithelial cells. This is generally not possible. The second best option is to use a molecule that has the same molecular weight and charge. If this is not possible, then the use of an established volume marker can be used to measure rate of appearance of the solute in the bathing fluid. If the rate of appearance of the volume marker is within established normal limits, then it can generally be concluded that the tubule is intact, and the rate of appearance of the solute in the bathing solution can be computed as the sum of the amount transported and the amount that normally leaks through the tight junctions. If the appearance of the volume marker in the bathing solution is greater than its normal rate of appearance, it can be assumed that the perfused tubular segment has been structurally compromised. In intact tubular segments, the leak of established volume markers is so minimal that its value can be considered to be equal to zero. The following equations compensate for increased leak, assuming that the leak is a bulk flow of luminal fluid into the bathing solution. The following equations are not valid if increased leak is due to an increase of a diffusive leak between the cells. This leak cannot be compensated for unless one knows if the leak is specific for the volume marker or general for all solutes. If one assumes that the increased leak of the volume marker is general, then the increase in solute leak can be calculated. Taking into account this assumption, the increased rate of appearance of a solute in the bathing solution will be proportional to the increased leak of the volume marker leak into the bathing solution.

The leak of luminal fluid (L_{VM}, nanoliters per minute per millimeter) in a tubular segment is measured by the rate of appearance of the volume marker in the bathing solution. This can be determined using Equation 9.

$$L_{VM} = J_{VM} \div ([VM]_P \times L) \tag{9}$$

where J_{VM} is the rate of flux (femtomoles per minute) of the volume marker across the tubular epithelium, $[VM]_P$ is the concentration (femtomoles per nanoliter) of the volume marker in the perfusing solution, and L is the length (millimeters) of the tubular segment. J_{VM} can be computed by using the following equation:

$$J_{VM} = [VM]_B \times V_B \tag{10}$$

where $[VM]_B$ is the concentration (femtomoles per milliliter) of the volume marker in the bathing solution and V_B is the rate at which the bathing solution is collected (milliliters per minute).

When a volume marker labeled with a radioisotope is used, a more simplified version of Equation 9 can be used to compute L_{VM}. This modification is presented below as Equation 11:

$$L_{VM} = \text{dpm}_{VM} \div (\text{sa}_{VM} \times T \times L) \tag{11}$$

where dpm_{VM} is the amount of disintegrations per minute of the radioisotope on the volume marker that appears in the bathing solution in T time (minutes), sa_{VM} is the specific activity of the radiolabel on the volume marker expressed per unit liquid volume (disintegrations per minute per nanoliter), and L is the length (millimeters) of the tubular segment.

Once the intercellular leak of fluid is determined, the expected leak of the solute being studied (L_{Solute}, femtomoles per minute per millimeter) can be calculated using Equation 12:

$$L_{Solute} = L_{VM} \times [Solute]_{MLC} \tag{12}$$

where L_{VM} is the magnitude of intercellular leak of fluid (nanoliters per minute per milliliter), $[Solute]_{MLC}$ is the mean luminal concentration (femtomoles per nanoliter) of the solute being studied, and L is the length (millimeters) of the tubular segment. The mean luminal concentration of the solute being studied can be determined using the following equation:

$$[Solute]_{MLC} = ([Solute]_P + [Solute]_C) \div 2 \tag{13}$$

where $[Solute]_P$ is the concentration (femtomoles per nanoliter) of the solute in the perfusing solution (perfusate) and $[Solute]_C$ is the concentration (femtomoles per nanoliter) of the solute in the collectate. This method of calculating the mean luminal concentration of the solute is only valid if the collectate solute concentration is greater than 30% of the perfusate solute concentration.[13,14] When the collectate concentration is below 30% of perfusate concentration, the decrease in luminal solute concentration along the tubule is not linear. This is controlled by matching the perfusion rate with the transport rate and the length of the tubule. If the rate of perfusion is too slow, or the length of the tubular segment is too long, then all of the solute within the tubular lumen will disappear at some point along the tubule, which causes the collectate solute concentration to be zero. Under these conditions, it is not known how much of the tubular segment actually participated in transporting the solute, and therefore the decrease in solute concentration along the perfused tubular segment is nonlinear, and the mean luminal solute concentration calculated with Equation 13 will be greatly overestimated. If the perfusion rate is too rapid for the length of the tubule, the difference between perfusate and collectate solute concentration will be so small that the disappearance rate of the solute from the lumen cannot be calculated. To avoid all these complications the investigator should keep the concentration of the solute in the collectate between 30 to 90% of the concentration of the solute in the perfusate.

Bulk flow leak of a solute into the lumen during the bath-to-lumen flux measurements can be calculated with the same equations used to determine the amount of lumen-to-bath leak except that one would substitute bathing solution parameters for luminal parameters.

8.4.12 Perfusion chamber

The perfusion chamber is milled out of the central region of a piece of Plexiglas (1/4 to 3/8″ thick) that has been cut to fit firmly on the stage of a microscope (Figure 2). The piece of Plexiglas should also be milled so that a copper heating jacket can be placed around the perfusion chamber (to heat the bathing solution) on the underside of the piece of Plexiglas (Figure 2). In general, we have found that a perfusion chamber that is about 1.0 cm in length and 0.6 cm in depth and width (which holds a volume of about 0.3 to 0.4 ml) works very nicely for isolated perfused tubule experiments. The heating jacket, which is made of 1/8″ copper tubing, is placed and sealed (with silicone sealant) around the perfusion chamber at a distance of not greater than about 1 to 2 mm from any of the sides of the chamber. In addition to the above mentioned milling, a small hole needs to be drilled diagonally from the top of the piece of Plexiglas, through one of the walls of the perfusion chamber just above the base of the chamber. The diameter of this hole should be just large enough to accommodate the insertion of the tip of the polyethylene tubing that carries bathing fluid to the perfusion chamber. Finally, the base of the perfusion chamber is made by adhering a thin coverslip (for a microscope slide) to the underside of the piece of Plexiglas with silicone sealant, insuring that the coverslip covers completely the base of the perfusion chamber.

During experiments, the copper tubing, used as the heating jacket, is supplied with warmed or cooled water from a recirculating pump to heat or cool the bathing fluid, which is pumped into the base of the perfusion chamber through polyethylene tubing with a peristaltic pump. The water in the heating jacket must be maintained at a sufficiently high enough temperature (around 55 to 60°C) to maintain the temperature of the bathing solution at 37 to 38°C. It is also necessary to heat the bathing solution prior to its being delivered to the perfusion chamber in order to efficiently keep the temperature of the bathing solution at 37 to 38°C. This is accomplished by wrapping the polyethylene tubing carrying the bathing fluid from a reservoir around a heat exchanger. This heat exchanger is simply made by wrapping the polyethylene tubing, which is carrying the bathing solution to the perfusion chamber, around the tubing which is supplying warm water to the copper tubing of the chamber heating jacket.

During bath-to-lumen flux experiments the tubule is bathed in a nonexchangeable bath that is covered with light mineral oil to prevent evaporation of water from the bathing solution. In these conditions, heat cannot escape, so the temperature of the water in the heating jacket must be kept at 38°C to maintain 38°C in the bathing solution.

In bath-to-lumen flux experiments unstirred layers in the bathing solution are prevented by the action of a reciprocating pump connected to the bathing solution through the oil layer with polyethylene tubing (I.D. 047″). Smaller tubing will not permit adequate undulating flow because of greater surface tension of the bathing solution on the inner surface of the tubing. The reciprocating action of the pump draws about 50 µl of bathing solution in and out of the chamber, resulting in a complete mixing of the bathing solution. It is important to place a small hole (needle puncture) in the polyethylene tubing connecting the bathing solution and the reciprocating pump. This allows for equilibration of air pressure between the ambient air and air confined inside the polyethylene tubing as the room temperature and pressure change during the course of an experiment; otherwise, air bubbles will be forced into the bathing solution, which will obscure viewing and may pull the tubule out of the pipettes.

8.5 Crafting pipettes used for perfusing segments of the nephron

To master the perfusion of isolated renal tubules one must learn to handcraft the glass pipettes used for mounting and perfusing segments of the nephron. This can be the rate-limiting step in learning how to perfuse isolated segments of the nephron *in vitro*. The following is a description of how to craft each of the following six pipettes: the holding pipette, the collection pipette, the perfusion pipette, the constant volume pipette, the transfer pipette, and the cleaning pipette.

8.5.1 Holding pipette

The holding pipette (Figures 6, 7, and 8) is made from borosilicate glass tubing (0.084″ O.D. by 0.064″ I.D. by 6″ in length, R-6 glass). This tubing is placed in a vertical pipette puller with the heating element positioned midway along the glass tube. The puller heats and pulls the glass tubing into two equal-length pipettes. Both of the pulled ends are checked for concentricity of the conical end. This is best accomplished by rotating the pipette and watching for wobbling of the tip. Usually one of the pulled pieces will be concentric and the other will be off center (non-concentric). The concentric pipette is used to make the holding pipette, while the non-concentric pipette is used to make the collection pipette. The holding pipette is finished on a microforge. On the microforge, the holding pipette is forged so that the terminal region of this pipette is 50 to 70 μm in length and 25 to 40 μm in diameter (Figures 6, 7, and 8). At the beginning of this terminal portion of the holding pipette, an alignment constriction is made by heating the glass under still-air conditions, which can be generated by placing the microforge in a 4-ft^2 box made of Plexiglas that is at least 2 ft in height and has a top.

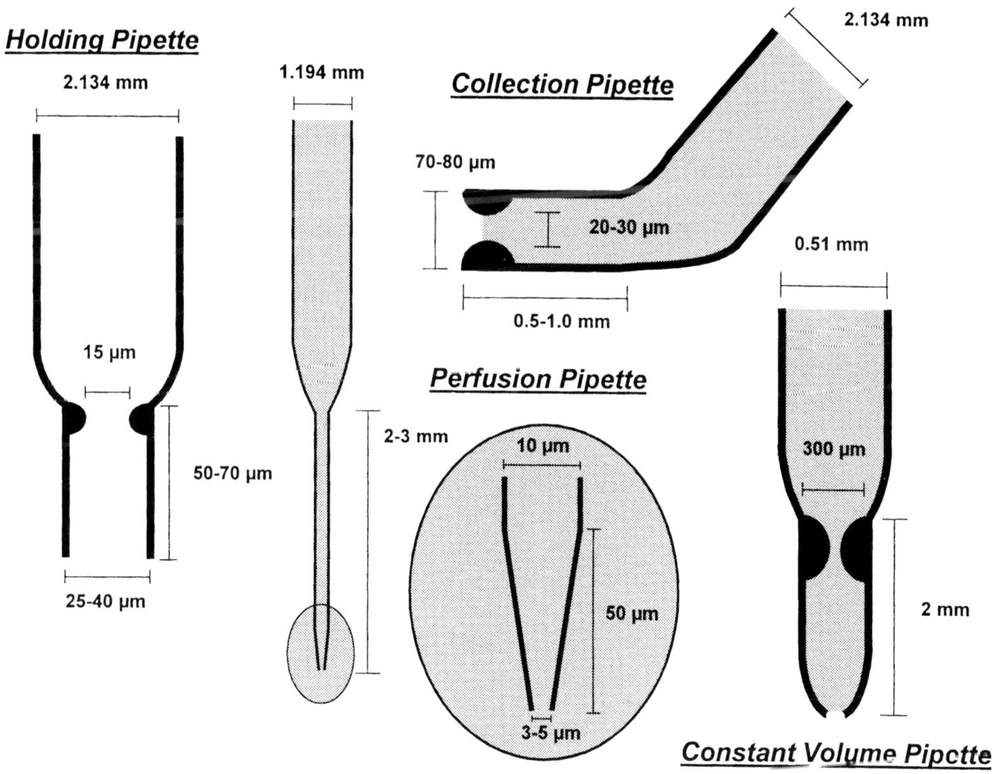

Figure 6 Schematic drawing showing some of the characteristics and dimensions of the four principal pipettes used to perfuse and study isolated segments of the nephron and collecting duct. The shapes of the pipettes are achieved by pulling borosilicate glass tubing on a vertical pipette puller and then forging the pulled glass on a mircoforge. See text for details.

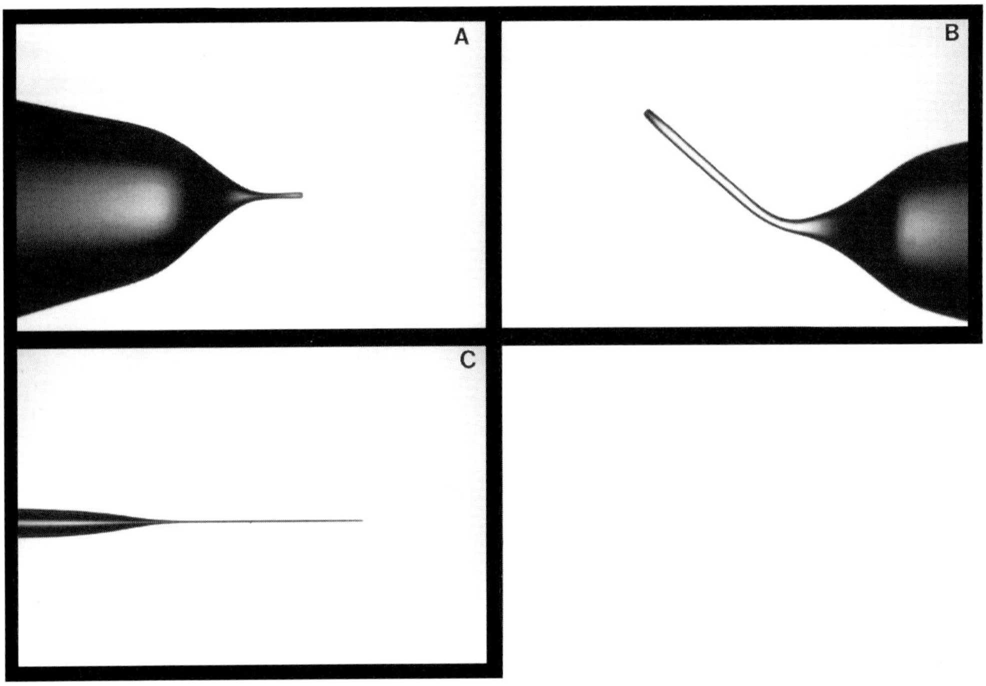

Figure 7 Low-power photomicrographs of a holding pipette (A), a collection pipette (B), and a perfusion pipette (C).

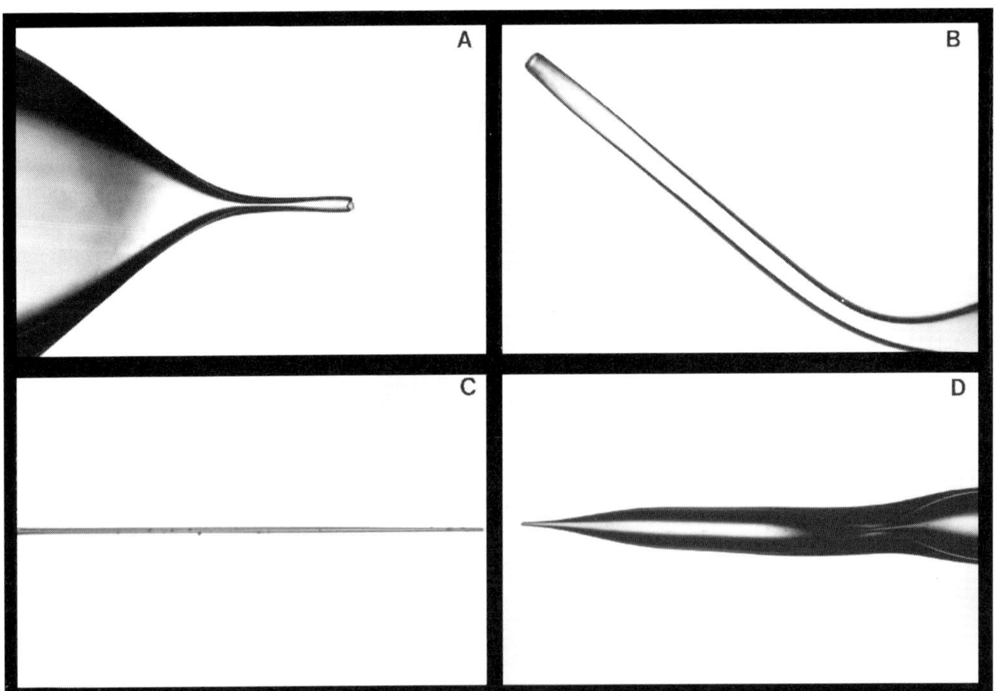

Figure 8 Photomicrographs showing the tip region of a holding pipette (A), a collection pipette (B), a perfusion pipette (C), and a constant volume or volumetric pipette (D).

8.5.2 Collection pipette

The initial steps for crafting the collection pipette (Figures 6, 7, and 8) are the same as those for the holding pipette. After obtaining the non-concentric end of piece of the borosilicate glass tubing (0.084″ O.D. by 0.064″ I.D. by 6″ in length, R-6 glass) that was pulled on the vertical pipette puller, the collection pipette is crafted on the microforge. The end of the pipette is pulled so that the terminal 0.5 to 1.0 mm of the pipette has a diameter of approximately 70 to 80 µm (Figures 6, 7, and 8). The end of the pipette is fire-polished so that the opening of the pipette is contricted to 20 to 30 µm in diameter. Once this is accomplished, the inside of the open tip is coated with catalyzed elastomer (Sylgard). This is accomplished by placing a mixture (1:1) of Sylgard and its catalyst in the first 100 µm of the pipette tip. Subsequently, the excess elastomer is blown out, leaving a thin coat of the mixture on the inside wall. Heat is then applied until the liquid elastomer becomes solid. This usually takes about 0.5 s. The final step in making this pipette is placing a 30° bend in the pipette at the junction between the conical portion and the portion of the pipette having a diameter of 80 µm. This is accomplished by bringing the heating element of the microforge near to the oustide of the pipette and heating slowly until the pipette is bent.

8.5.3 Perfusion pipette

The perfusion pipette is the simplest pipette to craft. It is crafted in a manner similar to that used to craft the holding and collection pipette. First, a smaller diameter borosilicate glass tube (0.47″ O.D. by 0.40″ I.D. by 6″ length, R-6 glass) is pulled in the vertical pipette puller, and then it is forged in the microforge. The tip of this pipette is made by starting as far along the conical shape as possible. The terminal 2 to 3 mm of the pipette is made to have a diameter of approximately 10 µm (Figures 6, 7, and 8). This is accomplished by using a light pulling weight (0.2 g). Subsequently, heat is applied to the tip of the pipette so as to constrict the opening of the pipette to a diameter of 3 to 5 µm.

8.5.4 Constant volume pipette

The constant volume (collection) pipette is made from borosilicate glass tubing having the smallest diameter of any of the other pieces of glass tubing used to make pipettes (0.020″ O.D. by 0.014″ I.D. by 6″, R-6 glass). This glass tubing is mounted vertically in the microforge with no initial molding in the vertical pipette puller. Using a weight (2 to 3 g), the end of the tube is pulled to reduce its diameter to about one half (300 µm) and is extended by about 2 to 3 mm (Figures 6 and 8). The end of this small region is then pulled to a point, and then the weight is removed and the heating element is placed 0.2 to 0.4 mm from the tip. With careful heating a constriction is formed 2 to 3 mm from the tip of the pipette. The excess glass is cut with small scissors leaving an opening of about 60 µm in diameter. The other end of the pipette is glued into a hypodermic needle. Calibration of the pipette volume is accomplished with a solution having a known concentration (disintegrations per minute per nanoliter) of a radioisotope suitable for this calibration.

8.5.5 Cleaning pipettes

Cleaning pipettes are made the same as the constant volume pipettes (see above), except the contriction is not made and the opening of the pipettes is three times larger than that of the constant volume pipettes.

8.5.6 Pipette holders

There is currently only one commercial source for pipette holders and left-sided and right-sided V-tracks used to mount the holders that are necessary for isolated perfused tubule experiments. This source is ITM, Inc., at 818 East Myrtle St., San Antonio, TX 78212, phone number (512) 227-9492. The left-sided V-track is used to guide the holding and perfusion pipettes, while the right-sided V-track is used to guide the collection and constant volume pipettes. In addition to the two precision V-tracks, an "A" pipette holder (used to hold the holding pipette), a "B" pipette holder (used to hold the perfusion pipette), and a "C" pipette holder (used to hold the collection pipette) are required. All these components can be puchased from ITM.

The V-track assemblies are attached to micromanipulators, which are suspended from the stage of the microscope by an aluminum bar assembly (Figures 1 and 2). This arrangment makes it possible to move the microscope stage and the perfusion apparatus in unison. The microscope should have a strong enough stage to support approximately 7 kg.

References

1. Burg, M., Grantham, J., Abramov, M., and Orloff, J., Preparation and study of fragments of single rabbit nephrons, *Am. J. Physiol.*, 210, 1293, 1966.
2. Barfuss, D. W., Robinson, M. K., and Zalups, R. K., Inorganic mercury transport in the rabbit proximal tubule, *J. Am. Soc. Nephrol.*, 1, 910, 1990.
3. Zalups, R. K., Robinson, M. K., and Barfuss, D. W., Factors affecting inorganic mercury transport and toxicity in the isolated perfused proximal tubule, *J. Am. Soc. Nephrol.*, 2, 866, 1991.
4. Robinson, M. K., Barfuss, D. W., and Zalups, R. K., Cadmium transport and toxicity in isolated perfused renal proximal tubules, *Toxicol. Appl. Pharmacol.*, 121, 103, 1993.
5. Zalups, R. K., Cherian, M. G., and Barfuss, D. W., Lack of luminal or basolateral uptake and transepithelial transport of mercury in isolated perfused proximal tubules exposed to mercury-metallothionein, *J. Toxicol. Environ. Health*, 44, 101, 1995.
6. Zalups, R. K. and Barfuss, D. W., Transport and toxicity of methylmercury along the proximal tubule of the rabbit, *Toxicol. Appl. Pharmacol.*, 121, 176, 1993.
7. Pirie, S. C. and Potts, D. J., A comparison of the relative effectiveness of three transplant preservation fluids upon the integrity and function of rabbit proximal convoluted tubules perfused *in vitro*, *Clin. Sci.*, 70, 443, 1986.
8. Barfuss, D. W. and Schafer, J. A., Collection and analysis of absorbate from the proximal straight tubules, *Am. J. Physiol.*, 241, F597, 1981.
9. Barfuss, D. W. and Schafer, J. A., Rate of formation and composition of absorbate from proximal nephron segments, *Am. J.Physiol.*, 247, F117, 1984.
10. Williams, J. C., Jr. and Schafer, J. A., A model of osmotic and hydrostatic pressure effects on volume absorption in the proximal tubule, *Am. J. Physiol.*, 253, F563, 1987.
11. Barfuss, D. W., McCann, W. P., and Katholi, R. E., Axial heterogeneity of adenosine transport and metabolism in the rabbit proximal tubule, *Kidney Int.*, 41, 1143, 1992.
12. Tune, B. M. and Burg, M. B., Glucose transport by proximal renal tubules, *Am. J. Physiol.*, 221, 580, 1971.
13. Barfuss, D. W. and Schafer, J. A., Flow dependence of nonelectrolyte absorption in the nephron, *Am. J. Physiol.*, 236, F163, 1979.
14. Barfuss, D. W. and Schafer, J. A., Difference in active and passive glucose transport along the proximal nephron, *Am. J. Physiol.*, 240, F322, 1981.

chapter nine

Suspensions of Rabbit Renal Proximal Tubules

Carlotta E. Groves and Rick G. Schnellmann

9.1 Introduction 147
9.2 Enzymatic method for isolation of rabbit renal proximal tubules 149
  9.2.1 Chemicals and media 149
  9.2.2 Supplies and equipment 150
  9.2.3 Procedures 150
9.3 Mechanical method for isolation of rabbit renal proximal tubules 151
  9.3.1 Chemicals and media 151
  9.3.2 Supplies and equipment 152
  9.3.3 Procedures 153
9.4 Characteristics of renal proximal tubules in suspension 155
9.5 Cytotoxicity assays for use with suspensions of rabbit renal proximal tubules 155
  9.5.1 Assay for determining amount of lactate dehydrogenase release 155
  9.5.2 Assay for determining intracellular content of potassium 157
  9.5.3 Assay for determining intracellular content of adenine nucleotides 158
  9.5.4 Assay for determining oxygen consumption 159
  9.5.5 Assay for determining accumulation of organic ions 159
References 160

9.1 Introduction

The renal proximal tubule is the primary site within the kidney involved in the active secretion and reabsorption of ions, metabolic substrates, and various xenobiotics.[1,2] One consequence of this high transport activity is the ability of renal proximal tubules (RPTs) to concentrate chemicals to high levels, resulting in the renal proximal tubule being a primary target along the nephron for injury. The study of physiological, biochemical, and toxicological mechanisms of the renal proximal tubule at the cellular level requires an appropriate *in vitro* model that eliminates the influence of other cell types and hormonal and hemodynamic effects. Various methods have been employed to isolate RPTs for the study of physiological, biochemical, and toxicological processes. One method that has proved to be useful is the microdissection of individual segments of the proximal tubule. Tubular segments isolated by this method are composed of one cell type and retain their

0-8493-3341-5/96/$0.00+$.50

normal tubular architecture and function; however, this technique is tedious, time consuming and results in a low yield of RPTs. Suspensions of RPTs have been employed extensively for *in vitro* studies since (1) their tubular morphology and polarity are maintained, (2) their oxidative metabolism and other cellular functions are maintained like those found *in vivo*, and (3) large quantities of quality RPTs can be obtained from a single animal.[3-8]

The use of collagenase treatment to isolate RPTs from rabbit kidneys was first employed by Burg and Orloff,[9] who used this model to measure the active transport of the organic anion *p*-aminohippurate. This suspension of cortical tubules resembled RPTs metabolically and morphologically but was contaminated with distal tubular fragments and glomeruli. Hence, subsequent methods for isolation of RPTs involved the use of density gradient centrifugation to further purify suspensions of cortical tubules.[3,6,7,10,11] Numerous metabolic properties of suspensions of rabbit RPTs prepared by the enzymatic method have been characterized and documented to be stable over a 24-h period.[7,11] One disadvantage of the enzymatic preparation is that the basement membrane is disrupted by the collagenase treatment, which results in the progressive loss of tubular structure, but not function, over time (Figure 1).[7]

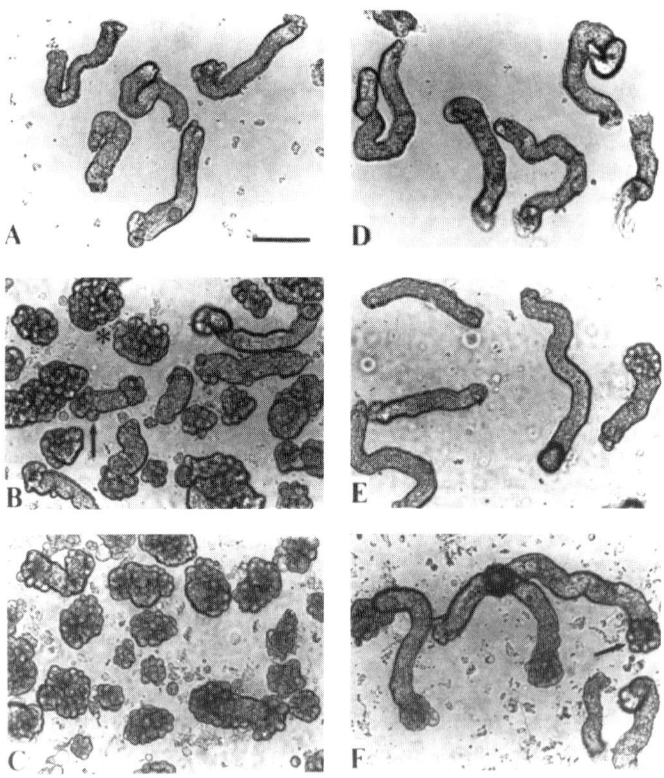

Figure 1 Photomicrographs of rabbit renal proximal tubules (RPTs) in suspension isolated by enzymatic and mechanical methods. RPTs isolated by the enzymatic method: (A) at 0 h; (B) at 6 h, cell clusters everted at the ends of tubules (arrow) and clusters of tubular cells (asterisk) were observed; and (C) at 24 h, less than 10% retained any tubular structure. RPTs isolated mechanically: (D) at 0 h; (E) at 6 h, tubules were unchanged from initial morphology; and (F) at 24 h, tubules with slightly everted ends (arrow) were observed. Bar equals 100 μm. (From Rodeheaver et al., *In Vitro Cell. Dev. Biol.*, 26, 899. Copyright© 1990 by the Tissue Culture Association. Reproduced with permission of the copyright owner.)

Mechanical (nonenzymatic) isolation methods have also been employed to isolate RPTs for study in suspensions.[7,8,12,13] In this method, the kidneys are perfused with iron oxide, which becomes trapped within the glomeruli. The renal cortex is then mechanically disrupted by homogenization, RPTs and glomeruli are isolated by differential sieving, and the iron oxide-filled glomeruli are separated from the RPTs using a magnet. Unlike RPTs isolated enzymatically, RPTs isolated by mechanical methods maintain their tubular morphology after 24 h of incubation (Figure 1).[7] However, RPT viability and various physiological processes of enzymatically isolated and mechanically isolated suspensions are similar over time.[7] In summary, both enzymatic and mechanical preparations are used extensively and serve as valuable tools for the *in vitro* study of renal physiology and toxicology. The objective of this chapter is to review the methods most commonly employed for the preparation of rabbit RPT suspensions and their use in *in vitro* toxicological studies.

9.2 Enzymatic method for isolation of rabbit renal proximal tubules

9.2.1 Chemicals and media

Alanine, bovine serum albumin (Fraction V) (BSA), deferoxamine, deoxyribonuclease (type I), dextrose, Dulbecco's Modified Eagle's/Ham's F–12 (50:50 mix with 15 m*M* *N*-2-hydroxyethyl-piperazine-*N*′-2-ethane sulfonic acid (HEPES) and L-glutamate, without sodium bicarbonate and phenol red) (DME/F–12), heptanoate, HEPES, lactate, malate, penicillin G (sodium salt), Percoll, and soybean trypsin inhibitor can obtained from Sigma Chemical Co. (St. Louis, MO). Collagenase (Type I) can be purchased from Worthington Biochemical Co. (Freehold, NJ). Heparin (1000 U/ml) and pentobarbital sodium (50 mg/ml) can be obtained from Elkins–Sinn Inc. (Cherry Hill, NJ) and Abbott Laboratories (North Chicago, IL), respectively. All other chemicals can purchased from standard sources and should be of the highest purity available.

Dissolve the powdered DME/F–12 medium (1-l vial or 15.6 g) in 800 to 900 ml of deionized H_2O (preferably cell culture grade). Add $NaHCO_3$, heptanoate, and penicillin G such that their final concentrations will be 15 m*M*, 2 m*M*, and 100 U/ml, respectively. Gas the medium with 95% O_2/5% CO_2 for 15 min, adjust the pH to 7.4 at 4°C using NaOH, and dilute to 1 l with deionized H_2O (315 mOsm/kg). For 2X-DME/F–12 (500 ml) dissolve a 1-l vial of DME/F–12 (15.6 g) in 400 ml of deionized H_2O. Adjust the media pH to 7.4 at 4°C with NaOH and dilute to 500 ml with deionized H_2O.

The incubation buffer used for cytoxicity studies contains the following: 1 m*M* alanine, 5 m*M* dextrose, 2 m*M* heptanoate, 4 m*M* lactate, 5 m*M* malate, 115 m*M* NaCl, 15 m*M* $NaHCO_3$, 5 m*M* KCl, 2 m*M* NaH_2PO_4, 1 m*M* $MgSO_4$, 1 m*M* $CaCl_2$, and 10 m*M* HEPES. Since HEPES interferes with the accumulation of organic anions by RPTs in suspensions (Groves, unpublished observations), a HEPES-free bicarbonate buffer is used for anion transport studies containing the following: 110 m*M* NaCl, 25 m*M* $NaHCO_3$, 5 m*M* KCl, 2 m*M* NaH_2PO_4, 1 m*M* $MgSO_4$, 1.8 m*M* $CaCl_2$, 10 m*M* sodium acetate, 8.3 m*M* D-glucose, 5 m*M* alanine, 0.9 m*M* glycine, 1.5 m*M* lactate, 1 m*M* malate, and 1 m*M* sodium citrate. To prepare the incubation buffer and HEPES-free buffer, add all reagents, except $CaCl_2$, in an appropriate volume of deionized H_2O and gas with 95% O_2/5% CO_2 for 15 min. Add $CaCl_2$ to the buffer while bubbling. Adjust the pH to 7.4 at 37°C with NaOH while bubbling and dilute to volume with deionized H_2O (295 mOsm/kg). Filter sterilize all media and buffers before use.

To prepare the 50% Percoll gradient for purification of RPTs, mix 40 ml of 2×-DME/F–12 with 40 ml of Percoll. Adjust the mixture to pH 7.4 with HCl. Prepare the enzymatic digestion media just prior to use by dissolving 150 U/ml collagenase, 70 U/ml deoxyribonuclease, 0.2% (w/v) BSA, and 1 m*M* deferoxamine (final concentrations) into 25 ml of DME/F–12. Filter sterilize the digestion media into a 125-ml Erlenmeyer flask and place on ice until used.

9.2.2 Supplies and equipment

Supplies needed for the enzymatic isolation of RPTs for suspensions include gloves, two 100-ml beakers, three 50-ml polypropylene centrifuge tubes, a glass petri dish with gauze, two single-edged razor blades, a scalpel blade and handle, surgical scissors, two sterile forceps, a 125-ml Erlenmeyer flask, a rubber stopper with gas ports, a 25-ml graduated cylinder, a 50-ml graduated cylinder, a 25-ml pipette, ice buckets, a 0.2-μm Nalgene syringe filter (25-mm surfactant free cellulose acetate membrane), pasteur pipettes, 23- to 25-gauge butterfly catheter, a tank of 95% O_2/5% CO_2 with regulator, tubing, and humidifying chamber, and 253 μm Nitex Swiss nylon monofilament screening fabric (Tetko Inc., Elmsford, NY). All supplies should be sterilized prior to use. The screening fabric can be held in place with embroidery hoops and sterilized in a container filled with 70% ethanol. Equipment needed includes a 37°C orbital shaking water bath, a laminar flow hood, and a Beckman J2-21 centrifuge with a JA-20 rotor.*

9.2.3 Procedures

The most commonly performed procedure for the enzymatic isolation and purification of rabbit RPTs is a modification of the Percoll method of Vinay et al.,[10] which has been described previously by Dickman and Mandel[11] and Rodeheaver et al.[7]

Insert a 23- to 25-gauge butterfly catheter into the ear vein of a 1.4- to 2-kg New Zealand White rabbit of either sex.** Inject 3000 U of heparin through the catheter and allow the heparin to circulate for 3 to 5 min. Euthanize the rabbit with an overdose of sodium pentobarbital (usually 150 mg). Working quickly, wet the hair on the abdominal area with 70% ethanol to minimize contamination with hair. Open the abdominal cavity with surgical scissors and expose the kidneys. Carefully remove the fat surrounding the kidneys and rapidly excise the kidneys and place them in ice-cold DME/F–12 medium. In a laminar flow hood, or suitable tissue culture hood, place the kidneys in a petri dish containing a piece of gauze and cover them with DME/F–12 medium.*** The petri dish should be placed on ice. Decapsulate the kidneys by placing one pair of sterile forceps at the pelvic inlet for stability while the second pair of forceps pierces (with minimal penetration of the cortex) and pulls the capsule from the kidney surface. Again, holding the kidney with a pair of forceps placed at the pelvic inlet, separate the renal cortex from the medulla with scissors, scalpel, or razor blade.**** After trimming the cortical tissue from both kidneys, mince the tissue into approximately 1-mm cubes with two single-edged razor blades held tightly together and suspend the tissue in the enzymatic digestion medium. Digest the cortical tissue in an orbital shaking water bath (200 rpm) at 37°C under 95% O_2/5% CO_2 (30 ml min^{-1} flow rate) for 30 to 40 min. To prevent excessive digestion, harvest dissociated tubules every 10 min by allowing the undigested tissue to settle and removing the dissociated tubular fragments by pipetting approximately 12 ml of the supernatant into a 50-ml conical tube. Centrifuge the conical tube for 2 min at 50 × g to pellet the tubules. Decant the supernatant back into the digestion flask for further

* Other centrifuges and fixed angle rotors will work following revolution-per-minute and time adjustments.

** The increased connective tissue in the kidneys of larger rabbits (>2.5 to 3 kg) makes digestion more difficult and generally results in lower yields of RPTs.

*** The use of a hood is not necessary when preparing suspensions of RPTs for short experiments (<6 h).

**** It is important to take only cortical tissue, using color and depth as cortical markers.

digestion of the remaining tissue. Resuspend the tubular pellet in 12 ml of fresh, ice-cold DME/F–12 medium and place on ice. Once the digestion is completed, add the previously harvested suspension of RPTs to a flask to stop the action of the enzymes. Filter the suspension through the 253-μm tissue sieve to remove undigested tissue and rinse the sieve with ice-cold DME/F–12 medium. Resuspend the filtered tissue in additional ice-cold DME/F–12 medium in two polypropylene centrifuge tubes and centrifuge at 50 × g for 2 min at 4°C. Aspirate and discard the supernatants and wash the pellets two more times with ice-cold DME/F–12 medium. Resuspend the last pellets in 50% Percoll and separate and purify the isolated RPTs by centrifugation at 37,000 × g for 30 min at 4°C.* Remove the proximal tubular band, located approximately 1/3 of the way up the side of the tube with a pasteur pipette, and place in a clean polypropylene centrifuge tube. Add DME/F–12 medium to the tube and pellet the tubules by centrifugation (50 × g for 2 min at 4°C). Wash the RPTs by resuspending the pellet and centrifugating at 50 × g for 2 min at 4°C in DME/F–12 and then wash twice with incubation buffer. Resuspend the tubules in incubation buffer at a final protein concentration of 1 mg protein per milliliter. Use a protein assay such as the Biuret, Lowry, or Bio-Rad to adjust the RPT concentration. The steps involved in the enzymatic isolation of rabbit RPTs are summarized in Figure 2.

This enzymatic procedure provides primarily a mixture of S1 and S2 segments of proximal tubules, with a very low yield of S3 segments due to their location in the outer medulla. The purity of preparation is 96 to 99% with the majority of the contamination being glomeruli and distal tubular segments. Other enzymatic methods involve the *in situ* perfusion of the kidneys with a collagenase solution and separation of proximal tubules on a Ficoll gradient.[3,14] The disadvantage of this Ficoll gradient method is the greater contamination with glomeruli and distal tubular fragments.[10,15]

The large yield of RPTs obtained by enzymatic isolation has made this technique useful for the growth and development of primary cultures of RPTs.[6,16,17] However, treatment with high concentrations of collagenase and the disruption of the basement membrane has been shown to decrease the ability of the RPTs to attach to the culture dish and grow.[18] The addition of various metabolic substrates such as butyrate to the culture medium or coating the culture dishes with collagen improves the seeding efficiency.[16,18]

Since some nephrotoxicants produce damage to selective segments of the proximal tubule, the ability to isolate S1 and S3 segments in bulk would allow for the investigation of the mechanisms involved in these effects. The enzymatic isolation technique has been modified by Ruegg and Mandel[19] to provide suspensions comprising S1 and S3 segments.[19,20] In this method, slices of renal tissue from the outer cortex (S1) and the outer stripe of the medulla (S3) are prepared using a Stadie–Riggs microtome, and tubular suspensions are prepared from the slices with a modification of the enzymatic digestion and Percoll gradient separation described above. This method provides greater than 98% pure populations of S1 and S3 segments, although the yields are relatively low compared with procedures that do not separate the different tubular segments.

9.3 Mechanical method for isolation of rabbit renal proximal tubules

9.3.1 Chemicals and media

Prepare 1 l of DME/F–12 as described above and an additional liter of DME/F–12 that contains 0.5 m*M* deferoxamine. Phosphate buffered saline (PBS) contains the following: 137 m*M* NaCl, 3 m*M* KCl, 2 m*M* KH_2PO_4, and 8 m*M* Na_2HPO_4 (pH 7.4). Prepare the iron oxide by the method of Cook and Pickering.[21] Gas 100 to 150 ml of deionized water with

* Do not use brake.

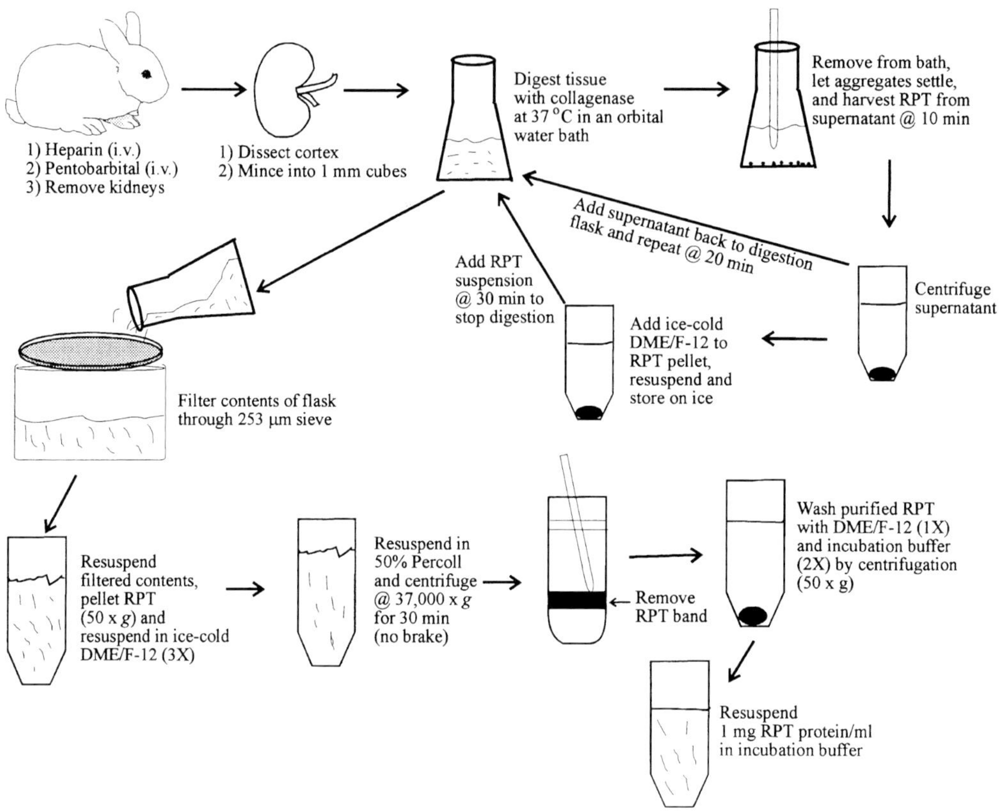

Figure 2 Flow diagram of the enzymatic method for the isolation of rabbit renal proximal tubules (RPTs). *Note:* Harvest the RPTs after 10 min of digestion by removing the flask from the water bath, allowing the aggregates to settle, and removing the supernatant. Centrifuge the supernatant to pellet the RPTs. Return the digestion medium to the digestion flask and resuspend the pellet of RPTs with ice-cold DME/F–12. Repeat this procedure after 20 min of digestion. After 30 min of digestion add the previously harvested RPTs suspension to the digestion flask to stop further digestion. Filter contents of digestion flask through a 253-μm sieve. The upper bands observed following centrifugation in Percoll contain distal tubules and cell debris.

95% O_2/5% CO_2 or 100% O_2 for 15 min to saturate the water with oxygen. Dissolve 1.3 g sodium hydroxide and 10 g KNO_3 (J. T. Baker Co., Phillipsburg, NJ) in 50 ml of the O_2 saturated water. Likewise, dissolve 4.5 g ferrous sulfate (J. T. Baker Co., Phillipsburg, NJ) in 50 ml of the O_2 saturated water. Add the ferrous sulfate solution to the NaOH/KNO_3 solution and boil for 20 min. Wash the resulting iron oxide precipitate 10 times with deionized water by placing a large stir bar or magnet on the bottom of the flask, decanting the water, and adding fresh water. After the final rinse, resuspend the iron oxide in 500 ml of PBS and autoclave. The incubation medium for cytotoxicity studies is the same as that described for the enzymatic isolation. See above for additional information concerning chemicals and solutions.

9.3.2 *Supplies and equipment*

The supplies required for the mechanical isolation preparation include three 100-ml beakers, two 50-ml conical centrifuge tubes, two petri dishes with gauze, one 50-ml glass syringe, a 15-ml Dounce homogenizer with a type A pestle, pasteur pipettes, three curved metal spatulas, a 1000-ml beaker, magnetic stir bars, two 18-gauge blunt-ended needles, two pairs of forceps, curved-nose scissors, surgical scissors, Bunsen burner, alcohol, heavy black suture, and 253-μm and 85-μm Nitex Swiss nylon monofilament screening fabric (Tetko Inc., Elmsford, NY) held in place with embroidery hoops. Different mesh sizes have been used successfully by other investigators for isolating rabbit RPTs (245 μm/105 μm;[22] 212 μm/63 μm;[23] and 210 μm/86 μm[13]). All supplies should be sterilized prior to use. Equipment needed includes a laminar flow hood and a Beckman GPR centrifuge with a GH 3.7 rotor.*

9.3.3 *Procedures*

The mechanical method was originally developed for the isolation of glomeruli, but was later modified for the isolation of RPTs.[12] The method of mechanical separation and purification of rabbit RPTs commonly used is based on this method as modified by Aleo et al.,[24] Rodeheaver et al.,[7] and Brendel et al.[8]

Euthanize the rabbit and expose the kidneys as described above. Carefully remove the fat surrounding the kidney and expose the renal artery and vein. Separate and cut the renal artery and vein leaving the artery as long as possible. Cut the ureter and remove the kidney and place it in a beaker containing ice-cold DME/F–12 medium. Repeat the procedure for the other kidney. In the laminar flow hood, remove the fat around the kidneys without damaging the capsule and rinse the kidneys with ice-cold DME/F–12 medium. Place the rinsed kidney in a clean petri dish with gauze and cover with ice-cold DME/F–12 medium. The petri dish should be placed on ice. Insert a blunted 18-gauge needle into the renal artery of each kidney and secure tightly with two heavy sutures. Attach a 50-ml glass syringe containing 50 ml of ice-cold DME/F–12 medium and perfuse the kidney using slow, steady pressure to clear the blood from the kidneys. Repeat the perfusion with 50 ml of ice-cold PBS. Fill the syringe with 40 to 45 ml of PBS and 5 to 10 ml of the iron oxide solution. Perfuse each kidney with enough iron oxide mixture to turn them a light-to-medium gray (usually 5 to 10 ml). Only clear fluid should exit the kidneys because the iron oxide is trapped within the glomeruli. Once suitably perfused with iron oxide, decapsulate the kidneys and place them in a clean petri dish with gauze and cover them with DME/F–12 medium containing 0.5 m*M* deferoxamine. Hold each kidney with a pair of forceps placed at the pelvic inlet and separate the cortex from the medulla with curved scissors, avoiding any areas that did not perfuse and contain blood or no iron oxide. Mince the cortical tissue into approximately 5- to 6-mm cubes.

Place the tissue sieves on top of a 1-l beaker (the 85-μm sieve on the bottom and the 253-μm sieve on the top) and rinse the ethanol from the sieves with PBS. Fill the Dounce homogenizer with 12 ml of DME/F–12 medium containing deferoxamine and add enough tissue to displace approximately 1 ml of medium. Disrupt the tissue with four to five strokes of the homogenizer, pour the homogenate over the sieves, and rinse with DME/F–12 medium containing deferoxamine. Repeat this step until all the tissue is homogenized. After all the tissue has been poured over the sieves, rinse the top sieve with 250 to 500 ml of PBS or DME/F–12 buffer containing deferoxamine and discard the top sieve. Using a curved spatula, collect the tissue on the 85-μm sieve, which contains the proximal tubules and glomeruli, and place into two 50-ml centrifuge tubes filled with 40 ml of DME/F–12 medium containing deferoxamine and a magnetic stir bar. Mix the suspension gently to allow greater contact between the magnet and the iron-filled glomeruli. After the tissue settles to the bottom, remove the iron oxide-coated magnet with the aid of a magnet on the outside of the tube. Repeat this process until the iron is no longer sticking to the magnet. Wash the purified RPTs once with DME/F–12 medium and twice with incubation buffer by centrifugating at $50 \times g$ for 2 min at 4°C and resuspending the

* Other centrifuges and rotors will work.

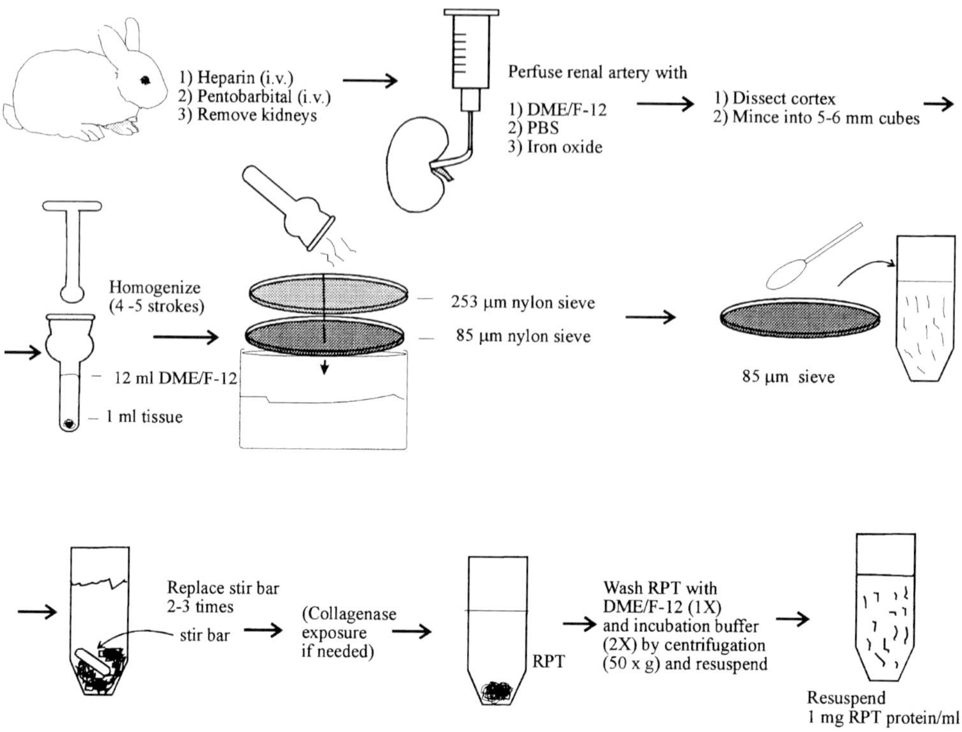

Figure 3 Flow diagram of the mechanical method for the isolation of rabbit renal proximal tubules. *Note:* Homogenize the tissue with four to five strokes of the homogenizer, pour the homogenate over the sieves, and rinse with DME/F–12 medium containing deferoxamine. Repeat this step until all the tissue is homogenized. After all the tissue has been poured over the sieves, rinse the top sieve with PBS or DME/F–12 buffer containing deferoxamine and then discard the top sieve. Using a curved spatula, collect the tissue on the 85-μm sieve, which contains the proximal tubules and glomeruli, and place into centrifuge tubes filled with 40 ml of DME/F–12 medium containing deferoxamine and a magnetic stir bar. Mix the suspension gently to allow greater contact between the magnet and the iron-filled glomeruli. After the tissue settles to the bottom, remove the iron oxide-coated magnet with the aid of another magnet on the outside of the tube. Repeat this process until the iron is no longer sticking to the magnet.

pellet. Resuspend the RPTs in incubation buffer at a final protein concentration of 1 mg/ml. The steps involved in the mechanical isolation of rabbit RPTs suspensions are summarized in Figure 3.

Mechanically isolated RPTs have been used extensively for the initiation of primary cultures of rabbit RPTs.[23-27] Unlike the enzymatic procedure, mechanically isolated RPTs adhere readily to the culture dish surface. However, mechanically isolated RPTs do not readily proliferate in culture. To promote proliferation and growth of RPTs, mechanically isolated RPTs can be briefly treated with collagenase in the presence of soybean trypsin inhibitor to disrupt the basement membrane and thereby facilitate cellular growth. Briefly, dissolve 2400 U of collagenase (Type I) and 0.6 mg of soybean trypsin inhibitor in 1 ml of DME/F–12 medium containing deferoxamine, filter sterilize, and add to 40 ml of RPT suspension. The collagenase step can be added either before or after the removal of glomeruli. However, collagenase treatment prior to the addition of the magnet may enhance glomeruli removal. Gently rock the RPTs suspension at room temperature for 15 min and wash the RPTs as described above. An additional advantage of briefly exposing mechanically isolated RPTs to collagenase is greater ease of removing the iron oxide-laden glomeruli and less clumping of RPTs during incubations.

Mechanically isolated rabbit RPTs retain an intact basement membrane, which results in the retention of tubular morphology over time.[7] Brendel et al.[8] reported that mechanically isolated RPTs had greater transport and metabolic function than enzymatically isolated tubules treated extensively with collagenase. However, Rodeheaver et al.[7] had previously reported that enzymatically isolated tubules treated conservatively with collagenase exhibited similar biochemical properties as mechanically isolated RPTs. The one biochemical difference that was observed in enzymatically isolated RPTs was an increase in ouabain-sensitive respiration. Both methods of isolation, however, provide a large yield of RPTs that are well-suited for *in vitro* studies of renal toxicology.

9.4 Characteristics of renal proximal tubules in suspension

There are many advantages of rabbit RPTs in suspensions from either method compared with freshly isolated RPT cells, renal cortical slices, primary cultures of RPT cells, and renal epithelial-like cell lines. For example, RPTs are composed primarily of one cell type, oxygen and metabolic substrate availability are not limited, they retain many physiological and biochemical functions at levels similar to those found *in vivo*, viability and physiological functions are excellent for at least 24 h, and they retain their tubular morphology and cellular polarity.[7] One disadvantage of RPTs prepared by either method is that the lumen of RPTs is mostly collapsed during the first few hours after incubation at 37°C.[7]

Cellular metabolism in RPTs has been studied extensively providing a large data base of information for toxicological studies. In particular, RPTs exhibit a high degree of oxidative phosphorylation, with very limited glycolysis, and a tightly linked relation exists among oxidative phosphorylation, ATP content, and membrane transport function.[3-4] Since RPTs derive their energy from oxidative phosphorylation, xenobiotics that affect mitochondrial function can have dramatic effects on the function and viability of RPTs.

Renal xenobiotic biotransformation is critical in mediating the renal toxicity and detoxification of various chemicals. RPTs in suspension are a good model system since the tubular fragments retain various enzymatic pathways such as glutathione conjugation and catabolism, cysteine conjugate β-lyase, cytochrome P-450, prostaglandin H synthase, glucuronosyltransferase, and sulfotransferase at levels similar to those found *in vivo*.[4,5,7,28-32]

Active transport of electrolytes and other plasma solutes such as glucose, amino acids, and organic ions is one of the primary functions of RPTs. Rabbit RPTs are capable of transporting many substrates as well as nephrotoxicants. Recently, Groves et al.[33] described the accumulation of the organic cation tetraethylammonium (TEA) by RPTs in suspension at times as short as 10 s. Furthermore, the kinetic characteristics for transport of TEA were quantitatively and qualitatively similar for enzymatically isolated rabbit RPTs in suspension and individually microdissected rabbit S2 segments. The rate of TEA efflux across the basolateral membrane of RPTs in suspension was equivalent to the rate of TEA efflux across the basolateral membrane of microdissected S2 segments with oil-filled lumina, suggesting that the lumina are initially collapsed in RPTs.[7,34] Our laboratory has also developed a fluorescent assay that directly measures the transport characteristics of the organic anion ochratoxin A in RPTs in suspension.[35] Thus, this model appears to be a valuable tool for the study of active transport of organic ions and nephrotoxicants.

9.5 Cytotoxicity assays for use with suspensions of rabbit renal proximal tubules

9.5.1 Assay for determining amount of lactate dehydrogenase release

The cellular injury produced by various nephrotoxicants often leads to cell death. This is primarily characterized by loss of integrity of the plasma membrane and cellular lysis. A number of markers have been used to measure cell death/lysis, such as exclusion of vital dyes (such as trypan blue); release of small endogenous or exogenous compounds (radiolabeled adenosine, radiolabeled chromium, neutral red, the fluorescent pH-sensitive dye BCECF); release of intracellular enzymes (lactate dehydrogenase [LDH], alanine aminotransferase, sorbital dehydrogenase); uptake of fluorescent dyes (propidium iodide); and/or mitochondrial dehydrogenase activity (MTT, XTT). A potential problem with exclusion of vital and fluorescent dyes is that these compounds can be taken up by uninjured cells, probably through one of the many transporters or endocytic mechanisms present in RPTs. Likewise, the release of small endogenous or exogenous compounds may be through a transporter or secondary to changes in the energy status of the RPTs and not due to cell death/lysis. Finally, alterations in mitochondrial dehydrogenase activity may occur without cell death/lysis. The release of LDH activity into the medium has proved to be a good reproducible marker of cell death/lysis in models of RPTs and renal cells in general. The premise of this assay is that increases in plasma membrane permeability extensive enough to result in the loss of large intracellular enzymes reflects cell death/lysis. The results of this assay are usually reported as the percentage of the total LDH activity that is found in the medium at a given time, indicating the percentage of the RPT cells that have died. The LDH assay can be performed quickly and easily; however, one disadvantage is that some toxicants can inactivate the enzyme. LDH release from rabbit RPTs in suspension has been described previously by Schnellmann and Mandel[36] and is based on the LDH assay of Bergmeyer et al.[37]

The chemicals required for the determination of LDH release from RPTs in suspension include β-NADH, sodium pyruvate, potassium phosphate monobasic and dibasic, dibutyl phthalate, and dioctyl phthalate and can be purchased from Sigma Chemical Co. (St. Louis, MO). Prepare a phthalate solution by mixing 20 ml of dibutyl phthalate with 10 ml of dioctylphthalate and aliquot into 1.5-ml microcentrifuge tubes (0.4 ml/tube). The 50 m*M* phosphate buffer is prepared by dissolving 4.38 g of K_2HPO_4 and 0.56 g of KH_2PO_4 in 400 ml of deionized water, adjusting the pH to 7.4, and diluting to 500 ml with deionized water. On the day of LDH analysis dissolve 21 mg of β-NADH in 120 ml of phosphate buffer (0.25 m*M*) and 25 mg of sodium pyruvate in 10 ml of phosphate buffer (22.7 m*M*). Place the β-NADH and pyruvate on ice until used.* Liquid nitrogen and a warm water bath are needed on the day of LDH analysis. A microcentrifuge (≥10,000 × g) is needed to separate the RPTs from the surrounding medium, and a UV-VIS spectrophotometer is needed for LDH analysis.

At the appropriate sampling time, remove a 0.5-ml aliquot of RPT suspension and place in a 1.5 ml-microcentrifuge tube. This tube represents total LDH activity (TOTAL). Remove a second aliquot (1.0 ml), carefully layer it on top of the phthalate layer (see above), and immediately centrifuge at 10,000 × g for 2 min. Remove 0.5 ml of the supernatant and place in a clean microcentrifuge tube (SUPE). Either determine LDH activity immediately upon completion of the experiment or freeze at –80°C until assayed.**

To release the LDH from the RPTs, subject all samples to at least three freeze–thaw cycles using liquid nitrogen and a warm water (≤37°C) bath. After the third freeze–thaw, the samples are centrifuged (10,000 × g) to sediment the tubular debris and placed on ice until assayed.

The measurement of LDH activity is based on the ability of LDH to convert pyruvate to lactate with the concomitant oxidation of β-NADH to β-NAD. The disappearance of β-NADH is followed spectrophotometrically at 25°C and 340 nm. Set up a series of 12 × 75 mm disposable test tubes, one for each TOTAL and SUPE. Add 0.75 ml of β-NADH

* β-NADH is light-sensitive.

** LDH activity is not stable at room temperature, 4°C or –20°C.

buffer to each SUPE tube and 0.9 ml to each TOTAL tube. Add 0.15 ml of pyruvate and 0.15 ml of sample to a SUPE tube, vortex immediately, and read the absorbance on the spectrophotometer every 10 s for eight readings.* Add 0.075 ml of pyruvate and 0.075 ml of sample to a TOTAL tube, vortex, and read the absorbance on the spectrophotometer as described for SUPE.

Disregard the first reading and determine the change in absorbance per minute.** If the absorbance is > 0.150/min, dilute the sample and run the sample again. The TOTAL values should be similar among the samples. If any TOTAL values are significantly decreased, determine whether the toxicant or experimental condition used has a direct effect on the LDH enzyme. Calculate percentage LDH release by dividing the value for the SUPE by the value for the TOTAL, dividing the result by 2, and multiplying the result by 100.

9.5.2 *Assay for determining intracellular content of potassium*

Toxicants can disrupt cellular ion homeostasis directly by altering the permeability of the plasma membrane and altering the transporters that normally regulate ion movement, and indirectly by altering cellular metabolism. Since there is a large concentration gradient across the plasma membrane (intracellular $\gg$ extracellular), K^+ content has been used frequently to monitor cellular ion homeostasis following toxicant exposure. The use of intracellular K^+ content as a marker of cellular viability is inappropriate since numerous reversible cellular events, such as decreases in ATP, the opening of potassium channels, and decreases in the activity of the Na^+, K^+-ATPase will result in the loss of intracellular K^+ without a loss of viability.[38] Cellular ion homeostasis, including intracellular K^+ content, should be determined prior to the onset of LDH release since it is difficult to draw conclusions concerning ion homeostasis when there is a significant amount of cell death. The determination of intracellular K^+ content in rabbit renal proximal tubules has been previously described by Mandel's laboratory.[15,38]

The chemicals required for the determination of intracellular K^+ content include a phthalate solution (described above), perchloric acid, and deionized water. A microcentrifuge ($\geq$10,000 × g) is needed to separate the RPTs from the surrounding medium, and a flame photometer or atomic absorption spectrophotometer is needed for K^+ analysis.

At the appropriate sampling time, remove a 1.0-ml aliquot of the suspension of RPTs and carefully layer it on top of the phthalate layer (0.4 ml, see above). Immediately centrifuge at 10,000 × g for 2 min.*** Carefully remove the supernatant, insuring the removal of liquid on the sides of the tube, and then the phthalate layer. Resuspend the pellet with 1 ml of a 6% perchloric acid solution to precipitate the RPTs protein and release the K^+. The samples may be frozen until analysis just prior to or after the addition of perchloric acid. Precipitate the renal proximal tubular protein by centrifugation (10,000 × g for 2 min). Alternatively, following the removal of the phthalate layer, the pellet can be resuspended with 1 ml of deionized water. Transfer a 0.4-ml aliquot of the homogenate of RPTs into a 5-ml tube and add 0.03 ml of a 70% perchloric acid solution to precipitate the protein. Precipitate the protein by centrifugation (10 min at 1480 × g at 4°C in a Beckman tabletop refrigerated centrifuge or equivalent).

Prepare a standard curve using potassium chloride in either 6% perchloric acid or 0.4 ml deionized water containing 0.03 ml of a 70% perchloric acid solution. Assay the

* Absorbance decreases with time.

** Check linearity.

*** The centrifugation of RPTs results in the dragging and trapping of some extracellular medium in the pellet. Due to the high concentration of the K^+ in the RPTs and the low concentration of potassium in the medium, it is not normally necessary to correct for this extracellular medium. However, extracellular fluid makers such as inulin, dextrans, or polyethylene glycol can be used if needed.

supernatants for K^+ using flame photometry or atomic absorption spectophotometry. Use a protein assay such as the Biuret, Lowry, or Bio-Rad to determine the protein concentration in the perchloric acid precipitates of the RPTs. Express intracellular K^+ content as nanomoles per milligram protein.

9.5.3 *Assay for determining intracellular content of adenine nucleotides*

The mitochondrion is the intracellular target for numerous nephrotoxicants.[39] A decrease in mitochondrial function results in the inhibition of a variety of cellular functions and ultimately cell death. The inhibition of numerous cellular functions in parallel makes it difficult to develop cause-and-effect relations, and studies must be completed carefully to temporally identify the sequence of events that occur following toxicant exposure. If mitochondrial dysfunction is a crucial event leading to cell death, then experiments should document that mitochondrial function (cellular respiration) and intracellular ATP content are decreased extensively prior to the initiation of cell death. Intracellular ATP content can be determined using the luciferin–luciferase assay [40]. While this method is capable of measuring ATP levels in a large number of samples quickly and easily, it does not give any information concerning the other adenine nucleotides in the RPTs. While the HPLC method requires additional instrumentation, a refrigerated autosampler can be used to process a large number of samples, and the levels of ATP, ADP, AMP, hypoxanthine, xanthine, and adenosine can be determined in a single run. Intracellular adenine nucleotide content is based on the method of Hull-Ryde et al.[41] and Mandel et al.[42]

The chemicals required for the determination of intracellular adenine nucleotide content include a phthalate solution (described above); ammonium phosphate; perchloric acid; potassium hydroxide; potassium carbonate; and HPLC-grade ATP, ADP, AMP, hypoxanthine, xanthine, adenosine, water, and methanol. Prepare a 6% perchloric acid solution using deionized water. Prepare a KOH/K_2CO_3 solution by dissolving 15 g of KOH and 15 g of K_2CO_3 in 70 ml of deionized water. Prepare a 0.01-m*M* solution of ATP, ADP, AMP, hypoxanthine, xanthine, and adenosine in water. A microcentrifuge ($\geq$10,000 × g) is needed to separate the RPTs from the surrounding medium and a gradient HPLC system with a UV detector (254 nm) is necessary to separate and quantify the adenine nucleotides. Use a 5-μm ODS-Hypersil (150 × 4.6 mm) HPLC column from Keystone Scientific (Bellefonte, PA).

At the appropriate sampling time, remove a 0.5-ml aliquot of the suspension containing the RPTs and place in a 1.5-ml microcentrifuge tube containing 0.5 ml ice-cold 6% perchloric acid. This tube represents total adenine nucleotides (TOTAL). Remove a second aliquot (1.0 ml), carefully layer it on top of the phthalate layer (see above), and immediately centrifuge at 10,000 × g for 2 min. Remove 0.5 ml of the supernatant and place in a microcentrifuge tube containing ice-cold 6% perchloric acid (SUPE). Vortex both samples and place on ice for 20 min. After 20 min, centrifuge the tubes as above and transfer 0.8 ml of the supernatants to new tubes. Neutralize the samples to pH 7.0 using the KOH/K_2CO_3 solution and place on ice for 2 min. Vortex both samples and centrifuge as above. Transfer the supernatant into new tubes and freeze at –80°C until assayed. Use a protein assay such as the Biuret, Lowry, or Bio-Rad to determine the RPT protein concentration in the perchloric acid precipitates.

To separate the adenine nucleotides, prepare a 100-m*M* ammonium phosphate buffer (pH 5.5) using HPLC-grade water (solution A). Use methanol for solution B. Set the flow rate to 1 ml/min with the mobile phase being 100% solution A/0% solution B. After 5.7 min change the mobile phase to 64% solution A/36% solution B rapidly. Quantify the eluted adenine nucleotides using UV detection (254 nm), an integrator, and known standards. The approximate times of elution are (in minutes): ATP 3.5, ADP 4, hypoxanthine

6, xanthine 6.5, AMP 7.5, and adenosine 9.5. Express results as nanomoles per milligram protein for TOTAL samples and SUPE samples. Subtract SUPE samples from TOTAL samples to obtain intracellular adenine nucleotide contents.

9.5.4 *Assay for determining oxygen consumption*

Determination of cellular oxygen consumption is one of the best ways to assess mitochondrial function. This method allows for direct and continual monitoring of mitochondrial function over time. Detailed methodology for the measurement of oxygen consumption in suspensions of RPTs has recently been described by Schnellmann.[43] Using several pharmacological tools, it is possible to examine several aspects of mitochondrial function/dysfunction within the RPTs. For example, using the Na^+,K^+-ATPase inhibitor ouabain, it is possible to determine the fraction of RPTs oxygen consumption that is associated with Na^+,K^+-ATPase activity and sodium transport vs. other cellular processes.

State 3 respiration of RPTs suspensions can be examined indirectly by measuring oxygen consumption in the presence of the monovalent ionophore nystatin.[4] Nystatin increases Na^+ influx, which stimulates Na^+,K^+-ATPase activity and results in the consumption of ATP and the formation of ADP. In general, the increase in ADP produces maximal mitochondrial ATP formation and thus maximal oxygen consumption (state 3 respiration). We have used nystatin as a stress test to uncover alterations in mitochondrial function prior to decreases in basal oxygen consumption. A decrease in nystatin-stimulated respiration may not always reflect a decrease in mitochondrial function since compounds may directly affect the Na^+,K^+-ATPase or decrease the adenine nucleotide pool. Thus, mitochondrial function can be probed directly in suspensions of RPTs by resuspending the RPTs in an intracellular-like buffer and selectively permeabilizing the plasma membrane to provide direct access to the mitochondrion. See Schnellmann[43] for details of the above procedures.

9.5.5 *Assay for determining accumulation of organic ions*

The transport of organic anions and cations such as *p*-aminohippurate (PAH), tetraethylammonium (TEA), and *N*-methylnicotinamide (NMN) is specifically a function of RPTs. Therefore, their accumulations have been used as markers of toxicant-induced injury in RPTs.[44] Organic anions and cations generally enter the renal proximal tubular cell by transport across the basolateral membrane and exit by apical membrane transport into the lumen. Since luminal access to RPTs in suspension appears to be limited,[7] basolateral uptake of organic anions and cations is evaluated using RPTs in suspension. A toxicant-induced decrease in organic anion and cation uptake may result from (1) a direct effect of the toxicant on the transporter, (2) increased plasma membrane permeability, (3) alterations in cellular metabolism, and/or (4) alterations in transmembrane electrochemical gradients. Thus, a decrease in organic ion accumulation can result from a variety of reversible cellular changes and cell death and is not a good marker for viability. However, the measure of organic ion transport can be a valuable tool in the assessment of transport and injury and of xenobiotic transport in RPTs.

The chemicals required for the determination of organic ion accumulation include ^{3}H- or ^{14}C-labeled TEA and PAH, probenecid, tetrapentylammonium, incubation buffer, and HEPES-free bicarbonate buffer (described above). An orbital shaking 37°C water bath is needed to incubate the RPTs, a Beckman tabletop refrigerated centrifuge or equivalent is necessary to separate the RPTs from the surrounding medium, and a liquid scintillation spectrometer is needed to quantify the radioactivity.

Preincubate RPTs in incubation buffer (TEA uptake) or HEPES free-bicarbonate buffer (PAH uptake) at an RPT protein concentration of 1 mg/ml for 15 to 20 min at 37°C in an orbital shaking water bath (150 rpm) under a 95% air/5% CO_2 atmosphere. This preincubation period allows the RPTs to regain their metabolic functions and ion gradients. Add radiolabeled ^{14}C-PAH or ^{14}C-TEA (0.1 μCi/ml, 1.8 μ*M*) to RPT suspensions treated with a toxicant or diluent. At timed intervals, remove a 0.5-ml aliquot of suspension of RPTs and transfer it to a 15-ml polypropylene tube containing 5 ml of ice-cold incubation buffer to stop uptake. Centrifuge the samples at 1480 × g for 20 to 30 s to pellet the RPTs. Aspirate the supernatant, resuspend the pellet with buffer, and centrifuge at 1480 × g for 20 to 30 s. To prevent the loss of accumulated radiolabel and to decrease the binding of radiolabel to the RPTs during processing of the sample, a saturating concentration of an organic anion inhibitor (2 m*M* probenecid for PAH) or organic cation inhibitor (1 m*M* tetrapentylammonium for TEA, Groves et al.[34]) is added to the ice-cold buffers used to stop uptake and wash the RPTs. Dissolve the pellet in 1 *N* NaOH, and determine the radioactivity in the solution by liquid scintillation spectrometry.* Use a protein assay such as the Biuret, Lowry, or Bio-Rad to determine the RPT protein concentration. Express organic ion uptake as picomoles per milligram protein at a given time.

While only a limited number of cytotoxicity assays are described in this chapter, many other physiological and biochemical parameters have been used as indicators of cell damage after nephrotoxicant exposure. Some of these parameters include lipid peroxidation, glutathione homeostasis, DNA damage, phospholipase A_2 activity, and altered Ca^{2+} homeostasis. Most important, the evaluation of damage to RPTs is best examined by the analysis of several parameters to provide a clear understanding of toxicity.

References

1. Leaf, A. and Coltran, R.S., Renal physiology: an introduction, in *Renal Pathophysiology*, Oxford University Press, New York, 1985, chap. 2.
2. Schrier, R.W. and Gottschalk, C.W., in *Diseases of the Kidney*, Little, Brown, Boston, 1993, 139.
3. Balaban, R.S., Soltoff, S.P., Storey, J.M., and Mandel, L.J., Improved renal cortical tubule suspensions: spectrophotometric study of O_2 delivery, *Am. J. Physiol.*, 238, F50, 1980.
4. Harris, S.I., Balaban, R.S., Barrett, L., and Mandel, L.J., Mitochondrial respiratory capacity and Na^+-K^+-dependent adenosine triphosphatase-mediated ion transport in the intact renal cell, *J. Biol. Chem.*, 256, 10319, 1981.
5. Hjelle, J.T., Hazelton, G.A., Klaassen, C.D., and Hjelle, J.J., Glucuronidation and sulfation in rabbit kidney, *J. Pharmacol. Exp. Ther.*, 236, 150, 1986.
6. Sina, J.F., Bean, C.L., Noble, C., and Bradley, M.O., Isolation and characterization of proximal tubule suspensions from rabbit for *in vitro* studies, *In Vitro Toxicol.*, 1, 5, 1986.
7. Rodeheaver, D.P., Aleo, M.D., and Schnellmann, R.G., Differences in enzymatic and mechanical isolated rabbit renal proximal tubules: comparison in long-term incubation, *In Vitro Cell. Dev. Biol.*, 26, 898, 1990.
8. Brendel, K., Hjelle, J.T., and Meezan, E., Proximal renal tubule preparations isolated from rat or rabbit kidneys without the use of collagenase, *Toxicol. Methods*, 3, 87, 1993.
9. Burg, M.B. and Orloff, J., Oxygen consumption and active transport in separated renal tubules, *Am. J. Physiol.*, 203, 327, 1962.
10. Vinay, P., Gougoux, A., and Lemieux, G., Isolation of a pure suspension of rat proximal tubules, *Am. J. Physiol.*, 241, F403, 1981.
11. Dickman, K.G. and Mandel, L.J., Glycolytic and oxidative metabolism in primary renal proximal tubule cultures, *Am. J. Physiol.*, 257, C333, 1989.
12. Brendel, K. and Meezan, E., Isolation and properties of a pure suspension of proximal kidney tubules obtained without collagenase treatment, *Fed. Proc. Fed. Am. Soc. Exp. Biol.*, 34, 803, 1975.
13. Hjelle, J.T., Morin, J.-P., and Trouet, A., Analytical cell fractionation of isolated rabbit renal proximal tubules, *Kidney Int.*, 20, 71, 1981.

* Samples generally require 6 to 12 h to completely dissolve.

14. Scholer, D.W. and Edelman, I.S., Isolation of rat kidney cortical tubules enriched in proximal and distal segments, *Am. J. Physiol.*, 237, F350, 1979.
15. Soltoff, S.P. and Mandel, L.J., Active ion transport in the renal proximal tubule, *J. Gen. Physiol.*, 84, 601, 1984.
16. Bello-Reuss, E. and Weber, M., Electrophysiological studies on primary cultures of proximal tubule cells, *Am. J. Physiol.*, 251, F490, 1986.
17. Tang, M.-J., Suresh, K.R., and Tannen, R.L., Carbohydrate metabolism by primary cultures of rabbit proximal tubules, *Am. J. Physiol.*, 256, C532, 1989.
18. Tang, M.-J. and Tannen, R.L., Metabolic substrates alter attachment and differentiated functions of proximal tubule cell culture, *J. Am. Soc. Nephrol.*, 41, 1908, 1994.
19. Ruegg, C.E. and Mandel, L.J., Bulk isolation of renal PCT and PST. I. Glucose-dependent metabolic differences, *Am. J. Physiol.*, 259, F164, 1990.
20. Ruegg, C.E., Preparation of precision-cut renal slices and renal proximal tubular fragments for evaluating segment-specific nephrotoxicity, *J. Pharmacol. Toxicol. Methods*, 31, 125, 1994.
21. Cook, W.F. and Pickering, G.W., A rapid method for separating glomeruli from rabbit kidney, *Nature*, 182, 1103, 1958.
22. Kanda, S., Nomata, K., Saha, P.K., Nishimura, N., Yamada, J., Kanatake, H., and Saito, Y., Growth factor regulation of the renal cortical tubular cells by epidermal growth factor, insulin-like growth factor–1, acidic and basic fibroblast growth factor, and transforming growth factor-β in serum free culture, *Cell Biol. Int. Rep.*, 13, 687, 1989.
23. Toutain, H., Vauclin-Jacques, N., Fillastre, J.-P., and Morin, J.-P., Biochemical, functional, and morphological characterization of a primary culture of rabbit proximal tubule cells, *Exp. Cell Res.*, 194, 9, 1991.
24. Aleo, M.D., Taub, M.T., Nickerson, P.A., and Kostyniak, P.J., Primary cultures of rabbit renal proximal tubules cells. I. Growth and biochemical characteristics, *In Vitro Cell. Dev. Biol.*, 25, 776, 1989.
25. Chung, S.D., Alavi, N., Livingston, D., Hiller, S., and Taub, M., Characterization of primary rabbit kidney cultures that express proximal tubule functions in a hormonally defined medium, *J. Cell. Biol.*, 95, 118, 1982.
26. Toutain, H., Vauclin-Jacques, N., Fillastre, J.-P., and Morin, J.-P., Isolation of a pure suspension of proximal tubular cells from the rabbit kidney: morphological, biochemical and metabolic assessment, *Cell Biol. Int. Rep.*, 13, 70, 1989.
27. Nowak, G. and Schnellmann, R.G., Improved culture conditions stimulate gluconeogenesis in primary cultures of renal proximal tubule cells, *Am. J. Physiol.*, 268, C1053, 1995.
28. Schnellmann, R.G., Gilchrist, S.M., and Mandel, L.J., Intracellular distribution and depletion of glutathione in rabbit renal proximal tubules, *Kidney Int.*, 34, 229, 1988.
29. Zenser, T.V., Mattammal, M.B., and Davis, B.B., Demonstration of separate pathways for drug metabolism in the rabbit kidney, *J. Pharmacol. Exp. Ther.*, 208, 418, 1979.
30. Groves, C.E., Lock, E.A., and Schnellmann, R.G., Role of lipid peroxidation in renal proximal tubule cell death induced by haloalkene cysteine conjugates, *Toxicol. Appl. Pharmacol.*, 107, 56, 1991.
31. Groves, C.E., Hayden, P.J., Lock, E.A., and Schnellmann, R.G., Differential cellular effects in the toxicity of haloalkene and haloalkane cysteine conjugates to rabbit renal proximal tubules, *J. Biochem. Toxicol.*, 8, 49, 1993.
32. Lock, E.A., Renal drug-metabolizing enzymes in experimental animals and humans, in *Mechanisms of Injury in Renal Disease and Toxicity*, Goldstein, R.S., Ed., CRC Press, Boca Raton, FL, 1994, 173.
33. Groves, C.E., Evans, K.K., Dantzler, W.H., and Wright, S.H., Peritubular organic cation transport in isolated rabbit proximal tubules, *Am. J. Physiol.*, 266, F450, 1994
34. Groves, C.E. and Wright, S.H., Tetrapentylammonium (TPeA): slowly dissociating inhibitor of the organic cation (OC) transporter, *Biochim. Biophys. Acta*, 1234, 37, 1995.
35. Groves, C.E., Morales, M.N., Rankin, D.R., and Wright, S.H. Peritubular transport of the nephrotoxic mycotoxin ochratoxin A in renal proximal tubule (RPTs) suspensions, *FASEB J.*, 8, 1995.
36. Schnellmann, R.G. and Mandel, L.J., Multiple effects of presumed glutathione depletors on rabbit renal proximal tubules, *Kidney Int.*, 29, 856, 1986.

37. Bergmeyer, H.-U., Bernt, E., and Hess, B., Lactate dehydrogenase, in *Methods of Enzymatic Analysis*, Bergmeyer, H.-U., Ed., Academic Press, London, 1963, 736.
38. Takano, T., Soltoff, S.P., Murdaugh, S., and Mandel, L.J., Intracellular respiratory dysfunction and cell injury in short-term anoxia of rabbit renal proximal tubules, *J. Clin. Invest.*, 76, 2377, 1985.
39. Schnellmann, R.G. and Griner, R.D. Mitochondrial mechanisms of tubular injury, in *Mechanisms of Injury in Renal Disease and Toxicity*, Goldstein, R.S., Ed., CRC Press, Boca Raton, FL, 1994, 247.
40. Lundin, A., Hasenson, M., Persson, J., and Ponsette, A., Estimation of biomass in growing cell lines by adenosine triphosphate assay, *Methods Enzymol.*, 133, 27, 1986.
41. Hull–Ryde, E.A., Cummings, R.G., and Lowe, J.E., Improved method for high energy nucleotide analysis of canine cardiac muscle using reversed phase high performance liquid chromatography, *J. Chromatogr.*, 275, 411, 1983.
42. Mandel, L.J., Schnellmann, R.G., and Jacobs, W.R., Intracellular glutathione in the protection from anoxic injury in renal proximal tubules, *J. Clin. Invest.*, 85, 316, 1988.
43. Schnellmann, R.G., Measurement of oxygen consumption, in *Methods in Toxicology: In Vitro Toxicity Indicators*, Tyson, C.A. and Frazier, J.M., Eds., Academic Press, San Diego, CA, 1994, 128.
44. Smith, M.A., Hewitt, W.R., and Hook, J.B., *In vitro* methods in renal toxicology, in *In Vitro Methods in Toxicology*, Atterwill, C.K. and Steele, C.E., Eds., Cambridge University Press, New York, 1987, 13.

chapter ten

Characterization and Use of Rabbit Renal Proximal Tubular Cells in Primary Culture for Toxicology Research

Michael D. Aleo and Paul J. Kostyniak

10.1 Introduction 163
10.2 Basic tissue isolation and cell culture methods 167
10.2.1 Reagent preparation 167
10.2.2 Materials 169
10.2.3 Isolation of renal proximal tubules 170
10.3 Optimization studies 173
10.3.1 Selected characteristics 173
10.3.2 Role of oxygenation and metabolic substrates 173
10.3.3 Role of glucose and insulin 174
10.3.4 Substratum 175
10.3.5 SV40 transformation 176
10.4 Applications for toxicological studies 176
10.4.1 Mercurials 178
10.4.2 Antibiotics 179
10.4.3 Antineoplastics 180
10.4.4 Cell injury and repair 181
10.5 Acknowledgment 182
References 182

10.1 Introduction

There are numerous experimental models to study the effects of chemicals on renal function, biochemical processes, and cellular integrity *in vitro*. Models that are used most extensively in renal physiological and toxicological studies include the isolated perfused kidney, precision-cut renal slices, *in situ* microperfused and *ex vivo* isolated perfused tubules, isolated tubular and cell suspensions, primary cultures of renal cells, established renal cell lines, isolated organelles, and preparations of brush border and basolateral membrane vesicles. Each model requires different technical skills and equipment to conduct research and has its own inherent advantages and disadvantages. Details regarding

0-8493-3341-5/96/$0.00+$.50

preparation and use of several of these models are presented elsewhere in this volume. The present chapter discusses the characteristics, technical aspects, and use of rabbit renal proximal tubular cells in primary culture for toxicological studies.

Mammalian cell culture is probably the most versatile model to study various toxicological, biochemical, and physiological processes within the kidney since specific cell types can be used from any animal source, including human. However, before using cultured cells for experiments, the cells should be evaluated to establish their cellular and biochemical characteristics. For instance, established cell lines typically express abnormal cellular functions, karyotypes, and biochemical characteristics since they are not cloned from a single parental cell. As such, they tend to express properties of multiple cell types in culture.[1] These deviations from expression of the parental cell phenotype may alter physiological and toxicological responses. For example, the porcine kidney-derived LLC-PK_1 cell line has long been used as a model for the renal proximal tubular cell because it expresses functions that are characteristic of the proximal tubule cell *in vivo*, such as Na^+-dependent amino acid, phosphate, phlorhizin-sensitive glucose, and organic cation transport.[2-10] LLC-PK_1 cells also express high activities of the brush-border enzymes alkaline phosphatase and γ-glutamyltranspeptidase (γ-GT).[11-13] However, this cell line has some aneuploid characteristics, comprises several morphologically and functionally distinct cell types, and expresses some differentiated functions that are unlike those of the proximal tubular cell *in vivo*.[14-16] For example, under normal culture conditions, LLC-PK_1 cells depend primarily on glycolytic metabolism to meet cellular energy demands rather than oxidative metabolism[17-18] and have an adenylate cyclase activity that is sensitive to arginine–vasopressin and calcitonin (distal tubular cell characteristics)[19] rather than to parathyroid hormone.[20] In addition, the brush border enzyme leucine aminopeptidase is absent,[12] the cells are not ammoniagenic,[21] and they lack an organic anion transporter.[10,22]

Although renal cell lines offer unique cellular characteristics in culture and are important models for renal research, it is important for some physiological and toxicological studies that highly differentiated functions that are characteristic of the parent cell type are maintained in culture. This is critical since expression of highly differentiated functions, such as transport characteristics, aerobic metabolism, biotransformation systems, and biochemical status can alter physiological and toxicological responses *in vitro*. For example, the primary pathway involved in *S*-(1,2,3,4,4′-pentachloro-1,3-butadienyl)-L-cysteine (PCBC) and *N*-acetyl-PCBC transport into the renal proximal tubular cell is via a probenecid-sensitive organic anion transporter on the basolateral membrane.[23] Nephrotoxicity *in vivo* can be prevented by prior administration of probenecid. Since LLC-PK_1 cells lack functional expression of an organic anion transport system,[10,22] conjugates of PCBC enter the cell via a Na^+-independent amino acid transport system.[24] Differences in cellular transport may in part explain why 25 μ*M* PCBC causes 50% cell death in suspensions of freshly isolated renal proximal tubules within 3 h of basolateral exposure,[25] whereas the same concentration of PCBC requires 16 h of basolateral exposure in LLC-PK_1 cells to produce 50% cell death.[24]

Although differences in cytotoxic potential of PCBC to LLC-PK_1 cells and suspensions of proximal tubules may be related to differences in uptake systems, they are most likely due to differences in cellular energy metabolism. For example, under normal culture conditions, LLC-PK_1 cells are glycolytic.[17,18] In contrast, since suspensions of renal proximal tubules are obtained directly from an animal, they are dependent on aerobic metabolism to meet cellular energy demands. Since mitochondrial dysfunction is an early event in the toxicity of PCBC to renal proximal tubules in suspension,[26] a model system that depends on aerobic metabolism may be more appropriate to study mechanisms of cellular injury caused by PCBC or other mitochondrial toxicants than a model system that depends on glycolytic metabolism. Furthermore, profound differences in sensitivity to mitochondrial inhibitors in cells cultured under different conditions have been demonstrated by Griner and Schnellmann.[27] They showed that rabbit renal proximal tubular cells cultured under standard (stationary) culture conditions were less sensitive to pure mitochondrial inhibitors, such as antimycin A, than cells cultured under conditions that minimize the induction of glycolytic metabolism *in vitro*.

Toxic responses can also be affected by the inability to maintain phase I biotransformation pathways in cultured cells at levels normally found *in vivo*. For example, the rank order cytotoxicity of a series of cephalosporins in LLC-RK_1 cells does not match their nephrotoxic potential *in vivo*.[28,29] The rank order of cytotoxicity *in vitro* can be restored to its *in vivo* order if an S9 microsomal fraction is added to the culture media to augment the lower than normal esterase activity found in these cultured cells.[28,29] Dramatic differences in toxicological responses can also exist between seemingly identical cell culture systems. For example LLC-RK_1 cells, which are derived from rabbit kidney, respond differently to cephalosporin and carbapenem antibiotics than rabbit renal proximal tubular cells (RPTC) in primary culture. Unlike rabbit RPTC in primary culture, LLC-RK_1 cells do not predict the rank order nephrotoxicity of carbapenem antibiotics *in vivo* and are generally more sensitive to cephalosporin and carbapenem cytotoxicity.[30]

Mechanisms of cellular injury can also be affected by differences in the biochemical status of the cells. For example, cephaloridine toxicity to rabbit proximal tubules in suspension changes in accordance with cellular glutathione content.[31,32] When glutathione levels are depressed, cephaloridine toxicity occurs by a lipid peroxidation-dependent mechanism. Conversely, when cellular glutathione levels are normal, toxicity proceeds through a lipid peroxidation-independent mechanism. These studies illustrate the importance of characterizing and then selecting cell model systems for toxicological studies that maintain differentiated functions, biotransformation pathways, and toxicological responses *in vitro* as close to *in vivo* as possible.

As illustrated in the previous examples, some inherent limitations of established cell lines can be overcome by using primary cultures, since these cells can be derived from a single cell type obtained directly from animal tissue. As such, they tend to retain many functional characteristics of the parent cell type in culture at levels that are comparable to or exceed those found in the other established renal cell lines, such as LLC-PK_1 and OK.[33,34] For example, primary cultures of rabbit RPTC express many functional attributes of proximal tubular cells *in vivo*, such as Na^+-dependent H^+ antiport, phosphate symport, and phlorhizin-sensitive glucose symport, a functional hexose monophosphate shunt, a renin–angiotensin system, and L-thyroxine metabolism.[35-42] The brush-border enzymes leucine aminopeptidase, alkaline phosphatase, and γ-GT are also present.[35,43] Unlike LLC-PK_1 cells, RPTC in primary culture have a parathyroid hormone-sensitive adenylate cyclase[35,44] and a probenecid-sensitive organic anion transporter.[45-47]

Although many differentiated functions of the parent cell type are retained in primary cell cultures, they still have limitations. Cellular energy metabolism quickly changes from aerobic to glycolytic metabolism under standard (stationary) culture conditions,[48,49] and the cells are unable to maintain normal levels of cytochrome P-450 mixed-function oxidase, brush-border membrane enzyme activities, succinic dehydrogenase, and acetylesterase activities.[43,50] The inability to maintain aerobic respiration rates and differentiated functions at *in vivo* levels using standard (stationary) culture conditions can limit RPTC in primary culture for some physiological and toxicological studies. Changes in cellular energy metabolism *in vitro* is of particular importance for highly aerobic tissues like RPTC,[51] since $(Na^+ + K^+)$-stimulated-ATPase activity regulates Na^+-dependent transport processes and is tightly coupled to mitochondrial respiration.[52]

Current strategies for alleviating some of these limitations have focused on several environmental factors, such as hypoxic culture conditions, which may promote induction of glycolytic metabolism and loss of differentiated functions in cultured cells.[53-55] Oxygen tension in the media used to grow cells under standard (stationary) culture conditions is extremely low, whether measured directly[54] or calculated by Fick's law.[56,57] Improving oxygenation by rocking culture plates enhances cellular metabolism and mitochondrial enzyme activity in LLC-PK_1 cells.[21,58] It also increases Na^+-dependent sugar transport and promotes dome formation (a morphological indication of vectorial solute transport across the cell monolayer) and the development of pH-modulated ammoniagenesis.[21,58] Rocking rabbit RPTC in primary culture, however, does not enhance mitochondrial respiration or prevent the induction of glycolytic metabolism.[48] This apparent inconsistency suggests that adequate oxygenation alone is insufficient to support aerobic respiration in primary cultures of rabbit RPTC.

The availability of proper metabolic substrates in the culture media also appears to regulate cellular energy metabolism *in vitro*.[59-61] The addition of a fatty acid to the culture media, as a preferential substrate for mitochondrial metabolism over glucose metabolism, maintains aerobic metabolism and viability in well-oxygenated suspensions of rabbit renal proximal tubules for 24 h without inducing glycolytic metabolism.[49] Therefore, oxygen tension in culture media and the presence of suitable metabolic substrates are at least two factors that modulate aerobic respiration and expression of differentiated functions *in vitro*.

The composition of the culture media also affects maintenance of differentiated functions *in vitro*. For example, cytochrome P-450 isozyme levels are affected by differences in the basal culture media, its supplements, and the presence or absence of cysteine.[63,64] In addition, LLC-PK_1 cells express gluconeogenic potential when grown in glucose-free media,[65] thereby illustrating how alterations in media formulations can alter expression of differentiated functions *in vitro*.

Cell-basement membrane interactions are also critical in maintaining normal cellular functions *in vitro*. Extracellular matrix materials, such as collagen, laminin, and fibronectin, have biological activity and modify cell growth, attachment, differentiation, and metabolism in cultured cells.[66-71] For example, even under standard culture conditions of limited oxygen supply MDCK cells,[72-74] cortical tubular cells from human kidney,[75] and rat proximal tubular cells[76] express differentiated functions and morphological characteristics that more closely resemble those of the parent cell type when these cells are grown on extracellular matrix proteins. Growing cells on a microporous membrane support also enhances cellular morphology and expression of differentiated functions in primary cultures of rabbit RPTC,[47] MDCK cells,[72-74] respiratory tract epithelial cells,[77] keratinocytes,[78] and Sertoli cells.[79] In MDCK cells, the microporous nature of the membrane support appears to be more important in altering the ultrastructural and protein synthetic activities and deposition of basement membrane than differences in extracellular matrix proteins.[72]

Since established cell lines and cells in primary culture have been used to study hypoxic cell injury,[80] to screen chemicals for cytotoxic potential,[81-83] and to study mechanisms of chemical-induced injury,[84-86] maintenance of aerobic metabolism and highly specific differentiated functions of the parent cell type in cultured cells is extremely important in the field of toxicology. Interpretation of toxicity-based mechanisms can be skewed by the induction of glycolytic metabolism and loss of important differentiated functions. Thus, *in vitro* models must be continually characterized, developed, and refined such that aerobic metabolism and differentiated functions of the parent cell type are maintained in culture. Only in this way can more accurate extrapolations be made from *in vitro* studies to *in vivo* studies. For rabbit RPTC in primary culture, the ideal culture conditions need to more closely resemble the extracellular environment of proximal tubular cells *in vivo*. This would include modifications to the culture conditions and media formulation that promote aerobic metabolism and, if desired, a suitable extracellular matrix protein and/or a porous basolateral membrane support surface for cell attachment.

Although the details of culturing RPTC have been published by several authors,[50,87,88] the present chapter describes the most current methods and culture conditions used for maintaining aerobic metabolism and some important differentiated functions in culture.

10.2 Basic tissue isolation and cell culture methods

10.2.1 Reagent preparation

High quality (pyrogen-free) deionized water should be used for tissue culture. The water should be obtained fresh from a system that prepares Type I grade water (e.g., Barnstead NANOpure ultrapure water system Model D4751) that has been previously processed by a reverse osmosis system (Barnstead ULTROpure).

1. *Preparation of iron oxide solution (500 ml).* Using a 250-ml beaker, dissolve 1.3 g of NaOH (Sigma No. S-0899) and 10.0 g of KNO_3 (Sigma No. P-6030) in 50 ml of oxygen-saturated, pyrogen-free deionized water. Using a 500-ml beaker, dissolve 4.5 g of $FeSO_4 \cdot 7H_2O$ (Sigma No. F-7002) in 50 ml of oxygen-saturated, pyrogen-free deionized water. Add the basic KNO_3 slowly to the $FeSO_4$ solution while stirring with a glass rod. Cover the mixture with a watch glass and boil for 20 min. After cooling to room temperature, the resulting precipitate of paramagnetic iron oxide is attracted to the bottom of the wash beaker with a strong magnet and is washed five to ten times by decanting, resuspending the precipitate each time with 400 ml of fresh, pyrogen-free deionized water. Remove the magnet after the last wash and resuspend the iron oxide in 500 ml of 0.9% NaCl (normal saline).[89] Dispense approximately 80 ml of a homogeneous suspension into 100-ml bottles with rubber-liner caps. The bottles containing the concentrated iron oxide solution are placed in an autoclavable tray filled with 0.5 in. of tap water and then autoclaved for 20 min on a liquid cycle for future use. Cool the tray containing the bottles to room temperature in a laminar flow hood. Tighten caps and store at room temperature.
2. *Preparation of sterile phosphate buffered saline (PBS) (2 l).* Dissolve 16.0 g of NaCl (Sigma No. S-5886), 4.32 g of $Na_2HPO_4 \cdot 7H_2O$ (Sigma No. S-9390), 0.4 g of KCl (Sigma No. P-5405), and 0.4 g of KH_2PO_4 (Sigma No. P-5655) in approximately 1.8 l of pyrogen-free deionized water. Adjust to pH 7.4 at 4°C and bring to final volume. Filter through a 0.45-μm pore size filter to remove particulate matter and dispense into four 500-ml glass bottles with rubber-liner caps. The bottles are placed in an autoclavable tray filled with 0.5 in. of tap water and then autoclaved for 20 min on a liquid cycle. Cool the tray containing the bottles to room temperature in a laminar flow hood. Tighten caps and store at room temperature. Refrigerate before using. If desired, one can substitute commercially available presterilized Dulbeccos PBS (Gibco No. 14190 series).
3. *Preparation of sterile preparation medium (1 l).* Dissolve 1.26 g of $NaHCO_3$ (Sigma No. S-5761), 100 U/ml of penicillin G (Sigma No. P-3032), and one 1-l bottle of Dulbeccos Modified Eagles Medium:Hams F12 (DMEM:F12) media mix (Sigma No. D-2906) in approximately 800 ml of pyrogen-free deionized water. Bubble with 95% O_2/5% CO_2 for 15 min. Add 283 μl of heptanoic acid (Sigma No. H-9378) and stir until dissolved. Adjust to pH 7.4 at 4°C and bring to 1 l. Adjust osmolality to 295 ± 5 mOsm/kg. Sterilize by filtration with a sterile, 0.2-μm pore size filter unit (Nalgene No. 300–4100 with Gelman Supor 200 membrane filter No. 60301). Store in refrigerator.
4. *Preparation of sterile deferoxamine medium (1 l).* Prepare as outlined for Reagent 3, but also dissolve 0.3284 g of deferoxamine mesylate (Sigma No. D-9533).
5. *Preparation of sterile, hormonally defined glucose-free culture medium (1 l).* The basal culture medium is a 50:50 DMEM:F12 special order media mix from Sigma Chemical Co. (St. Louis, MO) that does not contain phenol red, $NaHCO_3$, HEPES, glucose, or pyruvate. Before use, the dry mix for 1 l is supplemented with 1.26 g of $NaHCO_3$ (15 m*M*) (Sigma No. S-5761), 3.9045 g of HEPES (15 m*M*) (Sigma No.

H-0763), 0.5605 g of lactate (5 m*M*) (Sigma No. L-7022), and 39.2 mg of alanine (0.44 m*M*) (Sigma No. A-3534) and is dissolved in approximately 800 ml of pyrogen-free deionized water. (For experiments with growth factors like EGF, supplement the medium further with 5 m*M* glucose). Bubble with 95% O_2/5% CO_2 for 15 min. Adjust to pH 7.4 at 37°C and bring the volume to 1 l. Adjust osmolality to 295 ± 5 mOsm/kg. Sterilize by filtration with a sterile, 0.2-μm pore size filter unit (Nalgene No. 300–4100 with Gelman Supor 200 membrane filter No. 60301). Store in refrigerator.*

6. *Preparation of human transferrin (20 ml).* Gently dissolve 100 mg of human transferrin (Sigma No. T-1147) in 20 ml of glucose-free medium (Reagent 5). Sterilize by filtration using a 0.2-μm pore size filter (Gelman No. 4192) and dispense in 2-ml aliquots in sterile 12 × 75 mm tubes with caps (Falcon No. 2005). Freeze at -20°C until needed. Do not freeze/thaw each tube more than four times.
7. *Preparation of bovine insulin (20 ml).* Gently dissolve 5.7 mg of bovine insulin (Sigma No. I-6634) in 20 ml of 0.01 *N* HCl made with pyrogen-free deionized water. Sterilize by filtration using a 0.2-μm pore size filter (Gelman No. 4192) and dispense in 2-ml aliquots in sterile 12 × 75 mm tubes with caps (Falcon No. 2003). Store for up to one month at 4°C.
8. *Preparation of hydrocortisone (20 ml).* Dissolve 7.25 mg of hydrocortisone (Sigma No. H-4001) in 20 ml of absolute ethanol. Dispense in 1-ml aliquots in sterile 12 × 75 mm tubes with caps (Falcon No. 2005). Store for up to one month at 4°C.
9. *Preparation of sodium selenite (20 ml).* Dissolve 10.0 mg of sodium selenite (Sigma No. S-5261) in 20 ml pyrogen-free deionized water. Sterilize by filtration using a 0.2-μm pore size filter (Gelman No. 4192) and dispense in 2-ml aliquots in sterile 12 × 75 mm tubes with caps (Falcon No. 2005). Freeze at –20°C until needed. Refrigerate working solution.
10. *Preparation of ascorbic acid phosphate, magnesium salt*n-hydrate (20 ml).* Based on the formula weight of the ascorbate salt (Wako Chemicals, Richmond, VA, No. 013–12061), adjusted for water content, prepare a 100-m*M* stock solution in antibiotic- and glucose-free medium (Reagent 5). Sterilize by filtration using a 0.2-μm pore size filter (Gelman No. 4192) and dispense in 2-ml aliquots in sterile 12 × 75 mm tubes with caps (Falcon No. 2005). Store for up to two weeks at 4°C.
11. *Preparation of 0.1% (w/v) soybean trypsin inhibitor (100 ml).* Gently dissolve 0.1 g of soybean trypsin inhibitor (Sigma No. T-6522) into 100 ml of PBS (Reagent 2). Sterilize by filtration using a 0.2-μm pore size filter unit (Nalgene No. 120–0020) and dispense in 25-ml aliquots into sterile, 50-ml T-flasks (Falcon No. 3013). Freeze at –80°C until needed. For use, thaw rapidly in a water bath and store at 4°C.
12. *Preparation of digestion medium (4 ml).* Warm collagenase to room temperature (Worthington Biochemical Co., Freehold, NJ, Type IV, No. LS04188, stored desiccated at 4°C). Gently dissolve approximately 9600 U in 4 ml of sterile deferoxamine medium (Reagent 4) and sterilize by filtration using a 0.2-μm pore size filter (Nalgene No. 190–2520). Prepare fresh for each tubular cell isolation and store in refrigerator until use. Since collagenase lots vary in the balance of certain enzymatic/tryptic activities, different lots should be tested to determine which one promotes the best outgrowth.

* Before use, this medium is hormonally supplemented with 100 μl of human transferrin (5 μg/ml), 20 μl of bovine insulin (10 n*M*), 100 μl of selenite (5 ng/ml), 5 μl of hydrocortisone (50 n*M*), and 100 μl of ascorbic acid (100 μ*M*) for every 100 ml of medium. The hormonally defined medium should be changed every day to avoid substrate depletion.

Notes on reagent preparation. During our early work with rabbit RPTC in culture, we eliminated antibiotics from the culture medium for theoretical considerations and noticed some beneficial effects. RPTC appeared to reach confluence more quickly when grown in antibiotic-free medium as compared with medium supplemented with 1.1 mg/ml penicillin G and 92 U/ml streptomycin sulfate.[90] There is no real need for the antibiotics in the medium if the tissue culture facility is kept clean and good aseptic technique is always practiced. Dedicated equipment should be positioned away from doors, air vents, drafts, and overhangs, which can serve as a source of contamination from dust and airborne spores, and the area and equipment should be routinely and scrupulously cleaned. Antibiotics can be added to the media for novice tissue culture users in order to minimize contamination until aseptic/sterile technique is perfected.

Another important consideration is the presence or absence of phenol red as a pH indicator in culture medium. Since phenol red is a substrate for the organic acid transporter, its presence in culture medium can reduce uptake of organic anions (either metabolic substrates or xenobiotics of interest), in much the same way that probenecid reduces organic anion uptake and is used to reduce toxicity due to the active transport of nephrotoxic organic anions. Phenol red also inhibits growth of BSC-1 and MDCK cell lines[91] and can serve as a competitive substrate for glucuronidation in OK cells.[92] Although the relevance of these effects is dependent on the concerns of the investigator and the type of research being conducted, it is important to realize that phenol red does not act solely as a pH indicator in culture. It interacts with transport and metabolic processes within renal epithelial cells. Since culture media have been refined to minimize induction of glycolysis in cultured cells and the medium is changed every day, the utility of phenol red as a pH indicator is greatly diminished. Although Scheinman et al.[93] found the presence of phenol red in the media to be a convenient marker of confluence in cells grown on inserts, we still suggest that it be omitted from culture media for most applications.

Sodium bicarbonate should never be totally omitted from culture media in favor of a biological buffer. Bicarbonate and carbon dioxide are key solutes that regulate intracellular pH, urinary acidification, Na^+ reabsorption, and oxidative metabolism in RPTC. Its absence from culture media alters renal physiology and metabolism.[94]

10.2.2 Materials

The following items need to be individually covered, securely wrapped in aluminum foil, or enclosed in reusable autoclavable bags before autoclaving. Place contents in an autoclavable tray and autoclave for 30 min with a 15-min drying cycle. Cool to room temperature before use. There are enough materials and reagents for isolating both kidneys. Glassware should be clean (MICRO, VWR No. 21830–410) and free of detergent residues.

These items are autoclaved:

1. Two 1-liter beakers (Corning No. 1000–1L) used for filtering tubules.
2. One 250-ml beaker (Corning No. 1003–250) used to hold surgical instruments in laminar flow hood.
3. Two 100-ml beakers (Corning No. 1000–100) used to hold each kidney after removal from rabbit.
4. Two forceps. One blunt-tip serrated (VWR No. 25719–044) to hold renal pelvis and one curved serrated (VWR No. 25718–008) to remove fat and hair from kidney.
5. One pair curved dissecting scissors (VWR No. 25608–509) to remove renal cortex and mince tissue.
6. One pair straight dissecting scissors (VWR No. 25876–009).

7. Four 100-mm diameter, 20-mm deep petri dishes (Corning No. 3160–102), two containing 3 × 3 in. gauze sponges and two without.
8. Two 50-ml glass syringes with Luer-Lok Tip (BD2315).
9. Two 15-ml Dounce homogenizers (Wheaton No. 357544, Type A pestle).
10. Two blunt-end thin spatulas (VWR No. 57950–000) that have been bent to remove tubules from nylon mesh.
11. Eight 2-in. magnetic stir bars (VWR No. 58948–171), wrapped individually to remove iron-laden glomeruli from proximal tubules.
12. Four Luer-Lok stainless steel needles: Two 18-gauge (BD1097) and two 20-gauge (BD1075), previously filed down to a smooth blunt end and wrapped individually to cannulate renal artery.
13. Sutures (Ethicon 00 silk): Two packages wrapped with four loosely tied half knots.
14. Package containing a large pair of scissors (VWR No. 25608–316), small scissors (VWR No. 25878-048), and small serrated jaw forceps (VWR No. 25607–120).

These items are not autoclaved:

15. Nylon mesh screens (Tetko Inc., Depew, NY; 253-μm pore size (No. 3-253/46) and 85-μm pore size (No. 3–85/44)).
16. Four plastic embroidery hoops (4 in. diameter).
17. Two neodymium magnets (Adams Magnetic Products, Garland, TX; 35 MGO — 1/2″ × 3/8″ × 2″).

10.2.3 *Isolation of renal proximal tubules*

The isolation method originally described by Brendel and Meezan[95] has been further modified by Chung et al.[21] and Rodeheaver et al.[62] Proximal tubules isolated by this technique are essentially free from contaminating cells and structures[96] and retain their basement membrane.[97]

Allow the rabbits a one- to two-week acclimation period before use. Avoid using kidneys obtained from larger (i.e., older) rabbits, since this generally results in reduced tubular yields and outgrowth of epithelial cells. Prepare glassware, instruments, and buffers the day before the isolation procedure. On the morning of the isolation, place two sets of precut sieves in 70% (v/v) ethanol with the large mesh screen below the fine mesh screen. Prepare the digestion medium and keep cold until ready to use. Add 50 to 100 ml of absolute ethanol to a 250-ml beaker to hold surgical instruments. Flame surgical instruments between procedures.

Carefully restrain a male or female New Zealand White rabbit (2 to 2.5 kg) in a stainless steel cage (Lab Products Inc., Maywood, NJ, Model H–1428). Secure a piece of prefitted cardboard with tape to one ear. Using a butterfly infusion set (Abbott Laboratories, North Chicago, IL, No. 4506) connected to a three-way stopcock (Baxter Healthcare Corporation, Valencia, CA, No. K75), carefully cannulate ear vein and inject 3 to 5 ml of 1000 USP U/ml of heparin (Lyphomed, Deerfield, IL, No. 0468–2033–25) followed by 2 ml of normal saline (0.9%, w/v, NaCl). Wait 5 to 10 min before euthanizing the animal with an overdose (3 to 4 ml) of 65 mg/ml of sodium pentobarbital (The Butler Company, Columbus, OH, No. WAB10505). After the rabbit is euthanized, swab the abdomen with 70% (v/v) ethanol to minimize the amount of loose fur. Use a large pair of scissors to remove the fur coat from the abdomen. Rinse the exposed area with 70% (v/v) ethanol and open the abdominal cavity with another pair of scissors. Avoid contaminating the incision with rabbit hair or by cutting the intestines. Expose the left kidney and quickly, but gently, tease the fat away from the kidneys, being careful not to squeeze the kidney. Laying the kidney on your fingers, if necessary, expose the renal vein and artery with a pair of forceps and free the vein and artery from each other *in situ*. Cut the vein as close to the kidney as possible, while leaving as much of the ureter and renal artery intact. Cut the artery as close to the aorta as possible. Remove the kidney and place it in a 100-ml beaker containing ice-cold, antibiotic-supplemented medium and cover the beaker with foil. Repeat the procedure for the second kidney.

Transfer the kidneys to a laminar flow hood. Perform subsequent steps on a tray filled with chipped ice. Fill a 100-mm petri dish with antibiotic-supplemented medium (Reagent 3) and transfer the kidney from the beaker to a petri dish cover. Carefully remove hair and tease away fat without piercing the capsule. Lift kidney up by the ureter and wash with antibiotic-supplemented medium. Transfer the kidney to a clean, 100-mm petri dish bottom containing gauze with enough antibiotic-supplemented medium to soak the gauze. Using blunt-tip serrated forceps, cannulate the renal artery with a blunted 18-gauge needle. (Use a blunted 21-gauge needle if the renal artery is small in diameter). Remove the 00 suture (already half-knotted) and secure the two sutures to the cannulated artery. Tighten the knots and cut off excess suture. Ensure that the end of the needle is secured proximal to the bifurcation of the renal artery; otherwise only half of the kidney will be perfused.

Attach the outside part of the syringe to the needle and fill it with antibiotic-supplemented medium. Put the plunger in very slowly and apply slow, steady pressure to remove the blood from within the kidney. Avoid excessive pressure or the kidney will split apart. Separate the needle from the syringe and remove the plunger before the syringe is totally empty to avoid pushing air through the kidney. Aspirate excess medium from the petri dish. Reconnect the needle to the syringe and add another 50 ml of antibiotic-supplemented medium. Repeat the procedure above followed by 50 ml of PBS. The kidney should turn a pale brown or tannish color as the kidney is cleared of blood. Remove fluid from the petri dish after each perfusion. It usually takes about 100 ml of medium and 50 ml of PBS to clear the kidney of blood.

Resuspend concentrated iron oxide and flame the outer lip of the bottle in which the iron oxide is stored before use. Add 5 ml of concentrated iron oxide to the syringe containing 40 ml of PBS. Slowly force the diluted iron oxide through the kidney as done previously with the medium. As the kidney slowly turns a medium gray in color, clear liquid should come out of the ureter and renal vein. If iron oxide comes out of the ureter, too much pressure is being applied and the glomeruli will rupture. The kidney is completely perfused when the kidney becomes black in color and iron oxide comes out of the vein and resistance on the plunger increases. Aspirate fluid from the petri dish. Flame the outer lip of the iron oxide bottle and use it for the next perfusion. Reautoclave the bottle if necessary.

Wash the kidney with antibiotic-supplemented medium and transfer it to another petri dish. Add more medium. Cut off the needle, then cut off the ureter and artery. Gently peel off the capsule by holding onto the remaining stub of the ureter or some part of the capsule. Avoid holding the kidney itself. Wash the kidney again and transfer it to a clean petri dish containing deferoxamine-supplemented medium (Reagent 4) while cutting off the capsule. Repeat procedure for second kidney.

Carefully remove the cortex using a pair of curved scissors with the curved edge pointing toward the kidney. The renal cortex is grayish black in color while the medullary area is white. Do not include the medullary tissue in the preparation. The pieces of the cortex should be about 1 cm in size.

Take the screens out of the alcohol and set each pair on a separate sterile, 1-l beaker such that the fine mesh screen is placed below the large mesh screen. Wash down each set of screens with at least 500 ml of PBS, making sure that the sides and top of the screens are completely washed with PBS.

Without squeezing the tissue, carefully transfer about five to ten pieces of cortex to the Dounce homogenizer. Add approximately 5 to 7 ml of deferoxamine-supplemented medium to the homogenizer. Homogenize tissue with four to five slow, steady strokes of the pestle to avoid introducing air into the mixture. Pour the homogenate on top of the screen and rinse the homogenizer two times with deferoxamine-supplemented medium to remove the remaining cells. Repeat the procedure for the remaining tissue, being sure not to let the tissue on the screen dry out. After all of the homogenate has been added, rinse screens with about 500 ml of deferoxamine-supplemented medium.

Add a sterile stir bar to two 50-ml conical centrifuge tubes (Corning No. 25330–50). Add 40 ml of deferoxamine-supplemented medium to each tube. Discard the top screen and gently remove proximal tubules and glomeruli off the bottom screen with a sterile, curved metal spatula and evenly distribute them between two centrifuge tubes. Remove tubules that are stuck between the hoop and the screen. When all the tubules are off the screen, tighten the cap on the centrifuge tube, gently invert, and let stand for about 5 min. Carefully remove the stir bar inside the tube by placing another stir bar along the outside of the centrifuge tube and move the stir bar slowly up to the top. Aspirate the glomeruli that have been attracted to the stir bar. Repeat the procedure two to three times for each tube, using a new sterile stir bar each time.

Add 1 ml of 0.1% (w/v) soybean trypsin inhibitor (Reagent 12) and 1 ml of digestion medium (Reagent 13) to each centrifuge tube that contains tubules in 40 ml of medium. Keep tubules suspended for 15 min while warming the tube in the hands. Pellet tubules in a refrigerated centrifuge for 5 min at 50× g. The pellet should be packed tightly enough to be able to aspirate medium from the tube without disturbing the pellet, but not so tightly compressed that the tubules are difficult to resuspend. Aspirate the fluid and resuspend the pellet twice with antibiotic-, deferoxamine-, and glucose-free medium (Reagent 5). During each washing step, have a neodymium magnet taped to the outside of each centrifuge tube, resuspend the tubules, and let stand for 5 min. Carefully aspirate remaining glomeruli that have been attracted to the magnet from the inside of the tube. After the final spin, resuspend in 50 ml of antibiotic-, deferoxamine-, and glucose-free medium. Estimate protein yield by centrifuging 3 × 0.5-ml aliquots in a preweighed microcentrifuge tube (Sarstedt No. 72.690) using an Eppendorf 5415c centrifuge set to "high". The supernatant is completely removed from the protein pellet and, by difference, the average wet weight of the tissue (in milligrams) is divided by 2.2 and then multiplied by the total remaining volume (i.e., 48.5 ml) to obtain an estimate of total protein yield (in milligrams). Good protein yields are typically 150 to 200 mg/kidney, depending on the size of the rabbit and skill of the operator.

Assuming a 100-mg yield, add 200 μl of human transferrin (5 μg/ml), 40 μl of bovine insulin (10 n*M*), 200 μl of selenium (5 ng/ml), 10 μl of hydrocortisone (50 n*M*), and 200 μl of ascorbic acid (100 μ*M*) to 150 ml of antibiotic-, deferoxamine-, and glucose-free medium. Add 50 ml of suspension containing 100 mg of tubules to 150 ml of hormonally supplemented medium for a final protein concentration of 0.5 mg/ml. By trial and error and with further experience, this value may have to be adjusted higher to compensate for attachment of tubules to the inoculation bottle, in order to achieve an initial plating density of 1 mg/35-mm plate. Gently swirl the bottle each time before pipetting and place 2 ml of tubule suspension in either 35-mm plates (Falcon No. 3001) or microporous inserts. Try to do this step as rapidly as possible because the tubules will stick to the glass bottle. Place culture plates on an orbital shaker (BELLCO Glass, Inc., Vineland, NJ, No. 7744–01010) oscillating at 60 rpm in a standard humidified 95% air/5% CO_2 incubator at 37°C. Contrary to previous recommendations,[50,87,88] the complete hormonally supplemented medium should be changed daily to avoid depletion of important metabolic substrates so as not to adversely affect cell growth.

10.3 Optimization studies

10.3.1 Selected characteristics

A description of this model system was first published by Chung et al.,[35] who defined a serum-free hormonally defined medium that maintained higher levels of brush-border enzyme activities than cells cultured with serum and eliminated fibroblast overgrowth of the cultures. Under standard culture conditions (stationary cultures on plastic petri dishes grown in medium containing high glucose concentrations), these cells express many functional characteristics of proximal tubular cells *in vivo*,[33-47] but demonstrate dramatic declines in hormonal responsiveness, brush-border membrane enzyme activities, phase I biotransformation functions,[33,43,50,90] and changes in carbohydrate metabolism[33,38,48,49,90] as compared with freshly isolated proximal tubules. Morphologically, these cells maintain cellular polarity, but steadily dedifferentiate with age. They contain numerous autophagic vacuoles and glycogen granules[98,99] and retain only a rudimentary brush border. These ultrastructural findings supported an earlier recommendation[43] that these cultures are best used after achieving confluence through day 12 in culture. The growth of these cells under standard culture conditions is illustrated in Figure 1. The gradual realization of some of the initial limitations of this culture system for certain types of research studies prompted numerous investigations into cell culture to optimize the system for more representative physiological and toxicological studies.

10.3.2 Role of oxygenation and metabolic substrates

The induction of glycolytic metabolism in primary cultures of rabbit RPTC was first proposed to be a consequence of cellular proliferation, rather than a response to hypoxic culture conditions, the Pasteur effect, or the high concentration of glucose found in the media.[48,100] However, Dickman and Mandel[49] reported a rapid and profound reduction of oxidative metabolism (reduced transport-dependent and -independent oxygen consumption, respiratory capacity, and intracellular contents of ATP and K^+) with a corresponding increase in glycolytic metabolism (increased lactate production) within 6 h after placing freshly isolated proximal tubules under standard (stationary) culture conditions. The shift from oxidative metabolism occurred quickly after the initiation of culture, without any cell attachment or proliferation. Therefore, adequate oxygenation combined with the presence of a preferred fatty acid substrate (2 m*M* heptanoate) for mitochondrial oxidation, was critical for maintaining aerobic metabolism and preventing the induction of glycolysis during short-term (≤1 day) culture. The overall importance of meeting these two conditions was confirmed by Rodeheaver et al.[62] in 24-h suspension cultures of renal proximal tubules. However, Aleo and Schnellmann[101] showed that the full beneficial effects of adequate oxygenation in combination with heptanoate were not realized during long-term culture. The addition of 2 m*M* heptanoate did not prevent the induction of glycolytic metabolism in adequately oxygenated cultures of RPTC beyond the first 24 h in culture. As compared with stationary cultures, the primary benefit of reducing lactate production and lactate dehydrogenase activity occurred in shaken cultures in the absence of heptanoate. Other short-chain fatty acids were also without effect,[102] and higher concentrations of heptanoate reduced cell growth.[101] These findings suggest that the induction of glycolytic metabolism in primary cultures of RPTC cells is primarily controlled by the availability of oxygen. However, other environmental factors appear to be more important in minimizing and regulating the induction of glycolytic metabolism in culture besides the presence of a fatty acid substrate for mitochondrial oxidation.

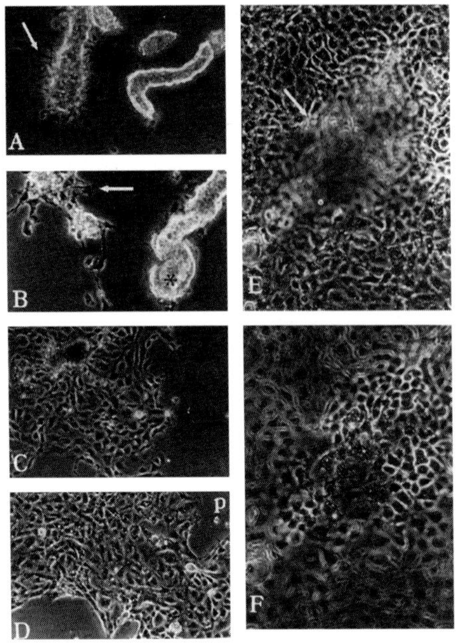

Figure 1 Phase contrast micrographs of rabbit RPTC in primary culture. A) Freshly isolated tubules 4 hr after initiation of culture. Note the distinction of proximal tubular lumina. The beginnings of epithelial cell migration from proximal tubules (arrow). x200. B) Proximal tubules 24 hr after initiation of cell culture. Some epithelial cells have fully migrated from remnant tubules (arrow) whereas other tubules show microscopic signs of degeneration (asterisk). x200. C) Proximal tubular cells after 3 days in culture. Colonies of cells have formed around explanted proximal tubules. Only a small portion of the remnant tubule is still visible. x100. D) Proximal tubular cells after 5 days in culture. Numerous large colonies of cells occupy the tissue culture plate and form connections. Some areas of the plate are still unoccupied by cell growth (p). x100. Dome formation in confluent cultures of proximal tubule cells. E) Dome in center of photograph (arrow) is distinctly out of focus with the cells attached to the culture plate. F) Cells that do not comprise the dome are not within the focal plane. x200. (From Aleo et al., *In Vitro Cell. Dev. Biol.*, 25, 776. Copyright © 1989 by the Tissue Culture Association. Reproduced with permission of the copyright owner.)

10.3.3 Role of glucose and insulin

Adequate oxygenation in combination with adjustments to glucose and insulin concentrations in culture media appear to be more critical in maintaining aerobic metabolism, gluconeogenesis, and expression of differentiated functions in primary cultures of rabbit RPTC. Although glucose is a substrate for transport by the proximal tubule, its presence at high concentrations in culture media may be deleterious for RPTC under standard (stationary) culture conditions. Compared with the metabolic and gluconeogenic properties of freshly isolated proximal tubules in suspension,[103] high glucose concentrations in media stimulate the high rate of glucose utilization seen in primary cultures of rabbit RPTC cultured under stationary conditions[38] and suppress gluconeogenic potential. Furthermore, use of mitogenic concentrations of insulin in the culture media appears to down regulate phosphoenolpyruvate carboxykinase, a key regulatory enzyme in the gluconeogenic pathway, in primary cultures.[104] Deleting glucose and insulin from the culture media, even under stationary culture conditions, can enhance expression of some representative marker enzyme activities, increase methyl glucose transport,[105,106] and reduce cellular glycogen content,[98] with no deleterious effects on the rate of cell growth or morphology.[106]

Enhanced expression of brush-border enzyme activities are correlated with a higher density of apical microvilli, as seen by scanning electron microscopy.[107] Although the cells can synthesize glucose from pyruvate and α-ketoglutarate,[107,108] deleting glucose and insulin from the culture media only delays the eventual decline in gluconeogenic enzyme activities.

Nowak and Schnellmann[109] considered the above observations and blended them into a singular experimental design in which primary cultures are constantly shaken to improve oxygenation, lactate and alanine are added to the media as respiratory and gluconeogenic substrates, glucose is deleted from the media, and insulin is provided at physiologic, rather than mitogenic, concentrations. Compared with standard culture conditions, their modifications maintain normal cellular energy metabolism, shifting glucose metabolism from glycolysis to gluconeogenesis and shifting lactate metabolism from net lactate production to net lactate consumption. Basal and ouabain-sensitive oxygen consumption are approximately two-fold higher in cultures that are shaken compared to cultures that are held stationary (Figure 2). Net glucose consumption, lactate production, and glycogen content decrease dramatically under shaken culture conditions as a function of decreasing concentrations of glucose. The presence of lactate stimulates net lactate consumption (Figure 3), while physiologic concentrations of insulin stimulate gluconeogenic capacity fourfold above that associated with cells exposed to mitogenic concentrations of insulin (Figure 4). The gluconeogenic capacity of the cells was retained despite a modest decrease in fructose-1,6-bisphosphatase activity. These combined changes to the culture conditions represent a major advance in maintaining aerobic metabolism and gluconeogenic capacity in primary cultures of rabbit RPTC.

10.3.4 Substratum

Utilizing microporous membrane supports offers additional benefits beyond independent access to the apical and basolateral membranes. They also appear to promote better retention of differentiated function even under standard culture conditions (stationary plates with high glucose and insulin levels). Rabbit RPTC grown on collagen-coated, polycarbonate Nucleopore filters expressed higher apical (14.3 ± 2.5 pmol/mg protein per minute) and basolateral uptake of *p*-aminohippuric acid (PAH) (42.4 ± 4.8 pmol/mg protein per minute) compared with cells grown on collagen-coated, plastic dishes (1.31 ± 0.08 pmol/mg protein per minute).[110] Despite an order-of-magnitude increase in total PAH uptake in cells grown on collagen-coated inserts compared with collagen-coated dishes, PAH uptake was still insensitive to 1 m*M* probenecid. However, when rabbit RPTC in primary culture are grown on Millicell-HA inserts under stationary conditions and are rocked during transport studies, PAH uptake is inhibited by 60% in cultures exposed to 70 μ*M* probenecid.[47] This apparent inconsistency is either the result of differences in the physicochemical nature of the different microporous membrane supports and/or the additional added benefit of rocking culture inserts.

Millicell-HA inserts have also been used to demonstrate preferential and inhibitable uptake of tetraethylammonium, methylglucopyranoside, and the adaptive response of transepithelial phosphate transport caused by phosphate deprivation.[47,93] Another study demonstrated a transepithelial pH gradient that was dependent on the polarized distribution of an apical Na^+-dependent H^+ antiporter and a basolateral Na^+-HCO_3^- cotransporter that was inhibitable by amiloride and 4-acetamido-4′-isothiocyanostilbene-2,2′-disulfonic acid (SITS).[111] Expression of this transport system was absent in cells grown on plastic dishes. Therefore, even without changes in content of lactate, alanine, glucose, and insulin in culture media, functional characteristics of these cells in culture may be enhanced further by utilizing microporous membrane inserts.

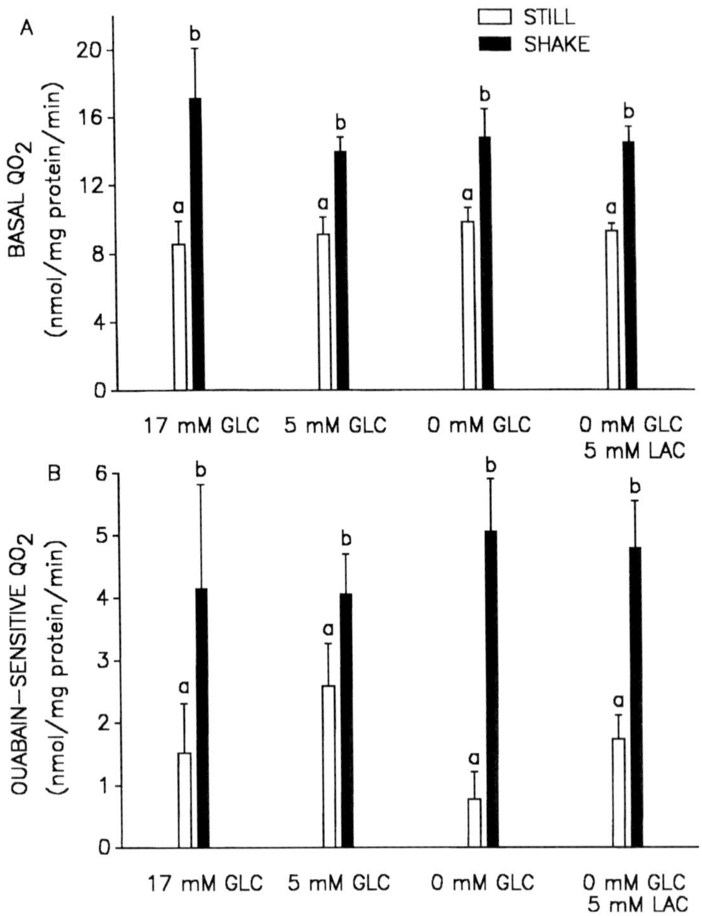

Figure 2 Effect of shaking and glucose (GlC) concentration and lactate (LAC) in culture medium on basal (A) and ouabain-sensitive (B) oxygen consumption (QO_2) in confluent (day 7) RPTC. Values with different superscripts are statistically different from each other (means ± SE, n = 4 to 6). (From Nowak, G. and Schnellmann, R.G., *Am. J. Physiol.*, 268, C1053, 1995. With permission.)

10.3.5 SV40 Transformation

Passaging rabbit RPTC has also been reported, but this apparently results in further loss of the brush-border membrane.[88,112] However, several investigators have transfected these cells with SV40 to produce a transformed cell line that has been sustained beyond 30 passages. While retaining several characteristic functions associated with proximal tubular cells *in vivo*,[113,114] these transformed cells begin to express Ca^{2+}-insensitive K^+ channels[115] and changes in sulfated proteoglycan composition.[116] While these transfected cells have the advantage of being immortalized in culture, they have not been characterized to the same extent as primary cultures, are typically grown under standard culture conditions, and, to our knowledge, have not been used for toxicological studies.

10.4 Applications for toxicological studies

Primary cultures of rabbit RPTC allow one to utilize a portion of the kidney that is a target for a number of toxicants as an *in vitro* model for toxicological studies. These cell cultures are indeed a useful tool for this purpose, since they have been relatively well characterized

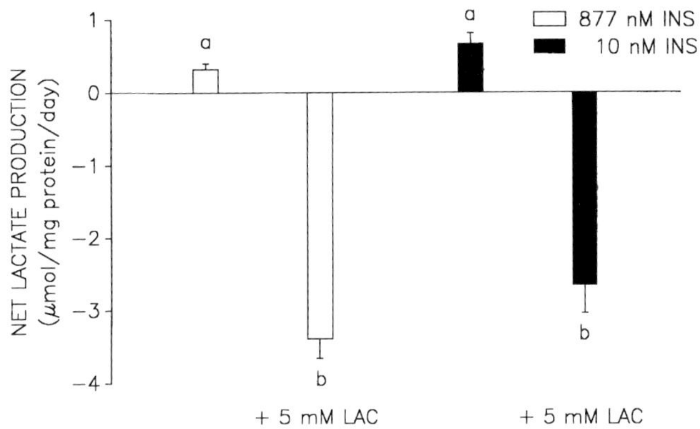

Figure 3 Effect of 5 m*M* lactate (LAC) and insulin (INS) on reorientation of lactate metabolism (net production vs. net consumption) in confluent shake cultures of RPTC grown in the presence of 5 m*M* glucose. Values with different superscripts are statistically different from each other (means ± SE, n = 8 to 11). (From Nowak, G. and Schnellmann, R.G., *Am. J. Physiol.*, 268, C1053, 1995. With permission.)

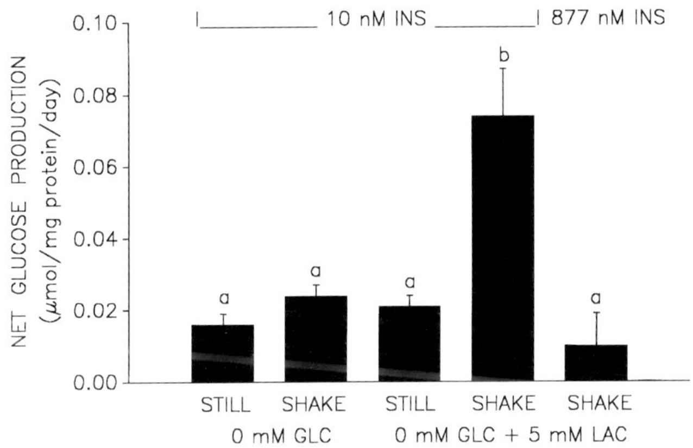

Figure 4 Effect of 5 m*M* lactate (LAC), insulin (INS), and culture [SHAKE vs. cultures held stationary (STILL)] on net glucose (GLC) production in confluent (day 7) cultures of RPTC grown in glucose-free media. Values with different superscripts are statistically different from each other (means ± SE, n = 4 to 8). (From Nowak, G. and Schnellmann, R. G., *Am. J. Physiol.*, 268, C1053, 1995. With permission.)

and maintain a number of intact functional characteristics, even under standard culture conditions, which are important when studying toxicant transport and toxicity. These functional properties include the presence of probenecid-sensitive organic anion transport; Na^+-dependent H^+ antiport; phosphate transport; phlorhizin-sensitive glucose transport; marker enzymes of the brush border; appropriate cellular redox status; drug metabolism and conjugation activities; and morphological evidence of solute transport.[35-47]

Because changes in culture conditions can alter cellular expression *in vitro*, any large deviations in functional expression from the *in vivo* condition in the *in vitro* model must be taken into consideration when interpreting results from the *in vitro* model. For example, alkaline phosphatase leakage into the culture medium would be a poor biomarker of cellular injury since less than 15% of the activity of freshly isolated tubules is retained in standard culture.[90] In contrast, lactate dehydrogenase leakage into the culture medium is an excellent biomarker of cellular injury since its activity is induced under standard culture conditions.[90] This emphasizes the importance of characterizing the *in vitro* model prior to applying it to a specific toxicological problem.

Specific toxicants affecting the proximal tubule include heavy metals such as mercury[117] and cadmium,[118] antibiotics such as gentamicin,[119] antineoplastics such as cisplatin,[120] and immunosuppressants such as cyclosporin A.[121] To understand the mechanism of action of a given toxicant, the kinetics of uptake and removal of the toxicant at its site of action, the interactions that occur with cellular and subcellular components, and the biochemical and physiological effects that result from those interactions must be considered. Primary cultures of RPTC have indeed been utilized to gain some insight into these processes[122,123] and to compare the relative effects of similar compounds or a series of drugs.[124,125] The examples selected below address the use of primary cultures of RPTC for studying mechanisms of toxicity of mercurials, antibiotics, antineoplastics, and mechanisms of cellular injury and repair processes.

10.4.1 Mercurials

The kidney has long been recognized as a target site for inorganic mercury, as typified by mercuric salts such as mercuric chloride. Acute exposures result in a dramatic loss of proximal tubular morphology and loss of function.[117] Organic forms of mercury, such as methylmercury, are recognized primarily for their central nervous system (CNS) effects. Nonetheless, repeated exposures can produce signs of proximal tubular dysfunction.[126,127] In comparing the two forms of mercury *in vivo*, vast differences are observed in the relative renal accumulation of the metals.[128,129] To add to the complexity of studying the comparative renal toxicity of these compounds, *in vivo* biotransformation of methylmercury to inorganic mercury can occur, leading to renal accumulation of *both* inorganic and organic mercury after repeated exposure to methylmercury. The accumulation of inorganic mercury has been hypothesized to be responsible for the proximal tubular effects seen with repeated methylmercury exposures.[130-133]

Rabbit RPTC in primary culture has been an extremely useful model to study the relative kinetics of uptake of mercurials, their relative toxicity to the proximal tubular cell, and their effects on cellular biochemical parameters, without the confounding effects that may result *in vivo* from differential effects of the compounds occurring at other target sites, including the CNS for methylmercury and the gastrointestinal tract for inorganic mercury. These effects at sites distant from the proximal tubule *in vivo* may nonetheless affect on the distribution and excretion of the metal and may also indirectly influence effects occurring in the kidney.

Aleo et al.[86] demonstrated differential toxicity of mercuric chloride and methylmercury chloride in primary cultures of RPTC. Inorganic mercury displayed an LC_{50} (defined as the concentration that produces lethality in 50% of the cells tested) of 34 μM compared with 6.1 μM for methylmercury. Although the kinetics of uptake for the two forms of mercury differed considerably (methylmercury showed a rapid uptake and equilibrium within 3 h, whereas inorganic mercury uptake was much slower and did not appear to have reached equilibrium at 24 h), the 24-h LC_{50} medium concentrations resulted in a greater cellular mercury content for cells exposed to inorganic mercury than to methylmercury (4.6 vs. 1.3 nmol/10^5 cells, respectively). Cellular uptake of methylmercury was linear as a function of initial medium concentration throughout a broad range of concentrations, whereas inorganic mercury demonstrated a less efficient uptake at higher media mercury concentrations. Thus, in this example, differences in the kinetics of uptake, which in one case showed considerable dose dependence, resulted in the establishment of different intracellular concentrations of mercury compared with what would be expected based on the LC_{50} media concentrations.

One can gain some insight into the mechanism of toxicity for methylmercury in the renal proximal tubular cell from these types of data. The lower LC_{50} value for methylmercury compared with mercuric chloride, together with the lower cellular concentration of mercury at the LC_{50} concentration argues against the notion that the nephrotoxicity of methylmercury results simply from its biotransformation to Hg^{2+}, the primary toxicant, as argued by some authors.[130-133] Although inorganic mercury may play a role in the toxic effects of methylmercury in the proximal tubule, it is likely that other factors come into play, including endogenous, acid-soluble thiol-containing compounds, such as glutathione and metallothionein. Cellular concentrations of these thiols can change in response to exposure to either form of mercury.

These cells in culture are an ideal system to study the role of endogenous thiols in mediating heavy metal uptake, intracellular binding, and toxicologic responses,[86] since even under standard culture conditions, this culture system maintains normal glutathione concentration and redox state[43] together with the ability for metallothionein induction.[134] The increase cytotoxic potential of methylmercury compared with mercuric chloride appears to be related to its intracellular distribution between acid-soluble binding sites (i.e., glutathione and metallothionein) and acid-insoluble binding sites (protein). As shown in Figure 5, intracellular binding and redistribution was affected by the physical form of the mercury (organic vs. inorganic) and the time of exposure. The toxicity of inorganic mercury appeared to be diminished by a shift in intracellular binding from acid-insoluble to acid-soluble binding sites at low concentrations of mercuric chloride in the media. This response was diminished as concentrations of inorganic mercury in the media approached the LC_{50} value and was nonexistent with the more potent cytotoxicant methylmercury. This suggests that the ability to shift cellular mercury from acid-insoluble to acid-soluble binding sites is an important adaptive response to inorganic mercury exposure that helps attenuate its toxic potential. Primary cultures of rabbit RPTC are more sensitive to methylmercury, not because a higher intracellular concentration of the metal is achieved, but because the cells do not redistribute the metal to innocuous (acid-soluble) binding sites.

10.4.2 *Antibiotics*

The aminoglycoside gentamicin is an antibiotic that, after repeated dosing, can accumulate in the kidney and produce proximal tubular damage[135] via alterations in phospholipid metabolism and accumulation of myeloid bodies in lysosomes.[136-138] Primary cultures of RPTC have provided a useful model for studying the mechanisms of aminoglycoside toxicity. This model displays a concentration-dependent uptake of gentamicin and manifestations of toxicity that are very closely related to biochemical, morphological, and functional changes observed after *in vivo* exposures. Biochemical changes in target organelle (lysosomal) enzyme activities include an increase in *N*-acetylglucosaminidase (NAG), a decrease in cathepsin B, and a decrease in sphingomyelinase. The stage of growth affects the response, with confluent cultures exhibiting a larger increase in NAG and smaller decreases in both cathepsin B and sphingomyelinase.[139] Functional changes due to gentamicin included a decrease in α-methyl glucopyranoside transport, and a decrease in protein and DNA synthesis. Morphological assessment indicated a targeted a[illegible]tion of myeloid bodies in the lysosomes and an increase in the lysosomal size and de[illegible] within the cell, similar to that after *in vivo* exposure.[139]

The role of alterations in phospholipid metabolism in gentamicin-induced myeloid accumulation in lysosomes has been studied in primary cultures of RPTC.[140] The parathyroid hormone-stimulated increase in the phosphoinositol cascade was inhibited by gentamicin. Gentamicin also inhibited the effects of other inositol triphosphate generation stimulators, including arginine vasopressin, bradykinin, and phenylephrine. The role of impaired phospholipase-mediated phospholipid degradation was implicated as a mechanism

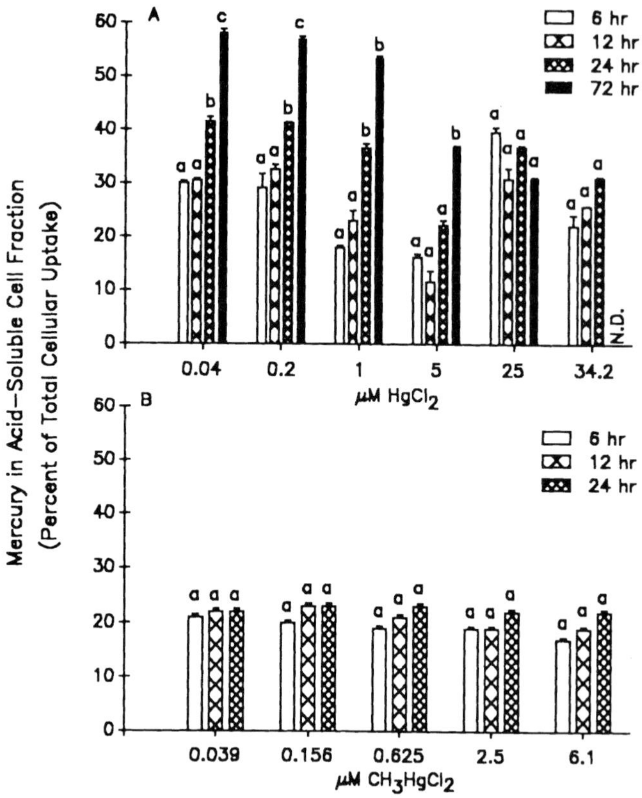

Figure 5 Cellular distribution of $HgCl_2$ and CH_3HgCl. Confluent cultures of rabbit RPTC were exposed to (A) $HgCl_2$ or (B) CH_3HgCl for 6 to 72 h. The percentage of inorganic mercury or methylmercury found in the acid-soluble cell fraction was determined by dividing the amount of mercury found in the acid-soluble fraction by the total cellular mercury accumulation multiplied by 100%. Data are means ± SD, n = 2 to 4. Values with different superscripts within the same exposure group are significantly different from one another ($p < 0.05$). N.D., not determined. (From Aleo, M. D., Taub, M. L., and Kostyniak, P. J., *Toxicol. Appl. Pharmacol.*, 112, 310, 1992. With permission.)

for gentamicin-induced toxicity.[141] In primary cultures of RPTC, gentamicin caused an increased incorporation of precursors into specific phospholipids and longer half-times for their removal from the cell.[141]

Manifestation of gentamicin toxicity is also dependent on phenotype expression in culture. Morin et al.[105] demonstrated that rabbit RPTC in primary culture was fivefold more sensitive to gentamicin in the absence than in the presence of glucose and insulin. This may have been due to a twofold increase in cellular accumulation of gentamicin shortly after exposure. Although no specific reasons were proposed for these differences, the cells maintained a more normal phenotype when grown in the absence of glucose and insulin, based on the activity of eight separate marker enzymes.

10.4.3 *Antineoplastics*

Primary cultures of rabbit RPTC have also been used to investigate the rank-order cytotoxicity and biochemical mechanisms of platinum-containing antitumor agents, such as *cis*-diamminedichloroplatinum (II) (cisplatin). The therapeutic use of cisplatin is limited due to its nephrotoxic potential, which is one of its most important dose-limiting side effects. Tay et al.[142] were the first to examine the *in vivo* effects of cisplatin in rabbits followed by a mechanistic study of the target cell type *in vitro*. Their work showed that cisplatin inhibited DNA synthesis (48 to 77%), RNA synthesis (36 to 77%), and protein synthesis (14 to 33%) within 6 h of exposure. Since these effects occurred before any effects on cellular viability or activities of (Na^+ + K^+)-stimulated-ATPase, alkaline phosphatase, or succinate dehydrogenase, this suggested that the effects of cisplatin on proximal tubular synthetic activity may be related to its nephrotoxic potential. A subsequent study by Courjault-Gautier et al.[143] investigated the effects of cisplatin on (Na^+ + K^+)-stimulated-ATPase activity in relation to Na^+-dependent transport functions. Cisplatin decreased (Na^+ + K^+)-stimulated-ATPase activity and Na^+-coupled glucose and phosphate uptake, but increased Na^+-coupled alanine uptake. Inhibition of these enzyme systems appeared to be independent phenomena, since the transient increase in alanine uptake suggested that the transmembrane Na^+ gradient was unaffected, although no intracellular measurements of Na^+ concentrations were made. These effects were present at 20- to 30-fold lower concentrations of cisplatin than for carboplatin. In a comparative study between primary cultures of rabbit RPTC and OK cells, Courjault et al.[144] reported that unlike OK cells, primary cultures retained the same rank-order toxicity of cisplatin, carboplatin, and transplatin *in vitro* as their rank-order nephrotoxicity *in vivo*, once again showing that primary cultures may be preferred over some renal cell lines for certain types of *in vitro* toxicity testing.

10.4.4 *Cell injury and repair*

The ability of renal proximal tubular cells to regenerate and differentiate *in vivo* after toxic insult is critical for the recovery of normal renal function (see Chapter 15 for a more detailed discussion and presentation of methods to study nephrogenic repair). Although autocrine- and paracrine-derived growth factors are thought to play an important role in these processes, it is not known how production of these important growth factors are affected by different nephrotoxicants. Primary cultures of rabbit RPTC have also been used to investigate these cellular repair processes after toxic injury *in vitro*. Kays et al.[145] first described a model of renal cell injury using confluent monolayer cultures. In their model, a 2-h exposure to *S*-(1,2-dichlorovinyl)-L-cysteine (DCVC) disrupted 60 to 70% of the monolayer within 2 days after exposure and regained 80% of the monolayer over the next 8 days. A subsequent study characterized the regenerative process after DCVC and *tert*-butylhydroperoxide (TBHP)-induced cell injury.[146] In this study, partial regeneration of the monolayer occurred after exposure without the addition of exogenous growth factors, but this was achieved by cellular hypertrophy and spreading rather than by cellular proliferation. This process was not mediated by interaction with integrins, but could be accelerated to completion by the addition of epidermal growth factor. Since complete regeneration of the monolayer only occurs after chemical injury in the presence of an exogenous growth factor but occurs after mechanical injury in the absence of exogenous growth factors,[147] the cell repair response has been altered by chemical injury.[147] This finding suggests that certain nephrotoxicants may contribute to and prolong renal dysfunction by impeding normal regenerative processes.

Although this is not an exhaustive review of the use of primary cultures of rabbit RPTC for physiological or toxicological experiments, it is hoped the examples above illustrate the versatility and utility of this *in vitro* model in studying mechanisms of proximal tubular damage from several commonly encountered metals and drugs. When used in conjunction with other *in vitro* and *in vivo* approaches, it provides an important experimental tool in assessing the nephrotoxic potential and mechanisms of toxicity of xenobiotics. It is anticipated that as research continues, better culture conditions will be defined that enhance maintenance of highly differentiated functions in culture. This will ultimately lead to better *in vitro* models for toxicological studies

10.5 Acknowledgment

The authors are indebted to Drs. Grazyna Nowak and Rick Schnellmann for sharing their modifications to the isolation procedure and most recent advances in culture conditions.

References

1 Grisham, J. W. and Smith, G. J., Predictive and mechanistic evaluation of toxic responses in mammalian cell culture systems, *Pharmacol. Rev.*, 36, 151S, 1984.
2. Rabito, C. A. and Karish, M. V., Polarized amino acid transport by an epithelial cell line of renal origin ($LLC-PK_1$), *J. Biol. Chem.*, 258, 2543, 1983.
3. Sepulveda, F. V. and Pearson, J. D., Characterization of neutral amino acid uptake by cultured epithelial cells from pig kidney, *J. Cell. Physiol.*, 112, 182, 1982.
4. Biber, J., Brown, C. D. A., and Murer, H., Sodium-dependent transport of phosphate in $LLC-PK_1$ cells, *Biochim. Biophys. Acta*, 735, 325, 1983.
5. Rabito, C. A., Phosphate uptake by a kidney cell line ($LLC-PK_1$), *Am. J. Physiol.*, 245, F22, 1983.
6. Mullin, J. M., Weibel, J., Diamond, L., and Kleinzeller, A., Sugar transport in the $LLC-PK_1$ renal epithelial cell line: similarity to mammalian kidney and the influence of cell density, *J. Cell. Physiol.*, 104, 375, 1980.
7. Rabito, C. A., Localization of the Na^+-sugar cotransport system in a kidney epithelial cell line ($LLC-PK_1$), *Biochim. Biophys. Acta*, 649, 286, 1981.
8. Fouda, A.-K., Fauth, C., and Roch-Ramel, F., Transport of organic cations by kidney epithelial cell line $LLC-PK_1$, *J. Pharmacol. Exp. Ther.*, 252, 286, 1990.
9. McKinney, T. D., DeLeon, C., and Speeg, K. V., Jr., Organic cation uptake by a cultured renal epithelium, *J. Cell. Physiol.*, 137, 513, 1988.
10. Fauth, C., Rossier, B., and Roch-Ramel, F., Transport of tetraethylammonium by a kidney epithelial cell line ($LLC-PK_1$), *Am. J. Physiol.*, 254, F351, 1988.
11. Rabito, C. A., Kreisberg, J. I., and Wight, D., Alkaline phosphatase and γ-glutamyltranspeptidase as polarization markers during the organization of $LLC-PK_1$ cells into an epithelial membrane, *J. Biol. Chem.*, 259, 574, 1984.
12. Perantoni, A. and Berman, J. J., Properties of wilms' tumor line (TuWi) and pig kidney line ($LLC-PK_1$) typical of normal kidney tubular epithelium, *In Vitro Cell. Dev. Biol.*, 15, 446, 1979.
13. Gstraunthaler, G., Pfaller, W., and Kotanko, P., Biochemical characterization of renal epithelial cell cultures ($LLC-PK_1$ and MDCK), *Am. J. Physiol.*, 248, F536, 1985.
14. Hull, R. N., Cherry, W. R., and Weaver, G. W., The origin and characteristics of a pig kidney cell strain, $LLC-PK_1$, *In Vitro Cell. Dev. Biol.*, 12, 670, 1976.
15. Wohlwend, A., Montesano, R., Vassalli, J-D., and Orci, L., $LLC-PK_1$ cysts: a model for the study of epithelial polarity, *J. Cell. Physiol.*, 125, 533, 1985.
16. Wohlwend, A., Vassalli, J-D., Belin, D., and Orci, L., LLC-PK1 cells: cloning of phenotypically stable subpopulations, *Am. J. Physiol.*, 250, C682, 1986.
17. Gstraunthaler, G., Pfaller, W., and Kotanko, P., Lack of fructose-1,6-bisphosphatase activity in $LLC-PK_1$ cells, *Am. J. Physiol.*, 248, C181, 1985.
18. Mullin, J. M., Cha, C-J. M., and Kleinzeller, A., Metabolism of *l*-lactate by $LLC-PK_1$ renal epithelia, *Am. J. Physiol.*, 242, C41, 1982.
19. Goldring, S. R., Dayer, J-M., Ausiello, D. A., and Krane, S. M., A cell strain cultured from porcine kidney increases cyclic AMP content upon exposure to calcitonin or vasopressin, *Biochem. Biophys. Res. Commun.*, 83, 434, 1978.
20. Malmstrom, K. and Murer, H., Parathyroid hormone inhibits phosphate transport in OK cells but not in $LLC-PK_1$ and JTC-12.P3 cells, *Am. J. Physiol.*, 251, C23, 1986.
21. Cole, L. A., Scheid, J. M., and Tannen, R. L., Induction of mitochondrial metabolism and pH-modulated ammoniagenesis by rocking $LLC-PK_1$ cells, *Am. J. Physiol.*, 251, C293, 1986.
22. Rabito, C. A., Occluding junctions in a renal cell line ($LLC-PK_1$) with characteristics of proximal tubule cells, *Am. J. Physiol.*, 250, F734, 1986.
23. Lock, E. A. and Ishmeal, J., Effect of the organic acid transport inhibitor probenecid on renal cortical uptake and proximal tubular toxicity of hexachloro-1,3-butadiene and its conjugates, *Toxicol. Appl. Pharmacol.*, 81, 32, 1985.

24. Mertens, J. J. W. M., Keukens, E. A. J., Appel, M., Spenkelink, B., Temmink, J. H. M., and van Bladeren, P. J., Cytotoxicity of *S*-(1,2,3,4,4′-pentachlorobutadienyl)-*L*-cysteine after apical and basolateral exposure of LLC-PK_1 monolayers. Involvement of an amino acid transport system, *Chem. Biol. Interact.*, 75, 119, 1990.
25. Groves, C. E., Schnellmann, R. G., Sokol, P. P., Steffens, T. G., and Lock, E. A., Pentachlorobutadienyl-*L*-cysteine (PCBC) toxicity: The importance of mitochondrial dysfunction, *J. Biochem. Toxicol.*, 6, 253, 1991.
26. Schnellmann, R. G., Lock, E. A., and Mandel, L. J., A mechanism of *S*-(1,2,3,4,4′-pentachloro-1,3-butadienyl)-*L*-cysteine toxicity to rabbit renal proximal tubules, *Toxicol. Appl. Pharmacol.*, 90, 513, 1987.
27. Griner, R. D. and Schnellmann, R. G., Decreasing glycolysis increases sensitivity to mitochondrial inhibition in primary cultures of renal proximal tubule cells, *In Vitro Cell. Dev. Biol.*, 30A, 30, 1994.
28. Williams, P. D., Laska, D. A., Tay, L. K., and Hottendorf, G. H., Comparative toxicities of cephalosporin antibiotics in a rabbit kidney cell line (LLC-RK_1), *Antimicrob. Agents Chemother.*, 32, 314, 1988.
29. Hottendorf, G. H., Laska, D. A., Williams, P. D., and Ford, S. M., Role of desacetylation in the detoxification of cephalothin in renal cells in culture, *J. Toxicol. Environ. Health*, 22, 101, 1987.
30. Ford, S. M., Laska, D. A., Hottendorf, G. H., and Williams, P. D., Correlation between the *in vitro* and *in vivo* nephrotoxicity of parenteral antibiotics in the rabbit, *Toxicol. Methods*, 3, 1, 1993.
31. Rush, G. F. and Ponsler, G. D., Cephaloridine-induced biochemical changes and cytotoxicity in suspensions of rabbit isolated proximal tubules, *Toxicol. Appl. Pharmacol.*, 109, 314, 1991.
32. Rush, G. F. and Ponsler, G. D., Biochemical mechanisms of cephaloridine nephrotoxicity in suspensions of isolated rabbit proximal tubules, *Toxicol. Lett.*, 53, 215, 1990.
33. Toutain, H., Courjault, F., Vauclin-Jacques, N., and Morin, J. P., Adenylate cyclase responses and biochemical characterization of primary rabbit renal proximal tubular cell cultures and LLC-PK_1 cells, *Renal Failure*, 12, 177, 1990.
34. Courjault, F., Gerin, B., Leroy, D., Chevalier, J., and Toutain, H., Morphological and biochemical characterization of the opossum kidney cell line and primary cultures of rabbit proximal tubule cells in serum-free defined medium, *Cell Biol. Int. Rep.*, 15, 1225, 1991.
35. Chung, S. D., Alavi, N., Livingston, D., Hiller, S., and Taub, M., Characterization of primary rabbit kidney cultures that express proximal tubule functions in a hormonally defined medium, *J. Cell Biol.*, 95, 118, 1982.
36. Alavi, N., Spangler, R. A., and Jung, C. Y., Sodium-dependent glucose transport by cultured proximal tubule cells, *Biochim. Biophys. Acta*, 899, 9, 1987.
37. Fine, L. G., Badie-Dezfooly, B., Lowe, A. G., Hamzeh, A., Wells, J., and Salehmoghaddam, S., Stimulation of Na^+/H^+ antiport is an early event in hypertrophy of renal proximal tubular cells, *Proc. Natl. Acad. Sci. U.S.A.*, 82, 1736, 1985.
38. Sakhrani, L. M., Badie-Desfooley, B., Trizna, W., Mikhail, N., Lowe, A. G., Taub, M., and Fine, L. G., Transport and metabolism of glucose by renal proximal tubular cells in primary culture, *Am. J. Physiol.*, 246, F757, 1984.
39. Waqar, M. A., Seto, J., Chung, S. D., Hiller-Grohol, S., and Taub, M., Phosphate uptake by primary renal proximal tubule cell cultures grown in hormonally defined medium, *J. Cell. Physiol.*, 124, 411, 1985.
40. Alavi, N., Brentjens, J., Geola, J., and Hershman, J., Further characterization of rabbit proximal tubule cells in culture, *Kidney Int.*, 25, 262, 1984.
41. Yanagawa, N., Capparelli, A. W., Jo, O. D., Friedal, A., Barrett, J. D., and Eggena, P., Production of angiotensinogen and renin-like activity by rabbit proximal tubular cells in culture, *Kidney Int.*, 39, 938, 1991.
42. Moe, O. W., Ujiie, K., Star, R. A., Miller, R. T., Widell, J., Alpern, R. J., and Henrich, W. L., Renin expression in renal proximal tubule, *J. Clin. Invest.*, 91, 774, 1993.
43. Aleo, M. D., Taub, M. L., Olson, J. R., and Kostyniak, P. J., Primary cultures of rabbit renal proximal tubule cells. II. Selected phase I and phase II metabolic capacities, *Toxicol. In Vitro*, 4, 727, 1990.

44. Wilson, P. D., Anderson, R. J., Breckon, R. D., Nathrath, W., and Schrier, R. W., Retention of differentiated characteristics by cultures of defined rabbit kidney epithelia, *J. Cell. Physiol.*, 130, 245, 1987.
45. Yang, I. S., Goldinger, J. M., Hong, S. K., and Taub, M., Preparation of basolateral membranes that transport *p*-aminohippurate from primary cultures of rabbit kidney proximal tubule cells, *J. Cell. Physiol.*, 135, 481, 1988.
46. Taub, M. L., Yang, I. S., and Wang, Y., Primary rabbit kidney proximal tubule cell cultures maintain differentiated functions when cultured in a hormonally defined serum-free medium, *In Vitro Cell. Dev. Biol.*, 25, 770, 1989.
47. Palmoski, M. J., Masters, B. A., Flint, O. P., Ford, S. M., and Oleson, F. B., Characterization of rabbit primary proximal tubule kidney cell cultures grown on Millicell-HA membrane filters, *Toxicol. In Vitro*, 6, 557, 1992.
48. Tang, M.-J., Suresh, K. R., and Tannen, R. L., Carbohydrate metabolism by primary cultures of rabbit proximal tubules, *Am. J. Physiol.*, 256, C532, 1990.
49. Dickman, K. G. and Mandel, L. J., Glycolytic and oxidative metabolism in primary renal proximal tubule cultures, *Am. J. Physiol.*, 257, C333, 1989.
50. Ford, S. M. and Williams, P. D., Primary proximal tubule cultures for screening nephrotoxicants, in *In Vitro Methods of Toxicology*, Watson, R. R., Ed., CRC Press, Boca Raton, FL, 1992, 123.
51. Mandel, L. J., Metabolic substrates, cellular energy production, and the regulation of proximal tubular transport, *Annu. Rev. Physiol.*, 47, 85, 1985.
52. Harris, S. I., Balaban, R. S., Barrett, L., and Mandel, L. J., Mitochondrial respiratory capacity and Na^+- and K^+-dependent adenosine triphosphatase-mediated ion transport in the intact renal cell, *J. Biol. Chem.*, 256, 10319, 1981.
53. Robin, E. D., Murphy, B. J., and Theodore, J., Coordinate regulation of glycolysis by hypoxia in mammalian cells, *J. Cell. Physiol.*, 118, 287, 1984.
54. Werrlein, R. J. and Glinos, A. D., Oxygen microenvironment and respiratory oscillations in cultured mammalian cells, *Nature*, 251, 317, 1974.
55. Wolfle, D. and Jungermann, K., Long-term effects of physiological oxygen concentrations on glycolysis and gluconeogenesis in hepatocyte cultures, *Eur. J. Biochem.*, 151, 299, 1985.
56. McLimans, W. F., Crouse, E. J., Tunnah, K. V., and Moore, G. E., Kinetics of gas diffusion in mammalian cell culture systems. I. Experimental, *Biotechnol. Bioeng.*, 10, 725, 1968.
57. Stevens, K. M., Oxygen requirements for liver cells *in vitro*, *Nature*, 206, 199, 1965.
58. Sahai, A., Cole, L. A., Clarke, D. L., and Tannen, R. L., Rocking promotes differentiated properties in LLC-PK_1 cells by improved oxygenation, *Am. J. Physiol.*, 256, C1064, 1989.
59. Paul, J., Carbohydrate and energy metabolism, in *Cells and Tissue in Culture*, Willmer, E. N., Ed., Academic Press, London, 1965, 239.
60. Reitzer, L. J., Wice, B. M., and Kennell, D., Evidence that glutamine, not sugar, is the major energy source for cultured HeLa cells, *J. Biol. Chem.*, 254, 2669, 1979.
61. Stanisz, J., Wice, B. M., and Kennell, D. E., Comparative energy metabolism in cultured heart muscle and HeLa cells, *J. Cell. Physiol.*, 115, 320, 1983.
62. Rodeheaver, D. P., Aleo, M. D., and Schnellmann, R. G., Differences in enzymatic and mechanical isolated rabbit renal proximal tubules: comparison in long-term incubation, *In Vitro Cell. Dev. Biol.*, 26, 898, 1990.
63. Steward, A. R., Dannan, G. A., Guzelian, P. S., and Guengerich, F. P., Changes in concentrations of seven forms of cytochrome P-450 in primary cultures of adult rat hepatocytes, *Mol. Pharmacol.*, 27, 125, 1985.
64. Grant, M. H., Melvin, M. A. L., Shaw, P., Melvin, W. T., and Burke, M. D., Studies on the maintenance of cytochromes P-450 and b5, monooxygenases and cytochrome reductases in primary cultures of rat hepatocytes, *FEBS Lett.*, 190, 99, 1985.
65. Gstraunthaler, G. and Handler, J. S., Isolation, growth, and characterization of a gluconeogenic strain of renal cells, *Am. J. Physiol.*, 252, C232, 1987.
66. Clayton, D. F., Harrelson, A. L., Darnell, J. E., Jr., Dependence of liver-specific transcription on tissue organization, *Mol. Cell. Biol.*, 5, 2623, 1985.
67. Grinnell, F., Cellular adhesiveness and extracellular substrates, *Int. Rev. Cytol.*, 53, 65, 1978.
68. Kleinman, H. K., Klebe, R. J., and Martin, G. R., Role of collagenous matrices in the adhesion and growth of cells, *J. Cell Biol.*, 88, 473, 1981.

69. Lee, E. Y-H. P., Lee, W-H., Kaetzel, C. S., Parry, G., and Bissell, M. J., Interaction of mouse mammary epithelial cells with collagen substrata: regulation of casein gene expression and secretion, *Proc. Natl. Acad. Sci. U.S.A.*, 82, 1419, 1985.
70. Mauchamp, J., Margotat, A., Chambard, M., Charrier, B., Remy, L., and Michel-Bechet, M., Polarity of three-dimensional structures derived from isolated hog thyroid cells in primary cultures, *Cell Tissue Res.*, 204, 417, 1979.
71. Wessells, N. K., Substrate and nutrient effects upon epidermal basal cell orientation and proliferation, *Proc. Natl. Acad. Sci. U.S.A.*, 52, 252, 1964.
72. Cook, J. R., Crute, B. E., Patrone, L. M., Gabriels, J., Lane, M. E., and Van Burskirk, R. G., Microporosity of the substratum regulates differentiation of MDCK cell *in vitro*, *In Vitro Cell. Dev. Biol.*, 25, 914, 1989.
73. Pitt, A. M., Gabriels, J. E., Badmington, F., McDowell, J., Gonzales, L., and Waugh, M. E., Cell culture on a microscopically transparent microporous membrane, *BioTech.*, 5, 162, 1987.
74. Karst, W. and Merker, H-J., The differentiation behavior of MDCK cells grown on matrix components and in collagen gels, *Cell Differ.*, 22, 211, 1988.
75. Yang, A. H., Gould-Kosta, J., and Oberly, T. D., *In vitro* growth and differentiation of human kidney tubular cells on a basement membrane substrate, *In Vitro Cell. Dev. Biol.*, 23, 34, 1987.
76. Mendrick, D. L., Chung, D. C., and Rennke, H. G., Heymann antigen GP330 demonstrates affinity for fibronectin, laminin, and type I collagen and mediates rat proximal tubule epithelial cell adherence to such matrices *in vitro*, *Exp. Cell. Res.*, 188, 23, 1990.
77. Whitcutt, M. J., Adler, K. B., Wu., R., A biphasic chamber for maintaining polarity of differentiation of cultured respiratory tract epithelial cells, *In Vitro Cell. Dev. Biol.*, 24, 420, 1988.
78. Bernstam, L. I., Vaughan, F. L., and Bernstein, I. A., Keratinocytes grown at the air-liquid interface, *In Vitro Cell. Dev. Biol.*, 22, 695, 1986.
79. Janecki, A., Jakubowiak, A., and Steinberger, A., Study of the dynamics of sertoli cell secretions in a new superfusion, two-compartment culture system, *In Vitro Cell. Dev. Biol.*, 23, 492, 1987.
80. Schwertschlag, U., Schrier, R. W., and Wilson, P. J., Beneficial effects of calcium channel blockers and calmodulin binding drugs on *in vitro* renal cell anoxia, *J. Pharmacol. Exp. Ther.*, 238, 119, 1986.
81. Williams, P. D., The application of renal cells in culture in studying drug-induced nephrotoxicity, *In Vitro Cell. Dev. Biol.*, 25, 800, 1989.
82. Wilson, P. D., Use of cultured renal tubular cells in the study of cell injury, *Miner. Electrolyte Metab.*, 12, 71, 1986.
83. Bruggeman, I. M., Mertens, J. J. W. M., Temmink, J. H. M., Lans, M. C., Vos, R. M. E., and Van Bladeren, P. J., Use of monolayers of primary rat kidney cortex cells for nephrotoxicity studies, *Toxicol. In Vitro*, 3, 261, 1989.
84. Smith, M. A., Acosta, D., and Bruckner, J. V., Development of a primary culture system of rat kidney cortical cells to evaluate the nephrotoxicity of xenobiotics, *Fd. Chem. Toxic.*, 24, 551, 1986.
85. Smith, M. A., Acosta, D., and Bruckner, J. V., Cephaloridine toxicity in primary cultures of rat renal cortical epithelial cells, *Toxicol. In Vitro*, 1, 23, 1987.
86. Aleo, M. D., Taub, M. L., and Kostyniak, P. J., Primary culture of rabbit renal proximal tubule cells. III. Comparative cytotoxicity of inorganic and organic mercury, *Toxicol. Appl. Pharmacol.*, 112, 310, 1992.
87. Taub, M. L., Primary culture of proximal tubule cells in defined medium, *J. Tissue Cult. Methods*, 9, 67, 1985.
88. Taub, M. L., Rabbit cortical epithelial cells, in *Methods in Toxicology*, Vol. 1, Part A, Tyson, C. A., and Frazier, J. M., Eds., Academic Press, San Diego, 1993, 366.
89. Cook, W. F. and Pickering, G. W., A rapid method for separating glomeruli from rabbit kidney, *Nature*, 182, 1103, 1958.
90. Aleo, M. D., Taub, M. L., Nickerson, P. A., and Kostyniak, P. J., Primary cultures of rabbit renal proximal tubule cells. I. Growth and biochemical characteristics, *In Vitro Cell. Dev. Biol.*, 25, 776, 1989.
91. Walsh-Reitz, M. M. and Toback, F. G., Phenol red inhibits growth of renal epithelial cells, *Am. J. Physiol.*, 262, F687, 1992.

92. Dickman, K. and Parrado, T., OK cells metabolize phenol red by glucuronidation, *J. Am. Soc. Nephrol.*, 4, 886, 1993.
93. Scheinman, S. J., Reid, R., Coulson, R., Jones, D. B., and Ford, S. M., Transepithelial phosphate transport in rabbit proximal tubular cells adapted to phosphate deprivation, *Am. J. Physiol.*, 266, C1609, 1994.
94. Dickman, K. G. and Mandel, L. J., Relationship between HCO_3^- transport and oxidative metabolism in rabbit proximal tubule, *Am. J. Physiol.*, 263, F342, 1992.
95. Brendel, K. and Meezan, E., Isolation and properties of a pure preparation of proximal kidney tubules obtained without collagenase treatment, *Fed. Proc. Fed. Am. Soc. Exp. Biol.*, 34, 803, 1975.
96. Hjelle, J. T., Morin, J-P., and Trouet, A., Analytical cell fractionation of isolated rabbit renal proximal tubules, *Kidney Int.*, 20, 71, 1981.
97. Carlson, E. C., Brendel, K., Hjelle, J. T., and Meezan, E., Ultrastructural and biochemical analyses of isolated basement membranes from kidney glomeruli and tubules and brain and retinal microvessels, *Ultrastruct. Res.*, 62, 26, 1978.
98. Koechlin, N., Pisam, M., Poujeol, P., Tauc, M., and Rambourg, A., Conversion of a rabbit proximal convoluted tubule (PCT) into a cell monolayer: ultrastructural study of cell dedifferentiation and redifferentiation, *Eur. J. Cell Biol.*, 54, 224, 1991.
99. Jung, J. C., Lee, S-M., Kadakia, N., and Taub, M., Growth and function of primary rabbit kidney proximal tubule cells in glucose-free serum-free medium, *J. Cell. Physiol.*, 150, 243, 1992.
100. Tang, M.-J. and Tannen, R. L., Relationship between proliferation and glucose metabolism in primary cultures of rabbit proximal tubules, *Am. J. Physiol.*, 259, C455, 1990.
101. Aleo, M. D. and Schnellmann, R. G., Regulation of glycolytic metabolism during long-term primary culture of renal proximal tubule cells, *Am. J. Physiol.*, 262, F77, 1992.
102. Griner, R. D., Aleo, M. D., and Schnellmann, R. G., The role of short chain fatty acid substrates in aerobic and glycolytic metabolism in primary cultures of renal proximal tubule cells, *In Vitro Cell. Dev. Biol.*, 29A, 649, 1993.
103. Klein, K. L., Wang, M. S., Torikai, S., Davidson, W. D., and Kurokawa, K., Substrate oxidations by isolated nephron segments of the rat, *Kidney Int.*, 20, 29, 1981.
104. Wang, Y. and Taub, M., Insulin and other regulatory factors modulate the growth and the phosphoenolpyruvate carboxykinase (PEPCK) activity of primary rabbit kidney proximal tubule cells in serum free medium, *J. Cell. Physiol.*, 147, 374, 1991.
105. Morin, J. P., Monteil, C., Glomot, R., and Fillastre, J. P., Rabbit kidney proximal tubule cells in primary culture: evaluation of the impact of expressed phenotype on toxic response, *Toxicol. In Vitro*, 5, 383, 1991.
106. Blais, A., Jalal, F., Crine, P., Paiemont, J., and Berteloot, A., Increased functional differentiation of rabbit proximal tubule cells cultured in glucose-free media, *Am. J. Physiol.*, 263, F152, 1992.
107. Monteil, C., Leclere, C., Fillastre, J. P., and Morin, J. P., Insulin and glucose impact on functional and morphological differentiation of rabbit proximal tubule cells in primary culture, *Renal Physiol. Biochem.*, 16, 212, 1993.
108. Courjault, F., Chevalier, J., Leroy, D., and Toutain, H., Effect of glucose and insulin deprivation on differentiation and carbohydrate metabolism of rabbit proximal tubular cells in primary culture, *Biochim. Biophys. Acta*, 1177, 147, 1993.
109. Nowak, G. and Schnellmann, R.G., Improved culture conditions stimulate gluconeogenesis in primary cultures of renal proximal tubule cells, *Am. J. Physiol.*, 268, C1053, 1995.
110. Miller, J. H., Sodium-sensitive, probenecid-insensitive *p*-aminohippuric acid uptake in cultured renal proximal tubule cells of the rabbit, *Proc. Soc. Exp. Biol. Med.*, 199, 298, 1992.
111. Ford, S. M., Williams, P. D., Grassl, W., and Holohan, P. D., Transepithelial acidification by cultures or rabbit proximal tubules grown on filters, *Am. J. Physiol.*, 259, C103, 1990.
112. Barron, E. T., O'Brien, A., and Ryan, M. P., Primary cultures of rat and rabbit renal proximal epithelium as models for nephrotoxicity investigations, *Toxicol. Lett.*, 53, 161, 1990.
113. Vandewalle, A., Lelongt, B., Geniteau-Legendre, M., Baudouin, B., Antoine, M., Estrade, S., Chatelet, F., Verroust, P., Cassingena, R., and Ronco, P., Maintenance of proximal and distal cell functions in SV40-transformed tubule cell lines derived from rabbit kidney cortex, *J. Cell. Physiol.*, 141, 203, 1989.

114. Fauth, C., Chabardes, D., Allaz, M., Garcia, M., Rossier, B., Roch-Ramel, F., and Claire, M., Establishment of renal cell lines derived from S_2 segments of the proximal tubule, *Renal Physiol. Biochem.*, 14, 128, 1991.
115. Teulon, J., Ronco, P. M., Geniteau-Legendre, M., Baudouin, B., Estrade, S., Cassingena, R., and Vandewalle, A., Transformation of renal tubule epithelial cells by simian virus-40 is associated with emergence of Ca^{2+}-insensitive K^+ channels and altered mitogenic sensitivity to K^+ channel blockers, *J. Cell. Physiol.*, 151, 113, 1992.
116. Lelong, B., Piedagnel, R., Chatelet, F., Baudouin, B., Brenchley, P. E. C., Verroust, P. J., Cassingena, R., Vandewalle, A., and Ronco, P. M., Dramatic changes of sulfated proteoglycans composition in a tumorigenic SV-40 transformed renal proximal-tubule cell line, *J. Biol. Chem.*, 267, 23815, 1992.
117. Ganote, C. E., Reimer, K. A., and Jennings, R. B., Acute mercuric chloride nephrotoxicity: an electron microscopic and metabolic study, *Lab. Invest.*, 31, 633, 1975.
118. Humes, H. D. and Weinberg, J. M., in *The Kidney*, Vol. 2, Brenner, B. M. and Rector, F. C., Eds., W. B. Saunders, Philadelphia, 1986, 1491.
119. Kosek, J. C., Mazze, R. I., and Cousins, M. J., Nephrotoxicity of gentamicin, *Lab. Invest.*, 30, 48, 1974.
120. Litterst, C. L., Cisplatinum: a review, with special reference to cellular and molecular interactions, *Agents Actions*, 15, 520, 1984.
121. Humes, H. D., Jackson, N. M., O'Connor, R. P., Hunt, D. A., and White, M. D., Pathogenic mechanisms of nephrotoxicity insights into cyclosporin nephrotoxicity, *Transplant. Proc.*, 27(Suppl. 1), 51, 1985.
122. Courjault, F., Leroy, D., Coquery, I., and Toutain, H., Platinum complex-induced dysfunction of cultured renal proximal tubule cells, a comparative study of carboplatin and transplatin with cisplatin, *Arch. Toxicol.*, 67, 338, 1993.
123. Sokol, P. P., Capodagli, L. C., Dixon, M., Holohan, P. D., Ross, C. R., Coulson, R., and Jones, D. B., Cyclosporin A and vehicle toxicity in primary cultures of rabbit renal proximal tubule cells, *Am. J. Physiol.*, 259, C897, 1990.
124. Courjault-Gautier, F., Hoet, D., Leroy, D., and Toutain, H. J., Dissimilar alterations of sodium-coupled uptake by platinum-coordination complexes in renal proximal tubular cells in primary culture, *J. Pharmacol. Exp. Ther.*, 270, 1097, 1994.
125. Legallicier, B., Leclere, C., Monteil, C., Morin, J. P., and Fillastre, J. P., Action toxique de deux agents antitumoraux derivés du platine, le cisplatine et l'oxaliplatine sur des cultures primaires de cellules tubulaires proximales de rein de lapin, *Pathol. Biol.*, 41, 873, 1993.
126. Fowler, B. A., The morphologic effects of dieldrin and methyl mercuric chloride on pars recta segments of rat kidney proximal tubules, *Am. J. Pathol.*, 69, 163, 1972.
127. Ware, R. A., Burkholder, P. M., and Chang, L. W., Ultrastructural changes in renal proximal tubules after chronic organic and inorganic mercury intoxication, *Environ. Res.*, 10, 121, 1975.
128. Magos, L., Webb, M., and Butler, W. H., The effect of cadmium pretreatment on the nephrotoxic action and kidney uptake of mercury in male and female rats, *Br. J. Exp. Pathol.*, 55, 589, 1974.
129. Magos, L. and Webb, M., The effect of selenium on the brain uptake of methylmercury, *Arch. Toxicol.*, 38, 201, 1977.
130. Klein, R., Herman, S. P., Bullock, B. C., and Talley, F. A., Methylmercury intoxication in rat kidneys, *Arch. Pathol.*, 96, 83, 1973.
131. Magos, L., Brown, A. W., Sparrow, S., Bailey, E., Snowden, R. T., and Skipp, W. R., The comparative toxicology of ethyl- and methylmercury, *Arch. Toxicol.*, 57, 260, 1985.
132. Fair, P. H., Dougherty, W. J., and Braddon. S. A., Methylmercury and selenium interaction in relation to mouse kidney γ-glutamyltranspeptidase, ultrastructure, and function, *Toxicol. Appl. Pharmacol.*, 80, 78, 1985.
133. Rodier, P. M., Kates, B., and Simons, R., Mercury localization in mouse kidney over time: autoradiography vs. silver staining, *Toxicol. Appl. Pharmacol.*, 92, 235, 1988.
134. Fine, L. G. and Sakhrani, L. M., Proximal tubular cells in primary culture, *Miner. Electrolyte Metab.*, 12, 51, 1986.
135. Morin, J. P. and Fillastre, J. P., Aminoglycoside-induced lysosomal dysfunctions in kidney, in *The Aminoglycosides: Microbiology, Clinical Use and Toxicology*, Whelton, A. and Neu, H. C., Eds., Marcel Dekker, New York, 1982, 303.

136. Tulkens, P. M., Nephrotoxicity of aminoglycoside antibiotics, *Toxicol. Lett.*, 46, 107, 1989.
137. De Broe, M. E., Paulus, G. J., Verpooten, G. A., Roels, F., Buyssens, N., Wedeen, R., Van Hoof, F., and Tulkens, P., Early effects of gentamicin, tobramycin and amikacin on the human kidney, *Kidney Int.*, 25, 643, 1984.
138. Morin, J. P., Viotte, G., Vandewalle, A., Van Hoof, F., Tulkens, P., and Fillastre, J. P., Gentamicin-induced nephrotoxicity: a cell biology approach, *Kidney Int.*, 18, 583, 1980.
139. Monteil, C., Leclere, C., Fillastre, J. P., and Morin, J. P., Characterization of gentamicin-induced dysfunctions *in vitro*: the use of optimized primary cultures of rabbit proximal tubule cells, *Renal Failure*, 15, 475, 1993.
140. Ramsammy, L. S., Josepovitz, C., and Kaloyanides, G. J., Gentamicin inhibits agonist stimulation of the phosphatidylinositol cascade in primary cultures of rabbit proximal tubular cells and in rat renal cortex, *J. Pharmacol. Exp. Ther.*, 247, 989, 1988.
141. Ramsammy, L. S., Josepovitz, C., Lane, B., and Kaloyanides, G. J., Effect of gentamicin on phospholipid metabolism in cultured rabbit proximal tubular cells, *Am. J. Physiol.*, 256, C204, 1989.
142. Tay, L. K., Bregman, C. L., Masters, B. A., and Williams, P. D., Effects of *cis*-diamminedichloroplatinum (II) on rabbit kidney *in vivo* and on rabbit renal proximal tubule cells in culture, *Cancer Res.*, 48, 2538, 1988.
143. Courjault-Gautier, F., Hoet, D., Leroy, D., and Toutain, H., Dissimilar alterations of sodium-coupled uptake by platinum-cooridination complexes in renal proximal tubular cells in primary culture, *J. Pharmacol. Exp. Ther.*, 270, 1097, 1994.
144. Courjault, F., Leroy, D., Coquery, I., and Toutain, H., Platinum complex-induced dysfunction of cultured renal proximal tubule cells: a comparative study of carboplatin and transplatin with cisplatin, *Arch. Toxicol.*, 67, 338, 1993.
145. Kays, S. E., Berdanier, C. D., Swagler, A. R., Lock, E. A., and Schnellmann, R. G., An *in vitro* model of renal proximal tubule cell regeneration, *J. Pharmacol. Toxicol. Methods*, 29, 211, 1993.
146. Kays, S. E. and Schnellmann, R. G., Regeneration of renal proximal tubule cells in primary culture following toxicant injury: response to growth factors, *Toxicol. Appl. Pharmacol.*, 132, 273, 1995.
147. Counts, R. S., Nowak, G., Wyatt, R. D., and Schnellmann, R. G., Nephrotoxicant inhibition of renal proximal tubule cell regeneration, *Am. J. Physiol.*, 269, F274, 1995.

chapter eleven

Use of Freshly Isolated and Primary Cultures of Proximal Tubular and Distal Tubular Cells from Rat Kidney

Lawrence H. Lash

11.1 Introduction 190

11.2 Isolation of epithelial cells from rat renal cortex and outer stripe of outer medulla 191

- 11.2.1 General considerations 191
- 11.2.2 Materials and reagents 191
  - 11.2.2.1 Equipment and supplies for isolation of epithelial cells from rat kidney 191
  - 11.2.2.2 Reagents 192
- 11.2.3 Cell isolation procedure 193

11.3. Purification of epithelial cell populations by Percoll density gradient centrifugation 195

- 11.3.1 Rationale 195
- 11.3.2 Materials and reagents 196
  - 11.3.2.1 Equipment and supplies for separation of renal PT and DT cells 196
  - 11.3.2.2 Reagents 196
- 11.3.3 Experimental design 196
- 11.3.4 Separation method 196
- 11.3.5 Identification of cell populations and assessment of purity 197
- 11.3.6 Incubation conditions and sampling methods 198
- 11.3.7 Selected biochemical properties of renal PT and DT cells 199

11.4 Primary cultures of proximal tubular and distal tubular cells from rat kidneys 201

- 11.4.1 Rationale 201
- 11.4.2 Cell culture media 203
  - 11.4.2.1 General media preparation instructions 205
  - 11.4.2.2 Preparation of media supplement stock solutions 205
- 11.4.3 General cell culture procedures 207
- 11.4.4 Assessment of growth and differentiated function 208

0-8493-3341-5/96/$0.00+$.50

11.4.4.1 Microscopy 208
11.4.4.2 Protein, DNA, and enzyme assays 209
11.4.5 Use of primary cultures of renal cells for toxicological studies 211
11.4.5.1 General comments 211
11.4.5.2 Acute cytotoxicity assay 211
11.5 Concluding remarks 213
11.6 Acknowledgments 214
References 214

11.1 Introduction

Suspensions of isolated renal epithelial cells have become a useful *in vitro* model for studying numerous biochemical, physiological, and toxicological processes. The nephron is composed of several populations of epithelial cells with distinct morphological, physiological, and biochemical characteristics.[1-4] As a consequence of this heterogeneity, each segment of the nephron exhibits a characteristic susceptibility to chemical and pathological injury.[5] In order to study mechanisms of toxicological and pathological responses of renal cells, it is necessary to be able to distinguish processes that occur in different cell populations along the nephron, because some exhibit marked cellular injury under a given set of conditions, whereas others are either not affected or much less affected.

In vitro systems are commonly employed models for biochemical studies of renal cellular function.[6-8] With the growing appreciation of cellular heterogeneity within the different populations of nephrons, it has become necessary to develop convenient methods to separate renal epithelial cells derived from specific nephron segments. The most convenient population of renal epithelial cells to isolate at near homogeneity is that from the segments of the proximal tubule (S_1, S_2, and S_3), the cells of which comprise approximately 80 to 85% of the tubular epithelia in the renal cortex and outer stripe of the outer medulla (OSOM).[6-8] In development of purification methods, advantage can be taken of the unique biochemical and physical properties of the proximal tubule. For example, the high content of microvilli, with their high content of negatively charged glycoproteins, allows efficient separation based on charge or carbohydrate content. Less specific features must generally be employed to enrich renal epithelial cell populations derived from other regions of the nephron.

Chief considerations in developing a process of enrichment or purification of renal epithelial cells are (1) purity, (2) yield, and (3) viability. Although a high degree of enrichment of proximal tubular (PT) cells can readily be obtained, enrichment of cells from other segments of the nephron is more difficult. The nature of the biochemical or physiological processes being studied determines the required degree of purity. Hence, certain investigations require an extremely high degree of cellular homogeneity, and for these studies, micropuncture or microperfusion techniques (see Chapter 5) or microtubular dissection techniques (see Chapter 6) are often necessary. For other purposes, however, enrichments and detailed definitions of biochemical and physiological properties of the different epithelial cell populations are sufficient. Even with suspensions of epithelial cells or tubular fragments from the PT region of the nephron, it is often necessary to further separate these cells or tubular fragments into those derived from S_1, S_2, and S_3 segments (see Chapter 8).[9] Yield is a concern for short-term studies with freshly isolated cells or tubular fragments, particularly from the rat. Hence, if procedures for purification have too many steps, final yield may be too small to allow biochemical studies with paired control and treated samples. Similarly, viability of the final material must be adequate to have a valid control sample to pair with samples treated with a xenobiotic. If the final, purified material is compromised significantly, the tissue will not continue to function during the course of experiments. This problem is particularly severe for isolated renal epithelial cells, possibly because the high basal metabolic rate of these cells makes them susceptible to energy depletion and injury during cell isolation and purification.

We have adapted methodology for the separation and enrichment of epithelial cell populations from rat renal cortex to provide cellular material with a high degree of enrichment and a reasonably high yield that is functionally competent. The methodology, which has been summarized in other recent publications,[10-12] is presented here with additional procedures that extend the use of these freshly isolated cells from short-term (acute) studies to longer term (chronic) processes by means of primary culture.

11.2 Isolation of epithelial cells from rat renal cortex and outer stripe of outer medulla

11.2.1 General considerations

Both the rat and rabbit have been used extensively as model species for the study of renal metabolism and physiology. In developing *in vitro* methods for study of renal toxicology, many investigators have chosen the rabbit as the model species because much more cellular material is available. However, there is and has been a large database on renal function in the rat. This has necessitated development of *in vitro* methods with this species to build on the available information. After selection of the animal species, the type of *in vitro* preparation must be chosen. Although several possibilities exist, as presented in this volume, we have chosen suspensions of single cells. Although isolation of single cells causes a loss of the luminal-to-basolateral cellular polarity that exists in the intact tissue, advantages of suspensions of single cells are that biological material with a high degree of homogeneity can be obtained; all membrane surfaces have equal access to metabolites or other chemicals in the suspending medium; adequate amounts of material can be obtained from a single animal to permit paired control and treated samples; and incubation conditions (i.e., pH, temperature, osmolarity, buffer and medium composition) can be controlled to a high degree, thereby eliminating some uncertainty in mechanistic studies. Consequently, medium pH, osmolarity, ionic composition, and nutrient supply can be altered within a certain range of values to permit study of the effects of these parameters on cellular function or cellular response to chemical toxicants.

Collagenase perfusion is employed to digest connective tissue to obtain suspensions of isolated cells from the renal cortex and OSOM. Since the renal inner medulla is poorly perfused, it can be removed with forceps. The process involves a two-step procedure whereby red blood cells and calcium ions are initially removed and then calcium ions are added back with collagenase to digest the connective tissue and release cells from the cortex and OSOM. Perfusion conditions are optimized to yield predominantly single cells rather than tubular fragments or multicellular aggregates. Any glomeruli, tubular fragments, or cell aggregates that are obtained are removed by filtration through polypropylene mesh. Any cellular debris is removed by centrifugation and resuspension of cells in fresh medium. The isolated renal epithelial cells can then serve as starting material for additional purification or enrichment steps to separate multiple epithelial cell populations (see below).

11.2.2 Materials and reagents

11.2.2.1 Equipment and supplies for isolation of epithelial cells from rat kidney

Temperature-controlled water bath
Peristaltic pump capable of a flow rate of 0.5 to 10 ml/min
pH meter

95% O_2/5% CO_2 gas tank
Tabletop clinical centrifuge
4–0 silk sutures
Surgical scissors
Angled, sharp forceps
19-gauge steel cannula
Tygon plastic tubing
Polypropylene or siliconized glass Erlenmeyer flasks
Polypropylene conical centrifuge tubes, 15-ml capacity
Hemacytometer for estimation of cell number
Light microscope

11.2.2.2 *Reagents*

Sodium pentobarbital (50 mg/ml saline [0.9%, w/v NaCl]) for anesthesia
Heparin (0.2%, w/v, in saline)
4-(2-Hydroxyethylpiperazine)ethanesulfonic acid (HEPES, free acid; Sigma Chemical Co., St. Louis, MO; No. H-3375)
Bovine serum albumin (fraction V; Sigma Chemical Co., St. Louis, MO; No. A-4503)
Collagenase (type I; Sigma Chemical Co., St. Louis, MO; No. C-0130)
Salts (see Tables 1 and 2) for preparation of buffers
Hank's 5× stock buffer (prepared at least monthly; stored at 0 to 4°C)
Krebs–Henseleit 2× stock buffer supplemented with $NaHCO_3$ and $CaCl_2$ (prepared at least monthly; stored at 0 to 4°C)
Trypan blue (0.2%, w/v, in saline): Filtered at least twice through Whatman No. 1 Filter Paper and stored at 0 to 4°C

Table 1 Composition of Buffer Used in Preparation of Epithelial Cells from the Rat Renal Cortex and OSOM

Component	Hank's buffer I	Hank's buffer II	Krebs–Henseleit buffer I
NaCl (m*M*)	137	137	118
KCl (m*M*)	5.4	5.4	4.8
$MgSO_4 \cdot 7H_2O$ (m*M*)	0.8	0.8	1.2
KH_2PO_4 (m*M*)	0.4	0.4	0.96
Na_2HPO_4 (m*M*)	0.4	0.4	—
$NaHCO_3$ (m*M*)	25	25	25
HEPES (m*M*)	25	—	25
$CaCl_2$ (m*M*)	—	4	2.5
EGTA (m*M*)	0.5	—	—
BSA (%, w/v)	2	—	2
Collagenase (%, w/v)	—	0.15	—

Note: Stock solutions are prepared in advance and are stored in polycarbonate bottles at 0 to 4°C for up to one month. Hank's 5× buffer stock: 0.5 l is normally prepared with the first six components. Krebs–Henseleit 2× buffer stock: dissolve indicated components except $CaCl_2$ and BSA in 1 l of deionized water, bubble the 2× solution with 95% O_2/5% CO_2 for 30 min, and then gradually add $CaCl_2$ with slow mixing. At the time of a cell preparation, stocks are diluted with deionized water, the extra components are added, the solutions are bubbled with 95% O_2/5% CO_2 for 30 min, pH values are adjusted to 7.36 with NaOH or HCl as needed, and the solutions are then continuously bubbled during cell isolation. Abbreviations: BSA, bovine serum albumin, fraction V; EGTA, ethylene glycol bis(β-aminoethyl ether)-*N,N,N′,N′*-tetraacetic acid; HEPES, 4-(2-hydroxyethylpiperazine)ethanesulfonic acid; OSOM, outer stripe of outer medulla.

Table 2 Composition of Krebs–Henseleit Buffer Used in Percoll Density Gradient Centrifugation Procedure to Fractionate Epithelial Cells from the Rat Renal Cortex and OSOM

Component	Concentration (m*M*)
NaCl	118
KCl	4.8
$MgSO_4{\cdot}7H_2O$	0.12
KH_2PO_4	0.96
$NaHCO_3$	25
HEPES	25
$CaCl_2$	0

Note: A 10× stock solution of the Ca^{2+}-free, low Mg^{2+} Krebs–Henseleit buffer is prepared in advance and is stored in a polycarbonate bottle at 0 to 4°C for up to one month. The Percoll mixture is prepared shortly before use by mixing (in order) 1 volume of 10× buffer stock, 4.5 volumes of deionized water, and 4.5 volumes of Percoll, to give a final Percoll concentration of 45% (v/v). This mixture is kept on ice until used. During this time, the Percoll mixture is bubbled with 95% O_2/5% CO_2, and the pH is adjusted to 7.36 with 1 *M* NaOH. Abbreviation: HEPES, 4-(2-hydroxyethylpiperazine)ethanesulfonic acid; OS-OM, outer stripe of outer medulla.

11.2.3 Cell isolation procedure

All perfusion steps are performed at 37°C. The basic procedure is that originally described by Jones et al.[6] and Ormstad et al.[7] and reviewed by Lash.[8] Several strains of rats have been used as the source for renal epithelial cells, including the Sprague–Dawley, the Fischer 344, and the Wistar strains, and the choice of strain for a particular study is dependent on those previously used and the types of processes being studied. Adult rats weighing 180 to 300 g are typically used, although the best results (i.e., yield, viability) are generally obtained with rats weighing less than 250 g. This is particularly true for Fischer 344 rats, which have a relatively high content of fat and connective tissue above 250 g body weight. Buffers are continuously bubbled with 95% O_2/5% CO_2 to assure adequate oxygenation of the kidney during perfusion. Before surgery, rats are anesthetized with an intraperitoneal injection of sodium pentobarbital (0.1 ml of a 50 mg ml^{-1} solution in saline per 100 g body weight, resulting in 50 mg nembutal per kilogram body weight). Blood clotting is prevented by injection of 0.2 ml of 0.2% (w/v) heparin into the tail vein just before beginning the surgery. Administration of heparin, although not essential, tends to hasten the removal of blood from the kidneys during the initial perfusion step.

Composition of buffers that are used in the isolation and implementation of epithelial cells from the kidney is given in Table 1. Once the water bath is warmed to 37°C, Hank's 1× and Krebs Henseleit 1× are prepared from stocks by dilution with deionized water. For each cell isolation procedure, 300 ml of Hank's 1× (for Hank's I + II) and 100 ml of Krebs–Henseleit 1× are placed in appropriately sized flasks or beakers. Additional components (i.e., HEPES, bovine serum albumin) are dissolved and solutions are bubbled for 30 min with 95% O_2/5% CO_2. After adjusting the pH of each buffer to 7.36, flasks are returned to the water bath for maintenance of temperature and for continuous bubbling with 95% O_2/5% CO_2. A pH value of 7.36 is used, rather than 7.40, to compensate for some loss of dissolved CO_2 that occurs, which causes the pH to rise slightly.

Once the animal is anesthetized and the heparin has been injected into the tail vein, the suspension of renal epithelial cells is prepared as follows:

1. The peritoneal cavity is opened by a midventral incision and the aorta is freed from the surrounding connective tissue and the adjacent inferior vena cava. Care should be taken when separating the aorta from the inferior vena cava to prevent puncturing the latter. If the vena cava is punctured, a hemostat should be clamped

around it to stop the blood flow, although its presence makes it difficult to complete the surgery.

2. A 4–0 silk ligature is placed around the aorta approximately 0.5 in. below the renal artery. A second ligature is placed around the aorta as high up in the abdomen as possible.
3. The celiac and superior mesenteric arteries are ligated to prevent diversion of perfusate.
4. Tubing connected to the peristaltic pump is filled with Hank's I buffer in preparation for the cannulation step.
5. An oblique incision is made through approximately 50% of the diameter of the aorta above the lower ligature; a cone-shaped, 19-gauge cannula is inserted into the aorta; and the cannula is secured with a new ligature. During insertion of the cannula, perfusate is allowed to drip out of the cannula at a slow rate (less than 0.5 ml/min) to prevent formation of air bubbles.
6. Once the cannula is secured, the perfusion flow rate is increased to 8 ml/min and *in situ* perfusion is allowed for approximately 1 min. At this time, both kidneys should become pale. If only one kidney becomes pale, it is likely that the other kidney did not perfuse due to insertion of the cannula above the level of the left renal artery. One can carefully adjust the position of the cannula if necessary.
7. The animal is sacrificed and the kidneys are removed from the posterior abdominal wall, and the kidneys with the attached cannula are transferred to the beaker containing the Hank's I perfusate. The kidneys undergo recirculating perfusion at 8 ml/min for approximately 10 min.
8. After 10 min, the perfusion assembly with cannula attached is transferred to a new beaker containing Hank's II buffer with collagenase. The kidneys undergo recirculating perfusion for 15 to 20 min at a flow rate of 5 ml/min. Kidneys that are adequately perfused and whose connective tissue has been digested appear pale and swollen.
9. Kidneys are removed from the perfusion apparatus, the renal capsule and adhering fat and connective tissue are removed, and cells are dispersed with a pair of forceps into 40 ml of the Krebs–Henseleit I buffer.
10. The dispersed cells are filtered through polypropylene gauze (210-μm pore size) to remove tissue fragments and multicellular aggregates.
11. The filtered cells are centrifuged in 15-ml polypropylene conical centrifuge tubes in a tabletop clinical centrifuge at $100 \times g$ for 30 s. Cell pellets are resuspended at concentrations of 5 to 8×10^6 cells/ml in either Krebs–Henseleit I buffer if subsequent purification steps are performed (see below) or Krebs–Henseleit I buffer supplemented with 5 m*M* glucose + 5 m*M* glutamate (= Krebs–Henseleit II) if the composite collection of cells is the final stage of cell isolation.
12. Concentration and cell viability are estimated by mixing a 50-μl aliquot of cells with 450 μl of 0.2% (w/v) trypan blue and counting the total number of cells and the fraction of cells that exclude the dye, respectively, on a hemacytometer.

As discussed above, perfusion conditions have been optimized to yield predominantly single cells in suspension rather than tubular fragments or aggregrates of cells. This is accomplished by having a collagenase concentration of 0.15% (w/v) and maintaining a perfusion flow rate for the Hank's II buffer containing the collagenase of no more than 5 ml/min. Higher concentrations of collagenase or higher perfusate flow rates cause less complete digestion of renal tissue, with release of aggregates and tubular fragments. Once a suspension of single cells is obtained, cells are stored in polypropylene or siliconized glass 25-ml Erlenmeyer flasks to prevent clumping of cells or attachment of cells to the surface of the flask. DNase (0.5 mg/ml) may also be added to the Hank's II perfusate to minimize clumping of cells due to DNA released from damaged cells.[13] A typical yield of composite cells from two kidneys of an adult rat is about 40 to 80 × 10^6 cells. Greater than 90% of these cells exclude trypan blue, indicating a high degree of intact cellular structure. The entire cell isolation procedure, including preparation of buffers, surgery, perfusion, and collection of cells requires approximately 2 h to complete.

11.3 Purification of epithelial cell populations by Percoll density-gradient centrifugation

11.3.1 Rationale

Although the preparation of renal epithelial cells from the cortex and OSOM comprises primarily PT cells, this cell preparation contains multiple cell populations, not all of which may exhibit the same biochemistry or physiology. Hence, the epithelial cells obtained by collagenase perfusion may serve as starting material for the further purification of PT cells and for the isolation of cell populations derived from other segments of the nephron. In order to study biological processes in specific segments of the nephron, investigators have developed separation techniques that take advantage of biochemical, morphological, or physical differences in the different nephron segments. As discussed above, any separation procedure to obtain enriched populations of renal epithelial cells must satisfy the following criteria: (1) the procedure must be relatively rapid; (2) any material used in the separation process must be biologically inert; (3) final yield must be high enough to enable performance of a sufficient number of paired control and test incubations; and (4) purity must be high enough to enable unambiguous conclusions regarding the tubular origin.

Tubular microdissection techniques have been used for several years to obtain renal epithelial cells derived from specific regions of the nephron. While this method provides material of extremely high purity, the procedure is not particularly useful for most typical biochemical or toxicological studies, especially those with the rat as the experimental animal, because of low yield. Similarly, electrophoretic techniques can be used to separate epithelial cell populations from the renal cortex. These techniques also suffer from low yield.

Differences in cell density are commonly used to separate a mixture of cell populations into individual components. Although these methods provide enrichment rather than absolute purification (since cell density is generally not a discrete parameter for a given cell population, but exhibits a range of values), they are relatively simple and quick to perform. Several methods involving density gradient centrifugation of renal tubular fragments or epithelial cells through biologically inert materials such as Ficoll or Percoll have been developed. Ficoll and Percoll spontaneously form density gradients when placed in a centrifugal field. Hence, specialized equipment to preform a density gradient is not required. Percoll is a liquid composed of microscopic, carbohydrate-coated beads.[14] Density marker beads can be purchased (Sigma Chemical Co., St. Louis, MO) for calibration of the gradient and optimization of centrifugation conditions. The beads are color coded and sediment at discrete densities in the Percoll gradient. Procedures have been developed to enrich PT and distal tubular (DT) fragments with Ficoll[15] and Percoll[16-18] and to enrich isolated PT cells from suspensions of renal epithelial cells with Ficoll.[19]

Percoll was developed after Ficoll and has the advantage of already being in liquid form, whereas Ficoll must be prepared from solid material. Accordingly, we developed a separation method based on previous methods of Percoll density gradient centrifugation and optimized it for separation of single cells from the rat kidney.[10-12] Optimal separation conditions were obtained by varying Percoll concentration (30 to 90%, v/v), centrifugation speed (1,000 × to 20,000 × g), centrifugation time (10 to 60 min), and the cell concentration layered on the Percoll (2 to 10 × 10^6 cells/ml).

11.3.2 Materials and reagents

In addition to the items listed above for the preparation of composite suspensions of renal epithelial cells from the cortex and OSOM, the following are required for the separation of PT and DT cells.

11.3.2.1 Equipment and supplies for separation of renal PT and DT cells

Refrigerated, low-speed centrifuge (e.g., Dupont/Sorvall RC2B)
Centrifuge rotor with slots for 50-ml centrifuge tubes
Polycarbonate, round-bottom centrifuge tubes, 50-ml capacity

11.3.2.2 Reagents

Percoll (Sigma Chemical Co., St. Louis, MO; No. P-1644); keep refrigerated
Krebs–Henseleit 10× stock solution for Percoll separation (prepared at least monthly)
Density marker beads (Sigma Chemical Co., St. Louis, MO; No. DMB-10)

11.3.3 Experimental design

Since Percoll is insoluble in the presence of high concentrations of divalent cations, a modified Krebs–Henseleit buffer is used that is nominally Ca^{2+}-free and has one tenth the Mg^{2+} concentration of the normal Krebs–Henseleit buffer used in suspending epithelial cells (Table 2). During the preparation of the Percoll mixture on which cells are layered, it is important to add the components of the mixture (i.e., 10× buffer stock, deionized water, Percoll) in a precise order, since variation of the order of addition can cause clumping of Percoll, and to keep the Percoll mixture on ice during oxygenation and pH adjustment. Additionally, we have found that addition of any other metabolites to the Krebs–Henseleit medium in which the cortical epithelial cells are suspended, even glucose or amino acids, alters the behavior of the Percoll during gradient formation. With these minor but critical points kept in mind, extremely consistent gradient formation is obtained from preparation to preparation and from day to day. This can be validated by the use of density marker beads or by fractionation of renal epithelial cells and measurement of the distribution of marker enzymes (see below).

11.3.4 Separation method

Isolated epithelial cells from rat renal cortex and OSOM, prepared by collagenase perfusion as described above, serve as the starting material for the enrichment of PT and DT cells. The cortical epithelial cells are suspended in Krebs–Henseleit buffer I, which contains only HEPES and BSA as supplements (Table 1). The following steps are performed in the separation of PT and DT cells from renal cortical epithelial cells:

1. At the stage when the kidneys with attached cannula are transferred to the beaker for the collagenase perfusion step (see step 8 above), the Percoll mixture is bubbled for 30 min with 95% O_2/5% CO_2 while kept on ice. The pH of the Percoll mixture is adjusted to 7.36 with 1 *M* NaOH. It is important to wait for any clumps of Percoll to dissolve in between dropwise additions of NaOH and to allow the pH meter to stabilize before further addition of NaOH.
2. Layer 5 ml of renal epithelial cells (5 to 8×10^6 cells/ml) on 35 ml of isosmotic Percoll mixture in 50-ml polycarbonate, round-bottom centrifuge tubes. Two tubes are normally prepared from each rat. Centrifuge at 0 to 4°C for 30 min at $20{,}000 \times g$ (12,900 rpm) in a Sorvall RC2B centrifuge in an SS34 rotor. During this centrifugation step, Krebs–Henseleit II (which is Krebs–Henseleit I with glucose and glutamine added; see Table 1) and Krebs–Henseleit III (which is the Ca^{2+}- free, low

Mg^{2+}-Krebs–Henseleit buffer; see Table 2) are bubbled with 95% O_2/5% CO_2 and their pH is adjusted to 7.36. It is important that the renal epithelial cells are in the range of cell concentration specified: if renal epithelial cells are layered on the Percoll at too high a cell concentration, the cells tend to clump; if they are layered on the Percoll at too low a cell concentration, poor recovery of cells is observed. Additionally, polycarbonate centrifuge tubes without scratches on their inside surface should be used, since cells tend to aggregate and bind to these indentations.

3. Cells are fractionated with an automatic pipettor. For analytical purposes, the gradient is fractionated from the top into 20 2-ml fractions. For preparative purposes, 5-ml fractions from the two gradients are collected from the top of the gradient as follows:

   Fractions 1 and 2: PT cells (save)
   Fractions 3 to 6: mixture of PT and DT cells, other cells (discard)
   Fractions 7 and 8: DT cells (save)

4. Pooled fractions representing PT and DT cells are placed in separate 50-ml polycarbonate or polystyrene centrifuge tubes, diluted 1:1 with Krebs–Henseleit III, and centrifuged in a tabletop clinical centrifuge at 500 × g for 5 min. This washing procedure is necessary to concentrate the PT and DT cells to the desired final cell concentrations and to remove the Percoll. Supernatants are carefully removed and the loose cell pellets are gently resuspended in Krebs–Henseleit II, generally at concentrations of 2 to 4×10^6 cells/ml. The only exception is when these enriched cells are used as seed material for primary cell culture (see below).
5. PT and DT cells are placed in 25-ml polypropylene Erlenmeyer flasks after estimation of cell concentration and yield and cell viability by trypan blue exclusion. Rubber serum bottle stoppers are placed in the flasks to seal them, and the atmosphere above the cells is equilibrated with 95% O_2/5% CO_2. Flasks are kept on ice until needed for experiments or for subsequent procedures (generally <30 min).

11.3.5 *Identification of cell populations and assessment of purity*

Centrifugation of renal epithelial cells (isolated from the cortex and OSOM) at 20,000 × g for 30 min through Percoll produces a continuous and concave density gradient, which ranges from a density of 1.016 to 1.120 g/ml, with an inflection point at 1.057 g/ml.[10] Two Gaussian distributions of cells are obtained, one near the top of the gradient (1.016 to 1.047 g/ml), and one near the bottom (1.076 g/ml to 1.120 g/ml). The middle region of the gradient contains few cells. Even with an epithelial cell population derived from a single region of the nephron, a range of densities is found, so that some overlap between cell populations is inevitable. Previous applications of density gradient methods for separation of renal epithelial cells showed that PT cells from the kidneys of rats had densities of 1.036 to 1.052 g/ml,[19] indicating that they should be recovered in the least dense portions of the gradient. In contrast, when tubular fragments are used as starting material for Percoll density gradient centrifugation, proximal tubules are recovered in the densest portions of the gradients and distal tubules are recovered in the least dense portions of the gradient,[15-17] which is the reverse order when suspensions of single cells are the starting material. Hence, the expectation is that the Gaussian distribution of cells found near the top of the Percoll gradient, which comprises the majority of the cells recovered, will be PT in origin, whereas the Gaussian distribution of cells found near the bottom of the Percoll gradient will be DT in origin.

The identity of the two cell populations is confirmed by measurement of marker enzyme activities in fractions from the Percoll gradient. Marker enzymes are so-named because they possess discrete cellular or subcellular localizations and can, therefore, be used to identify the presence of a given cell type or subcellular organelle. Furthermore, analysis of the presence of markers in different fractions allows one to estimate the purity or degree of enrichment of one cell type or subcellular fraction relative to another. For renal PT cells, several unique enzymatic markers are available due to the prevalence of the brush border membrane, which is rich in hydrolases, in that segment of the nephron. Alkaline phosphatase (AP; EC 3.1.3.1) and γ-glutamyltransferase (GGT; EC 2.3.2.2) are used as markers of PT cells. Since these enzymes (particularly GGT) are present at extremely high levels in brush border membranes of PT cells, one can readily detect the presence of contaminating PT cells in other renal cell populations. Carbohydrate metabolism shows marked heterogeneity along the mammalian nephron.[3,4] Thus, glycolytic activity is extremely low in PT cells, but occurs at very high levels in DT cells. Hexokinase (HK; EC 2.7.1.1) activity can therefore be used as a marker enzyme for the presence of DT cells.

Measurement of the distribution of the marker enzymes in fractions from the Percoll gradient confirmed that the cell population recovered near the top of the gradient is PT in origin, whereas that recovered near the bottom of the gradient is DT in origin. Of the total number of cells recovered from the gradient (total recovery = 80%), those identified as PT cells accounted for 57% of the total and those identified as DT cells accounted for 24% of the total, with the remaining 19% being found in the intermediate fractions and representing a heterogeneous mixture of epithelial cell populations. The degree of enrichment of the PT and DT cells can be calculated from the following equations:[10,11]

% Cell type A enrichment = 100% – [% Cells in starting material of type B origin × (Specific activity of cell type A marker in type B cells/Specific activity of cell type A marker in type A cells)] (1)

% Cell type B enrichment = 100% – [% Cells in starting material of type A origin × (Specific activity of cell type B marker in type A cells/Specific activity of cell type B marker in type B cells)] (2)

If we estimate that PT cells constitute 85% of the epithelial cells in the cortex and OSOM and the ratio of GGT activity in DT cells to that in PT cells is 0.17,[10] then the percentage of PT cell enrichment is calculated as 100% – (15% × 0.17) = 97%. For DT cells, if we assume that they comprise, at most, 15% of the epithelial cells in the same zones and use a ratio of HK activity in PT cells to that in DT cells of 0.13,[10] then the percentage of DT cell enrichment is calculated as 100% – (85% × 0.13) = 88%.

This analysis is at best an approximation, especially for DT cells. Two assumptions are made — namely, only two cell populations are present and each marker enzyme is distributed exclusively in one cell population. Although there are several discrete cell populations within the renal cortex and OSOM, PT cells (both straight and convoluted segments) comprise the vast majority of epithelial cells. Hence, the estimate of enrichment for PT cells is probably reasonably accurate. The DT cell population comprises a mixture of cells from distal convoluted tubules and cortical collecting ducts. Furosemide sensitivity of cellular oxygen consumption can be used as a marker for the presence of cortical thick ascending limb cells. By this method, cortical and outer medullary thick ascending limb cells were not detected in either the PT or, more important, in the DT cell fractions.[10]

11.3.6 *Incubation conditions and sampling methods*

Incubations can be performed with freshly isolated renal epithelial cells for up to 4 h. Cells are placed in 25-ml Erlenmeyer flasks made of siliconized glass or polypropylene to prevent cells from binding to the wall of the incubation vessel. Rubber serum stoppers are placed in the mouth of the Erlenmeyer flasks to seal them and regulate the oxygenation of the cells. Cells are oxygenated by gassing with 95% O_2/5% CO_2 for 30 s to 1 min. The CO_2 is required because of the presence of sodium bicarbonate in the buffer. Whenever samples are removed from flasks, the flasks are resealed and the atmosphere reequilibrated with the desired gas mixture. Total volume of cells in the 25-ml flasks should not exceed approximately 3 ml because increased volume decreases the rate of oxygen diffusion to the cells. Thus, use of higher incubation volumes could result in a significant portion of the cells becoming hypoxic. Flasks are placed in a shaking water bath (60 cycles/min) at 37°C. For most experiments, we have found it beneficial to preincubate cells for 15 min at 37°C prior to beginning any experimental incubations.[8,10-12] This brief preincubation period serves to stabilize the cell preparations, resulting in values of biochemical processes and levels of key parameters such as glutathione (GSH) and ATP that are closer to those that should be found in intact renal tissue. Additions to cell suspensions are usually made from concentrated stock solutions (10× to 100×) so that cells are minimally diluted.

A major advantage of the use of suspensions of isolated renal epithelial cells is that sampling is reproducible and simple. Contents of an intracellular metabolite of interest can be measured by mixing aliquots of the cell suspensions with acid (e.g., trichloroacetic acid [5%, w/v, final concentration] or perchloric acid [10%, v/v, final concentration]) and centrifugation (e.g., 10,000 × g × 2 min in a microcentrifuge). Acid-soluble supernatants are then processed according to the specific assay of interest. This simple, direct method works well if the chemical being measured is only present inside the cell. If, however, the objective is to quantitate metabolite transport, for example, it is necessary to separate the cells from the extracellular medium. A simple method to achieve this is to rapidly centrifuge cells through Percoll. Aliquots of cells (0.5 ml) are layered on 1.0 ml of 20% (v/v) Percoll in saline in 1.5-ml microcentrifuge tubes. The tubes are centrifuged in a microcentrifuge for 30 s at 10,000 × g, supernatants are removed, and cell pellets can be resuspended or treated with acid and processed for the assay of interest. Alternatively, we have also used rapid filtration under vacuum of aliquots of cells through 0.45-µm pore size filters (Gelman Sciences, GN-6 mixed cellulose esters filters). Cells are removed from the pellets by incubation in distilled water and are analyzed for the chemical of interest as above.

11.3.7 Selected biochemical properties of renal PT and DT cells

Examination of the isolated renal PT and DT cells by bright-field light microscopy (Figure 1) shows that the two cell populations exhibit some distinct morphological features. Although some clumping of the cells occurs, which is due to processing for microscopy, cells in the suspensions are generally obtained as individual cells with only a few clumps of two to five cells per clump. Note that when renal epithelial cells are placed in suspension, they tend to lose their characteristic cuboidal shape and assume a spherical appearance. A brush border is observed in the PT cells, but is absent from the DT cells; nuclei stain more intensely with toluidine blue in the PT cells; and the PT cells are generally larger than the DT cells, although both cell populations exhibit significant heterogeneity in their size.

Several key parameters of cellular function are summarized in Table 3 and show that the suspensions of renal PT and DT cells exhibit functional and biochemical integrity and are, therefore, useful *in vitro* model systems for toxicological studies. Cell viability, as assessed by either trypan blue exclusion or lactate dehydrogenase (LDH) release, should be >90% at the time of cell isolation (i.e., >90% of the cells should exclude trypan blue or <10% release of total cellular LDH activity should be observed). In incubations with buffer (= control cells) in 25-ml polypropylene Erlenmeyer flasks under the standard conditions described above, cell viability by either of these methods should exceed 80% for at least 2 h. Both PT and DT cells exhibit GSH/GSSG ratios >20; high intracellular contents of

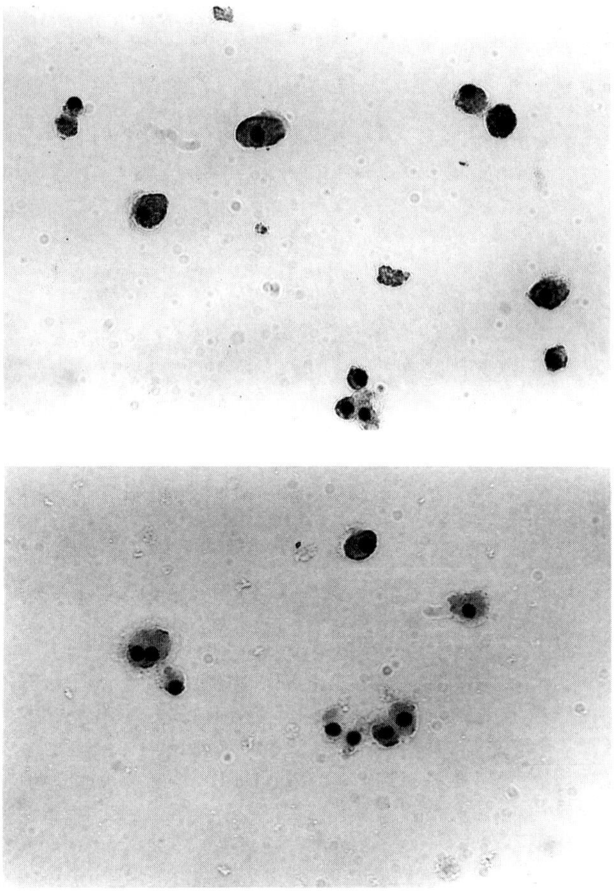

Figure 1 Bright-field light microscopy of toluidine blue-stained renal proximal tubular (PT; upper panel) and distal tubular (DT; lower panel) cells. Isolated renal PT and DT cells from male Fischer 344 rats were resuspended in 2% (w/v) bovine serum albumin in distilled water, were applied to microscope slides, and were fixed by a short application of heat (<1 min) and air-drying. Cells were stained with 0.01% (w/v) toluidine blue for 1 min, were rinsed with distilled water, and were sealed onto the slides with a coverslip. Bright-field light microscopy was performed on a Zeiss Axiophot microscope using a 40× objective with an ocular magnification of 2.5× and an optivar 1.25×, giving a total magnification of 125×. Pictures were taken with Panatomic X film (ASA 40, automatic exposure of 5.5 to 7.5 s; Kodak). Final magnification is 435×. (From Lash, L. H. and Tokarz, J. J., *Anal. Biochem.*, 182, 271, 1989. With permission.)

ATP, with cellular energy charge values (= [ATP + 0.5 ADP]/[ATP + ADP + AMP]) > 0.80; and rates of oxygen consumption that respond appropriately to addition of agents that modify cellular energetics. Specifically, addition of nystatin to uncouple the (Na^++K^+)-stimulated ATPase increases cellular ATP consumption and increases substrate-stimulated oxygen consumption. Conversely, addition of ouabain to inhibit the (Na^++K^+)-stimulated ATPase, which decreases cellular ATP consumption, decreases substrate-stimulated cellular oxygen consumption by >70%.

Nephron heterogeneity with regard to marker enzymes and enzymes involved in xenobiotic metabolism can be studied in these cell suspensions (Table 4). γ-Glutamyltransferase and alkaline phosphatase, which are used as PT cell markers, are found in PT cells at activities that are 8.0- and 3.4-fold higher, respectively, than those in DT cells. Hexokinase, which is used as a DT cell marker, in contrast, is found at activities that are 7.1-fold higher in DT cells than those in PT cells. Several GSH-dependent and other drug metabolism

Table 3 Biochemical Characteristics of Freshly Isolated Proximal Tubular (PT) and Distal Tubular (DT) Cells from the Rat Renal Cortex and OSOM

Parameter	PT cells	DT cells	*n*
Yield from one rat (× 10^6 cells)	30.1 ± 11.6	12.8 ± 5.1	29
Protein (mg/10^6 cells)	0.55 ± 0.05	0.90 ± 0.10	15
Cell viability			
Trypan blue exclusion (%)	94.5 ± 2.8	93.7 ± 2.9	20
LDH release (%)	9.9 ± 5.9	8.6 ± 5.6	11
Thiol status (nmol/10^6 cells)			
GSH	8.90 ± 0.96	12.0 ± 1.8	4
GSSG	0.37 ± 0.17	0.46 ± 0.16	4
PrSH	23.6 ± 3.3	34.9 ± 1.3	6
ATP (nmol/10^6 cells)	5.19 ± 0.77	10.6 ± 2.2	6
Mitochondrial respiration (nmol O_2/min per 10^6 cells)			3–7
Basal	16.7 ± 0.7	26.3 ± 0.7	
+ 5 m*M* succinate	37.5 ± 1.5	34.6 ± 0.9	
+ 5 m*M* glutamate	40.3 ± 3.2	69.5 ± 13.7	
+ 0.25 mg nystatin/ml	53.8 ± 7.5	91.9 ± 3.5	
+ 0.1 m*M* ouabain	9.58 ± 0.96	22.8 ± 2.4	

Note: Protein concentrations were determined by the Lowry method with Folin-phenol reagent. Lactate dehydrogenase (LDH) release was measured as NADH oxidation at 340 nm with pyruvate in the presence and absence of Triton X-100. Cellular contents of glutathione (GSH), glutathione disulfide (GSSG), and ATP were determined by HPLC. Protein sulfhydryl content (PrSH) of cells was determined with 5,5′-dithio-bis(2-nitrobenzoic acid). Rates of cellular oxygen consumption were measured polarographically with a Gilson 5/6H oxygen electrode. Results are the means ± SE of the indicated number of separate cell preparations.

enzymes that are critical for cellular defense against reactive species, such as oxidants, are also found in significantly higher amounts in PT cells than in DT cells. In particular, GSSG reductase, which is often the rate-limiting enzyme in the reduction of cytotoxic peroxides, is present in amounts that are 3.4-fold higher in PT cells than in DT cells. Catalase and DT-diaphorase, which are critical for detoxication of hydrogen peroxide and redox cycling quinones, are present in amounts that are severalfold higher in PT cells than in DT cells. From these findings and from investigations on the susceptibility of renal PT and DT cells to oxidants[5,20] and alkylating agents that target GSH and other soft nucleophiles,[5,21] we have concluded that isolated DT cells from the rat are more susceptible to these forms of chemically induced injury than isolated PT cells from the rat because they possess markedly diminished capacity to utilize GSH or other protective compounds for detoxication of reactive species.

11.4 *Primary cultures of proximal tubular and distal tubular cells from rat kidneys*

11.4.1 *Rationale*

Toxicological studies with suspensions of freshly isolated renal epithelial cells are limited to investigations of acute (i.e., minutes to hours) injury because the time period over which these cells can maintain functional integrity is on the order of only 4 h. Beyond this point, freshly isolated cells generally do not maintain adequate function, so that they cannot serve as valid controls for toxicological studies. Hence, for most of the types of responses that occur as a consequence of acute exposure to chemical toxicants, the survival time and

Table 4 Distribution of Marker Enzymes and Drug Metabolism Enzymes in Renal Proximal Tubular (PT) and Distal Tubular (DT) Cells

Enzyme	PT cells	DT cells
γ-Glutamyltransferase	1480 ± 280	186 ± 25
Alkaline phosphatase	403 ± 113	117 ± 34
Hexokinase	111 ± 48	785 ± 235
GSSG reductase	163 ± 30	47.4 ± 14.5
GSH peroxidase	1290 ± 360	571 ± 141
GSH *S*-transferase	144 ± 42	92.9 ± 23.7
Catalase	701 ± 99	287 ± 83
DT-diaphorase	102 ± 24	14.8 ± 0.9

Note: Results are total activity in nanomoles per minute and are the means ± SE of measurements from seven cell preparations. γ-Glutamyltransferase activity was measured with γ-glutamyl-*p*-nitroanilide and glycylglycine as substrates. Alkaline phosphatase activity was measured with *p*-nitrophenyl phosphate as substrate at pH 10. Hexokinase and GSSG reductase activities were measured by pyridine nucleotide-linked assays. GSH peroxidase activity was measured with H_2O_2 as substrate. Catalase activity was measured as H_2O_2 disappearance. DT-diaphorase (NADPH:quinone oxidoreductase) activity was measured as the dicumarol-sensitive reduction of 2,6-dichlorophenol indophenol in the presence of NADPH.

maintenance of function of suspensions of freshly isolated renal epithelial cells are adequate for observation of changes that can provide insight into biochemical mechanisms of action. For the examination of longer term or chronic effects of chemicals (i.e., effects that occur on the order of hours to days) in *in vitro* systems, cell culture methods are necessary.[22] A biological model system to study chronic responses in renal epithelial cells must meet two critical requirements. First, the model must consist of material whose renal cell type of origin can be unambiguously defined. Second, the model must be maintained in a viable state for at least 7 to 10 days. Normal *in vivo* properties of the tissue of origin must be maintained during the culture period. Otherwise, reliable conclusions relating to cell type specificity and mechanism of action cannot be made.

Two general types of renal cell culture systems have been used — established cell lines and primary cell culture. Although established cell lines that are originally derived from specific nephron segments are available and these cells are biochemically uniform and provide a reproducible model for toxicological studies, responses obtained with these cells may not always accurately reflect processes that occur *in vivo*. By becoming immortalized, cell lines may have undergone genetic transformation and thus may no longer resemble the cell type from which they were derived.[23] Cultured cells may dedifferentiate in culture, expressing some, but not all, properties of the original tissue. Additionally, cell lines from different nephron segments are not available from a single species but are derived from several species. Due to known and potential species-dependent differences in biochemical properties and susceptibility to toxic chemicals, ambiguity can arise from studies with these various cell lines.

Primary cell culture is an excellent model system, if applied properly, to investigate toxicological processes on a longer time scale. Advantages and limitations of the use of primary renal cell culture are summarized in Table 5. Two critical considerations in establishment of primary cell culture methodology are (1) cell type homogeneity and (2) stability of differentiated phenotype and function. Homogeneity relates to both the purity of the starting material and the tendency of minor populations of cells, particularly fibroblasts, to overgrow the major cell population. Stability of differentiated phenotype and function relates to the ability of cells to retain their biochemical, physiological, and morphological properties as they exist in the normal, *in vivo* state. These criteria are often difficult to satisfy with populations of renal epithelial cells. Taub and colleagues[24-26] (also see Chapters 10 and 12 in this volume) have pioneered the development and use of serum-free, hormonally defined media for primary culture of renal PT cells from rabbit. Much of the primary renal cell culture work has used rabbit as the experimental animal model, rather than the rat, because rabbit renal PT cells appear to have a greater capacity for growth as compared to cells from the rat.[27] It is important, however, to have such a primary cell culture model with renal cells from the rat because of the large database of renal studies using the rat.

Table 5 Advantages and Limitations to the Use of Primary Renal Cell Cultures

Advantages
Closely related to *in vivo* cells if differentiated function maintained; cell lines are often of ill-defined cellular origin
Precise definition of incubation conditions
Extended viability possible (up to two weeks in some cases)
Study cell type-specific processes
Maintenance of epithelial polarity if cells grown on appropriate matrix
Limitations
Difficult to maintain relative to cell lines (i.e., reproducibility can be difficult to achieve)
Dedifferentiation may occur during culture
Limited lifetime relative to immortalized cell lines

Several laboratories have recently developed procedures for primary culture of renal PT cells from the rat.[27-32] Much less work on development of primary cultures of renal cells from other nephron segments, however, has been reported. The rabbit, rather than the rat, has generally been the source of renal cells for primary culture.[33] The issue of homogeneity can be addressed readily by use of a procedure such as Percoll density gradient centrifugation,[10-12] as described above, to enrich specific cell populations from suspensions of isolated epithelial cells or tubular fragments. Use of either serum-free, hormonally defined medium or replacement of L-valine and L-arginine in culture medium with D-valine and L-ornithine, respectively,[31] can prevent fibroblast overgrowth. Serum functions to provide hormones and growth factors that are stimulatory for cell growth; attachment and spreading factors; and transport proteins carrying hormones, minerals, and lipids. However, the complexity of serum impairs definitive study of factors influencing differentiation and proliferation. The replacement strategy used by Boogaard and colleagues[31] for primary culture of rat renal PT cells takes advantage of the fact that the kidneys of the rodent and human contain D-amino acid oxidase and can therefore grow on D-amino acids, whereas fibroblasts do not have this enzymatic activity and therefore cannot grow in such media. With these defined media, fibroblast overgrowth is prevented and differentiated cellular function is maintained during culture to a greater extent than when serum-containing media are used. Much slower cell growth, however, is obtained with defined media.

This section describes an extension of our Percoll density gradient centrifugation method in which the suspensions of enriched PT and DT cells from the rat serve as seed material for primary cell culture.[34] A standard, serum-free, hormonally defined medium with inclusion of additional, specific hormones or growth factors is used to optimize growth and maintenance of differentiated phenotype for the two renal cell populations.

11.4.2 Cell culture media

The basal cell culture medium used for primary culture of renal PT and DT cells from rat is a 1:1 mixture of Dulbecco's Modified Eagle's Medium:Ham's F12 (DMEM:F12) (Table 6).

The basal medium contains all 20 amino acids, glucose and pyruvate, several vitamins and coenzymes, lipid derivatives, organic and inorganic ions, nucleic acid precursors, and a bicarbonate–CO_2 buffering system and can be purchased as a dry mixture of chemicals that is ready for reconstitution with doubly processed distilled water. All glassware used in the preparation of media is sterilized in an autoclave.

Table 6 Composition of Basal Cell Culture Medium for Primary Culture of PT and DT Cells from the Rat Renal Cortex and OSOM

Component	Concentration (*M*)	Component	Concentration (*M*)
Essential amino acids		Water-soluble vitamins and coenzymes	
Arg	7.00×10^{-4}		
CySH	1.00×10^{-4}	Biotin	1.50×10^{-8}
Half cystine	2.00×10^{-4}	Folic acid	6.05×10^{-6}
Gln	2.50×10^{-3}	α-Lipoic acid	5.00×10^{-7}
His	1.50×10^{-4}	Nicotinamide	1.66×10^{-5}
Ile	4.15×10^{-4}	Pantothenic acid	9.00×10^{-6}
Leu	4.50×10^{-4}	Pyridoxine	1.50×10^{-7}
Lys	5.00×10^{-4}	Pyridoxal	1.00×10^{-5}
Met	1.15×10^{-4}	Riboflavin	6.00×10^{-7}
Phe	2.15×10^{-4}	Thiamine	6.50×10^{-6}
Thr	4.50×10^{-4}	Vitamin B-12	5.00×10^{-7}
Trp	4.50×10^{-5}	Nucleic acid derivatives	
Tyr	2.15×10^{-4}	Hypoxanthine	1.50×10^{-5}
Val	4.50×10^{-4}	Thymidine	1.50×10^{-6}
Nonessential amino acids		Lipids and derivatives	
		Choline	6.45×10^{-5}
Ala	5.00×10^{-5}	*i*-Inositol	6.95×10^{-5}
Asn	5.00×10^{-5}	Linoleate	1.50×10^{-7}
Asp	5.00×10^{-5}	Bulk organic ions	
Glu	5.00×10^{-5}	Calcium	1.05×10^{-3}
Gly	2.50×10^{-4}	Magnesium	7.05×10^{-4}
Pro	1.50×10^{-4}	Potassium	4.20×10^{-3}
Ser	2.50×10^{-4}	Sodium	1.55×10^{-1}
Amino acid derivatives		Chloride	1.30×10^{-1}
Putrescine	5.00×10^{-7}	Nitrate	3.75×10^{-7}
Carbohydrates and derivatives		Phosphate	9.55×10^{-4}
		Sulfate	4.08×10^{-4}
Glucose	7.80×10^{-3}	Inorganic trace elements	
Pyruvate	1.00×10^{-3}	Cobalt	5.00×10^{-7}
Buffers and indicators		Copper	5.00×10^{-9}
Bicarbonate	2.90×10^{-2}	Iron	1.60×10^{-6}
CO_2 (gas phase, %)	5%	Zinc	1.50×10^{-6}
Phenol red	2.27×10^{-5}		

The dry DMEM:F12 powder is labile and should be refrigerated. The powder is normally an off-white powder, produces a clear solution when dissolved, has a pH in solution of 5.8 (without $NaHCO_3$) or 6.8 (with $NaHCO_3$), and has an osmolality of 279 mOsm/kg water (without $NaHCO_3$) or 299 mOsm/kg water (with $NaHCO_3$). Deterioration of the dry medium can be detected by the following: (1) color change, (2) granulation or clumping, (3) insolubility, (4) pH change, or (5) inability to promote cell growth when properly supplemented. If any of these occur, a new batch of dry media should be used.

11.4.2.1 General media preparation instructions

Media are prepared as follows:

1. Add 800 ml of doubly processed distilled water to a sterilized 1000-ml flask. The DMEM:F12 powder is added slowly with gentle stirring. In addition to this basal medium, a series of supplements is added to media for both cell populations (Table 7).
2. After dissolving the $NaHCO_3$, the pH of the media is adjusted to 7.2 with 1 *M* NaOH or 1 *M* HCl, as appropriate. Note that the desired pH is 7.4, but the pH is adjusted to a slightly lower value since pH generally rises slightly during filtration.
3. Volume of media is brought to 1 l with doubly processed distilled water.
4. Media are filtered through 0.22-µm pore size cellulose acetate filters for sterilization, and is dispensed into ten sterilized 100-ml bottles.
5. For each cell culture seeding, two sterilized 100-ml bottles of media are used. To each bottle, 48.69 ml of sterile media is added and the growth factor and hormonal supplements are added as shown in Table 8. One bottle is used for PT cells and one for DT cells.

Table 7 Complete Composition of Media for Primary Culture of Proximal Tubular (PT) and Distal Tubular (DT) Cells from the Rat Renal Cortex and OSOM

Basal medium: DMEM:F12 (1:1)
Standard supplementation
HEPES (15 m*M*, pH 7.4)
$NaHCO_3$ (20 m*M*)
Antibiotics (Day 0–3 only): penicillin (192 IU/ml) + streptomycin sulfate (200 µg/ml)
Amphotericin B (2.5 µg/ml)
Insulin (5 µg/ml) from bovine pancreas
Human transferrin (5 µg/ml)
Sodium selenite (30 n*M*)
Hydrocortisone (100 ng/ml)
Epidermal growth factor (100 ng/ml) from mouse submaxillary gland
Additional supplements
3,3′,5-Triiodo-DL-thyronine, T_3 (7.5 pg/ml): added to PT cells only
Thyrocalcitonin, CAL (5 ng/ml): added to DT cells only

Antibiotics are added to inhibit bacterial growth, but only through day 3; beyond this point of time in culture, PT cell growth is inhibited by penicillin. Amphotericin B is included to inhibit fungal growth. Although amphotericin B is a DT cell toxicant, the concentration used here is approximately three orders of magnitude below that which causes nephrotoxicity. A series of hormones was tested for their ability to promote growth and differentiated function; those tested included 3,3′,5-triiodo-DL-thyronine (T_3), prostaglandin E_1, prostaglandin $F_{2\alpha}$, isoproterenol, parathyroid hormone, thyrocalcitonin (CAL), and arginine vasopressin. Based on recoveries of cellular protein, DNA, and marker enzyme activities (described below) and known patterns of hormone responsiveness in different nephron cell populations, T_3 and CAL were chosen as the optimal supplements for PT and DT cells, respectively.

11.4.2.2 Preparation of media supplement stock solutions

1. *Insulin.* 1 mg/ml stock (200×); final concentration = 5 µg/ml. To prepare 3.0 ml of insulin stock solution:
   a. Weigh out 3 mg insulin in a 35-mm culture dish.
   b. Add 0.75 ml of 4 m*M* HCl (30 µl of concentration HCl in 100 ml distilled water; store at 0 to 4°C); bring to room temperature.

Table 8 Supplements Added to DMEM:F12 (1:1) Basal Medium for Primary Cell Culture of Proximal Tubular (PT) and Distal Tubular (DT) Cells from the Rat Renal Cortex and OSOM

Supplement	Final concentration	Stock concentration	Amount added per 100-ml medium (fold dilution)
Insulin (Sigma No. I 1882)	5 μg/ml	1 mg/ml	500 μl (200×)
Hydrocortisone (Sigma No. H 0888)	100 ng/ml	1 mg/ml	10 μl (10,000×)
Epidermal growth factor (EGF; Sigma No. E 4127)	100 ng/ml	0.1 mg/ml	100 μl (1,000×)
Human transferrin (Sigma No. T 1147)	5 μg/ml	1 mg/ml	500 μl (200×)
Sodium selenite (Sigma No. S 9133)	30 n*M*	0.3 m*M*	10 μl (10,000×)
Penicillin (Sigma No. P 3032) +	192 IU/ml	19,200 IU/ml	
Streptomycin (Sigma No. S 9137) +	200 μg/ml	20 mg/ml	1000 μl (100×)
Amphotericin B, solubilized; (Sigma No. A 9528)	2.5 μg/ml	0.25 mg/ml	
Triiodothyronine (T_3) (Sigma No. T 5516)	7.5 pg/ml	1.5 ng/ml	500 μl (200×) PT cells only
Thyrocalcitonin (CAL) (Sigma No. T 0522)	5 ng/ml	1 μg/ml	500 μl (200×) DT cells only

Note: Total volume added = 2.62 ml.

   c. Dilute with 2.25 ml of distilled water.
   d. Filter into snap cap tube (Falcon) using a 0.22-μm pore size cellulose acetate syringe filter.
   e. Store in freezer in 0.6-ml aliquots in microcentrifuge tubes.

2. *Hydrocortisone.* 1 mg/ml stock (10,000×); final concentration = 100 ng/ml. To prepare 2.0 ml of hydrocortisone stock solution:
   a. Weigh 2 mg of hydrocortisone in a 35-mm culture dish.
   b. Add 0.25 ml of ethanol and dissolve completely.
   c. Dilute with 1.75 ml of distilled water, making sure that no precipitation occurs.
   d. Filter into 35-mm culture dish using a 0.22-μm pore size cellulose acetate syringe filter.
   e. Store in freezer in 100-μl aliquots in microcentrifuge tubes.
3. *Epidermal growth factor (EGF).* 100 μg/ml stock (1000×); final concentration = 100 ng/ml. To prepare 1.0 ml of EGF stock solution:
   a. Material comes as 100 μg lyophilized EGF in a vial; add 1 ml distilled water to vial.
   b. Place 125-μl aliquots into sterile microcentrifuge tubes and store in freezer.
4. *Transferrin.* 1 mg/ml (200×); final concentration = 5 μg/ml. To prepare 3.0 ml of transferrin stock solution:
   a. Weigh out 3 mg transferrin in a 35-mm culture dish.
   b. Dissolve in 3.0 ml of distilled water.
   c. Filter in snap cap tube (Falcon) using a 0.22-μm pore size cellulose acetate syringe filter.
   d. Store in freezer in 0.6-ml aliquots in microcentrifuge tubes.
5. *Sodium selenite.* 0.3 m*M* (10,000×); final concentration = 30 n*M*. To prepare 2.0 ml of sodium selenite stock solution:
   a. Dissolve 1.0 mg sodium selenite in 5 ml of sterile basal medium (DMEM:F12, 1:1).
   b. Filter through a 0.22-μm pore size cellulose acetate syringe filter.
   c. Store in freezer in 100-μl aliquots in microcentrifuge tubes.

6. *Penicillin G–streptomycin–amphotericin B (100×).* Penicillin G (19,200 IU/ml stock; final concentration = 192 IU/ml); streptomycin (20 mg/ml stock; final concentration = 200 µg/ml); amphotericin B (0.25 mg/ml stock; final concentration = 2.5 µg/ml). To prepare 10 ml of antibiotic stock solution:
   a. Dissolve 115 mg of penicillin G, 200 mg of streptomycin, and 2.5 mg of amphotericin B in 10 ml of distilled water.
   b. Filter through a 0.22-µm pore size cellulose acetate syringe filter.
   c. Store in freezer in 1.1-ml aliquots in microcentrifuge tubes.
7. *Triiodothyronine (T_3).* Stock A = 20 µg/ml; stock B = 150 ng/ml; final stock = 1.5 ng/ml; final concentration in media = 7.5 pg/ml. To prepare stock solutions:
   a. Prepare a 20-µg/ml stock solution (stock A) by adding 1.0 ml of 1 *M* NaOH to container and gently swirl to dissolve contents; add 49 ml of sterile basal medium (DMEM:F12, 1:1).
   b. Filter stock A and store in freezer in 50-ml sterile centrifuge tubes after removing an aliquot for stock B.
   c. Prepare stock B by taking 10-µl stock A + 1.3233 ml of sterile basal medium (DMEM:F12, 1:1).
   d. Prepare final stock by mixing 50-µl stock B + 4.95 ml of sterile basal medium.
   e. Filter using a 0.22-µm pore size cellulose acetate syringe filter.
   f. Store in freezer in 0.6-ml aliquots in microcentrifuge tubes.
8. *Thyrocalcitonin (CAL).* Stock A = 50 µg/ml; final stock = 1 µg/ml; final concentration = 5 ng/ml. To prepare stock solutions:
   a. Prepare a 50-µg/ml stock (stock A) by dissolving contents of container in 20 ml of sterile basal medium (DMEM:F12, 1:1).
   b. Filter stock A with a 0.22-µm pore size cellulose acetate syringe filter and store in freezer in 50-ml sterile centrifuge tubes after taking aliquot for final stock.
   c. Prepare final stock by taking 0.2-ml stock A and adding 9.8 ml of sterile basal medium.
   d. Filter using a 0.22-µm pore size syringe filter.
   e. Store in freezer in 0.6-ml aliquots in microcentrifuge tubes.

11.4.3 General cell culture procedures

Epithelial cells from the renal cortex and OSOM are isolated from rats and the PT and DT cells enriched (essentially as described above) with the modification that precautions are taken to preserve sterility. Specifically, after animals are anesthetized, their torsos are shaved to prevent their fur from contaminating the cell preparation. Rat fur is a good source of bacteria and fungi, and it is imperative that no contamination occurs. All procedures are conducted while one is wearing latex gloves. After the animal is shaved, the torso is cleaned with 70% (v/v) ethanol to sterilize. All glassware and surgical tools used in the cell isolation and separation of cell populations are sterilized in an autoclave. Prior to the seeding of cells on dishes, the glassware and plasticware used in the culture process are exposed to ultraviolet light in the laminar flow hood for at least 30 min.

Suspensions of renal PT and DT cells are seeded onto 35-mm plastic tissue culture dishes at densities of 50 to 100 µg protein per square centimeter (= 1 to 2 × 10^5 cells per square centimeter or 0.5 to 1 × 10^6 cells per milliliter) in 1.5 ml of the appropriately supplemented media. Cultures are grown at 37°C in a humidified incubator under an atmosphere of 95% air/5% CO_2. This is defined as day 0 of cell culture. Cell attachment to dishes is monitored by means of an inverted microscope (e.g., Zeiss I.D. 02) under light or phase-contrast microscopy. After 24 h (= day 1), plates are washed with phosphate-buffered saline (PBS) to remove unattached cells (generally 50 to 60% of total seed population) and fresh medium is added to each dish. The medium is changed every 2 days thereafter, unless otherwise specified by the experimental protocol. After day 3, antibiotics are omitted from the medium because they inhibit cell growth. When necessary, cells can be harvested by either scraping the plates with a Teflon scraper or by incubating briefly (i.e., 15 min) with 0.05% (w/v) trypsin–0.02% (w/v) EDTA in a Ca^{2+}- and Mg^{2+}-free Hank's buffer. We have found that a more complete and consistent recovery of cells from dishes occurs with the scraping method, so we have adopted that one as our general harvesting procedure.[34]

11.4.4 *Assessment of growth and differentiated function*

11.4.4.1 *Microscopy*

Under a phase-contrast microscope (Figure 2), PT cells in primary culture exhibited epithelial morphology, and new cell growth was observed at the edges of colonies. No fibroblasts were detected at either day 3 or during the 9 days of culture, indicating that only epithelial cell growth is promoted. Similar photomicrographs of PT and DT cells grown for 3 days in optimized supplemented media, which contain the basal supplements and either T_3 (for PT cells) or CAL (for DT cells), demonstrate retention of epithelial morphology and new cell growth (cf. Figure 3). Since single cells in suspension rather than tubular fragments or tissue explants are used as seed material, cells attach to culture dishes and grow as colonies and generally do not form complete monolayers. By 5 days of primary culture, approximately 50 to 75% of the growth surface is covered with cells.

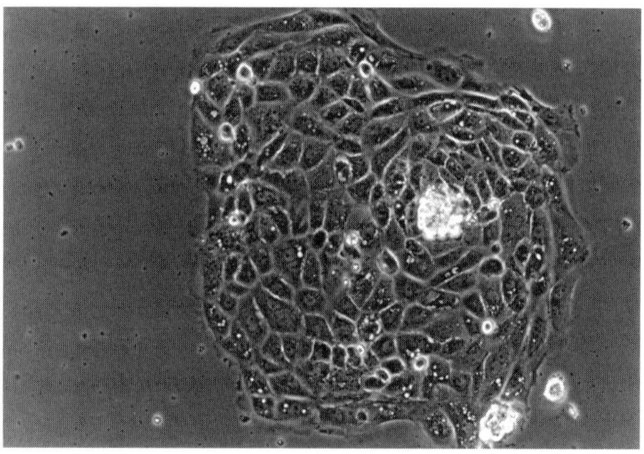

Figure 2 Phase-contrast photomicrograph of primary cultures of renal proximal tubular (PT) cells from rat kidney. Isolated PT cells from rat kidney (1.5 ml, 0.5 to 1.0 × 10^6 cells/ml) were seeded onto glass coverslips placed in 35-mm polystyrene dishes in basal supplemented media. Photomicrographs were taken of cells grown for 3 days. A Nikon diaphot camera with Kodak PX-125 black-and-white film (ASA = 125) was attached to a Nikon phase-contrast-2, ELWD 0.3 microscope. Final magnification = 98×. Cells retained epithelial morphology, growing as closely packed polygonal cells in monolayers. Outgrowth of the cells at the edges of colonies was observed, demonstrating new cell growth during culture. No fibroblasts were detected.

An additional means to demonstrate that primary cultures of renal PT cells retained epithelial markers and morphology is to stain for cytokeratins, which are cytoskeletal proteins that are characteristically expressed in these cells (Figure 4). Cytokeratins can be monitored by indirect immunofluorescent staining by the method described by Chopra et al.[35] The procedure is as follows:

1. Cells are cultured on glass coverslips coated with type I collagen and are placed in 35-mm polystyrene tissue culture dishes.

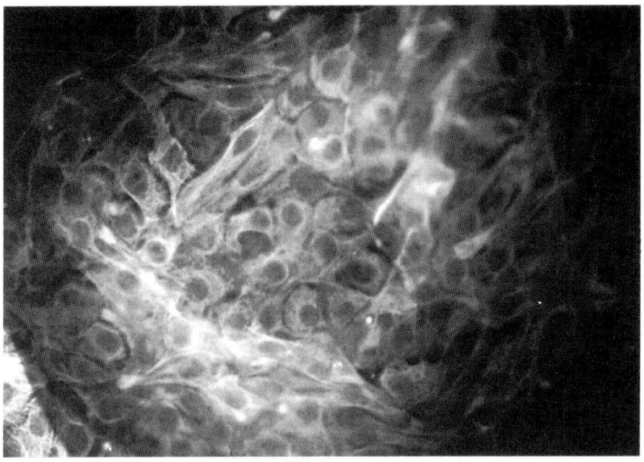

Figure 3 Indirect immunofluorescence staining of primary cultures of renal proximal tubular (PT) cells from rat kidney. Isolated PT cells from rat kidney (1.5 ml, 0.5 to 1.0 × 10^6 cells/ml) were cultured for 3 days on glass coverslips coated with type I collagen and placed in 35-mm polystyrene dishes in basal supplemented media. Cells were stained for cytokeratins by indirect immunofluorescence. Photomicrographs were taken with a Nikon FX-35WA camera using Kodak PX-125 black-and-white film (ASA = 125). Control cultures lacking the anti-α-keratin were negative for staining. Final magnification = 196×. (From Lash, L. H., Tokarz, J. J., and Pegouske, D. M., *Toxicology*, in press, 1995. With permission.)

2. Fix cells with 3.7% (v/v) formalin in PBS, wash several times with PBS, place in cold methanol, and dry.
3. Incubate dishes with α-keratin antiserum from guinea pig for 30 min.
4. Wash dishes with PBS and incubate with fluorescein isothiocyanate (FITC)-conjugated rabbit anti-guinea pig immunoglobulin G for 30 min.
5. Wash dishes with PBS, mount coverslips on slides, and view on a Nikon UFX-IIA fluorescence microscope.
6. Control samples lacking the anti-α-keratin are also prepared and should be negative for staining.

11.4.4.2 Protein, DNA, and enzyme assays

For all protein, DNA, and enzyme assays, media are removed from tissue culture dishes and cells are washed three times with PBS and then harvested with a Teflon tissue culture scraper into PBS containing 0.1% (v/v) Triton X-100.

Protein content of dishes is measured spectrophotometrically by the method of Lowry et al.[36] with bovine serum albumin as standard. A profile of protein concentration in PT and DT cell primary cultures over 5 days (Figure 5A) shows that both cell populations exhibit time-dependent increases in protein, particularly from day 3 to day 5.

DNA content of dishes is measured as the relative fluorescence of the DNA-diamidinophenylindole (DNA-DAPI) complex with 360-nm excitation and 450-nm emission according to Sorger and Germinario[37] using double-stranded calf thymus DNA as a standard. The DNA assay is performed as follows:

1. Solutions
   a. *DAPI stock.* 1 mg/ml in distilled water. Since DAPI is light-sensitive, tube is wrapped in aluminum foil and is stored at 0 to 4°C.
   b. *Assay buffer.* 18 m*M* Na_2SO_4, 50 m*M* HEPES, pH 7.0
   c. *DAPI working solution.* Add 1 ml of DAPI stock to 400 ml of assay buffer to give a final concentration of 2.5 μg/ml. This is wrapped in aluminum foil and is stored at 0 to 4°C for up to one month.

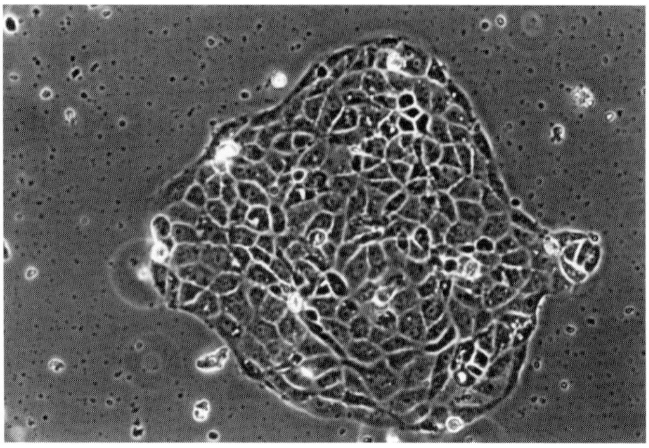

A

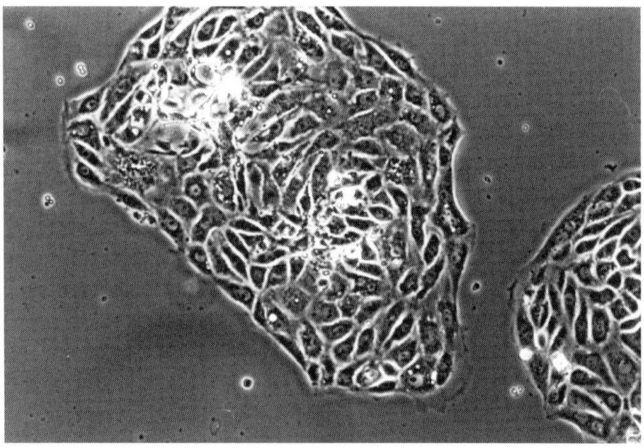

B

Figure 4 Phase-contrast photomicrographs of day 3 primary cultures of renal proximal tubular (PT) and distal tubular (DT) cells from rat. Isolated PT (A) and DT (B) cells from rat kidney (1.5 ml, 0.5 to 1.0 × 10^6 cells/ml) were seeded onto glass coverslips treated with type I collagen and placed in 35-mm polystyrene dishes in basal-supplemented media with either T_3 or CAL added to PT or DT cells, respectively. Final magnification = 98X. (From Lash, L. H., Tokarz, J. J., and Pegouske, D. M., *Toxicology*, in press, 1995. With permission.)

d. *DNA stock solution.* Prepare 1.0 to 1.2 mg double-stranded calf thymus DNA/ml in assay buffer containing 0.1 m*M* EDTA. Dilute 1:20 with assay buffer containing EDTA and determine absorbance at 260 nm. Solution is calibrated assuming that a 50 µg DNA/ml solution has an absorbance of 1.0 at 260 nm. The stock solution is stable for several months stored at 0 to 4°C.
e. *DNA working solution.* Prepare a 1:200 dilution of DNA stock solution with 0.2% (v/v) Triton X-100 in distilled water.
f. *DAPI reagent.* Prepare fresh daily by adding 0.4 volumes of DAPI working solution to 3.6 volumes of assay buffer and 6.0 volumes of distilled water.

2. Assay Method
   a. Solubilize cells (1 to 3 × 10^5 cells) by treatment for 15 min with 2.0 ml of 0.2% (v/v) Triton X-100 containing 10 µl/ml of 1 *M* NaOH.
   b. To a 0.2-ml aliquot of solubilized cells add 2.5 ml of DAPI reagent and mix.

c. After 90 min at room temperature, measure relative fluorescence with 360-nm excitation and 450-nm emission.
d. For DNA standards, use an appropriate volume of DNA working solution (5.0 μg/ml) to give a final DNA concentration in 0.2-ml sample of 0.25 to 2.5 μg/ml (10 to 100 μl). Add distilled water to give a total standard volume of 100 μl and add an additional 100 μl of 0.2 mg bovine serum albumin–10 μl of 1 *M* NaOH/ml–0.2% (v/v) Triton X-100. Standards are then processed as for samples.

To check that fluorescence is due solely to the presence of DNA, $MgSO_4$ is added to the DAPI reagent to a final concentration of 2.5 m*M* and DNase is added to the assay mixture to a final concentration of 50 μg/ml. The fluorescence of either standards or samples should be abolished by the inclusion of DNase. Measurement of DNA concentration in primary cultures of PT and DT cells (Figure 5B) shows that most of the net cell growth occurs between day 1 and day 3. After day 3, DNA content decreases in cultures of both cell populations. This does not necessarily mean that new cell growth is not occurring. Rather, visualization of cell culture dishes under the inverted microscope at the time that media are changed shows that a fraction of cells on dishes are dying and being sloughed off into the extracellular fluid. Hence, new cells are being produced to offset some of the cell turnover.

A variety of enzyme assays can be performed to quantitatively assess retention of differentiated function. Glutamate dehydrogenase (GDH; Figure 5C) and lactate dehydrogenase (LDH; Figure 5D) are measurements of mitochondrial and glycolytic activities, respectively. When renal PT cells are placed in culture, one of the common phenotypic changes that rapidly occurs is a loss of mitochondrial function and a large increase in glycolytic activity. Although there is a modest increase in LDH activity after day 3 (approximately twofold), this is much less than what is commonly observed (often >tenfold). Mitochondrial activity was maintained during at least 5 days of primary culture. Another common phenotypic change that occurs in primary culture of renal PT cells is a large drop (often >90%) in activities of brush border membrane enzymes during the first few days of culture. Both GGT (Figure 5E) and AP (Figure 5F) activities in primary cultures of renal PT cells either decreased by less than 30% from initial levels by day 5 or remained at initial levels, indicating that differentiated function was maintained during culture.

11.4.5 Use of primary cultures of renal cells for toxicological studies

11.4.5.1 General comments

The ability of PT and DT cells from rat renal cortex to grow for up to 9 days in primary culture enables assessment of numerous cytotoxic responses that are not possible with the freshly isolated PT and DT cells (Table 9). In addition to responses associated with acute cellular injury, responses that require several hours to several days to be expressed can be studied in primary cell culture. A key factor in this ability is that the primary cultures maintain differentiated function during the time course of culture.

11.4.5.2 Acute cytotoxicity assay

Cells are cultured as described above for 3 days. On day 3, media are changed and cells are incubated for up to 8 h with a chemical of interest by adding the chemical to fresh media. LDH release from cells is measured by determining LDH activity in the media and, after removal of media, washing cells with PBS, and solubilization of cells with 0.1% (v/v) Triton X-100, in total cells. The fraction of LDH release is defined by Equation 3:

$$\text{\% LDH Release} = \text{LDH activity in media}/(\text{LDH activity in media} + \text{LDH activity in total cells}) \times 100\% \quad (3)$$

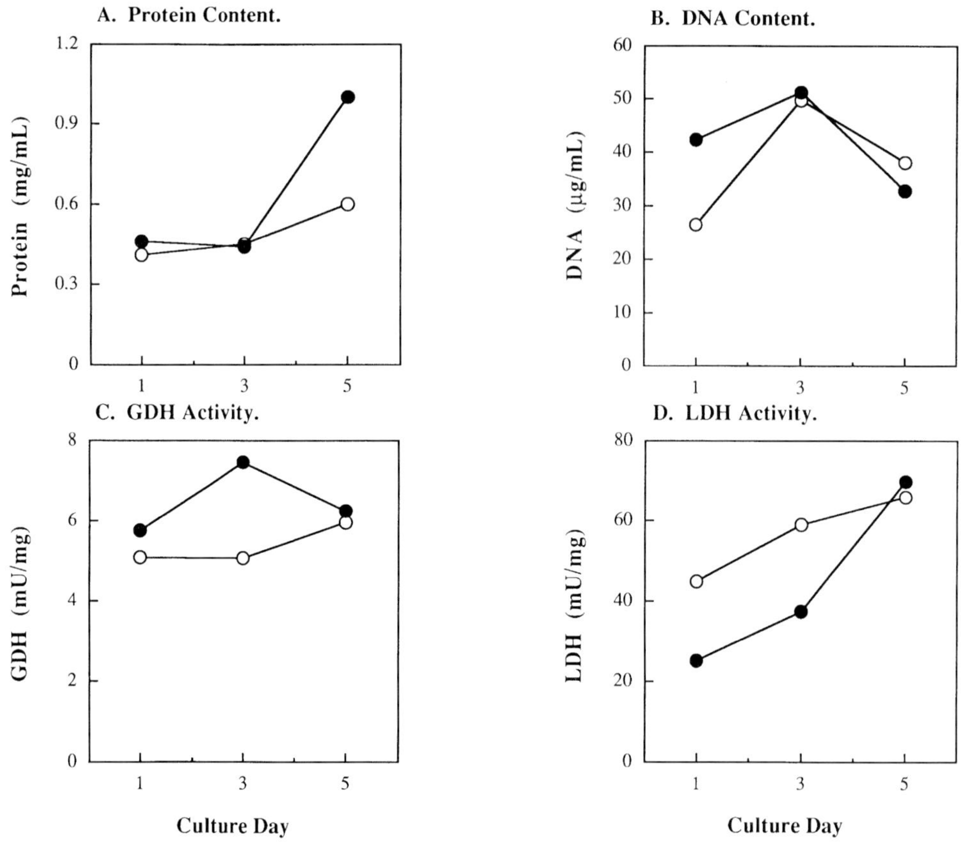

Figure 5 Time course of cellular protein and DNA contents and cellular activities of marker enzymes in primary cultures of renal proximal tubular (PT) and distal tubular (DT) cells. Isolated PT (filled circles) and DT (open circles) cells from rat kidney (1.5 ml; 0.5 to 1.0×10^6 cells/ml) were seeded onto 35-mm polystyrene tissue culture dishes. Cells were grown under conditions previously determined to be optimal (i.e., basal supplemented medium + T_3 [PT cells] or + CAL [DT cells]). Media were changed after 24 h (= day 1) and every second day thereafter. Parameters were measured in Triton X-100-solubilized samples, and results are means of measurements from three to five primary cultures, each assay being done in duplicate. Protein content was measured spectrophotometrically by the Lowry procedure. DNA content was measured fluorometrically using diamidinophenylindole. Glutamate dehydrogenase (GDH) and lactate dehydrogenase (LDH) activities were measured as NADH oxidation in the presence of 2-oxoglutarate or pyruvate, respectively, by following the decrease in absorbance at 340 nm. γ-Glutamyltransferase (GGT) activity was measured as formation of *p*-nitroanilide with γ-glutamyl-*p*-nitroanilide and glycylglycine as substrates by following the increase in absorbance at 410 nm. Alkaline phosphatase (AP) activity was measured as formation of *p*-nitrophenol with *p*-nitrophenyl phosphate as substrate by following the increase in absorbance at 410 nm.

Primary cultures of renal PT and DT cells incubated for up to 8 h with media alone (= control) exhibit less than 15% LDH release. Incubation of these cells with either *tert*-butyl hydroperoxide or methyl vinyl ketone — agents that alter intracellular thiol/disulfide status by oxidation or alkylation, respectively, for up to 8 h produces a time- and concentration-dependent increase in LDH release that is similar to the patterns observed previously in suspensions of freshly isolated PT and DT cells.[34] These data indicate that the cell type-specific patterns of chemical injury, such as the marked susceptibility of DT cells and the relative resistance of PT cells to oxidants,[5,20] are also observed in primary cultures of PT and DT cells. Hence, we can conclude that the primary cultures faithfully

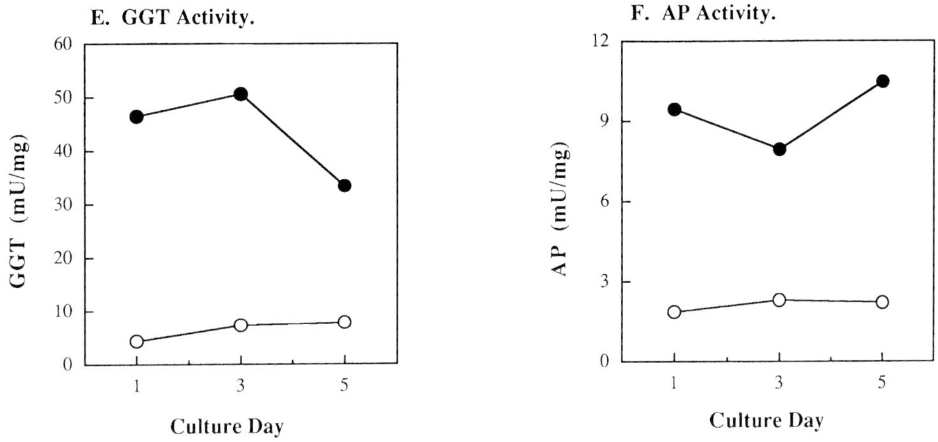

Figure 5 (continued)

Table 9 Experimental Protocols Performed with Primary Cultures for Toxicological Investigations

Parameter	Acute model	Chronic model
Dose	Low to high	Single or multiple, low
Exposure time	≤ 24 h	1 to as many as 10 days
Examples of processes measured	Intermediary metabolism	Gene expression
	Enzyme activities	Protein, DNA, RNA synthesis
	Respiration	Mutagenesis
	Active transport	DNA repair
	Metabolite concentrations	Processes measured in acute model (e.g., ATP, GSH)
	LDH release or trypan blue uptake	

reflect the toxicological susceptibilities that occur in freshly isolated cells and, presumably, in the whole animal.

11.5 Concluding remarks

This chapter describes methodology for the preparation of epithelial cells from rat renal cortex and OSOM by collagenase perfusion, the fractionation of these cells into two distinct populations (PT and DT cells) by Percoll density gradient centrifugation, and the use of these enriched cell populations as seed material for primary cell culture. Although epithelial cells from the rat kidney have been used in several investigations and can serve as a model of PT cellular function, since PT cells comprise >80% of the epithelial cells in the renal cortex and OSOM, nephron heterogeneity requires methods for analysis of cell type-specific processes. The advantage of the Percoll density gradient centrifugation method is that it is relatively simple, does not require any specialized equipment, is relatively fast, and provides a good yield of viable cells. Since cell population density is not a discrete property, but exhibits a range of values, enrichment rather than absolute purification is obtained.

Primary cell culture, while presenting many technological challenges, has several advantages over other *in vitro* models that are used for the study of chronic toxicity. For example, if proper culture conditions are used, cellular biochemistry and physiology of primary cultures of renal epithelial cells are generally better defined than those of cell lines. Recent advances in the development of immortalized cell lines have been achieved and are described by Taub in Chapter 12 of this volume. A distinct advantage of our methodological approach is that the use of PT and DT cell suspensions obtained by the Percoll method as seed material for primary culture is a logical continuation of our previous work on cell type-specific susceptibility to chemical and pathological injury. Simultaneous culturing of both PT and DT cells also provides for consistency in approach and allows for a more controlled and valid comparison of responses in different renal cell populations. This is important to improve understanding of mechanisms of both acute and chronic cytotoxic responses to nephrotoxicants and the relation between these types of responses.

11.6 Acknowledgments

Research from the author's laboratory was supported by a grant from the National Institute of Diabetes and Digestive and Kidney Diseases (Grant R01-DK40725). L.H.L. is a recipient of a Research Career Development Award from the National Institute of Diabetes and Digestive and Kidney Diseases (Grant K04-DK02090).

References

1. Jacobson, H. R., Functional segmentation of the mammalian nephron, *Am. J. Physiol.*, 241, F203, 1981.
2. Walker, L. A. and Valtin, H., Biological importance of nephron heterogeneity, *Annu. Rev. Physiol.*, 44, 203, 1982.
3. Guder, W. G. and Ross, B. D., Enzyme distribution along the nephron, *Kidney Int.*, 26, 101, 1984.
4. Ross, B. D. and Guder, W. G., Heterogeneity and compartmentation in the kidney, in *Metabolic Compartmentation*, Sies, H., Ed., Academic Press, London, 1982, 363.
5. Lash, L. H., Susceptibility to toxic injury in different nephron cell populations, *Toxicol. Lett.*, 53, 97, 1990.
6. Jones, D. P., Sundby, G.-B., Ormstad, K., and Orrenius, S., Use of isolated kidney cells for study of drug metabolism, *Biochem. Pharmacol.*, 28, 929, 1979.
7. Ormstad, K., Orrenius, S., and Jones, D. P., Preparation and characteristics of isolated kidney cells, *Methods Enzymol.*, 77, 137, 1981.
8. Lash, L. H., Isolated kidney cells in the study of chemical toxicity, in *In Vitro Toxicology: Model Systems and Methods*, McQueen, C. A., Ed., Telford Press, Caldwell, NJ, 1989, 231.
9. Ruegg, C. E. and Mandel, L. J., Bulk isolation of renal PCT and PST II. Differential responses to anoxia or hypoxia, *Am. J. Physiol.*, 259, F176, 1990.
10. Lash, L. H. and Tokarz, J. J., Isolation of two distinct populations of cells from rat kidney cortex and their use in the study of chemical-induced toxicity, *Anal. Biochem.*, 182, 271, 1989.
11. Lash, L. H., Nephrotoxicity studies with freshly isolated cells from rat kidney, in *In Vitro Methods in Toxicology and Pharmacology*, Watson, R. R., Ed., CRC Press, Boca Raton, FL, 1992, 115.
12. Lash, L. H., Purification of renal cell populations by Percoll density-gradient centrifugation, in *In Vitro Biological Systems: Preparation and Maintenance, Methods in Toxicology*, Vol. 1A, Tyson, C. A. and Frazier, J. M., Eds., Academic Press, San Diego, 1993, 397.
13. Aw, T. Y., Wilson, E., Hagen, T. M., and Jones, D. P., Determinants of mitochondrial O_2 dependence in kidney, *Am. J. Physiol.*, 253, F440, 1987.
14. Pertoft, H. and Laurent, T. C., Sedimentation of cells in colloidal silica (Percoll), in *Cell Separation: Methods and Selected Applications*, Vol. 1, Pretlow, T. G., II and Pretlow, T. P., Eds., Academic Press, New York, 1982, 115.
15. Scholer, D. W. and Edelman, I. S., Isolation of rat kidney cortical tubules enriched in proximal and distal segments, *Am. J. Physiol.*, 237, F350, 1979.

16. Cojocel, C., Maita, K., Pasino, D. A., Kuo, C.-H., and Hook, J. B., Metabolic heterogeneity of the proximal and distal kidney tubules, *Life Sci.*, 33, 855, 1983.
17. Gesek, F. A., Wolff, D. W., and Strandhoy, J. W., Improved separation method for rat proximal and distal renal tubules, *Am. J. Physiol.*, 253, F358, 1987.
18. Vinay, P., Gougoux, A., and Lemieux, G., Isolation of a pure suspension of rat proximal tubules, *Am. J. Physiol.*, 241, F403, 1981.
19. Kreisberg, J. I., Pitts, A. M., and Pretlow, T. G., II, Separation of proximal tubular cells from suspensions of rat kidney cells in density gradients of Ficoll in tissue culture medium, *Am. J. Pathol.*, 86, 591, 1977.
20. Lash, L. H. and Tokarz, J. J., Oxidative stress in isolated rat renal proximal and distal tubular cells, *Am. J. Physiol.*, 259, F338, 1990.
21. Lash, L. H. and Woods, E. B., Cytotoxicity of alkylating agents in isolated rat kidney proximal tubular and distal tubular cells, *Arch. Biochem. Biophys.*, 286, 46, 1991.
22. Handler, J. S., Studies of kidney cells in culture, *Kidney Int.*, 30, 208, 1986.
23. Wilson, P. D., Use of cultured renal tubular cells in the study of cell injury, *Miner. Electrolyte Metab.*, 12, 71, 1986.
24. Aleo, M. D., Taub, M. L., Nickerson, P. A., and Kostyniak, P. J., Primary cultures of rabbit renal proximal tubule cells. I. Growth and biochemical characteristics, *In Vitro Cell. Dev. Biol.*, 25, 776, 1989.
25. Chung, S. D., Alavi, N., Livingston, D., Hiller, S., and Taub, M., Characterization of primary rabbit kidney cultures that express proximal tubule functions in a hormonally defined medium, *J. Cell Biol.*, 95, 118, 1982.
26. Taub, M. L., Yang, I. S., and Wang, Y., Primary rabbit kidney proximal tubule cell cultures maintain differentiated functions when cultured in a hormonally defined serum-free medium, *In Vitro Cell. Dev. Biol.*, 25, 770, 1989.
27. Miller, J. H., Restricted growth of rat kidney proximal tubule cells cultured in serum-supplemented and defined media, *J. Cell. Physiol.*, 129, 264, 1986.
28. Rosenberg, M. R. and Michaelopoulos, G., Kidney proximal tubular cells isolated by collagenase perfusion grow in defined media in the absence of growth factors, *J. Cell. Physiol.*, 131, 107, 1987.
29. Chen, T. C., Curthoys, N. P., Lagenaur, C. F., and Puschett, J. B., Characterization of primary cell cultures derived from rat renal proximal tubules, *In Vitro Cell. Dev. Biol.*, 25, 714, 1989.
30. Hatzinger, P. B. and Stevens, J. L., Rat kidney proximal tubule cells in defined medium: the roles of cholera toxin, extracellular calcium and serum in cell growth and expression of γ-glutamyltransferase, *In Vitro Cell. Dev. Biol.*, 25, 205, 1989.
31. Boogaard, P. J., Zoetweij, J. P., van Berkel, T. J. C., van't Noordende, J. M., Mulder, G. J., and Nagelkerke, J. F., Primary cultures of proximal tubular cells from normal rat kidney as an *in vitro* model to study mechanisms of nephrotoxicity: toxicity of nephrotoxicants at low concentrations during prolonged exposure, *Biochem. Pharmacol.*, 39, 1335, 1990.
32. Elliget, K. A. and Trump, B. F., Primary cultures of normal rat kidney proximal tubule epithelial cells for studies of renal cell injury, *In Vitro Cell. Dev. Biol.*, 27A, 739, 1991.
33. Wilson, P. D, Anderson, R. J., Breckon, R. D., Nathrath, W., and Schrier, R. W., Retention of differentiated characteristics by cultures of defined rabbit kidney epithelia, *J. Cell. Physiol.*,130, 245, 1987.
34. Lash, L. H., Tokarz, J. J., and Pegouske, D. M., Susceptibility of primary cultures of proximal tubular and distal tubular cells from rat kidney to chemically induced toxicity, *Toxicology*, in press, 1995.
35. Chopra, D. P., Sullivan, J., Wille, J. J., and Siddiqui, K. M., Propagation of differentiating normal human tracheobronchial epithelial cells in serum-free medium, *J. Cell. Physiol.*, 130, 173, 1987.
36. Lowry, O. H., Rosebrough, N. J., Farr, A. L., and Randall, R. J., Protein measurement with the Folin phenol reagent, *J. Biol. Chem.*, 193, 265, 1951.
37. Sorger, T. and Germinario, R. J., A direct solubilization procedure for the determination of DNA and protein in cultured fibroblast monolayers, *Anal. Biochem.*, 131, 254, 1983.

chapter twelve

Immortalized Cell Lines of Renal Cells

Mary L. Taub

12.1 Introduction....217
12.2 Development of immortalized renal proximal tubular cell lines....220
12.2.1 Preparation of primary cultures....220
12.2.2 Transfection of primary cultures with plasmid DNA....221
12.2.3 Selection of immortalized transformants....222
12.2.4 Serial passaging....223
12.2.5 Characterization of immortalized cells....223
12.2.6 Possible problems and optimization of the procedure....224
12.2.6.1 Possible reasons for a lack of immortalized cells....224
12.2.6.2 Optimization of transfection....225
12.2.6.3 Optimization of culture conditions....226
12.3 Discussion....227
12.3.1 Characteristics of existing established renal epithelial cell lines....227
12.3.2 Strategies for the development of immortalized cell lines....229
12.3.2.1 Viral transformation....229
12.3.2.1.1 Temperature-sensitive viruses....229
12.3.2.1.2 The use of human papilloma virus for cell immortalization....230
12.3.2.1.3 The use of retroviruses for cell immortalization....230
12.3.3 Cell immortalization using plasmids with oncogenes....231
12.3.3.1 Immortalizing functions of adeno E1A oncogene....231
12.3.3.2 Immortalization using plasmids with the SV40 early region genes....231
References....232

12.1 *Introduction*

Methods have been established recently to develop "immortalized" animal cell lines from primary cultures. The development of immortalized cell lines generally involves the transfection of short-term cultures with plasmid or viral DNA containing an immortalizing gene (e.g., an oncogene). As a consequence, stable transformants may emerge that possess the capacity to divide indefinitely *in vitro* (unlike the parental primary, or short-term cultures). Prior to the use of such immortalizing genes, efforts to establish animal cell lines

0-8493-3341-5/96/$0.00+$.50

from primary cultures have been dependent, to a large extent, on chance. Some types of primary cultures can survive subculturing. The first-passage cultures may, in some cases, be passaged further. Most of these short-term cultures have a limited doubling potential and undergo what is called "a crisis of senescence" (i.e., the cells stop dividing *in vitro* and die, a process that is presumably distinct from apoptosis).[1] Whether the limited doubling potential of normal animal cells *in vitro* is an inherent property of the cells (due simply to programmed cell death), or whether the limited doubling potential of animal cells *in vitro* is due to imperfections in the tissue culture environment (e.g., a suboptimal nutrient medium) is not clearly understood. However, studies with serum-free, hormonally defined medium have clearly demonstrated that primary cultures of differentiated cells exhibit extended viability, without fibroblast overgrowth, as compared with cultures in serum-supplemented medium.[2,3]

During the initial development of serum-free medium, several reports were made concerning the establishment of differentiated parathyroid and testicular cell lines in hormonally defined culture conditions.[4,5] These results suggested that the serum in tissue culture medium was a factor that limited the life span of the normal animal cell *in vitro*. However, the generalized use of serum-free medium has not yet resulted in the development of large numbers of differentiated animal cell lines from primary tissue. Thus, the number of normal, differentiated animal cell lines is still limited.

In vitro studies with immortalized, or established, animal cell lines have particular advantages as compared with studies using intact tissue. When specifically considering the mammalian kidney, one must take into account that this large, complex organ is responsible for maintaining the overall homeostasis of the body's ionic and osmotic content. Homeostasis is maintained by the functioning of literally thousands of individual nephrons, each of which is composed of a renal corpuscle and tubules.[6] The blood is initially filtered by the glomerulus. The glomerular filtrate subsequently travels down the lumen of the nephron, where it is selectively reabsorbed by the numerous types of tubular epithelial cells present in the different segments of the nephron. The precise mechanisms by which these tubular epithelial cells reabsorb (and/or secrete) solutes is difficult to study, due to the heterogeneity found even within single segments of the nephron. However, single cell types present in immortalized (or established) kidney cell populations can be cloned, and large, homogenous populations of cloned cells can be grown for biochemical and genetic studies. Moreover, genetic variants and transformants can be obtained.

The use of renal tissue culture systems was first popularized for examining the mechanisms responsible for the establishment and the maintenance of cellular polarity. Renal tubular epithelial cells *in vivo* possess a polarized morphology, with an apical surface that faces the luminal space and a basolateral surface that faces the renal interstitium (i.e., the blood side) (Figure 1). Solutes are selectively transported into the tubular epithelial cells from the luminal space by means of specific transport systems localized on the apical membrane and are transported out of the cells (to the blood side) by means of transport systems localized on the basolateral membrane. In addition, a proportion of the solutes diffuse through the tight junctions that exist between cells. These properties of polarized cells have been retained by renal tubular epithelial cell lines *in vitro*, and extensive studies concerning the polarized orientation of these cells have been conducted.[7,8]

In addition to their use for polarity studies, *in vitro* renal cell culture systems have been important for studies concerning the mechanisms by which hormones and growth regulatory factors control the growth and the expression of differentiated transport systems.[9] Such *in vitro* studies are particularly advantageous, because cell culture systems can be maintained over a prolonged period in a steady state situation, unlike, for example, tissue slices. For this reason, *in vitro* studies concerning the mechanism of action of hormones, drugs, and nutrients with isolated tissue have been impeded. The use of serum-free, hormonally defined medium has largely alleviated these problems.

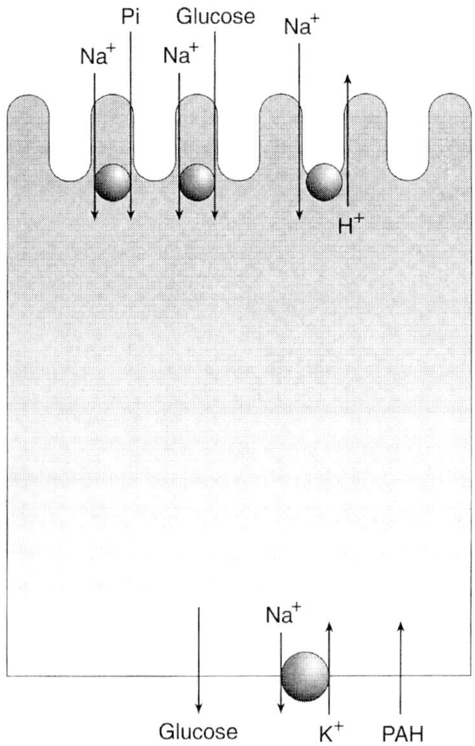

Figure 1 Polarized proximal tubular epithelial cells. Renal proximal tubular cells, like other epithelial cells, have a polarized morphology, with an apical surface that faces the luminal space and a basolateral surface that faces the blood side. Sodium is reabsorbed from the luminal side of the cells via a Na^+/H^+ antiport system, localized on the apical surface of the cells, and leaves cells via the (Na^+ + K^+)-stimulated ATPase, which is localized on the basolateral surface of the cell. Glucose and other sugars in the lumen of the nephron are reabsorbed with sodium, via a Na^+/glucose cotransport system. Subsequently, glucose leaves the cells via a facilitated diffusion system for glucose localized on the basolateral surface. Organic anions, including drugs that are present in the interstitial space enter the renal proximal tubular cells via the *p*-aminohippurate transport system and subsequently leave the cells via another mechanism.

A more recent use of renal cell cultures is for toxicological studies. A major need exists for toxicological studies with renal cells, because nephrotoxicity is a major concern in drug design and usage.[10] The mammalian kidney is exposed to much higher concentrations of many drugs and other chemicals due to its reabsorptive capacities. The kidney receives 25% of the cardiac output and filters much of this cardiac output into the nephrons. Thus, the cells lining the renal vasculature, and the tubular epithelial cells, particularly those in the initial segments of the nephron (the proximal tubule), are extensively exposed to substances that are potential toxicants.

For many years, the nephrotoxicity of drugs and chemicals has been evaluated primarily by means of whole animal studies. Such whole animal studies are costly and time consuming. In addition, whole animal studies are at best an indirect means of studying the mechanism of action of nephrotoxicants. Freshly isolated renal cells have been used as an alternative. Such studies have been impaired by the limited viability of freshly isolated cells and by the lack of a steady state condition.

The mechanisms by which nephrotoxicants act on renal cells to cause damage and/or cell death are still not clearly understood. A number of different routes of toxicity very likely occur, because several classes of nephrotoxicants clearly exist. In one class of drugs and chemicals are those that are directly toxic to renal proximal tubular cells *in vivo*, such as mercuric chloride.[11] In another class are those that must be appropriately metabolized by renal cells in order to exert their toxic effects.[10,12] Included among this latter group of nephrotoxicants are drugs such as acetaminophen.[10,12] The beta-lactam antibiotics, such as the cephalosporins, similarly require activation by mixed-function oxidases such as cytochrome P-450 in order to exert their toxic effects.[10,12,13] The role of cytochrome P-450 in activation of certain nephrotoxicants is a matter of controversy.

In order to study the mechanism of action of nephrotoxicants *in vitro*, appropriate cell culture systems must exist. The renal proximal tubule is a major target of a number of nephrotoxic agents, including cephaloridine and mercuric chloride. However, other types of toxic agents target other nephron segments. Thus, *in vitro* model systems of renal tubular epithelial cells that are representative of a number of different nephron segments, including the renal proximal tubule, are needed for *in vitro* toxicology studies.

Presently, a limited number of well-characterized, established renal cell lines are available for such *in vitro* nephrotoxicity studies. Included among the best-characterized established renal cell lines are the Madin Darby canine kidney (MDCK) cell line, which in many respects is representative of distal tubular cells, and the LLC-PK_1 cell line, which in some respects is representative of renal proximal tubular cells.[7,9] Additional *in vitro* model systems are therefore needed, particularly *in vitro* systems derived from animals in which extensive toxicology studies have been conducted.

One means of fulfilling this need for additional *in vitro* model systems is through the use of primary renal cell cultures. Primary renal cell cultures that retain differentiated functions typical of tubular epithelial cells have been developed using serum-free, hormonally defined medium.[14-16] Serum-free, hormonally defined medium has been particularly important in these regards, because such media can permit the growth of differentiated epithelial cells in the absence of fibroblast overgrowth.[14-16] The advantages of such primary culture systems are not only that one can develop differentiated cell culture systems typical of particular types of normal renal cells, but also that *in vitro* studies can be conducted using renal cells derived from animal models of interest. The limitation of such primary cultures is that clonal populations of renal cells are not being studied. Genetic variants and stable transformants cannot generally be isolated.

Additional established (or immortalized) cell lines are needed for these purposes. However, no systematic method has yet been devised for developing established cell lines from normal tissues without the use of transforming (or immortalizing agents). The development of immortalized cell lines, using plasmids with oncogenes, has been reasonably successful with a variety of tissues. In this chapter, a method for developing immortalized renal proximal tubular cell lines using the pRSVT plasmid, which possesses the SV40 early region genes, is described.

12.2 Development of immortalized renal proximal tubular cell lines

12.2.1 Preparation of primary cultures

Primary cultures of proximal tubular cells from rabbit kidney are prepared for cell culture by a modification of the method of Chung et al.[14] An adult male New Zealand White rabbit (5 to 6 lb) is killed by CO_2 inhalation followed by puncture of the diaphragm. The kidneys are removed with the renal artery and vein intact (the left kidney has the larger of the two arteries) and are placed in a sterile, 50-ml conical tube with medium on ice. In the tissue culture hood, a kidney is removed, placed within a sterile, 100-mm petri dish, and washed several times with serum-free medium. A sterile, blunt-ended 19-gauge needle is inserted into the renal artery and sutured in place (a hemostat may also be used). A sterile, glass 50-ml syringe is attached to the needle. The kidney is then perfused with PBS, followed by iron oxide in PBS (prepared as described in Table 1).

Table 1 Preparation of Iron Oxide Solution for Purification of Glomeruli and Proximal Tubules

	Preparative procedure
1.	Sodium hydroxide (2.6 g) and potassium nitrate (20 g) are dissolved in 100 ml of oxygen-saturated water.
2.	Ferrous sulfate (9 g) is dissolved in 100 ml of oxygen-saturated water. The ferrous sulfate solution is mixed with the sodium hydroxide/potassium nitrate solution made in step 1 above.
3.	The mixture is boiled for 20 min.
4.	The resulting precipitate of magnetic iron oxide is washed five to ten times. The precipitate is then resuspended in water and is then attracted to the bottom of the wash flask by a strong magnet (placed underneath the flask). The wash water is then decanted.
5.	The iron oxide is resuspended in several liters of 0.9% NaCl. This concentrated iron oxide solution is then autoclaved for future use. Immediately prior to use, the iron oxide solution is diluted in PBS, as detailed by Cook and Pickering.[66]

The initial perfusion with PBS removes the blood, whereas the second perfusion with iron oxide is designed to eventually permit removal of glomeruli. During this perfusion step, iron oxide particles, which are large, become associated with the glomeruli and do not enter the lumen of the nephrons. The kidney, which becomes gray-black in color, is decapsulated, and slices of the cortex are removed using sterile scissors. The cortical slices are transferred into a sterile, 7-ml Dounce homogenizer containing medium and are disrupted by means of four to five strokes with a type A (loose) pestle.

The nephron segments are subsequently separated by using two 9-cm diameter sieves, placed in series (i.e., a 253-μm pore size nylon mesh sieve placed over a sieve made of 83-μm pore size nylon mesh). The tubular suspension is poured over the upper 253-μm pore size sieve and is washed through the upper sieve by 500 to 700 ml of medium poured through the sieves. Distal tubules and loops of Henle also pass through the lower sieve during this process, because they are narrower in diameter than other nephron segments. Using a sterile spatula, the proximal tubules and glomeruli, which are present on the lower sieve, are then removed and transferred into a sterile, 50-ml tube containing 40 ml of serum-free medium and a sterile stir bar. The stir bar, which contains glomeruli with iron oxide, is removed. This procedure is repeated with another sterile stir bar. Large, 2-in. stir bars with a large magnet are preferable for this purpose.

The tubular suspension is treated for 2 min at 23°C with 0.05 mg/ml soybean trypsin inhibitor (Life Technologies), Gaithersburg, MD and 0.05 mg/ml collagenase (Class IV, Worthington). The tubules are washed twice by centrifugation at low speed (5 min) in a tabletop centrifuge. The tubules are suspended at approximately 0.5 mg protein per milliliter into serum-free, Dulbecco's Modified Eagle's Medium: Ham's F12 (DMEM:F12) medium supplemented with 5 μg/ml insulin, 5 μg/ml transferrin, and 5×10^{-8} *M* hydrocortisone (Table 2). The tubular suspension is then distributed into 60-mm culture dishes, and the culture dishes are maintained at 37°C in a 5% CO_2/95% air environment. The medium is changed the next day (to remove debris) and every 2 days thereafter.

12.2.2 *Transfection of primary cultures with plasmid DNA*

When the primary cultures approach 50% confluence, the cells are used for transfection studies by the strontium phosphate method.[17] On the day of the transfection, the cultures are first refed. Two to four hours later, strontium phosphate precipitates of plasmid DNA are prepared and added to the cultures.

To prepare strontium phosphate precipitates, 0.25 ml sterile 2× HEPES-buffered saline with low phosphate (HBSLP) (prepared as described in Table 3) is added to a sterile, 4-ml polypropylene tube, followed by 218 μl of sterile water and 10 μl of pRSVT plasmid

Table 2 Serum-Free Medium for Proximal Tubular Cells

Medium supplements	Final dosage in medium	Stock solution	
		Concentration	Storage
Insulin	5 μg/ml	5 mg/ml in 0.01 *M* HCl	4°C
Transferrin	5 μg/ml	5 mg/ml in water	–20°C
Hydrocortisone	5×10^{-8} M	10^{-3} *M* in 100% ethanol	4°C

Note: The supplements are added to the medium immediately prior to use for cell culture. The basal medium utilized is a 50:50 mixture of Ham's F12 and Dulbecco's Modified Eagle's Medium (DMEM) (with high glucose, and lacking sodium pyruvate) supplemented with 15 m*M* HEPES buffer, 1.2 mg/ml sodium bicarbonate, 1192 IU/ml penicillin, and 200 μg/ml streptomycin. The medium is brought to pH 7.4 and is sterilized by filtration. Individual bottles of medium are stored frozen, are thawed, and are maintained at 4°C for up to two weeks. Individual sterile aliquots of insulin, transferrin, and hydrocortisone are stored as described above. Aliquots of transferrin are frozen and thawed up to four times. Hydrocortisone stock solutions are kept for up to three to four months in polypropylene tubes.

DNA (at a concentration of 0.5 μg/μl).[17] Subsequently, 31 μl of a sterile, 2.0 *M* $SrCl_2$ solution is added and the tube is mixed gently at 37°C for 30 s. The precipitate is then pipetted onto the cells, and the dish is rocked gently to distribute the precipitate over the entire monolayer. The tissue culture dish is incubated at 37°C in a 5% CO_2/95% air environment for 2 to 4 h.

At the end of the incubation period with the strontium phosphate–DNA precipitate, the cells are subjected to a glycerol shock. The culture medium is removed by aspiration, and the monolayer is washed twice with 2 ml of serum-free, basal medium. Subsequently, 0.5 ml of glycerol-1× HBSLP (Table 3) is added to the culture for 30 s at room temperature and immediately removed by aspiration. The monolayer is washed three times with 2.5 ml of serum-free, basal medium and incubated overnight with 2.5 ml of normal growth medium in a 37°C, 5% CO_2/95% air environment. The medium is changed the next morning to 5 ml of normal growth medium.

Table 3 Solutions for Strontium Phosphate Transfection Procedure

Solution	Composition
2.0 m*M* $SrCl_2$	Spectrosol, BDH Chemicals, Ltd., Poole, England
2× HEPES-buffered saline with low phosphate (2X HBSLP)	42 m*M* HEPES, pH 7.3, 274 m*M* NaCl, 10 m*M* KCl, 1.4 m*M* Na_2HPO_4–2 H_2O, 11 m*M* glucose
15% (w/v) glycerol in 1X HBSLP (gly-HBSLP)	15 g glycerol + 50 ml of 2× HBSLP in 100 ml of H_2O
Serum-free DMEM/F12 medium	
Water	

Note: All solutions are sterilized by filtration through a 0.22-μm pore size filter and are stored at 4°C.

12.2.3 *Selection of immortalized transformants*

After transfection of the cells with the pRSVT plasmid, 24 to 72 h are allowed for expression of plasmid cDNA. The primary cultures may then be subjected to a selection procedure to enrich for transformants containing pRSVT DNA. As the pRSVT plasmid does not itself possess selectable markers, selection of transformants in primary cultures would require either cotransfection with a plasmid containing a selectable marker (such as neomycin resistance) or simply extended passaging. In the former case, transformants would be selected by their resistance to G418 (in the case where the neomycin resistance gene is used). G418 (Geneticin) is the mammalian homologue of neomycin and may be obtained commercially (Life Technologies). A G418 concentration of 200 to 400 μg/ml can be used for selection. Several different concentrations can be tested.

Stable transformants are further selected by their ability to survive numerous passages and by continued G418 resistance (in the case where such a selectable marker is used). Simple selection, based on the ability of immortalized transformants to be subcultured continuously, is feasible with proximal tubular cells from rabbit kidney. Normal proximal tubular cells from rabbit kidney can be passaged only once (or twice) in serum-free, DMEM:F12 medium, supplemented with insulin, transferrin, and hydrocortisone. The majority of the cells do not survive a second passage. Thus, the cell population is rapidly enriched with respect to the proportion of "immortalized" cells. If the cells are plated appropriately, clonal isolates can be obtained.

Following the second passage, only a small portion of the cells still divide. If these cells are present at a low enough density, individual clones can be isolated using cloning cylinders, and they are removed from the culture dish by the use of a 0.05% (w/v) trypsin/0.53 m*M* EDTA solution. After incubation with trypsin/EDTA at 37°C in a 5% CO_2/95% air environment, the clonal isolates are examined under an inverted microscope. When the cells appear rounded, trypsin action is inhibited by the addition of a 0.1% (w/v) soybean trypsin inhibitor solution (in PBS) to the cloning cylinders. Using sterile, cotton-stuffed pasteur pipettes, the clonal isolates are transferred to other culture dishes to grow to confluence. When considerable cell growth has occurred, the cells are passaged. The monolayers are washed twice with PBS, and the cells are removed from the culture dish by incubation with trypsin/EDTA at 37°C. Trypsin action is inhibited with a solution of 0.1% (w/v) soybean trypsin inhibitor, and the cells are washed by centrifugation in a tabletop centrifuge (at 500 rpm). The cell pellet is resuspended in growth medium and transferred to new, 60-mm culture dishes containing growth medium.

12.2.4 Serial passaging

The successful serial passaging of immortalized cells may depend on the composition of the basal medium and the growth supplements, as well as the cell adhesion molecules on the culture dish. Primary cultures of proximal tubular cells from rabbit kidney can grow to confluence in serum-free, DMEM:F12 medium, supplemented with 5 μg/ml insulin, 5 μg/ml transferrin, and 5×10^{-8} *M* hydrocortisone.[14] However, the cells can also grow in response to other growth regulatory supplements, including epidermal growth factor (EGF) and fibroblast growth factor (FGF), which may be added to the medium in addition to insulin, transferrin, and hydrocortisone, to promote growth.

During the process of serial passaging, portions of the subcultured cells are removed by trypsinization for freezing in liquid nitrogen. Trypsin action is inhibited by means of soybean trypsin inhibitor. The cells are washed by centrifugation and are resuspended in serum-free, DMEM:F12 medium containing 10% (v/v) glycerol. The cells are transferred into sterile freezing ampoules and gradually cooled using a biological freezer. Finally, the ampoules are placed on freezing canes and transferred into a liquid nitrogen freezing tank. By these means, we have obtained a number of immortalized clones of proximal tubular cells from rabbit kidney in serum-free culture medium.

12.2.5 Characterization of immortalized cells

Primary cultures of proximal tubular cells from rabbit kidney have been transfected with the pRSVT plasmid and subsequently passaged.[18] The immortalized cells have been grown for more than 24 months in serum-free medium supplemented with insulin, transferrin, hydrocortisone, EGF, bovine pituitary extract, heparin, and bovine serum albumin. Normal renal cells from rabbit do not survive for more than two passages under these conditions. However, four independently transformed populations of rabbit renal proximal tubular (RRPT) cells have survived more than 23 passages in serum-free medium. Clonal populations have also been obtained.

The possibility was examined initially that the immortalized RRPT cells retain differentiated functions typical of the renal proximal tubule. Renal proximal tubular cells *in vivo* possess a polarized morphology, with a brush border and brush border enzymes. Several clones, RRPT clone 8 and clone E, were found to possess considerable activities of three brush border enzymes, alkaline phosphatase, leucine aminopeptidase, and γ-glutamyl transpeptidase. The activities of the brush border marker enzymes alkaline phosphatase and leucine aminopeptidase can be readily assayed with intact monolayers in 35-mm dishes using *p*-nitrophenylphosphate and *l*-leucine *p*-nitroanilide as substrates, respectively. Their products, *p*-nitrophenol and *p*-nitroanilide, are measured spectrophotometrically.[19,20] The γ-glutamyltranspeptidase assay requires the use of crude, detergent-solubilized membrane preparations. The substrate for the γ-glutamyltranspeptidase assay is L-γ-glutamyl-*p*-nitroanilide, and the acceptor molecule is glycylglycine. The reaction product, *p*-nitroanilide, is read at 405 nm (E_{405} = 9600), whereas *p*-nitrophenol is read at 420 nm (E_{420} = 18,300). The activities of these enzymes were retained with extended passages. Higher γ-glutamyltranspeptidase activity was observed in serum-free, rather than in serum-supplemented, growth conditions.

A Na^+/glucose cotransport system is a distinctive characteristic of proximal tubular cells, as compared with cells in other nephron segments.[26] The Na^+/glucose cotransport system is localized in the renal brush border membrane and is involved in the reabsorption of sugars by the renal proximal tubule *in vivo*.[22] The presence of this transport system can be determined by means of uptake studies into intact cells, using ^{14}C-alpha-methyl-D-glucoside (alpha MG), a nonmetabolized sugar.[14] Previously, we observed a high rate of sodium-dependent ^{14}C-alpha MG uptake into primary cultures of proximal tubular cells from rabbit kidney.[14]

When using a modified Kreb's Ringer buffer system in the uptake studies,[14] we detected significant alpha MG uptake into RRPT clone 8. The rate of sodium-dependent alpha MG uptake into RRPT clone 8 was 23% of the rate we previously reported with primary cultures of proximal tubular cells from rabbit kidney (0.15 nmol alpha MG per minute per milligram protein).[14] The observation of this transport system is critical to the argument that immortalized proximal tubular cells possess the appropriate phenotype (i.e., that of the renal proximal tubule). Sodium-dependent sugar uptake only occurs via the Na^+/glucose cotransport system. This transport system is a marker that is only observed in renal cells originating from the renal proximal tubule.

The immortalized renal proximal tubular cell from rabbit also retains the sensitivity to various nephrotoxicants. Three different cephalosporin drugs rank similarly with regard to their cytotoxicity *in vitro* and *in vivo* (i.e., cephaloridine > cefazolin > cephalothin). Methylmercury is significantly more toxic than inorganic mercury in primary renal cell cultures.[23]

12.2.6 *Possible problems and optimization of the procedure*

12.2.6.1 *Possible reasons for a lack of immortalized cells*

A number of possible explanations may be given if immortalized cells are not obtained at the end of the transfection period. First, the transfection was not performed under optimal conditions. Most of the transformants obtained immediately after transfection are unstable. In only a small fraction of instances is an "immortalizing" gene integrated into the genome of the host cell, resulting in a stable transformant. Furthermore, not all immortalizing genes (which generally speaking are oncogenes) are appropriate for the immortalization of particular cell types. Although a normal karyotype is desirable, secondary genetic changes may also be required in order for immortalization to occur successfully.

Second, if transformants are initially isolated using a drug selection procedure, the selection procedure may be a limiting factor. For example, mammalian cells transfected with a plasmid containing the neomycin resistance gene can be initially selected using G418.[24] The use of too high of a concentration of G418 may kill a substantial portion of potential transformants, whereas G418 levels that are too low may prevent effective selection. Immortalized transformants may be particularly difficult to isolate from these short-term cell culture systems that can undergo a substantial number of passages before senescing, unless an appropriate selection procedure following transformation with plasmid DNA is used.

Finally, suboptimal culture conditions may be prohibitive to the isolation of immortalized cells. Immortalized cells may constitute only a small proportion of the cell population. Thus, only a small number of immortalized cells may be present in the culture situation. If the cells cannot readily grow at a low density under the culture conditions used, then immortalized transformants may never be obtained. The ability of cells to grow at a low density is a function of the culture conditions.

12.2.6.2 Optimization of transfection

The single most important factor to consider when optimizing transfection efficiency is the transfection protocol. A number of different methods for transfection of animal cells are available, including calcium phosphate precipitation, the use of DEAE–dextran, electroporation, and liposome-mediated transfection.[25] Although the calcium phosphate method has generally been successful for many different types of animal cells, the calcium phosphate precipitate that forms may cover the cells and have toxic effects, especially in serum-free culture conditions. Similar problems with toxicity have been encountered with the DEAE–dextran method. In general, the use of liposomes to deliver DNA to animal cells in culture has been extremely successful, resulting in higher efficiencies of transformation without undesired, toxic side effects.

The wide use of electroporation (made possible by the use of commercial apparatuses) has generally been successful with cells in suspension (a notable example is human lymphocytes). However, the use of this procedure with primary cultures essentially requires a passage. The electroporation procedure has not been utilized extensively for fresh tissue, but does have potential applications for tubular suspensions prepared from tissue for primary culture purposes.

When optimizing specific transfection procedures, a number of variables must be considered. With respect to the strontium phosphate method, the amount of DNA (100 to 250 μg/60-mm dish) in the precipitate, the length of time the precipitate is left on the cultures (2 to 4 h), and the duration of the glycerol shock (0 to 3 min) are important variables. In order to obtain reproducible results, cell cultures of a similar density and age should be used.

Similar factors influence the efficiency of calcium phosphate transfection. With regard to the DEAE–dextran method, the cell number and the concentration of DNA and DEAE–dextran are important variables. A calcium phosphate precipitate and DEAE–dextran can be cytotoxic, particularly in excess, preventing the effective use of these procedures on particular cell types.

Liposome-mediated transfection is a convenient new method that is often used in obtaining permanent transformants. Liposome preparations sold by such companies as Life Technologies permit high transfection efficiencies to be obtained, using minimal quantities of DNA (3 to 6 μg/60-mm dish). In this case, the concentration of lipid and DNA and the incubation time with the liposome–DNA complex are important variables. Generally, increasing concentrations of liposomes permit increased transfection efficiencies, which may in turn increase the probability of obtaining immortalized transformants. The use of very high concentrations of liposomes, however, can be quite costly. Using

DNA at too high of a concentration can reduce the efficiency of transfection in this procedure. Finally, the incubation time with liposome–DNA complex is a critical variable.

If no immortalized clones are obtained, this result may possibly be attributed to a low efficiency of transfection and/or a lack of stability of the foreign DNA within the cells over a long time interval. The initial efficiency of transfection can be assessed by a number of methods. If the pRSVT plasmid, which lacks a selectable marker, is used, the initial transfection can be conducted with pRSVT and another plasmid, such as pMC1neo Poly A (Stratagene), which contains the gene for neomycin phosphotransferase and confers neomycin resistance. The number of transfected cells can then be assessed by determining the number of cells or colonies that survive treatment with G418 (G418 is added several days after transfection to permit gene expression). Alternatively, the cells can be cotransfected with an expression vector containing the beta-galactosidase gene, such as pSVbetagal (Promega). Subsequently, colonies that express beta-galactosidase can be identified by the X gal staining technique, which causes cells expressing beta-galactosidase to turn blue.[26] The percentage of stained cells can be determined by observation under an inverted microscope at 100× magnification.

12.2.6.3 *Optimization of culture conditions*

Serum-free, hormonally defined medium has been an important tool for the growth of primary cultures of differentiated cells, as well as in the development of established lines of differentiated cells.[2] Animal cells derived from various tissues require different groups of hormones, growth factors, cell attachment factors and transport binding proteins in order to grow in serum-free medium.[2] In addition, the use of an appropriate basal medium has been an important means of promoting the growth of animal cells.[27,28]

Serum-free medium has proved to be especially important for primary cultures of normal cells. Not only can serum-free medium promote the growth of the differentiated cells of interest, but the use of an appropriate serum-free medium can prevent fibroblast overgrowth of the differentiated cells. A good example is the case of primary cultures of renal tubular epithelial cells from baby mice, which grow without fibroblast overgrowth in Medium K-1 (the defined medium for MDCK cells).[16] The primary cultures of renal cells from baby mice exhibit a growth response to each of the five growth supplements in this particular serum-free medium (5 μg/ml insulin, 5 μg/ml transferrin, 5×10^{-12} *M* triiodothyronine, 5×10^{-8} *M* hydrocortisone, and 25 ng/ml prostaglandin E_1).[15] Thus, in normal mouse kidneys, cells exist that exhibit growth responses to hormones that are very similar to those observed with the MDCK epithelial cell line.

Not all normal renal epithelial cells, however, exhibit growth responses to all five supplements, as exemplified by primary cultures of renal proximal tubular cells from rabbit, which only exhibit growth responses to three of the five factors — insulin, transferrin, and hydrocortisone.[14]

Short-term cultures of renal tubular epithelial cells derived from normal tissue have not yet been successfully immortalized in a serum-free medium without the use of a transforming agent. However, this feat has been successfully accomplished with epithelial cell cultures derived from other tissues. Notable examples include the establishment of the FRTL rat thyroid epithelial[29] and the TM_4 rat Sertoli cell lines,[5] which were both successfully immortalized in a serum-free, hormonally defined medium without undergoing a crisis of senescence.

The use of serum-free, hormonally defined medium for long-term passaging has only been successful with a few different types of normal cells. Presumably, appropriate culture conditions have not been identified for the long-term culturing of many types of normal, differentiated cells. If appropriate growth regulatory factors are not added to the culture medium, cell longevity may be limited. Appropriate growth regulatory factors may include previously identified growth factors, such as either EGF or FGF and hormones such as parathyroid hormone (PTH) or aldosterone, as well as vitamins such as retinoic acid.[2] The basal medium may also be a limiting factor for long-term growth of normal cells.[27,28] Optimized basal media have been developed for such cell types as human epidermal keratinocytes (MCDB 151), Chinese hamster ovary cells (MCDB 301), and mouse neuroblastoma cells (MCDB 411). This subject has been reviewed in detail by Ham and colleagues.[27,28]

The use of an appropriate substratum is an important factor to consider in cell immortalization studies. Renal proximal tubular cells from rabbit can be passaged readily only once. Continuous passage is limited, at least in part, by the ability of trypsinized cells to adhere to the new culture dish after passaging. The ability of the cells to attach to a substratum and to grow following a passage can be affected by the substratum itself, as well as the growth supplements in the culture medium. Defined substrata which can be utilized to promote attachment (and growth) include fibronectin,[30] laminin,[31] collagen IV, type I collagen (rat-tail collagen), as well as synthetic peptides. Included among synthetic peptides are poly-D-lysine[32] and RGDS- and YIGSR-related peptides.[33,34] In addition, more complex substrata, such as matrigel, may be utilized.[35] For example, substrata such as laminin may be added to the culture dishes either individually or in combination with collagen IV.

An adhesion mixture that is especially simple to apply is the BFN coating mixture, which contains fibronectin and vitrogen collagen. The BFN mixture is applied to the dish and immediately removed or is incubated at 37°C for 2 h to gel. The BFN coating mixture has been used in the development of immortalized human epithelial cells derived from the bronchus and the prostate.[36]

The use of appropriate hormones, growth factors, cell attachment factors, and basal media should prolong the life span of normal animal cells in culture. A limited life span in culture may be explained by the fact that appropriate culture conditions have not yet been identified. Alternatively, normal cells may indeed have a limited doubling potential. The introduction of appropriate oncogenes into the cultured animal cells may conceivably result in immortalization by altering the environmental requirements of the cell in tissue culture or by actually introducing an immortalizing function, or both.

12.3 *Discussion*

12.3.1 *Characteristics of existing established renal epithelial cell lines*

A limited number of well-characterized renal tubular epithelial cell lines that retain properties characteristic of the transporting epithelial cells in renal tubules are available for study. The MDCK cell line, isolated from the kidney of a normal cocker spaniel in 1958, still retains growth and functional properties typical of normal renal tubular epithelial cells.[7,9] MDCK cells retain the polarized morphology typical of cells in the distal tubule of the kidney. The apical (or luminal) surface of the cells uniformly faces the tissue culture medium, and their basolateral surface uniformly faces the culture dish. At confluence, adjacent MDCK cells are interconnected by tight junctions, such that a continuous sheet forms like that of a frog skin or toad bladder. Multicellular domes or hemicysts can be observed in such confluent monolayers. Domes consist of portions of the monolayer that are slightly elevated from the tissue culture dish due to transepithelial salt and water transport. The salt and water that are transported across the monolayer from the apical surface through the basolateral surface may become trapped between the monolayer and the culture dish. The resulting hydrostatic pressure leads to dome formation.

That dome formation is indeed indicative of transepithelial salt and water transport across the monolayer has been firmly established by the Ussing chamber studies of Misfeldt et al.[37] and Cereijido et al.[38] MDCK cells exhibit both a spontaneous potential difference across the monolayer and an electrical resistance. The electrical resistance observed across MDCK monolayers by these researchers was approximately 100 ohm cm^{-2}, which is typical of leaky epithelial cells such as those present in the renal proximal tubule. Another strain of MDCK cell, which has a considerably higher transepithelial electrical resistance (4000 ohm cm^{-2}), has been identified and designated as "high resistance" MDCK cells (as opposed to the "low resistance" MDCK cells of Misfeldt et al. and Cereijido et al.).[39] However, MDCK cells do not possess a resistance as high as that observed with cells *in vivo*, which has placed serious limitations on *in vitro* electrophysiologic studies. Whether the lack of cultured epithelial cells with a truly high resistance is due to changes that occur due to the tissue culture environment or due to difficulties in culturing tubular epithelial cells that possess a truly high resistance is unclear.

In other respects, MDCK cells exhibit properties typical of distal tubular cells, including an arginine vasopressin-sensitive adenylate cyclase, an amiloride sensitive Na^+/H^+ antiport system, and a furosemide-sensitive Na^+, K^+, Cl^- cotransport system.[7,9] These transport systems play important roles in transepithelial solute transport. Sodium enters MDCK cells via such an amiloride-sensitive Na^+/H^+ antiport system (localized on the apical surface) and leaves the cells via the (Na^+ + K^+)-stimulated ATPase (localized on the basolateral surface). In addition, high resistance MDCK cells possess the capacity for chloride secretion. Chloride enters the cells via the Na^+, K^+, Cl^- cotransport system (localized on the basolateral surface), and leaves the cells via a chloride channel localized on the apical membrane. The (Na^+ + K^+)-stimulated ATPase provides the driving force for such polarized transport.

Major questions in epithelial cell biology focus on the mechanisms by which the polarized morphology of epithelial cells is established and maintained.[8] Plasma membrane proteins are localized on either the apical or the basolateral membrane of epithelial cells. The MDCK cell line has been used to study the mechanisms by which such proteins are inserted into particular domains of the plasma membrane. A significant number of these studies use enveloped viruses that may bud from either the apical membrane (in the case of Influenza virus) or the basolateral membrane (in the case of VSV). Other studies concerning the polarity question have dealt with the (Na^+ + K^+)-stimulated ATPase, which becomes localized to the basolateral membrane of MDCK cells at confluence. The polarized orientation of the (Na^+ + K^+)-stimulated ATPase has been attributed to the association of the enzyme with a complex containing fodrin and ankyrin.

MDCK cells are particularly useful for *in vitro* studies concerning hormones, growth factors, and signal transduction. The cell line can be grown at the same rate (1.5 doublings per day), both in a serum-free, hormonally defined medium and in medium supplemented with 10% (w/v) fetal calf serum.[16] The serum-free medium contains 5 μg/ml insulin, 5 μg/ml transferrin, 5×10^{-8} *M* hydrocortisone, 5×10^{-12} *M* triiodothyronine (T_3), and 25 ng/ml prostaglandin E_1 (PGE_1).[16] Similarly, primary cultures of renal cells from baby mice grow in response to each of the five supplements, suggesting that the growth responses are physiologically significant.[15] Indeed, each of these five supplements are used at physiologic concentrations, with the exception of insulin. This latter observation can be explained by the fact that insulin is interacting with receptors for insulin-like growth factors (MDCK cells lack insulin receptors). In addition, MDCK cells grow in response to numerous other effector molecules, including EGF, FGF, arginine vasopressin, dopamine, and norepinephrine. Of particular interest in these regards, several classes of clonal isolates of MDCK cells have been identified, which either have both alpha and beta adrenergic receptors, or simply beta adrenergic receptors.[40]

The LLC-PK_1 epithelial cell line from pig kidney retains a number of the differentiated transport systems typical of the renal proximal tubule, unlike MDCK cells.[7,9] The Na^+/glucose cotransport system, an apical transport system, is responsible for the initial reabsorption of glucose from the lumen of the renal proximal tubule. Labeled flux studies indicate that confluent LLC-PK_1 monolayers possess the capacity for Na^+-dependent sugar transport.[41] Sodium-dependent sugar uptake was inhibited by phlorizin (an inhibitor of the Na^+/glucose cotransport system) rather than phloretin. Similarly, in Ussing chamber studies with the LLC-PK_1 cell line, the addition of phlorizin to the apical bath caused a decrease in the transepithelial potential difference (PD) across the monolayer.[42] The PD (2.8 mV) and the resistance (211 ohm/cm^2) were dependent on the presence of glucose in the apical bath. The LLC-PK_1 cell line also possesses the capacity for polarized amino acid transport[43] and organic cation secretion[44] like renal proximal tubular cells. However, the LLC-PK_1 cell line does not possess the PTH-sensitive adenylate cyclase typical of the renal proximal tubule. The opossum kidney (OK) cell line, which exhibits PTH responsiveness,[46] has been used instead for *in vitro* studies concerning the regulation of phosphate transport by PTH. Rather than exhibiting PTH responsiveness, LLC-PK_1 cells exhibit responsiveness to arginine vasopressin and calcitonin, which is typical of epithelial cells in more distal segments of the nephron.[45] LLC-PK_1 cells also lack the gluconeogenic capacity that is typical of renal proximal tubular cells.[47]

12.3.2 *Strategies for the development of immortalized cell lines*

Previously, established renal tubular epithelial cell lines have been developed from normal tissue without the use of an immortalizing agent. Examples include MDCK cells, which were derived from the kidney of a normal cocker spaniel and the OK cell line, which was derived from an opossum kidney. A problem with these cell lines is that they are derived from animals that are not inbred strains. Thus, experimental studies cannot be conducted readily to examine the physiologic significance of *in vitro* studies. An ideal of tissue culturists is to perform investigations in which one can go back and forth from the *in vitro* to the *in vivo* situation. However, difficulties have been encountered in developing, at will, established cell lines from normal tissues of the species of interest, due to imperfections in the *in vitro* environment and/or a limited life span of normal cells.

12.3.2.1 *Viral transformation*

An approach to overcome these limitations is the transformation of normal cells either with whole, intact viruses or with plasmids containing viral oncogenes. A notable example of a cell line established using an intact virus is the 293 human embryonic renal cell line, which was established following transfection with adenovirus DNA.[48] The 293 renal cell line exhibits several apical marker enzymes, but is, to a large extent, uncharacterized with regard to its differentiated functions.[48]

A major problem with this type of transformation approach is that the differentiated cells may undergo a variety of alterations that are often associated with malignant transformation, such as (1) a loss of anchorage dependence and the formation of multilayers in culture; (2) an altered cellular morphology, including a loss of polarity and junctional complexes; (3) an increased growth rate and saturation density; (4) the loss of the requirement for serum, and/or altered growth requirements of cells in serum-free medium; and (5) the acquisition of the ability of the cells to form tumors in nude mice.[1]

12.3.2.1.1 *Temperature-sensitive viruses.* An approach that has been taken to overcome these problems is to use temperature-sensitive viruses. An example is the SV40 virus, which possesses a temperature-sensitive mutation in the viral A gene (tsA mutants).[49] In those cells that can be transformed by SV40, the expression of the A gene is required for the maintenance of the transformed phenotype. Animal cells that are transformed with SV40 virus possessing a tsA mutation are conditionally transformed cells. That is, the cells express the transformed phenotype only at the permissive temperature (33°C), while at the nonpermissive temperature (40°C), the cells revert to a normal nontransformed phenotype. Initially, the use of a tsA mutant of SV40 to develop immortalized cell lines was demonstrated for rat liver cells.[49] Two well-characterized fetal rat liver cell lines, RLA255-4 and RLA209-15, were established by infecting the cells with virus at the permissive temperature (33°C). Subsequently, clonal isolates were switched to the nonpermissive temperature and were screened for the ability to produce alpha fetoprotein (AFP), albumin, and transferrin. The isolated clones are invaluable for studying the expression of differentiated function. Precise studies can be conducted by means of temperature shift experiments, in which the temperature is shifted from 33°C to 40°C and vice versa.

This temperature-sensitive SV40 virus has been successfully used to develop cell lines from other tissues, including kidney. An SV40 tsA-transformed collecting duct cell line from rabbit has been established.[50] This tsA transformant exhibits arginine vasopressin-responsive adenylate cyclase at the nonpermissive temperature, but not at the permissive temperature, and is a valuable tool for studying the action of arginine vasopressin.

12.3.2.1.2 The use of human papilloma virus for cell immortalization. Human papilloma virus (HPV) has been recently used to immortalize normal human cells in culture. Both HPV16 and HPV18 form nonmalignant growths in the larynx, trachea, and bronchus. When normal human bronchial epithelial cells were transformed *in vitro* with either the HPV16 or the HPV18 virus, immortalized cell lines were obtained that were nontumorigenic in nude mice.[51] Both the BEP3 cell line (immortalized with HPV16) as well as the BEP2 and the BEP1 cell lines (immortalized with HPV18), expressed HPVE6 and HPVE7 mRNAs (which encode for proteins involved in early viral transforming functions).[51] The cells exhibited a lower degree of squamous differentiation, which is typically induced when the normal cells achieve a confluent state.

Similarly, HPV16 was used to successfully immortalize human endocervical cells[52] and rat embryo fibroblasts.[53] In the latter case, the E7 ORF, but not the E6 ORF, was sufficient to immortalize this cell type in primary culture. In HPV16-immortalized human keratinocytes, E7-dependent immortalization was associated with modifications of E2F multiprotein complexes.[54] In particular, complexes between E2F and pRB were disrupted, while complexes between E2F and cyclin A were maintained. The E6 gene was also sufficient to immortalize epithelial cells from human mammary gland and to reduce their growth factor requirements.[55] In such HPV16-immortalized human mammary cells, the Rb protein was found to be normal while the level of p53 protein was reduced. Presumably, the observed modifications of E2F multiprotein complexes could be attributed to a change in pRb.

12.3.2.1.3 The use of retroviruses for cell immortalization. Retroviral vectors are another invaluable tool for obtaining immortalized renal cells. A case in point is the use of a retrovirus construct to immortalize renal proximal tubular cells from rabbit.[56] Proximal convoluted tubules (S_1 segment) from rabbit kidney were microdissected and cocultured with irradiated PA 317-SV40-6 cells (an amphotropic producer line for Molony murine leukemia virus, which had been infected with the replication-defective retrovirus construct containing the genes for neomycin phosphotransferase and SV40 large T antigen under the control of a common promoter). Both vEPT cell lines (cocultured with virus-producing feeder layers) and EPT cell lines (cocultured with feeder layers without virus) were obtained. The cells were routinely passaged six times with nonproliferating fibroblast feeder layers.[56] Subsequently, the monolayers were passaged (on a 1/6 basis) without feeder layers. The cells possessed a polarized morphology with junctional complexes. PTH and angiotensin II both caused an increase in intracellular calcium levels. A phlorizin-sensitive, short-circuit current was detected in glucose-containing medium, suggesting the presence of a Na^+/glucose cotransport system. However, the presence of SV40 T antigen was not detected, and thus the continued presence of the SV40 large T antigen gene was unclear.

12.3.3 *Cell immortalization using plasmids with oncogenes*

Oncogenic DNA viruses, such as polyoma (Py) and human adenovirus (Ad), possess the ability to transform both primary and established cell lines *in vitro*. Transformation of primary cells requires both an establishment function, which is concerned with cell immortalization, and a transformation function, which is required for full expression of an oncogenic phenotype.[57]

12.3.3.1 *Immortalizing functions of adeno E1A oncogene*

The adeno E1A gene possesses establishment function(s), which when used in combination with another viral gene (e.g., adeno E1B), result in phenotypic changes that are characteristic of oncogenic transformation.[57] In the classic paper by Ruley,[57] primary cultures of renal epithelial cells from baby rat were transformed by the t24 Harvey *ras* 1 gene or the polyoma virus middle-T gene only if the adenovirus E1A gene was present.

More recently, additional oncogenes have been tested in combination with adeno E1A for their transforming ability. The product of a naturally occurring, dominant negative mutation in WT1 was found to cooperate with E1A to induce the fully transformed malignant phenotype.[58] However, the overexpression of the Wilms' tumor gene WT1 had no effect on immortalization of primary cultures of renal epithelial cells from baby rat by E1A or on transformation by E1A and E1B.[58] In contrast, two other tumor-suppressor genes, RB1 and p53, have a dramatic growth-suppression effect when transfected into primary cells transformed by E1A and Ha-*ras* (a growth-suppressive effect that has been found to vary with the recipient cell type).[58]

The differentiated functions of adeno E1A-transformed renal cells in primary culture have not been determined. However, retention of differentiated function may be a problem when using the adeno E1A oncogene. When differentiated F9 cells are infected with wild-type adenovirus, a decline is observed in the levels of collagen IV mRNA and plasminogen activator mRNA.[59] The decline in expression of these markers of differentiation could be attributed to negative regulation by the viral E1A gene.

Similarly, transfection of BCH_3 myoblasts with an expression vector containing the Ad5 E1A gene, resulted in suppression of the expression of the muscle-specific genes creatine kinase, the nicotinic acetylcholine receptor subunits, and alpha actin.[60] Transfection of PC12 pheochromocytoma cells with a vector containing the Ad5 E1A gene resulted in a loss of the ability of the cells to form neurites in response to nerve growth factor (NGF) and forskolin.[61] This defect was associated with a loss of NGF and EGF receptors, as well as the mRNAs for chromaffin, tyrosine hydroxylase, and peripherin in the E1A-transformed PC12 cells.

12.3.3.2 *Immortalization using plasmids with the SV40 early region genes*

A number of differentiated cells that are derived from normal tissues have been successfully immortalized using plasmids containing the SV40 early region genes, which include genes for the large T and the small T antigens. A good example is the use of the pRSVT plasmid for the immortalization of primary cultures of normal human bronchial epithelia (NHBE) cells in serum-free medium.[17] The frequency of stable transfection by the strontium phosphate method was greater than 10^{-4}. Southern analysis indicated that stable transformants possessed the SV40 early region genes in the cellular genomic DNA. Indirect immunofluorescence studies indicated that the SV40 large T antigen was expressed in immortalized NHBE cells. The immortalized normal human bronchial epithelial cells have been used to study the effects of transformation with other oncogenes, such as Ha-*ras* and c-*erbB*-2, as well as the effects of treatment with such carcinogens as benzo(a)pyrene. The human bronchial epithelial cell line BEAS-ZB, which is nontumorigenic, has been especially useful in these types of studies.[62]

Other types of normal differentiated epithelial cells have similarly been immortalized using the pRSVT plasmid. Immortalized normal human mesothelial cells are of potential importance in studies of the effects of asbestos exposure.[63] Human fetal prostate epithelial cells that are transformed with pRSVT (i.e., the 267B1 cell line) are both immortal and nontumorigenic.[64] These cells, like immortalized bronchial epithelial cells, can be further malignantly transformed *in vitro* using chemicals or oncogenes, such as activated Ki-*ras*.[65,66] In this manner, the immortalized cells have been used to study the process of multistep transformation.

References

1. Taub, M., The biology of cultured cells, in *Fundamentals of Medical Cell Biology,* Bitter, E., Ed., JAI Press, Greenwich, CT, 1991, 323.
2. Taub, M., The use of defined medium in cell and tissue culture, *Toxicol. In Vitro,* 4, 213, 1990.
3. Sato, G. H., The role of serum in cell culture, in *Biochemical Actions of Hormones, Vol. 3,* Litwack, G., Ed., Academic Press, New York, 1975, 391.
4. Brandi, M. L., Fitzpatrick, L. A., Coon, H. G., and Aurbach, G. D., Bovine parathyroid cells: cultures maintained for more than 140 population doublings, *Proc. Natl. Acad. Sci. U.S.A.,* 83, 1709, 1986.
5. Mather, J. P., The establishment and characterization of two distinct mouse testicular epithelial cell lines, *Biol. Reprod.,* 23, 243, 1980.
6. Brenner, B. M. and Rector, F. C., Eds., 3rd ed., *The Kidney,* W.B. Saunders, Philadelphia, 1986.
7. McRoberts, J., Taub, M., and Saier, M. H., Jr., The Madin Darby canine kidney (MDCK) cell line, in *Functionally Differentiated Cell Lines,* Sato, G., Ed., Alan R. Liss, New York, 1981, 117.
8. Taub, M., Viruses in the study of the polarity of epithelial membranes, in *Tissue Culture of Epithelial Cells,* Taub, M., Ed., Plenum Press, New York, 1985, 127.
9. Taub, M., Importance of hormonally-defined, serum-free medium for *in vitro* studies concerning epithelial transport, in *Tissue Culture of Epithelial Cells,* Taub, M., Ed., Plenum Press, New York, 1985, 255.
10. Kluwe, W. M., The nephrotoxicity of low molecular weight halogenated alkane solvents, pesticides and chemical intermediates, in *Toxicology of the Kidney,* Hook, J. B., Ed., Raven Press, New York, 1981, 176.
11. Aleo, M. D., Taub, M. L., Olson, R. R., Nickerson, P. A., and Kostyniak, P. J., Primary cultures of rabbit renal tubule cells. II. Selected phase I and phase II metabolic capacities, *Toxicol. In Vitro,* 4, 727, 1990.
12. Kluwe, W. M. and Hook, J. B., Effects of environmental chemicals on kidney metabolism and function, *Kidney Int.,* 18, 648, 1980.
13. Tune, B. M. and Hsu, C. Y., Mechanisms of beta-lactam antibiotic nephrotoxicity, *Toxicol. Lett.,* 53, 81, 1990.
14. Chung, S. D., Alavi, N., Livingston, D., Hiller, S., and Taub, M., Characterization of primary rabbit kidney cultures that express proximal tubule functions in a hormonally defined medium, *J. Cell Biol.,* 95, 118, 1982.
15. Taub, M. and Sato, G., Growth of functional primary cells of kidney epithelial cells in defined medium, *J. Cell. Physiol.,* 105, 369, 1980.
16. Taub, M., Chuman, L., Saier, M. H., Jr., and Sato, G., Growth of Madin Darby canine kidney epithelial cell (MDCK) line in hormone-supplemented, serum-free medium, *Proc. Natl. Acad. Sci. U.S.A.,* 76, 3338, 1979.
17. Brash, D. E., Reddel, R. R., Quanrud, M., Yang, K, Farrell, M. P., and Harris, C. C., Strontium phosphate stable expression of the Simian Virus 40 Large-T-antigen gene in primary human bronchial epithelial cells, *Mol. Cell. Biol.,* 7, 2031, 1987.

18. Taub, M., Allen, C., Han, H. J., and Park, J. H., Immortalization of rabbit kidney proximal tubule cells in serum-free medium, *In Vitro Cell. Dev. Biol.*, 30A, 43, 1994.
19. Bessey, O. A., Lowry, O. H., and Brock, M. L., A method for the rapid determination of alkaline phosphatase with five cubic millimeters of serum, *J. Biol. Chem.*, 164, 321, 1946.
20. Green, M. N., Tsou, K. C., Bressler, R., and Seligman, A. M., The colorimetric determination of leucine aminopeptidase activity with L-leucyl-beta-naphthylamide hydrochloride, *Arch. Biochem. Biophys.*, 57, 458, 1955.
21. Tate, S. S. and Meister, A., Interaction of γ-glutamyl transpeptidase with amino acids, dipeptides and derivatives of glutathione, *J. Biol. Chem.*, 249, 7593, 1974.
22. Kinne, R. H., Murer, E., Kinne-Saffron, E., Thies, M., and Sachs, G., Sugar transport by renal plasma membrane vesicles, *J. Membr. Biol.*, 21, 375, 1975.
23. Aleo, M. D., Taub, M. L., and Kostyniak, P. J., Primary cultures of rabbit renal proximal tubule cells. III. Comparative cytotoxicity of inorganic and organic mercury, *Toxicol. Appl. Pharmacol.*, 112, 310, 1992.
24. Colbere-Garapin, F., Horodinceanu, F., Kourilsky, P., and Garapin, A., A new dominant hybrid selective marker for higher eukaryotic cells., *J. Mol. Biol.*, 150, 1, 1981.
25. Kingston, R. E., Chen, C. A., and Okayama, H., Transfection of DNA into eukaryotic cells, in *Current Protocols in Molecular Biology*, Ausubel, F. M., Brent, R., Kingston, R. E., Moore, D. D., Seidman, J. G., Smith, J. A., and Struhl, K, Eds., John Wiley & Sons, New York, 1989, Section 9.1.9.
26. Cepko, C., X gal staining of cultured cells, in *Current Protocols in Molecular Biology*, Ausubel, F. M., Brent, R., Kingston, R. E., Moore, D. D., Seidman, J. G., Smith, J. A., and Struhl, K., Eds., John Wiley & Sons, New York, 1989, Section 9.11.9.
27. Bettger, W. J. and Ham, R. G., The nutrient requirements of cultured mammalian cells, in *Advances in Nutritional Research 4*, Draper, H. H., Ed., Plenum Press, New York, 1982, 249.
28. Ham, R. G., Survival and growth requirements of nontransformed cells, in *Handbook of Experimental Pharmacology*, Vol. 57, Baserga, R., Ed., Springer-Verlag, Berlin, 1981, 13.
29. Ambesi-Impionbato, F. S., Parks, L. A. M., and Coon, H. G., Culture of hormone dependent functional epithelial cells from rat thyroids, *Proc. Natl. Acad. Sci. U.S.A.*, 77, 3455, 1980.
30. Orly, J. and Sato, G., Fibronectin mediates cytokinesis and growth of rat follicular cells in serum-free medium, *Cell*, 17, 295, 1979.
31. Kleinman, H. K., McGoodwin, E. B., Rennard, S. L., and Martin, G. R., Preparation of collagen substrata for cell attachment: effect of collagen concentration and phosphate buffer, *Anal. Biochem.*, 94, 308, 1979.
32. Shipley, G. D. and Ham, R. G., Improved medium and culture condition for clonal growth with minimal serum protein and enhanced serum free survival of Swiss 3T3 cells, *In Vitro*, 17, 671, 1981.
33. Buck, C. A. and Horwitz, A. F., Cell surface receptors for extracellular matrix molecules, *Annu. Rev. Cell. Biol.*, 3, 179, 1987.
34. Graf, J., Iwamoto, Y., Sasaki, M., Martin, C. R., Kleinman, H. K., Robey, F. A., and Yamada, Y., Identification of an amino acid sequence in laminin mediating cell attachment, chemotaxis and receptor binding, *Cell*, 48, 989, 1987.
35. Kleinman, H. K., McGarrey, M. C., Hassell, R. R., Star, V. C., Cannon, F. B., Laurie, G. W., and Martin, G. R., Reconstituted basement membrane: a defined supramolecular complex with biological activity, *Biochemistry*, 25, 312, 1989.
36. Lechner, J., Haugen, A., McClendon, I. A., and Pettis, E. W., Clonal growth of normal adult human bronchial epithelial cells in a serum-free medium, *In Vitro*, 18, 633, 1982.
37. Misfeldt, D. S., Hamamoto, S. T., and Pitelka, D. R., Transepithelial transport in cell culture, *Proc. Natl. Acad. Sci. U.S.A.*, 73, 1212, 1976.
38. Cereijido, M., Robbins, E. S., Dolan, W. J., Rotunno, G. A., and Sabatini, D. D., Polarized monolayers formed by epithelial cells on a permeable and translucent support, *J. Cell Biol.*, 77, 853, 1978.
39. Simmons, N. L., Ion transport in "tight" epithelial monolayers of MDCK cells, *J. Membr. Biol.*, 59, 105, 1981.

40. Meier, K. E., Snavely, M. D., Brown, S. L., Brown, J. H., and Insel, P. A., Alpha$_1$- and beta$_2$-adrenergic receptor expression in the Madin-Darby canine kidney epithelial cell line., *J. Cell Biol.*, 97, 405, 1983.
41. Mullin, J. M., Weibel, J., Diamond, L., and Kleinzeller, A., Sugar transport in the LLC-PK$_1$ renal epithelial cell line: similarity to mammalian kidney and the influence of cell density, *J. Cell. Physiol.*, 104, 375, 1980.
42. Misfeldt, D. S. and Sanders, M. J., Transepithelial transport in cell culture: D-glucose transport by a pig kidney cell line (LLC-PK$_1$), *J. Membr. Biol.*, 59, 13, 1981.
43. Sepulveda, F. V. and Pearson, J. D., Amino acid transport in cultured kidney tubule cells, in *Tissue Culture of Epithelial Cells*, Taub, M., Ed., Plenum Press, New York, 1985, 87.
44. Fouda, A. K., Fauth, C., and Roch-Ramel, F., Transport of organic cations by kidney epithelial cell line LLC-PK$_1$, *J. Pharmacol. Exp. Ther.*, 252, 286, 1990.
45. Goldring, S. R., Dayer, J. M., Ausiello, D. A., and Krane, S. M., A cell strain cultured from porcine kidney increases cyclic AMP content upon exposure to calcitonin or vasopressin, *Biochem. Biophys. Res. Commun.*, 83, 434, 1978.
46. Segal, J. H. and Pollock, A. S., Transfection-mediated expression of a dominant cAMP-resistant phenotype in the opossum kidney (OK) cell line prevents parathyroid hormone-induced inhibition of Na-phosphate cotransport, *J. Clin. Invest.*, 86, 1442, 1990.
47. Gstraunthaler, G. and Handler, J. S., Isolation, growth and characterization of a gluconeogenic strain of renal cells, *Am. J. Physiol.*, 252, C232, 1987.
48. Robinson, P. S. and Goochee, C.F., Kidney-specific enzyme expression by human kidney cell lines generated through oncogene transfection, *J. Cell. Physiol.*, 148, 54, 1991.
49. Chou, J. Y., Establishment of rat fetal liver lines and characterization of their metabolic and hormonal properties: use of temperature-sensitive SV40 virus, *Methods Enzymol.*, 109, 385, 1985.
50. Prie, D., Ronco, P. M., Baudouin, B., Geniteau-Legendre, M., Antoine, M., Piedagnel, R., Estrade, S., Lelong, B., Berroust, P. J., Cassingena, R., and Vandewalle, A. K., Activation of the Simian Virus 40 (SV40) genome abrogates sensitivity to AVP in a rabbit collecting tubule cell line by repressing membrane expression of AVP receptors, *J. Cell Biol.*, 113, 951, 1991.
51. Willey, J. C., Broussoud, A., Sleemi, A., Bennett, W. P., Cerutti, P., and Harris, C. C., Immortalization of normal human bronchial epithelial cells by human papilloma viruses 16 or 18, *Cancer Res.*, 51, 5370, 1991.
52. Sun, Q., Tsutsumi, K., Kelleher, M. B., Pater, A., and Pater, M. M., Squamous metaplasia of normal and carcinoma *in situ* of HPV 16-immortalized human endocervical cells, *Cancer Res.*, 52, 4254, 1992.
53. Inoue, H., Kondoh, G., Kamakurah, C. R., Yutsudo, M., and Hakura, A., Progression of rat embryo fibroblast cells immortalized with transforming genes of human papilloma virus type 16, *Virology*, 180, 191, 1991.
54. Pagano, M., Durst, M., Joswig, S., Draetta, G., and Jansen-Durr, P., Binding of the human E2F transcription factor to the retinoblastoma protein but not to cyclin A is abolished in HPV-16-immortalized cells, *Oncogene*, 7, 1681, 1992.
55. Band, V., De Caprio, J. A., Delmolino, L., Kulesa, V., and Sager, R., Loss of p53 protein in human papilloma virus type H E6-immortalized human mammary epithelial cells, *J. Virol.*, 655, 6671, 1991.
56. Romero, M. F., Douglas, J. G., Eckert, R. L., Hopfer, U., and Jacobberger, J. W., Development and characterization of rabbit proximal tubular epithelial cell lines, *Kidney Int.*, 42, 1340, 1992.
57. Ruley, H. E., Adenovirus early region 1A enables viral and cellular transforming genes to transform primary cells in culture, *Nature*, 304, 602, 1983.
58. Haber, D. A., Timmers, H. T. M., Pelletier, J., Sharp, P. A., and Housman, D. E., A dominant mutation in the Wilms tumor gene in transformation of primary kidney cells, *Proc. Natl. Acad. Sci. U.S.A.*, 89, 6010, 1992.
59. Young, K. S., Weigel, R., Hiebert, S., and Nevins, J. R., Adenovirus E1-A-mediated negative control of genes activated during F9 differentiation, *Mol. Cell. Biol.*, 9, 3109, 1989.
60. Mymryk, J. S., Lee, R. W. H., and Bayley, S. T., Ability of adenovirus 5 E1A proteins to suppress differentiation of BC$_3$H$_1$ myoblasts correlates with their binding to a 300 kDa cellular protein, *Mol. Biol. Cell.*, 3, 1107, 1992.

61. Heasley, L. E., Benedict, S., Gleavy, J., and Johnson, G. L., Requirement of the adenovirus E1A transformation domain 1 for inhibition of PC12 cell neuronal differentiation, *Cell Regul.*, 2, 479, 1991.
62. Noguchi, M., Murakami, M., Bennett, W., Lupu, R., Hui, F., Jr., Harris, C. C., and Gerwin, B. I., Biological consequences of overexpression of a transfected c-erb B-2 gene in immortalized human bronchial epithelial cells, *Cancer Res.*, 53, 2035, 1993.
63. Gabrielson, E. W., Van der Meeren, A., Reddel, R. R., Reddel, H., Gerwin, B. I., and Harris, C. C., Human mesothelioma cells and asbestos-exposed mesothelial cells are selectively resistant to amosite toxicity: a possible mechanism for tumor promotion by asbestos, *Carcinogenesis*, 13, 1359, 1992.
64. Kaighn, M. E., Reddel, R. R., Lechner, J. F., Peehl, D. M., Camalier, R. F., Brash, D. E., Saffiotti, U., and Harris, C. C., Transformation of human neonatal prostate epithelial cells by strontium phosphate transfection with a plasmid containing SV40 early region genes, *Cancer Res.*, 49, 3050, 1989.
65. Parda, D. S., Thraves, P. J., Kuettal, M. R., Lee, M. S., Arnstein, P., Kaighn, M. E., Rhim, J. S., and Dritschilo, A., Neoplastic transformation of a human prostate epithelial cell line by the v-Ki-ras oncogene, *Prostate*, 23, 91, 1993.
66. Cook, W. F. and Pickering, G. W., A rapid method for separating glomeruli from rabbit kidney, *Nature*, 182, 1103, 11958.

chapter thirteen

Methods in Renal Carcinogenesis and Mutagenesis

R. Rita Misra, Bhalchandra A. Diwan, Deborah E. Devor, Jerrold M. Ward, and Michael P. Waalkes

13.1 Introduction 237
13.2 Renal anatomy 238
13.3 Descriptive histomorphology of rodent renal tumors 239
13.4 Experimental induction of renal tumors in rodents 239
 13.4.1 Induction of renal cell tumors 240
 13.4.2 Induction of renal transitional cell tumors 242
 13.4.3 Induction of nephroblastomas 243
 13.4.4 Induction of mesenchymal tumors 243
13.5 Renal mutagenesis 244
 13.5.1 Cytogenetic analysis 244
 13.5.2 Southern blot–restriction fragment length polymorphism analysis 244
 13.5.3 Polymerase chain reaction based techniques 244
  13.5.3.1 Single-strand conformation polymorphism analysis 245
  13.5.3.2 Denaturing gradient gel electrophoresis 245
  13.5.3.3 RNase a cleavage 246
  13.5.3.4 Chemical mismatch cleavage 247
  13.5.3.5 Direct sequencing 247
 13.5.4 Summary of renal mutagenesis 247
13.6 Necropsy and associated techniques in renal pathology 248
 13.6.1 Enzyme histochemistry/immunohistochemistry 248
 13.6.2 DNA and RNA isolation techniques 249
References 249

13.1 Introduction

Many chemical and physical agents can affect the intricate process of heredity, and clearly one of the most important results of this type of effect is carcinogenesis. Mutations, the probable basis to this effect, occur when the cell either inserts incorrect nucleotides, omits nucleotides, or adds unnecessary nucleotides within DNA. Mutational alterations inducing inactivation or overexpression of critical genes may result in a variety of disorders, including cancer. The probability that a particular chemical will cause genetic damage leading to cancer inevitably depends on a series of interdependent variables, including

0-8493-3341-5/96/$0.00+$.50

organism exposure level, tissue distribution and retention, activities of biotransformation systems, the ability of the affected cell to either repair or amplify genetic damage, and the ability of the body to recognize and suppress the multiplication of transformed cells.

The kidney may be particularly sensitive to pathologic insult for a variety of reasons.[1] Being the major excretory organ with a high blood flow, the kidney is exposed to any number of possibly noxious chemicals. The concentrating mechanisms found in the kidney for urine formation can also favor concentration of potential toxicants. Intrarenal xenobiotic metabolism, though quantitatively minor compared to the liver, is significant and can result in the local formation of toxic reactive metabolites, including electrophiles and free radicals.[1] The kidney is an extremely complex organ with a wide variety of functions, ranging from waste elimination to hormone production, and contains many specialized cell populations that likely have an extensive range of individual sensitivities to potential toxicants.

Probably the most reliable approach to predicting the human carcinogenic potential of a given chemical, in the absence of direct data, is the carcinogenicity bioassay.[2] In combination with mechanistic studies on the organ at both the cellular and molecular levels, rodent tumor data can prove invaluable in predicting risk. In this regard, nearly all the pathologic types of renal tumors observed in man have been duplicated experimentally in rodents using various chemical or physical means.[2-4] The pattern of tumor development, where tumors of epithelial origin predominate, is similar in humans and experimental animals,[2] indicating similar or comparable etiologies.

In this chapter we discuss the methods that are currently being used to investigate renal carcinogenesis and mutagenesis. The discussion focuses on determination of renal mutagenesis and induction of renal tumors in experimental animals. Necropsy techniques directed at proper renal dissection and descriptive histomorphology of rodent renal tumors are also included.

13.2 Renal anatomy

Rodent kidneys are unique paired organs in terms of location, which is remarkably consistent among mammals. While often considered as visceral organs of the abdominal cavity, they, their associated lymph nodes, and the adrenals actually lie outside the cavity, i.e., retroperitoneal, dorsal to the liver and stomach. In addition to the peritoneum separating the organs from the rest of the abdominal contents, each kidney is encased in a relatively tough renal capsule. Both organs are supplied with blood via the renal arteries and veins branching off the abdominal aorta and the inferior vena cava, respectively. In healthy, nonobese animals, fat accumulation occurs laterally and around the hilus and is unusual on the ventral or dorsal surfaces. There are age and sex differences in organ size and weight within species.

The right kidney rests higher than the left, and its apical pole may actually lie in the thoracic cavity, level with the first lumbar vertebra. It is largely obscured by the right lateral lobes of the liver and the intestines and mesenteries in a typical ventral dissection. One of the vital considerations in the removal of the right kidney is the proximity of some major blood vessels that lie in tight conjunction to the ventral surface, frequently forming adhesions to the renal capsule. These include the hepatic and superior mesenteric arteries and the portal veins. While either organ can be exposed using a dorsal incision, the left kidney is considered a more attractive choice for nephrectomy, cannulation, and other procedures requiring manipulation of a single organ.

The left kidney sits lower relative to the right by about one fourth to one to half its length, but there can be great variation between animals. Access to the left kidney, in a normal ventral approach, is straightforward compared to the right organ, requiring only the shifting of the spleen, stomach, and intestines to expose it. The left renal artery and vein are occasionally longer, as measured from the branching off the aorta and vena cava, and more prominent due to the lack of interference or overshadowing by other structures.

Internally, the kidney is composed of three major areas or zones that are grossly discernible in a good medial cross or longitudinal section. The outermost layer is the cortex, which contains the glomeruli and the renal corpuscles, the proximal and distal convoluted tubules, and the peritubular capillary beds. Beneath the cortex is the outer medulla, which consists of two bands of tissue — the outer and inner stripe — that are fairly well demarcated in larger organs. The outer stripe of the medulla contains the straight portions of both proximal and distal tubules and collecting ducts, and the inner stripe is made up of thin descending limbs and thick ascending limbs of the loops of Henle and collecting ducts. The transition from the pars recta of proximal tubules to the descending thin limb of the loop of Henle occurs at the junction of the inner and outer stripes. The inner medulla, also known as the renal papilla, contains descending and ascending thin limbs of Henle's loops of juxtamedullary nephrons and collecting tubules. Glomeruli, segments of the nephron, and collecting ducts are epithelial structures[5-8] and give rise to the more common renal tubular and, rarely, to transitional cell tumors.[4]

The amount of interstitial tissue increases from the cortex inward such that approximately one third of the volume of the papilla is composed of interstitial cells (primarily monocytes, pericytes, and stellate cells), stroma, and mucopolysaccharides.[5-8] The less common renal mesenchymal tumors and sarcomas are derived from these tissues.[4] Nephroblastomas may also arise from the interstitium, probably from undifferentiated mesonephric remnants.[4]

13.3 *Descriptive histomorphology of rodent renal tumors*

Spontaneous renal tumors are uncommon in most strains of rats and mice except for the Eker rat, a strain with a high incidence of hereditary renal tumors and nephropathy.[9] Tumors may arise in the kidney(s) of rodents from various cell types.[4,10–12] Most commonly, renal tumors arise from renal tubular epithelium. In the renal tubules, the origin may occur from the S2 or S3 segment of the proximal tubules or from distal tubules, the former being much more common. The earliest lesions induced by carcinogens or found spontaneously are renal tubular dysplasias (atypical hyperplasias). Renal tubular adenomas are well-circumscribed nodules composed of well-differentiated cells forming one of several morphological patterns. These patterns include solid, tubular (Figure 1), and papillary types. Solid tumors may be basophilic, eosinophilic, clear, or oncolytic. Renal tubular carcinomas may arise from adenoma or *in situ* and are invasive and malignant in appearance. They may also have the same solid patterns as adenomas (Figure 2) and may also be anaplastic. They invade adjacent tissues and have morphological characteristics of carcinoma. Metastatic renal tubular carcinomas are often of the anaplastic type (Figure 3), but are uncommon except when induced by certain carcinogens, including lead.

Other renal tumors may arise from the pelvic transitional epithelium (transitional cell papillomas and carcinomas) and renal mesenchyme (lipoma, liposarcoma, fibrosarcoma, nephroblastoma, and renal mesenchymal tumors in rats). Mesenchymal tumors are most often seen in rats after exposure to specific carcinogens (Figure 4) and are composed of varying populations of mesenchymal elements. They rarely occur spontaneously and rarely metastasize. Spontaneous lipomatous tumors are occasionally seen in certain strains of rats and, when they occur, can metastasize in high incidence.

13.4 *Experimental induction of renal tumors in rodents*

A wide variety of chemicals have been shown to be capable of inducing malignant renal tumors in rodents. A brief description of studies related to the experimental induction of

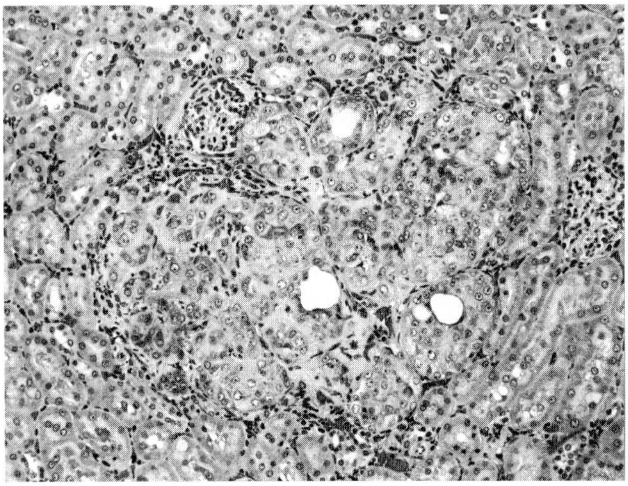

Figure 1 Renal tubular cell adenoma showing some tubule formation (H&E; original magnification × 150).

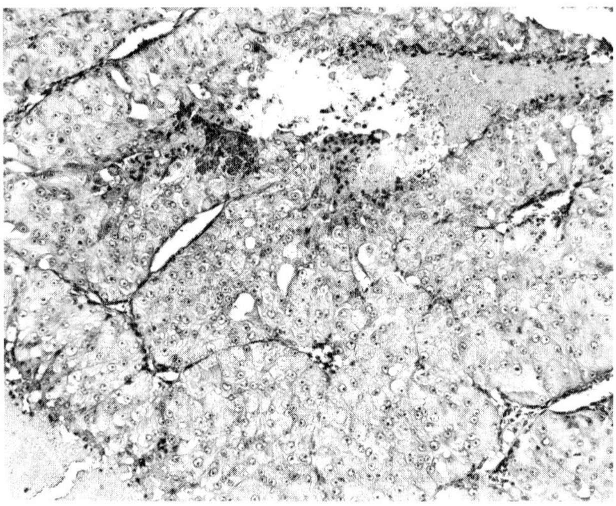

Figure 2 Well-differentiated renal tubular cell adenocarcinoma showing cells with abundant cytoplasm (H&E; original magnification × 150).

major types of renal tumors will be reviewed here. Greater details are available in several recent comprehensive reviews.[1,3,13] For precise technical details, readers should direct themselves to the original source work.

13.4.1 Induction of renal cell tumors

Renal cell tumors (adenomas and adenocarcinomas) are derived from renal tubular epithelial cells and constitute 90% of the total renal tumors diagnosed in rats, mice, and other mammals, including humans.[1,3,13–17] Renal cell tumors are induced by a variety of agents including nitrosoureas, nitrosamines, some inorganic reagents (including transition metals), mycotoxins, and some solvents (Table 1).[1,3,13,18-26] The most widely used agents for sequential observations on the appearance of neoplastic lesions in rats and mice include

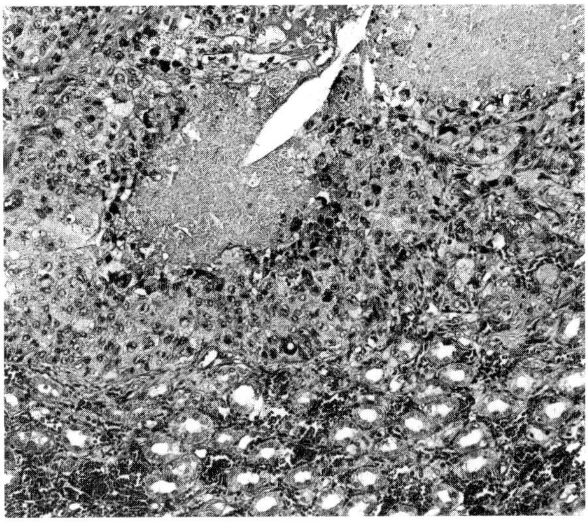

Figure 3 Poorly differentiated renal tubular cell carcinoma with prominent central necrosis (H&E; original magnification × 150).

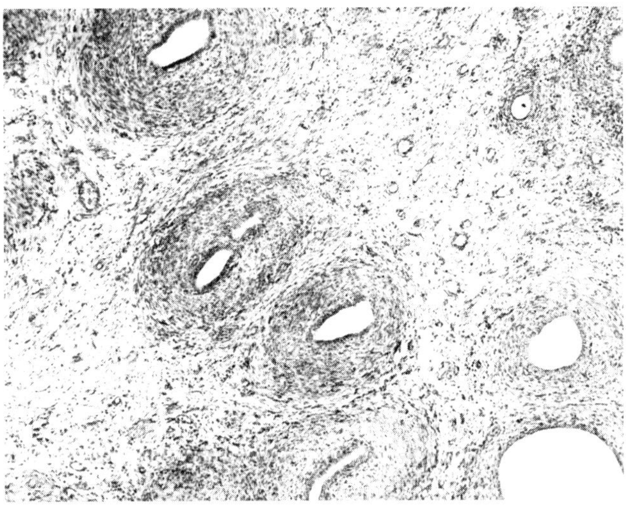

Figure 4 Malignant mesenchymal tumor of rat kidney with variable patterns of growth (H&E; original magnification × 75).

strong carcinogens such as *N*-nitrosoethylurea (ENU); *N*-nitrosomorpholine (NNM); *N*-4-(4´-fluorobiphenyl)acetamide (FBPA); diethylnitrosamine (NDEA); and dimethylnitrosamine (NDMA). These carcinogens have been shown to induce renal cell tumors after a single administration or limited exposure period in rats and mice. Thus, induction of renal cell tumors in mice has been achieved by injecting them with a single dose of ENU or streptozotocin.[18,19] Similarly, a high incidence (60 to 78%) of renal tubular cell tumors had been induced in rats given 1000 to 2000 ppm of *N*-ethyl-*N*-hydroxyethylnitrosamine (EHEN) in the diet for two weeks.[1,3,20]

The two-stage carcinogenesis phenomenon described first in the skin of mice has also been demonstrated in renal cell carcinogenesis. Thus, there are several reports in the literature that illustrate modification of renal tumorigenesis by a variety of chemicals

Table 1 Induction of Renal Cell Tumors

Species	Chemical	Treatment	Incidence	Ref.
Rat	EHEN	Diet (2000 ppm for 2 wks)	78%	1, 20
Rat	FBPA	Diet (400 ppm for 36 wks)	50%	21
Rat	LA	Diet (10,000 ppm for 72 wks)	98%	22
Rat	$KBrO_3$	Diet (500 ppm for 96 wks)	88%	23
Mouse	Phenacetin	Diet (12,500 ppm for 104 wks)	67%	24
Rat	4NQO	Diet (10 mg/kg for 72 wks)	66%	55
Mouse	DCA	Inhalation (9 ppm for 48 wks)	76%	26

Note: EHEN, *N*-ethyl-*N*-hydroxyethylnitrosamine; FBPA, *N*-4-(4′-fluorobiphenyl)-acetamide; LA, lead acetate; $KBrO_3$, potassium bromate; 4NQO, 4-hydroxyaminoquinoline *N*-oxide; DCA, dichloroacetylene.

including β-cyclodextrin, DL-serine, lead acetate, trisodium nitrilotriacetate monohydrate, potassium bromate, nicotinamide, carbon tetrachloride, sodium barbital, and its metabolite 5-ethyl-phenyl acetylurea.[1,3,27,28] Table 2 shows the initiation–promotion studies in rats that result in a 50 to 100% incidence of renal cell tumors. Many nongenotoxic agents that enhance renal cell carcinogenesis have been shown to be nephrotoxins and cause degenerative and regenerative hyperplasia (cell proliferation) in proximal convoluted tubules.[1,3,28-30] Most of these modifiers of renal cell tumorigenesis when administered alone can also induce renal cell tumors in both mice and rats.[1-3] However, in contrast to genotoxic renal carcinogens they are effective only when administered at high doses and over prolonged periods of time. For example, repeated injections of iron–nitrilotriacetate complex (Fe-NaNTA) induce renal cell tumors in rats,[31] while chronic administration of potassium bromate and lead acetate in either diet or drinking water induces a high incidence of renal cell tumors in several strains of rats.[1-3]

Table 2 Promotion of Renal Cell Tumors in Rats

Initiator	Promoter	Incidence	Ref.
EHEN (1000 ppm, p.o.; in diet for 2 wks)	β-c (450 mg/k, s.c.; daily for 1 wk)	100%	1, 3
	DL-serine (1000 mg/kg, s.c.; biweekly for 6 wks)	100%	1, 3
	LA (1000 ppm, p.o.; in diet for 30 wks)	100%	1, 3
	Kbro3 (500 ppm, p.o.; in diet for 30 wks)	47%	1, 3
	Na3NTA (1000 ppm, p.o.; in diet for 30 wks)	100%	1, 31
NDEA (75 mg/kg, i.p.; single dose)	NaBB (500 ppm, p.o.; in diet for 70 wks)	50%	27
	EPAU (500 ppm, p.o.; in diet for 70 wks)	50%	28

Note: p.o., per os; s.c., subcutaneous; i.p., intraperitoneal; EHEN, *N*-ethyl-*N*-hydroxyethylnitrosamine; NDEA, *N*-nitrosodiethylamine; β-c, β-cyclodextrin; LA, lead acetate; Kbro3, potassium bromate; Na3NTA, trisodium nitrilotriacetate; NaBB, sodium barbital; EPAU, ethylphenylacetylurea.

13.4.2 *Induction of renal transitional cell tumors*

Renal transitional cell tumors are induced in rats by a variety of nongenotoxic and genotoxic chemicals (Table 3).[1,3,32,33] In addition, a low incidence of pelvic transitional cell tumors is induced in rats by genotoxic carcinogens such as *N*-nitrosomethylurea (NMU), di-isopropanolamine, and *N*-[4-(5-nitro-2-furyl)-2-thiazolyl]formamide.[1-3] NaBB promotes pelvic tumors of transitional cell origin initiated by NDEA in rats.[27,28] Some nongenotoxic compounds, including phenacetin, paracetamol, caffeine, and phenazone, may also induce transitional cell neoplasm in rats.[1,3,34]

Table 3 Induction of Renal Transitional Cell Tumors

Species	Chemical	Treatment	Incidence	Ref.
Rat	DHPN	Water (2000 ppm for 3 wks)	50%	1, 3
Rat	NFTA	Diet (2000 ppm)	50%	32
Rat	OPP-Na	Diet (4000 ppm)	50%	1
Rat	DIPN	Single dose (s.c. for 20 wks)	41%	33

Note: DHPN, *N*-bis(2-hydroxypropyl)nitrosamine; NFTA, *N*-[4-(5-nitro-2-furyl)-2-thiazolyl]acetamide; OPP-NA, methylazoxymethanol-beta-D-glucosiduronic acid; DIPN, di-isopropanolnitrosamine.

13.4.3 *Induction of nephroblastomas*

Nephroblastomas have been induced in rats and mice after treatment with several chemical agents (Table 4).[1,3,35-38] They are predominantly found in offspring of rats and mice exposed transplacentally or neonatally to ENU, NMU, and dimethylbenz(*a*)anthracene (DMBA).[1,3,35] Some strains of rats (e.g., Noble rats) and rabbits are particularly susceptible to the induction of nephroblastomas after transplacental treatment with ENU.[35,38]

Table 4 Induction of Nephroblastoma

Species	Chemical	Treatment	Incidence	Ref.
Rat NB	ENU	Single dose (i.p., transplacental, 60 mg/kg)	47–50%	35
Rat	NMU	Single dose (s.c., 2–4 days after birth, 50 mg/kg)	42%	36
Opossum	ENU	Single dose (s.c., 1–6 wks after birth, 100 mg/kg)	30%	37
Rabbit	ENU	Single dose (i.p., transplacental, 60 mg/kg)	80%	38

Note: ENU, ethylnitrosourea; NMU, methylnitrosourea.

13.4.4 *Induction of mesenchymal tumors*

Renal mesenchymal tumors are induced in mice and rats by a variety of chemical carcinogens, including NDMA, NMU, cycasin, ethyl methanesulfonate, dimethylhydrazine, and streptozotocin (Table 5).[1,3,39-41] They are also induced by transplacental treatment with ENU in rats.[39] The compound most widely used to induce mesenchymal tumors in rats is NDMA. These tumors occur in a high incidence in rats exposed to NDMA at a very young age.[40] Direct injections of some nickel compounds have also been shown to induce a high incidence of malignant renal mesenchymal tumors in adult rats.[42]

Table 5 Induction of Renal Mesenchymal Tumors

Species	Chemical	Treatment	Incident	Ref.
Rat	DMN	Single dose (i.p., 30 mg/kg at 4 wks of age)	70%	40
Rat	DHPN	Water (2000 ppm for 3 wks)	50%	1, 3
Rat	Cycasin	Single dose (s.c., 408 mg/kg)	38%	1, 3
Rat	DMH	Two doses (s.c., 120 mg/kg)	90%	41
Rat	NMU	Single dose (s.c., 2–4 days after birth, 50 mg/kg)	42%	36
Rat	Ni_3S_2	Two doses (intrarenal, 5 mg per dose)	60%	42

Note: DMN, dimethylnitrosamine; DHPN, *N*-bis(2-hydroxypropyl)nitrosamine; DMH, 1,2-dimethylhydrazine; NMU, methylnitrosourea; Ni_3S_2, nickel subsulfide.

13.5 Renal mutagenesis

In recent years a variety of molecular methods have been used to detect and characterize mutations in renal tumors from humans and rodents. In most cases the objective of such studies has been (1) to identify particular oncogenes or tumor suppressor genes involved in tumor initiation or progression or (2) to understand better how a particular carcinogenic agent interacts with the genetic material to induce disease. Using the methods described below investigators have thus far analyzed DNA collected from spontaneous and chemically induced renal tumors and generated mutational spectra for *ras* proto-oncogenes[43-45] and the tumor suppressor genes p53,[46,47] WT1,[48,49] and VHL.[50,51]

In reviewing the literature it immediately becomes apparent that the method used for mutation screening is best determined by the expected nature of the mutation, the size and sequence of the gene in question, the degree of sensitivity required, and perhaps most important, the experimental resources available.

13.5.1 Cytogenetic analysis

Extremely large (> 1 million bases) insertions, deletions, and translocations can often be detected by high-resolution cytogenetics and the use of fluorescent *in situ* hybridization (FISH).[52] According to this method, fluorescently labeled DNA probes are hybridized to metaphase chromosome or interphase chromatin preparations to detect the presence, absence, or translocation of the region of the chromosome corresponding to the target gene. One advantage of this technique is that multiple probes labeled with different fluorescent dyes can be hybridized and analyzed simultaneously. The most obvious disadvantage of this technique is its lack of sensitivity.

13.5.2 Southern blot–restriction fragment length polymorphism analysis

Southern blot–restriction fragment length polymorphism (RFLP) analysis[53] is one of the fastest ways to screen for certain types of mutations and may therefore be an ideal starting point in any experimental scheme (Figure 5). The main advantage of this method is that detailed knowledge of the sequence of a gene is not required; analysis can begin as soon as a probe for the target gene has been isolated. According to this technique, DNA is isolated from the tumor tissue and cut with appropriate restriction endonucleases. The DNA fragments are then separated according to their size by agarose gel electrophoresis, transferred by capillary transfer to nylon or nitrocellulose membranes, and subsequently hybridized to a labeled probe. After autoradiographic visualization, relatively large insertions and deletions can be detected by the presence of novel fragments and/or changes in band intensities. Point mutations may also be detected if they inactivate or create new restriction sites and thus change the fragment pattern observed. The main disadvantages of this method include the requirement for relatively large amounts of DNA ($\geq 10\ \mu g$) and a size limitation for the genes that can be analyzed (i.e., portions of very large genes will escape analysis due to restriction sites contained within the gene).

13.5.3 Polymerase chain reaction based techniques

The ability to accurately replicate DNA *in vitro* via the polymerase chain reaction (PCR)[54] has revolutionized mutation detection technology by obviating the requirement for large amounts of DNA. The methods described below all employ PCR amplification prior to mutation analysis.

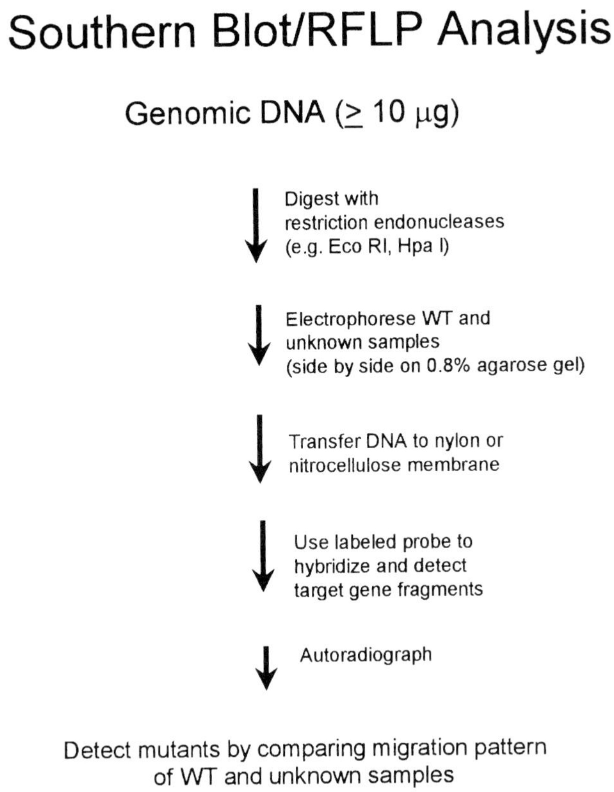

Figure 5 Southern blot–restriction fragment length polymorphism (RFLP) analysis. For further details see Southern.[53] WT = wild type.

13.5.3.1 Single-strand conformation polymorphism analysis

Analysis of single-strand conformation polymorphisms (SSCP) to detect mutations in particular genes was first reported by Orita et al. in 1989.[55] Since then it has become the most widely used method for mutation screening. In this technique (Figure 6), labeled oligonucleotide primers are used to PCR-amplify particular segments, typically individual exons, of the target gene. Amplified samples of wild-type and mutant DNA are subsequently denatured and then electrophoresed side by side through a non-denaturing polyacrylamide gel. During migration, the two single-stranded DNA molecules from each denatured PCR product assume a three-dimensional conformation that is dependent on the primary sequence of each strand and the temperature during electrophoresis. If a mutation exists, it usually results in differential migration of one or both of the mutant strands. Once an altered migration pattern has been identified, the corresponding PCR product is sequenced to determine the exact nature and location of the mutation observed. One big advantage of the SSCP method is the fact that multiple samples can be analyzed simultaneously. Regarding the sensitivity of the method, it has been estimated that 85% of mutations in a given gene segment of up to 400 bp in length can be routinely detected.[56,57]

13.5.3.2 Denaturing gradient gel electrophoresis

Another analytical method that relies on differential migration of wild-type and mutant fragments of DNA is denaturing gradient gel electrophoresis (DGGE). According to this technique, PCR-generated fragments of labeled double-stranded DNA are electrophoresed through a gradient of a denaturing agent (urea and formamide) in a polyacrylamide gel.

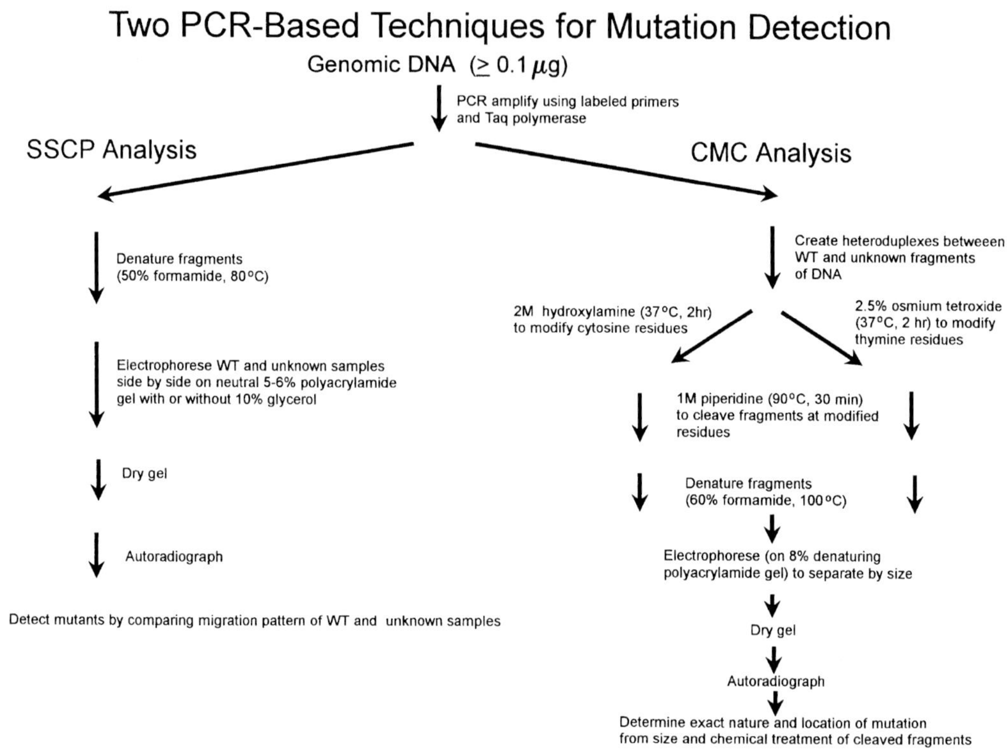

Figure 6 Two examples of polymerase chain reaction PCR-based techniques for the detection of mutations: single-strand conformation polymorphism (SSCP)[55] analysis and chemical mismatch cleavage (CMC).[62] WT = wild type.

During migration the strands dissociate in discrete sequence-dependent domains of low melting temperature. This partial melting of duplex strands leads to abrupt decreases in mobility. For example, molecules differing by only a single base substitution have been shown to migrate differently in DGGE gels.[58] The sensitivity of DGGE is also greatly enhanced if heteroduplexes, formed by mixing potential mutant and wild-type DNA fragments, are used for analysis. Since the initial development of this technique investigators have discovered that mutations are most easily detected when they fall within a domain of relatively low melting temperature. This can be achieved for almost any sequence of interest by adding a 40-mer "GC clamp" to one of the PCR primers used for fragment amplification, thereby creating a domain with a very high melting temperature at one end of the fragment.[59] Although it is possible that mutations in high GC rich regions may present a problem, it is estimated that DGGE can routinely detect up to 100% of mutations in gene fragments up to 600 bp in length.[55,57] Again, once an altered pattern of migration has been identified, the corresponding PCR product is sequenced to determine the exact nature and location of the mutation.

13.5.3.3 *RNase A cleavage*

In the RNase A cleavage method, radioactive RNA probes (complementary to the gene of interest) and PCR-amplified mutant DNA are mixed together to form RNA–DNA heteroduplexes. RNase A is then used to recognize and cleave single-strand RNA at the points of mismatch with the DNA strand, and the samples are subsequently analyzed by electrophoresis and autoradiography.[60] On the gels, the presence and location of a mutation are indicated by a labeled band of shortened size. The main disadvantage of the RNase A cleavage technique is the fact that RNase A routinely detects only 50% of all mismatches. This makes it considerably less sensitive than SSCP or DGGE.

13.5.3.4 Chemical mismatch cleavage

The principle behind the chemical mismatch cleavage (CMC) technique, as illustrated in Figure 6, also involves creating heteroduplexes, but in this case, the heteroduplexes are between wild-type and mutant DNA. Maxam–Gilbert sequencing chemistry is then used to modify mismatched bases at sites where melting occurs. The labeled heteroduplexes are cleaved by piperidine at the mismatch sites, and the samples are subjected to denaturing polyacrylamide gel electrophoresis and autoradiography. According to this technique, osmium tetroxide is used to modify mispaired thymines, and hydroxylamine is used for mismatched cytosines.[61] It is estimated that this method can detect up to 100% of mismatches when both wild-type and mutant DNA are labeled.[56,57] Furthermore, PCR products greater than 1 kb can be successfully examined,[56] and the precise location and nature of the mutation can usually be determined by the size of the cleaved fragment and the cleaving reagent used.

13.5.3.5 Direct sequencing

Although each of the methods described above is capable of detecting mutations in DNA, with the exception of chemical mismatch cleavage, none is capable of determining the precise nature of the genetic alteration. DNA sequencing, therefore, often becomes the necessary last step in mutation characterization. The Sanger dideoxy chain termination method is most commonly used for direct sequencing,[62] and either radioactive (using ^{32}P or ^{35}S) or fluorescence detection may be employed. According to the standard direct sequencing method, double-stranded PCR products must first be converted into single-stranded sequencing templates. This can be accomplished in one of two ways: in the first technique, "asymmetric PCR,"[63] the PCR product is reamplified in a reaction in which one of the oligo primers is present in 100-fold excess of the other primer. In the second technique, one of the PCR primers is biotinylated so the double-stranded PCR product can be captured on avidin-coated magnetic beads. The nonbiotinylated strand is subsequently removed from the beads with NaOH, and the immobilized strand is collected for sequencing.[64] The sequencing process itself involves DNA polymerase and dideoxy and arabinonucleoside analogs of normal deoxynucleoside triphosphates, which act as specific chain-terminating inhibitors of the enzyme — for example, when primer and template are incubated with DNA polymerase in the presence of dideoxyTTP (ddTTP) as well as the other three normal nucleotides (one of which is labeled), a mixture of fragments all having the same 5′ end with ddTTP at the 3′ ends is obtained. When this mixture is separated by electrophoresis on denaturing polyacrylamide gels, the pattern of bands shows the distribution of deoxythymidines in the newly synthesized DNA. By using terminators for the other nucleotides in separate incubations and running the samples in parallel on a gel, a pattern of bands is obtained from which the entire sequence of the DNA fragment can be determined. A modification of the Sanger sequencing technique termed "cycle sequencing"[65] has also recently been developed. In this modification, the template is simultaneously amplified and sequenced by adding terminators directly to the PCR reaction. Cycle sequencing has the distinct advantage of requiring very small amounts of template. However, when radioactive or fluorescent detection is used, the technique requires that the sequencing primer be end-labeled. A variety of sequencing kits based on these principles (e.g., Sequenase, United States Biochemical, Cleveland, OH) are also commercially available and widely used.

13.5.4 Summary of renal mutagenesis

Although all of the methods described above may detect genetic alterations, they do not provide any information on the biological significance of particular mutations. While some DNA sequence alterations, such as those causing frame shifts or chain terminations may be expected to impair protein function, other changes such as those leading to single amino acid substitutions or changes in introns or untranslated regions of the gene may be phenotypically irrelevant. In many cases, functional assays after *in vitro* expression may be required in order to determine the significance of a genetic change.

13.6 Necropsy and associated techniques in renal pathology

Before the actual dissection, it is important to remember why the tissue is being taken in the first place and to have all necessary procedures, instruments, and fixatives present. For routine light microscopy and some immunohistochemical analyses, there may be little more to do than remove and preserve the organs in the fixative appropriate for the morphological structure(s) and/or tissue markers. If DNA is to be isolated, aseptic technique and cryopreservation may be necessary. There is no single procedure that can be applied to cover all potential uses of tissue that will give optimal results in all analyses. The most frequent methods of tissue analysis are discussed briefly in subsequent sections.

The easiest way to remove the kidneys is to do so after the abdominal organs have been taken out. The organ should not be grasped directly with forceps because the tissue is not as firm as it appears and has a friable texture that is easy to tear and puncture. Instead, forceps should be used to lift up on the caudal fat or the renal vessels near the hilus (avoiding the renal papilla, which may be obscured by fat and connective tissues), and scissors should be slid beneath to sever attachments. For optimal fixation and accurate examination and weight, the renal capsule should be removed. This can be accomplished without damage to the organ itself by puncturing the membrane at the hilus where there is some slack, inserting closed scissor points into the opening, and opening the points to spread the capsule off the surface to where it can be gently peeled away.[66] Once removed and denuded of capsule the organ(s) can be preserved for routine microscopy or further manipulated for special techniques such as histochemistry or DNA/RNA extraction. It should be emphasized that whatever other methods are used to evaluate the kidney, equivalent H&E sections are necessary to serve as morphological and diagnostic guides.

13.6.1 Enzyme histochemistry/immunohistochemistry

Enzyme histochemistry can be used to investigate the characteristic alterations in cellular enzymes that occur in nephropathies and tumorigenesis. There is often little difference, other than the substrate and end point, between enzyme analysis and immunohistochemistry, which involves the selective binding of antibodies raised to specific cellular constituents. They are valuable adjuncts to routine histology and to molecular techniques and have the advantage of showing the *in situ* location and rough quantification of the substrate in paraffin- or plastic-embedded slide-mounted sections,[67] as well as indicating tumor histogenesis. While all commercial kits available include fairly detailed instructions that tend to infer a "cookbook" approach, good and consistent enzyme/immunohistochemistry requires working knowledge of the disciplines that make up the names. Many factors influence the outcome of histochemical staining, first and foremost being the tissue itself and the preservative.[68,69] Autolytic tissue is not suitable for immunohistochemistry due to the degradation of both cellular structure and biochemical integrity. Neutral buffered formalin and Bouin's solution may be the most widely used fixatives that give good-to-excellent results for light microscopy and can be used for a wide range of immunological targets, but are not suitable in every instance. Tissues preserved in these fixatives may require digestion or microwaving to expose protein antigens optimally.[70] Other determining factors are the species from which the tissue was obtained, the effects of any *in vivo* experimental treatments on the tissues in question, the length of time in fixative or paraffin storage, the specificity and quality of the reagents, the conditions under which the tissue is incubated with immune markers, and the method of visualization of the conjugated moiety.[71-75]

13.6.2 DNA and RNA isolation techniques

The examination and analysis of normal and tumor DNA and RNA for mutations, translational products, and characterization is becoming a routine procedure in carcinogenesis assays. Fresh and frozen specimens are preferred, but are not always available. Both DNA and RNA are extractable from paraffin sections as well as from fresh, wet fixed, and frozen tissues.[76] At least one group has reported retrieval DNA fragments from highly degraded autolytic samples from a limited number of tissues.[77]

Many of the factors that determine the quality of enzyme and immunohistochemistry are equally important for purification of DNA/RNA.[78,79] If the analysis of nucleic acids is an end point, the necropsy procedure should be modified to incorporate aseptic technique, since contamination with foreign DNA is not only easy but highly likely if adequate precautions are not taken. Amplification by PCR is only primer-specific. If extraneous DNA contains binding sites compatible to the primer sequences used, it will be amplified as well. In some cases, "foreign" material may include normal or abnormal, tumorous or nontumorous, portions of the same organ.[80,81]

Fresh tissues, rinsed or perfused free of blood and other extraneous components, are immediately usable for purification of nucleic acids. Frozen tissues need only to be thawed and rinsed, if necessary. Various methods have been reported for DNA/RNA isolation and purification from preserved, paraffin-embedded tissue. In general, most practices involve removal of paraffin and the digestion of protein cross-links induced by most formalin-based fixatives. Noncross-linking fixatives such as ethanol, acetone, Omnifix, and AMeX (acetone/methyl benzoate/xylene) have been shown to increase the yields of high molecular DNA;[78,79,82] the AMeX method has also been shown to preserve RNA as well as a considerable number of antigens normally lost in formalin.[6]

References

1. Dietrich, D. R. and Swenberg, J. A., Renal carcinogenesis, in *Toxicology of the Kidney*, Hook, J. B. and Goldstein, R. S., Eds., Raven Press, New York, 1993, 495.
2. Hewitt, W. R., Goldstein, R. S., and Hook, J. B., Toxic responses of the kidney, in *Toxicology, The Basic Science of Poisons*, Amdur, M. O., Doull, J., and Klaassen, C. D., Eds., McGraw-Hill, New York, 1991, 354.
3. Hiasa, Y. and Ito, N., Experimental induction of renal tumors, *CRC Crit. Rev. Toxicol.*, 17, 279, 1987.
4. Konishi, N. and Hiasa, Y., Renal carcinogenesis, in *Carcinogenesis*, Waalkes, M. P. and Ward, J. M., Eds., Raven Press, New York, 1994, 123.
5. Alden, C. L. and Frith, C. H., Urinary system, Part 1, Kidney, in *Handbook of Toxicologic Pathology*, Haschek, W. M. and Rousseau, C. G., Eds., Academic Press, San Diego, 1991, 315.
6. Corman, B. J. and Owen, R. A., Normal development, growth, and aging of the kidney, in *Pathobiology of the Aging Rat, Vol. 1*, Mohr, U., Dungworth, D. L., and Capen, C. C., Eds., ILSI Press, Washington, D.C. 1992, 195.
7. Hummel, K. P., Richardson, F. L., and Fekete, E., Anatomy. Urinary system, in *Biology of the Laboratory Mouse, 2nd ed.*, Staff of the Jackson Laboratory, Eds., Dover, New York, 1966, 285.
8. Hebel, R. and Stromberg, M. W., *Anatomy of the Laboratory Rat*, Williams & Wilkins Co., Baltimore, 1976, 62.
9. Everitt, J. I., Goldsworthy, T. L., Wolf, D. C., and Walker, C. L. Hereditary renal cell carcinoma in the Eker rat: a rodent familial cancer syndrome, *J. Urol.*, 148, 1932, 1992.
10. Hard, G. D., Tumours of the kidney, renal pelvis and ureter, in *Pathology of Tumours in Laboratory Animals, Vol. 1*, Turusov, V. and Mohr, U., Eds., IARC Scientific, Lyon, 1990, 301.

11. Hard, G. C., Alden, C. L., Stula, E. F., and Trump, B. F., Proliferative lesions of the kidney in rats, Washington, D.C., Armed Forces Institute of Pathology (in press).
12. Frith, C. H., Terracini, B., and Turusov, V. S., Tumours of the kidney, renal pelvis and ureter, in *Pathology of Tumours in Laboratory Animals, Vol. 2*, Turusov, V. and Mohr, U., Eds., IARC Scientific, Lyon, 1994, 357.
13. Huff, J., Cirvello, J., Haseman, J., and Bucher, J., Chemicals associated with site-specific neoplasia in 1394 long-term carcinogenesis experiments in laboratory animals, *Environ. Health Perspect.*, 93, 247, 1991.
14. Baskin, G. B. and De Paoli, A., Primary renal neoplasm of the dog, *Vet. Pathol.*, 14, 591, 1977.
15. Sandison, A. T. and Anderson L. J., Tumors of kidney in cattle, sheep, and pigs, *Cancer Res.*, 21, 727, 1968.
16. Mostofi, F. K., Tumors of renal parenchyma, in *Kidney Disease; Present Status, vol. 1*, Churg, J., Spargo, B. H., Mostofi, F. K., Abell, M. R., Eds., Williams & Wilkins, Baltimore, 1979, 356.
17. Jones, S. R. and Casey, H. W., Primary renal tumors in nonhuman primates, *Vet. Pathol.*, 18, 89, 1981.
18. Lombard, L. S., Rice, J. M., and Vesselinovitch, D. S., Renal tumors in mice; light microscopic observation of epithelial tumors induced by ethylnitrosourea, *J. Natl. Cancer Inst.*, 53, 1677, 1974.
19. Hard, G. C., Identification of a high-frequency model for a renal carcinoma by the induction of renal tumors in the mouse with a single dose of streptozotocin, *Cancer Res.*, 45, 703, 1985.
20. Hiasa, Y., Ohshima, M., Iwata, C., and Tanikake, T., Histopathological studies on renal tubular cell tumors in rats treated with *N*-ethyl-*N*-hydroxyethylnitrosamine, *Gann*, 70, 817, 1979.
21. Reuber, M. D., A model for carcinoma of the kidney in Buffalo strain rats ingesting *N*-4-(4′-fluorobiphenyl)-acetamide, *Gann*, 65, 389, 1974.
22. Boyland, E., Dukes, C. E., Grover, P. L., and Mitchley, B. C. V., The induction of renal tumors by feeding lead acetate to rats, *Br. J. Cancer,* 16, 283, 1962.
23. Kurokawa, Y., Hayashi, Y., Maekawa, A., Takahashi, M, and Kokubo, T., Induction of renal cell tumors in F-344 rats by oral administration of potassium bromate, a food additive, *Gann*, 73, 335, 1982.
24. Nakanishi, K., Kurata, Y., Oshima, M., Fukushima, S., and Ito, N., Carcinogenicity of phenacetin: long-term feeding study in B6C3F1 mice, *Int. J. Cancer,* 29, 329, 1982.
25. Tucker, M. J., Carcinogenic action of quinoxaline 1,4-dioxide in rats, *J. Natl. Cancer Inst.*, 55, 137, 1975.
26. Reichert, D., Spengler, U., Romen, W., and Henschler, D., Carcinogenicity of dichloroacetylene: an inhalation study, *Carcinogenesis*, 5, 1411, 1984.
27. Diwan, B. A., Ohshima, M., and Rice, J. M., Promotion by sodium barbital of renal cortical and transitional cell tumors, but not intestinal tumors in F344/NCr rats given methyl(acetoxymethyl)nitrosamine and lack of effect of phenobarbital, amobarbital or barbituric acid on development of either renal or intestinal tumors, *Carcinogenesis,* 10, 183, 1989.
28. Diwan, B. A., Nims, R. W., Ward, J. M., Hu, H., Lubet, R. A., and Rice, J. M., Tumor promoting activities of ethylphenylacetylurea and diethylacetylurea, the ring hydrolysis products of barbiturate tumor promoters phenobarbital and barbital, in rat liver and kidney initiated by *N*-nitrosodiethylamine, *Carcinogenesis*, 10, 189, 1989.
29. Swenberg, J. A. and Short, B. G., Influence of cytotoxicity on the induction of tumors, in *Banbury Report: Nongenotoxic Mechanism of Carcinogenesis*, Butterworth, B. E. and Slaga, T. J., Eds., Cold Spring Harbor Laboratory Press, Cold Spring Harbor, NY, 1987, 151.
30. Hagiwara, A., Diwan, B. A., and Ward, J. M., Barbital sodium, a tumor promoter for kidney tubules, urinary bladder, and liver of the rat, induces persistent increases in levels of DNA synthesis in renal tubules but not urinary bladder epithelium or hepatocytes, *Fundam. Appl. Toxicol.*, 13, 332, 1989.
31. Ebina, Y., Okada, S., Hamazaki, S., Ogino, F., Jia-li, L., and Midorikawa, O., Nephrotoxicity and renal cell carcinoma after use of iron- and aluminium-nitrilotriacetate complexes in rats, *J. Natl. Cancer Inst.*, 76, 107, 1986.
32. Cohen, S., Erturke, E., Von Esch, A., Corvetti, A., and Bryan, G., Carcinogenicity of 5-nitrofurans and related compounds with amino-heterocyclic substituents, *J. Natl. Cancer Inst.*, 54, 841, 1975.

33. Reznick, G. and Mohr, U., Induction of renal pelvis tumors in Sprague–Dawley rats by di-isopropanolnitrosamine, *Cancer Lett.*, 2, 87, 1976.
34. Johanson, S. L., Carcinogenicity of analgesics: long-term treatment of Sprague–Dawley rats with phenacetin, phenazone, caffeine, and paracetamol(acetaminophen), *Int. J. Cancer*, 27, 521, 1981.
35. Hard, G., Comparative oncology. I. Nephroblastoma in laboratory animals, in *Wilms Tumor, Clinical and Biological Manifestations*, Pochedly, C. and Baum, E. S., Eds., Elsevier, New York, 1984, 147.
36. Sharma, P. M., Bowman, M., Yu, B.-F., and Sukumar, S., A rodent model for Wilms tumors: embryonal kidney neoplasms induced by *N*-nitroso-*N*′-methylurea, *Proc. Natl. Acad. Sci. U.S.A.*, 91, 9931, 1994.
37. Jurgelski, W., Hudson, P. M., and Falk, H. L., Embryonal neoplasms in the opossum: a new model for solid tumors of infancy and childhood, *Science*, 193, 328, 1976.
38. Fox, R. R., Diwan, B. A., and Meier, H. Transplacental induction of primary renal tumors in rabbits treated with 1-ethyl-1-nitrosourea, *J. Natl. Cancer Inst.*, 54, 1439, 1975.
39. Hard, G., Mesenchymal tumor, kidney, rat, in *Monographs on Pathology of Laboratory Animals, Urinary System*, Jones, T. C., Mohr, U., and Hunt, R. D., Eds., Springer-Verlag, New York, 1986, 61.
40. Hard, G. C., Effect of age at treatment on incidence and type of renal neoplasm induced in the rat by a single dose of dimethylnitrosamine, *Cancer Res.*, 39, 4965, 1979.
41. Sunter, J. P. and Senior, P. Y., Induction of renal tumors in rats by the administration of 1,2-dimethylhydrazine, *J. Pathol.*, 140, 69, 1983.
42. Kasprzak, K. S., Diwan, B. A., and Rice, J. M., Iron accelerates while magnesium inhibits nickel-induced carcinogenesis in the rat kidney, *Toxicology*, 90, 129, 1994.
43. Ohgaki, H., Kleihues, P., and Hard, G. C., Ki-ras mutations in spontaneous and chemically induced renal tumors of the rat, *Mol. Carcinog.*, 4, 455, 1991.
44. Higinbotham, K. G., Rice, J. M., and Perantoni, A. O., Activating point mutation in Ki-ras codon 63 in a chemically induced rat renal tumor, *Mol. Carcinog.*, 5, 136, 1992.
45. Higinbotham, K. G., Rice, J. M., Buzard, G. S., and Perantoni, A. O., Activation of the K-*ras* gene by insertion mutations in chemically induced rat renal mesenchymal tumors, *Oncogene*, 9, 2455, 1994.
46. Ohgaki, H., Hard, G. C., Hirota, N., Maekawa, A., Takahashi, M., and Kleihues, P., Selective mutation of codons 204 and 213 of the p53 gene in rat tumors induced by alkylating *N*-nitroso compounds, *Cancer Res.*, 52, 2995, 1992.
47. Reiter, R. E., Anglard, P., Liu, S., Gnarra, J. R., and Linehan, W. M., Chromosome 17p deletions and p53 mutations in renal cell carcinoma, *Cancer Res.*, 53, 3092, 1993.
48. Pelletier, J., Bruening, W., Kashtan, C. E., Mauer, S. M., Manivel, J. C., Striegel, J. E., Houghton, D. C., Junien, C., Habib, R., Fouser, L., Fine, R. N., Silverman, B. L., Haber, D. A., and Housman, D., Germline mutations in the Wilm's tumor suppressor gene are associated with abnormal urogenital development in Denys–Drash syndrome, *Cell*, 67, 437, 1991.
49. Diwan, B. A., and Rice, J. M., Effect of the stage of development on the frequency and pathogenesis of kidney tumors induced in Noble (Nb) rats exposed prenatally or neonatally to N-nitrosoethylurea, *Carcinogenesis*, 16, 2023, 1995.
50. Gnarra, J. R., Tory, K., Weng, Y., Schmidt, L., Wei, M. H., Li, H., Latif, F., Liu, S., Chen, F., Duh, F-M., Lubensky, I., Duan, D. R., Florence, C., Pozzatti, R., Walther, M. M., Bander, N. H., Grossman, H. B., Brauch, H., Pomer, S., Brooks, J. D., Isaacs, W. B., Lerman, M. I., Zbar, B., and Linehan, W. M, Mutations of the VHL tumor suppressor gene in renal carcinoma, *Nat. Genet.*, 7, 85, 1994.
51. Shuin, T., Kondo, K., Torigoe, S., Kishida, T., Kubota, Y., Hosaka, M., Nagashima, Y., Kitamura, H., Latif, F., Zbar, B., Lerman, M. I., and Yao, M., Frequent somatic mutations and loss of heterozygosity of the von Hippel-Lindau tumor suppressor gene in primary human renal cell carcinomas, *Cancer Res.*, 54, 2852, 1994.
52. Lee, W., Han, K., Harris, C. P., and Meisner, L. F., Detection of aneuploidy and possible deletion in paraffin-embedded rhabdomyosarcoma cells with FISH, *Cancer Genet. Cytogenet.*, 68, 99, 1993.

53. Southern, E. M., Detection of specific sequences among DNA fragments separated by gel electrophoresis, *J. Mol. Biol.*, 98, 503, 1975.
54. Mullis, K. B. and Faloona, F. A., Specific synthesis of DNA in vitro via a polymerase-catalyzed chain reaction, *Methods Enzymol.*, 155, 335, 1987.
55. Orita, M., Suzuki, Y., Sekiya, T., and Hayashi, K., Rapid and sensitive detection of point mutations and DNA polymorphisms using the polymerase chain reaction, *Genomics*, 5, 874, 1989.
56. Condie, A., Eeles, R., Borresen, A-L., Coles, C., Cooper, C., and Prosser, J., Detection of point mutations in the p53 gene: comparison of single-strand conformation polymorphism, constant denaturant gel electrophoresis, and hydroxyamine and osmium tetroxide techniques, *Hum. Mutat.*, 2, 58, 1993.
57. Grompe, M., The rapid detection of unknown mutations in nucleic acids. *Nat. Genet.*, 5, 111, 1993.
58. Myers, R. M., Maniatis, T., and Lerman, L. S., Detection and localization of single base changes by denaturing gradient gel electrophoresis, *Methods Enzymol.*, 155, 501, 1987.
59. Sheffield, V. C., Fishman, G. A., Beck, J. S., Kimura, A. E., and Stone, E. M., Identification of novel rhodopsin mutations associated with retinitis pigmentosa by GC-clamped denaturing gradient gel electrophoresis, *Am. J. Hum. Genet.*, 49, 699, 1991.
60. Myers, R. M., Fischer, S. G., Lerman, L. S., and Maniatis, T., Nearly all single base substitutions in DNA fragments joined to a GC-clamp can be detected by denaturing gradient gel electrophoresis, *Nucleic Acids Res.*, 13, 3131, 1985.
61. Sanger, F., Nicklen, S., and Coulson, A. R., DNA sequencing with chain-terminating inhibitors, *Proc. Natl. Acad. Sci. U.S.A.*, 74, 5463, 1977.
62. Cotton, R. G., Rodrigues, N. R., and Campbell, R. D., Reactivity of cytosine and thymine in single-base-pair mismatches with hydroxylamine and osmium tetroxide and its application to the study of mutations, *Proc. Natl. Acad. Sci. U.S.A.*, 85, 4397, 1988.
63. Gyllensten, U. B. and Erlich, H. A., Generation of single-stranded DNA by the polymerase chain reaction and its application to direct sequencing of the HLA-DQA locus, *Proc. Natl. Acad. Sci. U.S.A.*, 85, 7652, 1988.
64. Syvanen, A. C., Aalto, S. K., Kontula, K., and Soderlund, H., Direct sequencing of affinity-captured amplified human DNA: application to the detection of apolipoprotein E polymorphism, *FEBS Lett.*, 258, 71, 1989.
65. Ruano, G. and Kidd, K. K., Coupled amplification and sequencing of genomic DNA, *Proc. Natl. Acad. Sci. U.S.A.*, 88, 2815, 1991.
66. Devor, D. E., Henneman, J. R., Kurata, Y., Rehm, S., Weghorst, C. M., and Ward, J. M., Pathology procedures in laboratory animal carcinogenesis studies, in *Carcinogenesis*, Waalkes, M. P. and Ward, J. M., Eds., Raven Press, New York, 1994, 429.
67. Tsuda, H. and Krieg, K., Neoplastic lesions in the kidney, in *Pathobiology of the Aging Rat*, Mohr, U., Dungworth, D. L., and Capen, C. C., Eds., ILSI Press, Washington, D.C., 1992, 227.
68. Roholl, P. J. M., Dullens, H. F. J., Dubbink, E. J., and Den Otter, W., Acid ethanol fixation and polyester wax embedding combines preservation of antigenic determinants with good morphology and enables simultaneous bromodeoxyuridine (BrdU) labeling, in *Biotechnic & Histochemistry*, Williams & Wilkins, Baltimore, 1991, 55.
69. Ward, J. M., Perantoni, A. O., and Santos, E., Comparative immunohistochemical reactivity of monoclonal and polyclonal antibodies to H-*ras* p21 in normal and neoplastic tissues of rodents and humans, *Oncogene* 4, 203, 1989.
70. von Wasielewski, R., Werner, M., Nolte, M., Wilkens, L., and Georgii, A., Effects of antigen retrieval by microwave heating in formalin-fixed tissue sections on a broad panel of antibodies, *Histochemistry*, 102, 165, 1994.
71. Sternberger, L. A., *Immunocytochemistry*, 3rd ed., John Wiley & Sons, New York, 1986, 210.
72. Kuhlmann, W. D., *Immuno Enzyme Techniques in Cytochemistry*, Verlag Chemie, Weinheim, Germany, 1984, 71.
73. Wada, T., Shimabukuro, T., Matsuyama, H., Naito, K., Skog, S., and Tribukait, B., Optimal conditions of fixation for immunohistochemical staining of proliferating cell nuclear antigen in tumour cells and its cell cycle related immunohistochemical expression, *Cell Prolif.*, 27, 541, 1994.

74. Elias, J. M., Gown, A. M., Nakamura, R. M., Wilbur, D. C., Herman, G. E., Jaffe, E. S., Battifora, H., and Brigati, D. J., Special report: quality control in immunohistochemistry. Report of a workshop sponsored by the Biological Stain Commission, *Am. J. Clin. Pathol.*, 92, 836, 1989.
75. Baak, J. P. A., Noteboom, E., and Koevoets, J. J. M., The influence of fixatives and other variations in tissue processing on nuclear morphometric features, *Anal. Quant. Cytol. Histol.*, 11, 219, 1989.
76. Heller, M. J., Robinson, R. A., Burghart, L. J., TenEyck, C. J., and Wilke, W. W., DNA extraction by sonication: a comparison of fresh, frozen and paraffin-embedded tissues extracted for use in polymerase chain reaction assays, *Mod. Pathol.*, 5(2), 203, 1992.
77. Goodyear, P. D., MacLaughlin–Black, S., and Mason, I. J., Purification of highly degraded DNA by gel filtration for PCR, *Biotechniques*, 15(2), 235, 1994.
78. Greer, C. E., Wheeler, C. M., and Manos, M. M., Sample preparation and PCR amplification from paraffin-embedded tissues. *Manual supplement to PCR Methods and Applications,* Cold Spring Harbor Laboratory, ISSN 1054–9805, 3, S113, 1994.
79. Crisan, D. and Mattson, J. C., Retrospective DNA analysis using fixed tissue specimens, *DNA Cell Biol.*, 12(5), 455, 1993.
80. Bohm, M., Wieland, I., and Totzeck, B., Detection of tumor-specific homozygous deletions in human biopsies by polymerase chain reaction, *Cancer Genet. Cytogenet.*, 65, 83, 1993.
81. Sundaresian, V., Ganly, P., Haselton, P., Bleehen, N. M., and Rabbitts, P., Paraffin wax-embedded material as a source of DNA for the detection of somatic genetic changes, *J. Pathol.*, 169, 43, 1993.
82. Sato, Y., Mukai, K., Furuya, S., Kameya, T., and Hirohashi, S., The AMeX method: a multipurpose tissue-processing and paraffin-embedding method. Extraction of protein and application to immunoblotting, *Am. J. Pathol.*, 140, 775, 1992.

chapter fourteen

Measurement of Reactive Oxygen Species, Oxidative Damage, and Antioxidant Systems in the Kidney

Norishi Ueda and Sudhir V. Shah

14.1 Introduction 257
14.2 Assay for reactive oxygen species 258
14.2.1 Measurement of superoxide anion 258
14.2.1.1 Superoxide dismutase-inhibitable cytochrome *c* reduction assay 258
14.2.1.1.1 Principle 258
14.2.1.1.2 Reagents 258
14.2.1.1.3 Procedure 258
14.2.1.1.4 Calculation of data 259
14.2.1.2 Chemiluminescence assay for reactive oxygen metabolites 259
14.2.1.2.1 Principle 259
14.2.1.2.2 Preparation of glomeruli and tubules 259
14.2.1.2.3 Reagents 259
14.2.1.2.4 Procedure 259
14.2.1.2.5 Comments 260
14.2.2 Measurement of intracellular hydrogen peroxide 260
14.2.2.1 Aminotriazole-inhibitable catalase assay 260
14.2.2.1.1 Principle 260
14.2.2.1.2 Sample preparation 261
14.2.2.1.3 Animal treatment 261
14.2.2.1.4 Preparation of tissue homogenates 261
14.2.2.1.5 Reagents 261
14.2.2.1.6 Procedure 261
14.2.2.1.7 Comments 262
14.2.2.2 Fluorometric assay for intracellular hydrogen peroxide 263
14.2.2.2.1 Principle 263
14.2.2.2.2 Reagents 263
14.2.2.2.3 Procedure 263
14.2.3 Measurement of hydroxyl radical 265
14.2.3.1 Aromatic hydroxylation assay using phenylalanine as a detector molecule 265
14.2.3.1.1 Principle 265
14.2.3.1.2 Reagents 265

0-8493-3341-5/96/$0.00+$.50

14.2.3.1.3 Procedure 265
14.2.3.1.4 HPLC analysis 266
14.2.3.1.5 Comments 266
14.3 Measurement of oxidative damage 266
14.3.1 Measurement of lipid peroxidation 266
14.3.1.1 Thiobarbituric acid reaction 267
14.3.1.1.1 Principle 267
14.3.1.1.2 Reagents 267
14.3.1.1.3 Procedure 267
14.3.1.1.4 Comments 267
14.3.1.2 Measurement of conjugated dienes 268
14.3.1.2.1 Principle 268
14.3.1.2.2 Reagents 268
14.3.1.2.3 Lipid extraction from tissue samples 268
14.3.1.2.4 Determination of conjugated dienes by simple UV spectrophotometry 268
14.3.1.2.5 Comments 268
14.3.1.2.6 Determination of conjugated dienes by second-derivative UV spectrophotometry 268
14.3.2 Measurement of reduced glutathione (GSH) and glutathione disulfide (GSSG) 268
14.3.2.1 DTNB-GSSG reductase recycling assay for GSH and GSSG 269
14.3.2.1.1 Principle 269
14.3.2.1.2 Tissue preparation 269
14.3.2.1.3 Reagents 269
14.3.2.1.4 Procedure 269
14.3.2.2 DTNB-GSSG reductase recycling assay for GSSG 270
14.3.2.2.1 Principle 270
14.3.2.2.2 Reagents 270
14.3.2.2.3 Procedure 270
14.3.2.2.4 Comments 270
14.4 Bleomycin-detectable iron assay 270
14.4.1 Principle 270
14.4.2 Tissue preparation 271
14.4.2.1 Renal cortex 271
14.4.2.2 Glomeruli and tubules 271
14.4.2.3 Reagents 271
14.4.2.4 Procedure 272
14.4.2.5 Comments 272
14.5 Assay for antioxidant enzymes 272
14.5.1 Measurement of superoxide dismutase 272
14.5.1.1 Acetylated cytochrome *c* reduction assay 272
14.5.1.1.1 Principle 272
14.5.1.1.2 Tissue preparation 273
14.5.1.1.3 Reagents 273
14.5.1.1.4 Procedure 274
14.5.1.1.5 Definition of unit 275
14.5.1.1.6 Calculation of data 275
14.5.1.1.7 Comments 275
14.5.2 Measurement of catalase 275
14.5.3 Measurement of glutathione peroxidase (GSH-Px) 275

14.5.3.1 Glutathione peroxidase (GSH-Px) assay 275
14.5.3.1.1 Principle 275
14.5.3.1.2 Tissue preparation 276
14.5.3.1.3 Total GSH-Px activity assay 276
14.5.3.1.4 Calculation of data 276
14.5.3.1.5 Selenium-dependent GSH-Px activity assay 277
14.5.3.1.6 Selenium-independent GSH-Px activity 277
References 277

14.1 Introduction

A large body of evidence accumulated over the last decade indicates that partially reduced oxygen metabolites are important mediators of ischemic, toxic, and immune-mediated tissue injury.[1-6] The role of reactive oxygen metabolites in various forms of renal injury has been recently reviewed.[7-9]

Oxygen normally accepts four electrons and is converted directly to water. However, partial reduction of oxygen can and does occur in biological systems leading to the generation of partially reduced and potentially toxic reactive oxygen intermediates.[10,11] Thus, sequential reduction of oxygen along the univalent pathway leads to the generation of superoxide anion, hydrogen peroxide, hydroxyl radical, and water:[10,11]

$$\text{Oxygen} \rightarrow \underset{\text{(free radical)}}{\text{Superoxide}} \rightarrow \text{Hydrogen Peroxide} \rightarrow \underset{\text{(free radical)}}{\text{Hydroxyl Radical}} \rightarrow \text{Water} \quad (1)$$

Superoxide and hydrogen peroxide appear to be the primary species generated; these may then play a role in the generation of additional and more reactive oxidants, including the highly reactive hydroxyl radical (or a related highly oxidizing species) in which iron salts play a catalytic role in a reaction, commonly referred to as the metal-catalyzed Haber–Weiss reaction.[12]

$$Fe^{3+} + O_2^{\cdot-} \rightarrow Fe^{2+} + O_2 \quad (2)$$

$$Fe^{2+} + H_2O_2 \rightarrow Fe^{3+} + \cdot OH + OH^- \quad (3)$$

$$O_2^{\cdot-} + H_2O_2 \rightarrow O_2 + \cdot OH + OH^- \quad (4)$$

These oxygen metabolites — the free radical species, superoxide and hydroxyl radical, and other metabolites such as hydrogen peroxide and hypohalous acids — are often collectively referred to as reactive oxygen metabolites. The role of reactive oxygen metabolites in cell biology and injury has been examined by demonstrating enhanced production of reactive oxygen metabolites; examining the effect of increasing or decreasing the level of antioxidant defenses; and examining the effect of enzymatically generated reactive oxygen metabolites on biological processes. While most of the studies have emphasized enhanced generation of reactive oxygen metabolites, antioxidant defenses are likely to be equally important as determinants of injury.

In this chapter we describe methods to measure the superoxide anion, hydrogen peroxide (emphasizing intracellular generation), and hydroxyl radical in renal systems. Because of the difficulty in measuring reactive oxygen metabolites, lipid peroxidation is often used as an index of free radical mediated injury. Since iron appears to be critical in the generation of powerful oxidant species, we detail the assay for the measurement of catalytic iron in renal systems. Finally, we describe measurement of major enzymatic antioxidant defenses and one of the major intracellular, nonenzymatic defenses, glutathione, in renal tissues.

14.2 Assay for reactive oxygen species

14.2.1 Measurement of superoxide anion

Several methods have been used to measure superoxide anion, including cytochrome *c* reduction,[13] irreversible oxidation of epinephrine to adrenochrome,[14] electron spin resonance with spin-trapping,[15-17] and chemiluminescence from the reaction of oxidized luciferin.[18] Reduction of cytochrome *c* by superoxide is a rapid, single-electron process that can be monitored with great sensitivity and specificity. Because of its simplicity, this assay has been most widely used in biological samples.

14.2.1.1 Superoxide dismutase-inhibitable cytochrome c reduction assay

14.2.1.1.1 Principle. The production of superoxide anions (O_2^-) can be monitored by their ability to reduce chemically an electron-accepting compound. The reduction of cytochrome *c* by O_2^-, w,ith and without superoxide dismutase, and the reduction of superoxide dismutase-inhibitable cytochrome *c* can be used to monitor the production of O_2^-.[13,19] When samples of organelles from renal tissue (such as mitochondria, microsomes, or nuclei) contain cytochrome *c* reductase and cytochrome oxidase, it is suitable to use acetylated cytochrome *c* (see superoxide dismutase assay).[20]

14.2.1.1.2 Reagents. All reagents are prepared in buffer except superoxide dismutase, which is dissolved in water.

Buffer. Phosphate-buffered saline or Hank's balanced salt solution (HBSS) without phenol red.
Cytochrome *c* (0.15 m*M*; horse heart, type III or IV, superoxide dismutase-free). A stock solution (1.5 m*M*) is prepared in buffer and then filtered through a micropore membrane.
Superoxide dismutase (200 μg/ml; SOD; bovine erythrocyte). A stock solution (20 mg/ml) is prepared in deionized water.

14.2.1.1.3 Procedure. Cells are washed two times with phosphate buffer or HBSS. Place 1 ml of the buffer used to culture cells in wells (approximately 1×10^5 to 2×10^7 cells/well) or 1 ml cell suspension in plastic tubes. Add 10 μl of SOD (final concentration, 200 μg/ml) to one tube and 10 μl of deionized water to the other. After 10 min of incubation at 37°C in a water bath with mixing, 100 μl of 1.5 m*M* cytochrome *c* (final concentration, 0.15 m*M*) and the agent that enhances the production of O_2^- is added to the incubation mixture. Fifteen minutes after the addition of cytochrome *c*, incubations are terminated by placing the tubes on ice. Cells are removed by centrifugation at 1500 × g for 10 min or 14,000 × g for 30 s at 4°C. Aliquots of the supernatants are kept on ice or stored at –20°C before being assayed. For the determination of reduced cytochrome *c*, 400 μl of supernatant is diluted with 800 μl of phosphate buffer or HBSS, and the absorption of the SOD-free supernatant is determined at 550 nm using a spectrophotometer against the SOD-containing supernatant as the reference. The cytochrome *c* in each sample is fully oxidized by the addition of a few grains of sodium ferricyanide so that the observed A_{550} represents the absorbance due only to the reduced cytochrome *c*, and the difference between the two readings is used to calculate the amount of cytochrome *c* reduced.

14.2.1.1.4 Calculation of data. The A_{550} of the supernatant is converted to nanomoles of cytochrome *c* reduced using the extinction coefficient of $2.1 \times 10^4\ M^{-1}cm^{-1}$.[21] With a 1-cm light path and 1-ml reaction mixture, the observed A_{550} should be multiplied by 47.6 to yield the number of nanomoles of superoxide measured because 1 mol of superoxide reduces 1 mol of ferricytochrome *c*. The results can be expressed as nanomoles of superoxide per minute per milligram protein. Time of incubation may be varied, and the reduction of cytochrome may be followed by continuous measurements.

14.2.1.2 Chemiluminescence assay for reactive oxygen metabolites

14.2.1.2.1 Principle. Although not specific, chemiluminescence provides a very sensitive method for the detection of reactive oxygen metabolites. For example, it can be readily utilized to detect the generation of reactive oxygen metabolites by freshly isolated glomeruli.

The most common luminescent reagents as detectors of superoxide anion are luminol (5-amino-2,3-dihydro-1,4-phthalazinedione)[22-24] or lucigenin (9,9′-bis-*N*-methylacridinium nitrate).[25,26] Other luminescent probes such as 2-methyl-6-phenyl-3,7-dihydroimidazol[1,2-*a*]pyrazin-3-one (CLA) or 2-methyl-6-(*p*-methoxyphenyl)-3,7-dihydroimidazol[1,2-*a*]pyrazin-3-one (MCLA) have also been used to measure reactive oxygen metabolites.[18] It is generally assumed that univalent oxidation of luminol or univalent reduction of lucigenin can react with superoxide anion yielding unstable endoperoxide or dioxetane.[23,27] The decomposition of these compounds by electronic excitation leads to release of photons and thus emitted luminescence can be monitored. It is, thus, generally believed that when these probes are utilized to monitor chemiluminescence (as opposed to monitoring native chemiluminescence), it is a measure of superoxide production.

14.2.1.2.2 Preparation of glomeruli and tubules. Glomeruli and tubules are isolated from perfused kidneys by a combination of differential sieving and centrifugation[28] and resuspended in Hank's balanced salt solution (HBSS) without phenol red.

14.2.1.2.3 Reagents

HBSS without phenol red.

Luminol. Stock solution (30 m*M*) is made in DMSO and stored in the dark. Dilute the stock solution to give a final concentration of 30 μ*M* with HBSS.

Lucigenin. An alternative luminescent probe, used at a final concentration of 100 μ*M* prepared in HBSS.

14.2.1.2.4 Procedure. Chemiluminescence measurements are carried out at ambient temperature, in a dark room illuminated with red light. Reactions are carried out in dark-adapted glass scintillation vials. Chemiluminescence is measured with a Beckman liquid scintillation system (Model 9000) or equivalent, operated in the out-of-coincidence summation mode as described.[23,29]

A reaction mixture consists of 2 ml HBSS without phenol red containing 30 μ*M* luminol (or 100 μ*M* lucigenin). Background chemiluminescence is measured in vials containing the reaction mixture without cells. Under these conditions the background chemiluminescence of vials containing luminol range between 8000 and 12,000 cpm. Then, to each vial isolated glomeruli or tubules prepared in HBSS (prewarmed at 37°C for 15 min) are added, and a second measurement is carried out. The incubation is initiated by addition of an agent that enhances superoxide anion production, and chemiluminescence is measured for the desired period of time. The results are calculated as counts per minute (cpm) minus the background cpm.

14.2.1.2.5 Comments. Although the chemiluminescence assay using luminol or lucigenin is not specific for superoxide anion because luminescent probes are also oxidized by hydrogen peroxide or hydroxyl radical, it provides a very sensitive way of monitoring the generation of reactive oxygen metabolites in biological samples.[24] Luminol has a disadvantage for the detecting reactive oxygen metabolites within living cells because of its poor solubility,[23] ability to generate superoxide anion when its univalently oxidized form autoxidizes, and poor quantum yield in the neutral pH.[27] Lucigenin or other luminescent reagents (CLA or MCLA) may be better probes because of their solubility and a greater specificity for superoxide anion. preferred

14.2.2 *Measurement of intracellular hydrogen peroxide*

A number of methods have been reported to measure hydrogen peroxide in living cells.[30] They include direct monitoring of catalase intermediate (catalase compound I), measurement of substrate oxidation by the catalase–H_2O_2 intermediate or of hydrogen peroxide release using cytochrome *c* peroxidase or horseradish peroxidase coupled with oxidation of hydrogen donors, oxygen formation by the catalatic reaction, myoglobin conversion, aminotriazole inhibition of catalase, or fluorescent analysis.[30] Most of the methods are a measure of extracellular generation of hydrogen peroxide. We describe the two methods that allow the measurement of intracellular generation of hydrogen peroxide using aminotriazole-inhibitable catalase assay and a fluorescence indicator.

14.2.2.1 *Aminotriazole-inhibitable catalase assay*

14.2.2.1.1 Principle. Aminotriazole-inhibitable catalase assay has been recently used to measure normal[31] and enhanced intracellular generation of hydrogen peroxide *in vivo*.[32,33] The method employed is based on the inhibition of endogenous catalase by 3-amino-1,2,4-triazole. Catalase is inactivated by aminotriazole only in the presence of hydrogen peroxide, because aminotriazole reacts with the catalase intermediate, compound I, to form an inactive covalent complex with the protein.[34,35] The inactivation of tissue catalase by aminotriazole can, therefore, be interpreted as a qualitative measure of hydrogen peroxide production.[31-35] The reaction sequence is shown in Equations 5 and 6:

$$\text{catalase} + \text{hydrogen peroxide} \rightarrow [\text{catalase-hydrogen peroxide}]\ \text{compound I} \quad (5)$$

$$\text{compound I} + \text{aminotriazole} \rightarrow \text{irreversibly inhibited catalase} \quad (6)$$

Both the *in vitro* and *in vivo* inactivation of catalase can be prevented by ethanol because ethanol rapidly reduces compound I and effectively competes with the aminotriazole reaction.[31-35]

$$\text{compound I} + \text{hydrogen peroxide} \rightarrow \text{catalase} + O_2 + 2H_2O \quad (7)$$

(catalatic activity)

$$\text{compound I} + \text{ethanol} \rightarrow \text{catalase} + \text{acetaldehyde} + 2H_2O \quad (8)$$

(peroxidatic activity)

Based on the aminotriazole-induced inhibition of catalase, coupled with the prevention of the aminotriazole-induced inhibition by ethanol, generation of intracellular hydrogen peroxide can be measured in *in vitro*[28,31] and *in vivo* renal systems.[32]

14.2.2.1.2 Sample preparation. Kidneys are perfused with ice-cold Hank's balanced salt solution (HBSS, pH 7.4) to remove blood as a contaminating source of hydrogen peroxide. Glomeruli are isolated by a combination of differential sieving and centrifugation.[31] Glomeruli are resuspended in ice-cold HBSS and distributed randomly in order to have approximately 0.5 mg protein per tube. Following preincubation for 15 min at 37°C in a shaking water bath, aminotriazole is added to the tubes. When the effect of ethanol (0.17 *M*), to prevent aminotriazole-induced inhibition of catalase, is assessed, ethanol should be added to the tubes 10 min prior to the addition of aminotriazole. The final volume of each suspension is 1 ml, with final concentration of aminotriazole ranging from 2.5 to 50 m*M* (see below). The tubes are incubated with the agent that enhances hydrogen peroxide production for the desired period of time. Tubes are then centrifuged at 700 × g at 4°C for 5 min, the supernatant is removed, and glomeruli are washed once with ice-cold HBSS. The glomeruli are then resuspended in 1 ml of cold 50 m*M* phosphate buffer (pH 7.0) containing 0.1% (v/v) Triton X-100, 0.1 m*M* EDTA, and 0.17 *M* ethanol. The addition of ethanol at the end of the incubation period prevents any further effect of aminotriazole present within the cells. The glomeruli are disrupted three times by sonication for every 5 s on ice at a power output of 40 W, and the samples are centrifuged at 700 × g for 10 min. Aliquots of the supernatants are used for the assay. Since ethanol and Triton X-100 are already present in the sonication buffer, they are not added, as recommended by Cohen,[36] to the samples before performing the catalase assay.

14.2.2.1.3 Animal treatment. Control and experimental rats are subdivided into two groups — one receiving intraperitoneal injection of ethanol (2 g/kg) in saline (1:1, w/v) (in order to verify that the inhibition by aminotriazole is due to inhibition of compound I) and the other injected with the same volume of saline. The rats are then injected intraperitoneally with aminotriazole (0.1 g/kg). Rats are killed at the desired time points (e.g., 30, 60, and 90 min) after aminotriazole injection to obtain tissue for measurement of catalase activity.

14.2.2.1.4 Preparation of tissue homogenates. Perfused renal cortex is minced and homogenized in 1:10 (w/v) cold 50 m*M* potassium phosphate (pH 7.0) containing 0.1% (v/v) Triton X-100 and 0.1 m*M* EDTA using a Potter–Elvehjem homogenizer with a motor-driven Teflon pestle. The homogenates are centrifuged at 700 × g and 4°C for 10 min, and the supernatants are used for the assay.

14.2.2.1.5 Reagents

Phosphate buffer (50 m*M*, pH 7.0). Dissolve (a) 6.81 g KH_2PO_4, and (b) 8.90 g $Na_2HPO_4 \cdot 2H_2O$ in deionized water and make up to 1 l each. Mix the two solutions (a) and (b) in the proportion 1:1.55 (v/v).

3-Amino-1,2,4-triazole (2.5 to 50 m*M*) prepared in the buffer used for the experiment.

Hydrogen peroxide (50 m*M*; H_2O_2). Solution is standardized spectrophotometrically at 240 nm, using a molar extinction coefficient of $E_{240} = 43.6\ M^{-1}cm^{-1}$.[37,38]

Ethanol (0.17 *M*).

14.2.2.1.6 Procedure. Catalase activity in samples is measured by the method according to Aebi.[37,38] The samples are diluted with cold 50 m*M* phosphate buffer without Triton X-100 to achieve a fourfold dilution. Each 0.8 ml of the diluted samples are then placed in reference and test cuvettes. In the reference cuvette, 0.2 ml of phosphate buffer is added. The reaction is started by adding 0.2 ml of 50 m*M* H_2O_2 (final concentration, 10 m*M*) in the test cuvette. The decrease in absorbance at 240 nm against the reference is followed for 15 or 30 s using a spectrophotometer. The dilution makes it easy to obtain sufficient sample for the assay and to achieve a stable rate of decrease of optical density between 0.04 and 0.20/30 s.[37,38] Under the conditions employed, the decomposition of H_2O_2 by catalase in the samples follows a first-order kinetic as given by the equation:

$$k = 2.3/t \times \log A_0/A_t \tag{9}$$

where k is the first-order kinetic rate constant, t is the time over which the decrease of H_2O_2 due to catalase activity is measured (15 or 30 s), A_0 and A_t are the absorbance at time 0 and at the time of measurement, respectively. Data are expressed as k per milligram protein or k per gram wet weight tissue.

Adriamycin, an anthracycline antibiotic, undergoes a one-electron reduction to a free radical and thus generates reactive oxygen metabolites. In Adriamycin-treated glomeruli, aminotriazole (2.5 m*M*, 45-min incubation) results in a much greater inhibition of catalase activity, and this effect is reversed by ethanol (Figure 1), indicating that Adriamycin enhances intracellular generation of H_2O_2 by rat glomeruli. When glucose/glucose oxidase and menadione, which generate H_2O_2, are used, similar results are obtained.[28]

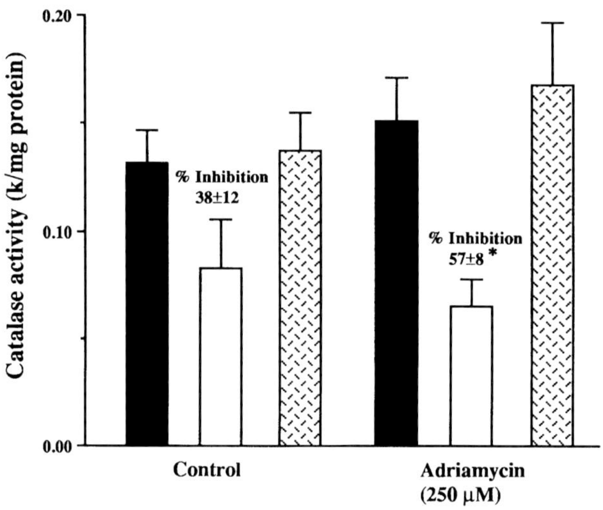

Figure 1 Effect of Adriamycin on intracellular generation of hydrogen peroxide in rat glomeruli. After 15 min incubation with or without Adriamycin (250 μ*M*), glomeruli (■) were incubated with 2.5 m*M* aminotriazole (AT) for 45 min with (▨) or without (□) 0.17 *M* ethanol. Results are means ± SE, *n* = 4. *P < 0.01, compared to control glomeruli + AT. (From Ueda, N., Guidet, B., and Shah, S. V., *Kidney Int.*, 45, 788, 1994. With permission.)

An example of an *in vivo* measurement is shown in Table 1, which demonstrates that aminotriazole also causes a greater inhibition of compound I generation in the glycerol-treated rats as compared with controls, indicating enhanced generation of H_2O_2.

14.2.2.1.7 *Comments*

Dose and incubation time of aminotriazole in the assay. It is extremely important to obtain appropriate dose and incubation time under specified conditions because if the catalase activity is maximally inhibited by aminotriazole, it would not be possible to demonstrate increased inhibition of catalase activity. The inhibitory effect of aminotriazole is time- and dose-dependent (Figure 2), and thus preliminary

Table 1 Effect of Aminotriazole on Renal Cortical Catalase Activity and Renal Function in Control and Glycerol-Treated Rats

		Control			Glycerol-treated		
	n	Ethanol (+)	Ethanol (−)	Inhibition (%)	Ethanol (+)	Ethanol (−)	Inhibition (%)
Catalase, k/mg protein	12	0.77 ± 0.03	0.42 ± 0.05	45 ± 6	0.61 ± 0.04[a]	0.18 ± 0.02[b]	70 ± 3[b]
Plasma urea nitrogen, mg/dl	9	16 ± 1	15 ± 1		82 ± 7[b]	85 ± 7[b]	
Plasma creatinine, mg/dl	12	0.40 ± 0.04	0.40 ± 0.02		1.80 ± 0.27[b]	1.90 ± 0.24[b]	

Note: Values are means ± SE. Rats were dehydrated for 24 h, injected with glycerol, and then allowed free access to water. Control animals were dehydrated as above, except no injections were made. Eighteen hours after glycerol injection, control and glycerol-treated rats were subdivided into two groups, one group receiving intraperitoneal injections of ethanol (2 g/kg) in saline (1:1 w/v) and the other injected with same volume of saline. All rats were then injected intraperitoneally with 3-amino-1,2,4-triazole (0.1 g/kg), and at 90 min, tissue was obtained for measurement of catalase activity, and a sample of heparinized blood was obtained for measurement of creatinine and plasma urea nitrogen. Inhibition of compound I by aminotriazole was calculated as follows: [ethanol (+) – ethanol (–)/ethanol (+)] × 100, where ethanol (+) is renal cortical catalase activity in rats injected with ethanol and ethanol (–) is catalase activity in rats injected with saline.

[a] $P < 0.01$ (unpaired *t*-test) compared with corresponding values in control rats.

[b] $P < 0.005$ or greater level of significance (unpaired *t*-test) compared with corresponding values in control rats.

From Guidet, B. and Shah, S. V., *Am. J. Physiol.*, 257, F440, 1989. With permission.

experiments are necessary to determine the right dose and incubation time at which aminotriazole does not maximally inhibit catalase under each condition.

Sensitivity of catalase–aminotriazole system. A linear relation is observed between the amounts of H_2O_2 added and catalase inhibition (Figure 3). This assay system can detect nanomole concentrations of H_2O_2 and has a fairly broad pH optimum (pH 6.8 to 7.5).[28,34,37,38] Thus, this assay is sensitive and has general applicability for the measurement of intracellular H_2O_2 in biological settings.

14.2.2.2 *Fluorometric assay for intracellular hydrogen peroxide*

14.2.2.2.1 Principle. Keston and Brandt[39] first described a fluorometric assay for the detection of intracellular production of H_2O_2 using 2′,7′-dichlorofluorescin-diacetate (DCFH-DA) as a fluorescent probe. This compound readily diffuses into cells and is hydrolyzed by intracellular esterases to the nonfluorescent derivative 2′,7′-dichlorofluorescin (DCFH). In the presence of intracellular H_2O_2, DCFH is rapidly oxidized to the highly fluorescent compound, 2′,7′-dichlorofluorescein (DCF), and the reaction is markedly enhanced by peroxidase.[40] Cellular fluorescence intensity is proportional to the level of DCF formed intracellularly, and thus intracellular H_2O_2 generation can be monitored by spectrofluorometry[41] or flow cytometry.[40] Because of its simplicity and high sensitivity, this method has been recently used in a variety of biological systems.[40,42-44]

14.2.2.2.2 Reagents

2′,7′-Dichlorofluorescin-diacetate (1 mg/ml; DCF-DA; Molecular Probes) in ethanol.

14.2.2.2.3 Procedure. Cultured renal cells in wells (1×10^5 to 2×10^7 cells/well) are washed and preincubated with phosphate-buffered saline or a modified Gey's buffer

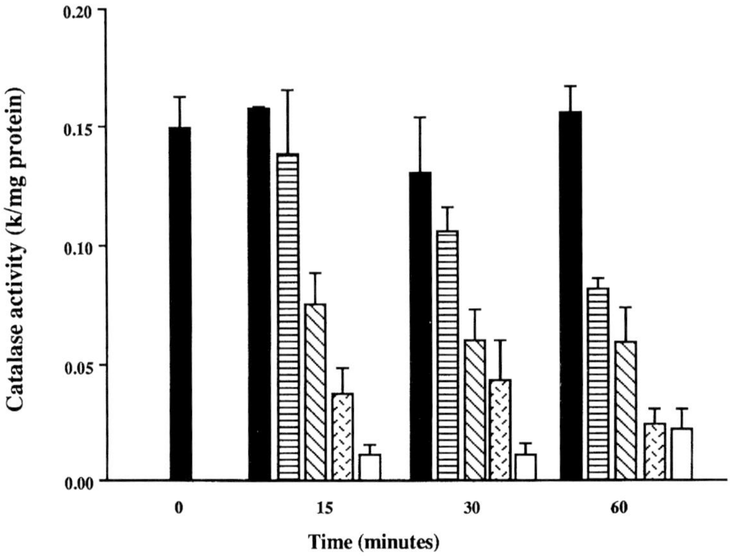

Figure 2 Effect of different doses of aminotriazole on catalase activity at various time points in rat glomeruli under normal conditions. After 30 min incubation, glomeruli (■) were incubated with various doses of aminotriazole (AT; (▤) 5 m*M*; (▧) 10 m*M*; (▨) 20 m*M*; (□) 50 m*M*) for variable periods (15 to 60 min). Results are means ± SE, $n = 5$. Inhibition of glomerular catalase activity was proportional to the dose of aminotriazole used and incubation period. (From Ueda, N., Guidet, B., and Shah, S.V., *Kidney Int.*, 45, 788, 1994. With permission.)

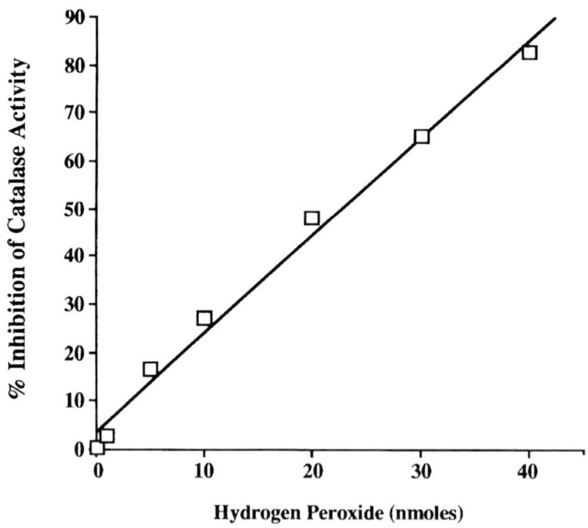

Figure 3 Sensitivity of the catalase–aminotriazole system for measuring hydrogen peroxide. The various amounts of hydrogen peroxide (1, 5, 10, 20, 30, and 40 nmol) were added to the reaction mixture containing phosphate buffer (pH 7.0), 0.1% (v/v) Triton X-100, 0.25 mg/ml catalase, and 2.5 m*M* aminotriazole in a total volume of 1 ml. Results are expressed as % inhibition of catalase compared to that in the absence of hydrogen peroxide, $n = 2$. (From Ueda, N., Guidet, B., and Shah, S. V., *Kidney Int.*, 45, 788, 1994. With permission.)

(145 m*M* NaCl, 5 m*M* KCl, 1 m*M* Na_2HPO_4, 10 m*M* HEPES, 1 m*M* $CaCl_2$, 0.5 m*M* $MgSO_4$, pH 7.4) containing DCF-DA (1 to 10 µg/ml, final concentration) for 30 to 60 min at 37°C. The final concentration of ethanol should be 0.1% or less to avoid artifactual effects on

fluorescence.[40] Cells are washed three times with the same buffer without DCF-DA to remove free DCF-DA. The reagent that enhances intracellular H_2O_2 production is added and incubated for the desired time period at 37°C. When a spectrofluorometer for microtiter plate or fluorescence microscope is available, the fluorescence intensity is read every 15 min with an excitation wavelength of 488 nm and an emission wavelength of 525 nm.[42] If such equipment is not available, cells can be scraped and the cell suspension transferred to 3-ml quartz cuvettes with a magnetic stirring bar, and the fluorescence intensity is measured using a spectrofluorometer with the same wavelengths of excitation and emission.

14.2.3 *Measurement of hydroxyl radical*

Measurement of hydroxyl radicals in renal systems is difficult because they are highly reactive with most organic molecules (with rate constants of 10^9 to 10^{10} $M^{-1}s^{-1}$) and their lifetime is extremely short (<1 nsec). Although a number of assays have been developed to measure hydroxyl radicals in biological samples,[45] no convenient and satisfactory method is currently available. The most reliable assays are probably electron spin resonance with spin trapping[16,46,47] and aromatic hydroxylation.[45,48-50] We describe the latter assay using biological samples.

14.2.3.1 *Aromatic hydroxylation assay using phenylalanine as a detector molecule*

14.2.3.1.1 Principle. Formation of 2,3- and 2,5-dihydroxybenzoates from salicylate (2-hydroxybenzoate), mediated by hydroxyl radicals, has been utilized to detect hydroxyl radicals in biological systems.[45,51,52] However, salicylate has a serious disadvantage as a detector molecule because of its high affinity for iron (III), which might perturb iron-dependent hydroxyl radical formation, its inhibitory effect on cyclooxygenase, and its toxicity. Thus, there is a limitation of its use for *in vivo* measurements.

An alternative aromatic detector of the hydroxyl radical is the amino acid phenylalanine.[48,49,53] When L-phenylalanine is administered to animals, it is hydroxylated into L-*p*-tyrosine. Attack of hydroxyl radicals on L-*p*-tyrosine results in formation of three isomeric tyrosines — *o*-,*m*-, and *p*-tyrosines.[48] Thus, formation of these tyrosines from phenylalanine has been used as an index of hydroxyl radical formation in biological systems. In whole animals or organs, *p*-tyrosine is not particularly useful as a marker of hydroxyl radicals because it is a normal metabolite of phenylalanine produced by phenylalanine hydroxylase.[53] However, *o*- and *m*-tyrosines are not normal metabolites of phenylalanine, so the formation of *o*- and *m*-tyrosines can be used as an index of hydroxyl radical formation.[48,49,53]

14.2.3.1.2 Reagents

L-Phenylalanine, 5 m*M*.

Standard mixture containing *o*-, *m*-, and *p*-tyrosines (70 μ*M* each) and phenylalanine (3.5 m*M*).

14.2.3.1.3 Procedure. Renal cells are washed in Krebs–Ringer–phosphate buffer (120 m*M* NaCl, 4.8 m*M* KCl, 10 m*M* KH_2PO_4, 1.3 m*M* $CaCl_2$, 1.2 m*M* $MgSO_4$, pH 7.4) and freed of iron contamination by the transferrin method.[54] Cells are incubated with the buffer containing L-phenylalanine at a final concentration of 5 m*M* for 60 min at 37°C. The agent that enhances hydroxyl radical formation is then added, and the mixture is incubated for the desired time period. The reaction is stopped by chilling in ice. The cells are scraped and transferred to a new clean tube and sonicated for 20 s. Samples are centrifuged at 14,000 × g for 15 min, and supernatants are ultrafiltered through an Amicon Centrifree Micropartition device at 4000 × g for 1 h at 4°C. Samples are stored at –70°C until use. The filtrates are analyzed by injecting 20 μl onto the high-performance liquid chromatography (HPLC) column as described below.

14.2.3.1.4 HPLC analysis. HPLC separation of hydroxylated products and metabolites of L-phenylalanine is carried out on HPLC technology Nucleocil 5 μm C-18 column (25 × 4.6 mm) with a guard column. The eluant is 500 m*M* KH_2PO_4/H_3PO_4 (pH 3.0) with 10% (v/v) methanol at a flow rate of 1 ml/min and the ultraviolet detector set at 274 nm (sensitivity 0.02). A standard mixture (20 μl) should also be separated under the same conditions to confirm each corresponding peak in the test sample.

14.2.3.1.5 Comments. It is important to exclude iron contamination from the reagents as much as possible. The addition of 0.5 μ*M* apotransferrin will minimize contamination of iron in the reaction mixture.[54] Iron bound to transferrin does not participate in the formation of hydroxyl radicals. Alternatively, contaminating iron can be removed from the reagents by treatment with Chelex resin (see bleomycin-detectable iron assay).

The disadvantage of using phenylalanine may be a low rate constant for reaction with hydroxyl radicals (1.9×10^9 $M^{-1}s^{-1}$), which is five times less than that of salicylate.[50] To verify the specificity of the assay, it should be confirmed that scavengers of hydroxyl radicals, such as mannitol, prevent the generation of tyrosine metabolites under specified conditions.

14.3 Measurement of oxidative damage

Biological membranes have a high content of polyunsaturated fatty acids and are also constantly bathed in oxygen-rich fluids; as a result, they are particularly susceptible to peroxidative attack by oxygen-derived oxidants.[3,5,30] Lipid peroxidation can alter membrane structure and function.[30] Despite this, it has not always been possible to implicate this process directly as the cause of tissue injury. Nonetheless, a number of investigators have recently attempted to demonstrate that oxygen-derived products are generated in tissues by detecting the products of their action, such as lipid peroxides.[55-58] Thus, while uncertainty remains about lipid peroxidation as a cause of tissue injury, detection of enhanced lipid peroxidation in a particular tissue serves as an important marker of oxygen-mediated tissue injury and provides additional support for oxygen-mediated injury in a particular model of tissue injury.

Glutathione (GSH), a tripeptide, occurs in high concentrations in virtually all mammalian cells and is the most prevalent intracellular thiol with many diverse functions.[59,60] The importance of the glutathione redox cycle as a defense against hydrogen peroxide and other agents that cause oxidative injury is well recognized. Under normal conditions, very little glutathione is present in tissues in the disulfide form (GSSG). Oxidant-mediated tissue injury results in increased amounts of GSSG and altered GSSG/GSH ratios.[61,62] In addition to increased content of GSSG in the tissue, oxidant-induced injury is accompanied by an efflux of GSSG from several (though not all) isolated cell systems and isolated perfused organs.[63,64] In the kidney, the decreased content of GSH and/or increased content of GSSG has been shown in models of acute renal failure[65-67] and has been used as an index of free radical-mediated injury.

14.3.1 Measurement of lipid peroxidation

A number of methods have been used to detect lipid peroxidation, including measurement of loss of lipid substrate, increase in oxygen uptake, and products of lipid peroxidation such as malondaldehyde (MDA), diene conjugates, lipid hydroperoxides, hydroxyaldehydes, hydroxy fatty acids, and alkenes and alkanes (ethene or pentane).[68] We describe here several methods that have been most widely used for their simplicity and satisfactory specificity.

14.3.1.1 Thiobarbituric acid reaction

14.3.1.1.1 Principle. MDA is the most abundant aldehyde product of lipid peroxidation. One molecule of MDA reacts with two molecules of thiobarbituric acid (TBA) and yields a pink chromogen that can be detected spectrophotometrically. The reaction should be carried out under acidic conditions, which enables maximal reaction of MDA with TBA.[69]

14.3.1.1.2 Reagents

Trichloroacetic acid (10%, w/v).
TBA (0.67%, w/v).

14.3.1.1.3 Procedure. To prevent any lipid peroxidation from occurring during sample processing, 0.01 volumes of 2% (w/v) butylated hydroxytoluene (as an antioxidant) in ethanol and 1 m*M* EDTA at a final concentration to chelate iron should be added to the tissue sample.[70,71] The sample is mixed with 2 volumes of cold 10% (w/v) trichloroacetic acid and placed in ice for 15 min, and then centrifuged at $3000 \times g$ for 15 min to precipitate protein.[72] The resulting supernatant is mixed with an equal volume of 0.67% (w/v) TBA and incubated in a boiling water bath for 10 min. The sample is cooled in ice for 5 min, and then the absorbance is read at 532 nm. The concentration of MDA can be calculated based on a molar extinction coefficient 159,200[73] or from standards of MDA as described.[70]

14.3.1.1.4 Comments. This assay has been widely used to measure lipid peroxidation because it is simple and easy to perform. However, it is not specific for MDA because a variety of other substances can form TBA complexes, especially substances derived from acid-catalyzed or thermally decomposed precursors, such as other aldehydes, protein–MDA complexes, oxidized lipids, amino acids, or sialic acid.[70,74] To improve the specificity of the assay, most of the potential MDA precursors, such as protein–MDA complexes or oxidized lipids, should be removed from tissue samples by trichloroacetic acid precipitation in the cold before the assay.[70] Although other TBA-reactive substances, such as aldehydes, amino acids, sugars, and fatty acid hydroperoxides, could be present in the deproteinized supernatant, they give a very weak color in the standard TBA assay.[70]

The following conditions or procedures should be avoided: the use of whole tissues without deproteination, sample preparation with various acids other than trichloroacetic acid or without antioxidants or metal chelators, high pH of the reaction mixture, prolonged reaction time in the presence of TBA, preparation of TBA reagent in strong acid solutions, or high concentrations of iron or sugars.[70,74] For example, the modifications with 1% (w/v) phosphoric acid instead of trichloroacetic acid results in detection of significantly elevated levels of TBA-reactive substances.[75] Heating the test sample with TBA in acidic solution is a common process in the assay. This causes various errors if only absorption at 530 to 535 nm is measured, because yellow chromogen with maxima at 450 to 490 nm are often formed, leading to overestimates of MDA formation. Thus, the spectrum in the 430- to 600-nm range should be recorded to prove the existence of the 532- to 535-nm maximum typical for the MDA–TBA complex and to correct for the background absorption by interpolation.[76]

In any case, it is appropriate to refer to the data as TBA-reactive substances using this assay. The exact amount of MDA in tissues can be determined using the HPLC method.[69,76,77]

14.3.1.2 *Measurement of conjugated dienes*

14.3.1.2.1 Principle. Abstracting a hydrogen atom from unsaturated fatty acids by a free radical results in rearrangement of the double bond to form conjugated dienes and, in the presence of O_2, the formation of fatty acid hydroperoxides. The conjugated dienes that are generated give a characteristic absorption at 233 nm using UV spectroscopy.[78]

14.3.1.2.2 Reagents

Chloroform–methanol (2:1, v/v)
Cyclohexane (spectrophotometric grade)

14.3.1.2.3 Lipid extraction from tissue samples. Renal tissue or cells are homogenized with 20 volumes of chloroform–methanol mixture (2:1, v/v).[79] Allow the mixture to stand at room temperature for 10 min with mixing. The sample is centrifuged at 260 × g for 10 min to sediment the insoluble material. Add 0.25 volumes of water to the supernatant and mix gently by inversion only. The sample is centrifuged again for 10 min, and the upper phase is removed. Transfer the lower phase (chloroform phase) into a clean tube and place at 40°C under vacuum. The dried pellet is resuspended in 3 ml of cyclohexane.

14.3.1.2.4 Determination of conjugated dienes by simple UV spectrophotometry. Absorbance of extracted lipids from samples is recorded at 233 nm (1-cm light path) against a cyclohexane blank. After the measurements, the concentration of extracted lipids is measured, as described.[78,80] Correct the absorbance to a uniform base of 1 mg lipid.

14.3.1.2.5 Comments. Although this assay is simple and easy to perform, sensitivity is limited because the absorption of conjugated dienes occurs as a rather imprecise shoulder on the strong absorption peak of unperoxidized fatty acid.

14.3.1.2.6 Determination of conjugated dienes by second-derivative UV spectrophotometry. In second-derivative spectra, two sharp and distinct signals are seen, with minima at 242 nm and 232 nm, due to absorption by *cis–trans* and *trans–trans* conjugate dienes. Using a second-derivative UV spectrophotometer, record the absorbance spectra between 220 and 300 nm. The heights of the two signals with a minimum at 233 and 242 nm are measured and added together, and the concentration of conjugated dienes in the sample is determined based on the standard curve, as described.[80] Data are expressed as nanomoles of conjugated diene equivalents per milligram of lipid.

14.3.2 *Measurement of reduced glutathione (GSH) and glutathione disulfide (GSSG)*

Glutathione exists predominantly in two forms within cells — one is a reduced glutathione (GSH) and the other is glutathione disulfide (GSSG). More than 99.5% of tissue "total glutathione" (GSH + GSSG) is in the form of GSH, due to the action of the widely distributed enzyme glutathione reductase.[81]

There are a number of procedures (e.g., chemical, enzymatic, chromatographic) for measurement of GSH and GSSG in biological samples.[82] We describe the enzymatic methods to measure total glutathione and GSSG contents, as described by Tietze[81] with modification.[83]

14.3.2.1 DTNB-GSSG reductase recycling assay for GSH and GSSG

14.3.2.1.1 Principle. DTNB-GSSG reductase recycling assay was first described by Owens and Belcher[84] and modified later by Tietze.[81] We describe the modification by Griffith.[83] This assay is a sensitive and specific enzymatic procedure. As shown in the reactions below, oxidation of GSH by 5,5′-dithiobis(2-nitrobenzoic acid) (DNTB) results in the formation of GSSG and 5-thio-2-nitrobenzoic acid (TNB). GSSG is then reduced to GSH by GSSG reductase and NADPH. The rate of TNB formation is monitored at 412 nm and is proportional to the sum of GSH and GSSG present:

$$2\text{GSH} + \text{DTNB} \rightarrow \text{GSSG} + \text{TNB} \tag{10}$$

$$\text{GSSG} + \text{NADPH} + \text{H}^+ \xrightarrow{\text{GSSG reductase}} 2\text{GSH} + \text{NADP}^+ \tag{11}$$

GSSG content is determined with the same assay after binding of the GSH by 2-vinylpyridine.[83] Thus, the ratio of [GSSG/GSH + GSSG] can be calculated.

14.3.2.1.2 Tissue preparation. Since GSH rapidly oxidizes nonenzymatically, and GSH and GSSG are degraded by γ-glutamyl transpeptidase, which is abundant in the kidney, biological samples must be acidified quickly to reduce oxidation of GSH to GSSG and to inactivate γ-glutamyl transpeptidase. The kidney should not be frozen and thawed because γ-glutamyl transpeptidase cleaves GSH as the tissue is warmed.[85] Although various acids have been used for deproteination, metaphosphoric, trichloroacetic, and perchloric acids may not prevent oxidation of GSH to GSSG, and thus 5-sulfosalicylic acid (5%, w/v) or picric acid (1%, w/v) is preferable.[85]

The perfused kidney is rapidly removed and the medulla is cut out. The renal cortex is rinsed in the buffer and homogenized in 5 volumes of cold 5% (w/v) 5-sulfosalicylic acid (SSA). The homogenates are centrifuged at 10,000 × g for 10 min at 0 to 4°C and the resulting supernatant is stored at –80°C until use.

14.3.2.1.3 Reagents

Sodium phosphate (125 m*M*, pH 7.5) containing 6.3 m*M* EDTA.
NADPH (0.3 m*M*) in the sodium phosphate buffer (prepared fresh).
5,5′-Dithiobis-(2-nitrobenzoic acid) (DTNB; 6.0 m*M*) prepared in sodium phosphate buffer.
Glutathione reductase (50 U/ml; type IV from yeast).
GSH standard solution prepared in 5% (w/v) 5-sulfosalicylic acid (SSA). Standards (0, 10, 25, 50, 75, 100 nmol/ml) are diluted daily in 5% (w/v) SSA from frozen stock solution (100 m*M* GSH).

14.3.2.1.4 Procedure. Place 0.1 ml of 6.0 m*M* DTNB, 0.7 ml of 0.3 m*M* NADPH, 0.18 ml of H_2O, and 10 μl of test sample. Mix the mixture and incubate for 10 to 15 min at 30°C in a water bath. Then add 10 μl of glutathione reductase to the reaction mixture to initiate the reaction. The formation of TNB is monitored against the sample blank, which contains only 5% (w/v) SSA, by recording the absorbance at 412 nm until it exceeds 2.0. The linear portion of the curve is usually between 1 and 2 absorbance units. The GSH content in the test sample is determined from a standard curve in which the GSH equivalents present (0, 0.1, 0.25, 0.5, 0.75, 1.0 nmol) are plotted against the rate of change in absorbance at 412 nm.

14.3.2.2 DTNB-GSSG reductase recycling assay for GSSG

14.3.2.2.1 Principle. The determination of GSSG in biological samples is difficult because of the low levels of GSSG in cells and because GSH is easily oxidized. Thus, GSSG content is determined with the same assay but where GSH is bound by 2-vinylpyridine.[83]

14.3.2.2.2 Reagents

2-Vinylpyridine. (If the reagent becomes brown or viscous it may be purified by vacuum distillation.)
Triethanolamine (50%, v/v) in deionized water.
Standard solutions. GSSG (50 m*M* stock solution) is diluted in 5% (w/v) SSA.

The other reagents are the same as described for the DNTB-GSSG reductase recycling assay for GSH and GSSG.

14.3.2.2.3 Procedure. The 2-vinylpyridine derivatization should be carried out in a hood because it has a low vapor pressure and exposure may be irritating. Add 2 μl of 2-vinylpyridine per 100 μl of sample (prepared in SSA) with mixing. Triethanolamine (6 μl) is added to the side of the tube and the solution is vigorously mixed. The final pH should be 7 to 7.5, as determined by use of pH paper. Allow the samples to stand at room temperature for 60 min to derivatize GSH. The samples are assayed as in the DNTB-GSSG reductase recycling assay. GSSG standards and sample blank containing the same amount of 2-vinylpyridine and triethanolamine are also run. The GSSG content in the test sample is determined based on the absorbance using 10 μl of standard solution of GSSG (0, 1.0, 2.5, 5.0, 7.5, 10 nmol/ml) prepared in 5% (w/v) SSA. Standard solutions should be treated with 2-vinylpyridine and triethanolamine like the sample, and the change in absorbance should be read at 412 nm for 2 min using 10 μl aliquot.

14.3.2.2.4 Comments. Acidic solutions must be neutralized before GSH and 2-vinylpyridine react.[83] If tissues are homogenized in five volumes of 1% (w/v) picric acid, 2-vinylpyridine can be added directly to the protein-free supernatant (2 μl per 100 μl of sample) and the final pH will be 7 to 7.5. If 5% (w/v) SSA is used to prepare the sample, additional bases, such as triethanolamine, should be added to increase the pH to the point where autooxidation is rapid.

14.4 Bleomycin-detectable iron assay

14.4.1 Principle

Bleomycin, a glycopeptide antibiotic, chelates metal ions through its secondary amide groups and binds to guanosine residues of DNA, resulting in DNA strand breaks and degradation of deoxyribose.[86] The degradation products of deoxyribose further break down to release the three-carbon aldehyde, MDA. Since MDA reacts with TBA to give a pink chromogen, DNA degradation by bleomycin can be followed by measuring TBA reactants. This degradation requires transition metal ions within the DNA–bleomycin complex, and chromogen development is proportional to iron concentration.[87]

The DNA damage by bleomycin appears to be site specific and involve ferryl species, a ferric peroxide, bleomycin–Fe(III)O_2H^-, formed from a bleomycin–Fe(III)O_2^{2-} complex. A DNA-degrading bleomycin–Fe(II) complex can be generated by adding Fe(II) salts to bleomycin or by reducing a bleomycin–Fe(III) complex with reducing agents such as ascorbate. Thus, the assay can measure both ferrous and ferric iron. The bleomycin assay is a highly sensitive measure of iron that catalyzes free radical reactions so that it easily detects a trace amount of iron in most biological samples.[12,88]

14.4.2 Tissue preparation

14.4.2.1 Renal cortex

Kidneys are perfused with ice-cold Chelex-treated 0.9% (w/v) NaCl.[88] Perfused kidneys are removed, decapsulated, and immediately kept on ice. The renal tissues are weighed after the medulla is removed. Tissues are minced in 1/10 (w/v) of Chelex-treated pyrogen-free water in specially cleaned glassware and homogenized by six to ten cycles at 600 rpm using a Potter–Elvehjem homogenizer at 0°C. The homogenates are loaded into a Centriprep-30, which has a cutoff of 3000 mol wt and centrifuged at 4°C for 30 min at 1500 × g. The clear ultrafiltrate is collected and used for the assay.

14.2.2.2 Glomeruli and tubules

Glomeruli and tubules are isolated using Chelex-treated 0.9% (w/v) NaCl by a combination of differential sievings and centrifugation, as described.[28] Isolated glomeruli and tubules are pelleted by centrifugation at 4°C and 700 × g for 10 min and resuspended in 1 ml of Chelex-treated deionized water. They are sonicated three times for 5 s on ice at a power output of 40 W and are centrifuged at 14,000 × g for 15 min. The supernatants are used for the iron and protein measurement.

14.4.2.3 Reagents

All reagents are made up in pyrogen-free, Chelex-treated water (5 g of Chelex per 100 ml H_2O, leave overnight, then centrifuge 3000 × g for 10 min to remove Chelex). All reagents are stored in iron-free plastic containers rather than glassware and are stable for about one month when stored at 4°C, except the ascorbic acid, bleomycin, and iron standards, which must be freshly prepared.

Bleomycin sulfate (1U/ml). Dissolve 15 unit of Blenoxane (Mead Johnson) in 15 ml of pyrogen-free and Chelex-treated deionized water and treated with Chelex (50 mg of Chelex per 1 ml solution of bleomycin) for 30 min with mixing. The solution is centrifuged at 3000 × g for 10 min at 4°C, and the supernatant is carefully removed. The pH of the solution is neutral, and it should be used within 24 h.

Calf thymus DNA (1 mg/ml; type I, Sigma). Dissolve 50 mg DNA in 50 ml of pyrogen-free and Chelex-treated water and leave it overnight at 4°C. Add 20 g of Chelex in the DNA solution, mix gently by inversion, and leave it overnight at 4°C. Centrifuge at 3000 × g for 10 min to remove Chelex.

$MgCl_2$ (50 m*M*). Add 0.1 g of $MgCl_2$ in 10 ml of pyrogen-free and Chelex-treated water. Add 0.3 g of Chelex per 1 ml of $MgCl_2$ and leave it for 30 min with mixing, then centrifuge at 3000 × g to remove Chelex.

Ascorbic acid (free acid). Dissolve 0.7 g of ascorbic acid in 10 ml of Chelex-treated water and shake with 0.4 g Chelex for 30 min. The solution is centrifuged at 3,000 × g for 10 min. Dilute ascorbic solution 1:50 with Chelex-treated, pyrogen-free water. *Do not* treat the diluted ascorbate with Chelex again.

HCl (50 m*M*). The solution should be prepared in Chelex-treated water but should *not* be treated with Chelex.

NaOH (20 m*M*). Add 80 mg of NaOH to 100 ml of Chelex-treated water, and 5 g of Chelex again. Leave it for 30 min with mixing, then centrifuge at 3000 × g for 10 min. Addition of NaOH (30 to 200 µl) may be necessary to adjust to pH 7.4 in the reaction mixture.

EDTA (0.1 M) in Chelex-treated water.

Thiobarbituric acid (TBA; 1%, w/v) in 50 m*M* NaOH (prepared fresh).

HCl (25%, v/v).

n-Butanol.

14.4.2.4 Procedure

1. The reaction mixture is as follows:

DNA (1 mg/ml)	0.5 ml
Bleomycin (1 U/ml)	0.05 ml
$MgCl_2$ (50 m*M*)	0.1 ml
HCl/NaOH	amount varies with assay
Sample or standard	0.1 ml
Diluted ascorbic acid	0.1 ml

   Before running the assay, the pH of the reaction mixture must be adjusted to 7.2 to 7.8 using a pH electrode. If the pH of the reaction mixture is acidic, add an appropriate amount of 20 m*M* NaOH (usually 30 to 200 μl) since the optimum pH of the reaction mixture is in this range (critical for reaction). The pH of the reaction mixture containing iron standard should also be checked in a similar manner. Sample or standard blanks are identical except that bleomycin is omitted.
2. Tubes are mixed before and after addition of ascorbate and then incubated at 37°C for 2 h with shaking. The reaction is stopped by adding 0.1 *M* EDTA and mixed with 1 ml of TBA (1%, w/v, in 50 m*M* NaOH) and 1 ml of HCl (25%, v/v). This reaction mixture is then heated at 100°C for 15 min, followed by cooling to room temperature. The chromogen is extracted with 3 ml of *n*-butanol per tube followed by centrifugation of 2500 × g for 20 min. The absorbance of the upper organic layer is read at 532 nm using a spectrophotometer against the sample or standard blank, which contains all reagents and samples or standards except bleomycin. The iron concentration in the samples is calculated based on the standard curve.
3. A standard curve is prepared using various concentrations of ferric chloride (0, 3.125, 6.25, 12.5, 25, and 50 nmol per 0.1 ml) in Chelex-treated, pyrogen-free water. Each standard also has a corresponding blank that is identical except that bleomycin is omitted. The absorbance of the zero standard (which contains only Chelex-treated, pyrogen-free water), reflecting iron contamination in the reagents, etc., is subtracted from all standards to construct the standard curve. A typical standard curve is shown in Figure 4. Results can be expressed either per wet weight of tissue or protein concentration.

14.4.2.5 Comments

Some iron contamination can be removed by treatment with Chelex resin, which binds both iron and copper salts. The Chelex treatment leaves the solution with an alkaline pH and restricts the treatment of most biological buffers. Thus, the assay is often carried out in unbuffered solution. After Chelex treatment, the solutions must be carefully removed to avoid contamination by resin, which could bind iron in the samples and lead to errors. Problems often encountered are (1) failure to develop any color at all due to the wrong pH in the reaction mixture, and (2) high absorbance in all tubes due to insufficient removal of contaminant iron from the reagents.

14.5 Assay for antioxidant enzymes

14.5.1 Measurement of superoxide dismutase

14.5.1.1 Acetylated cytochrome c reduction assay

14.5.1.1.1 Principle. Superoxide dismutases (SOD) are found in all oxygen-utilizing organisms[89] and catalyze the following reaction with diffusion being limiting:

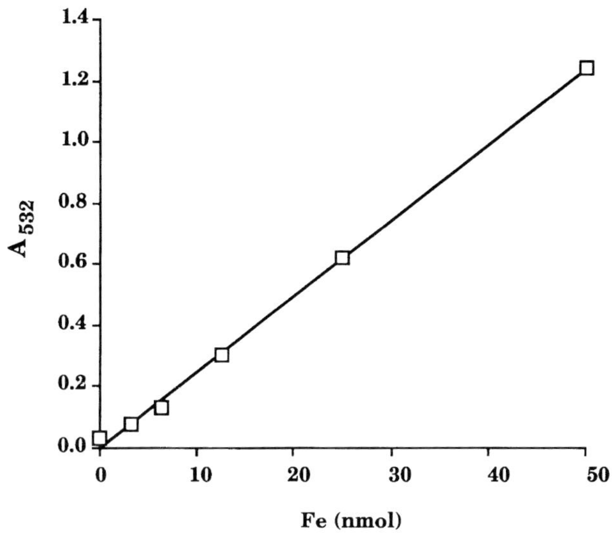

Figure 4 Bleomycin standard. Representative standard curve relating iron concentration and A_{532} for the bleomycin-detectable iron assay.

$$2\,O_2^{\cdot -} + 2H^+ \rightarrow H_2O_2 + O_2 \tag{12}$$

Although direct assays have been used,[90-92] most of these methods are not applicable to biological samples or need special equipment. Thus, the method to detect superoxide dismutase in biological systems is generally indirect because of its unstable substrate, the superoxide anion.[93] Superoxide is generated chemically or enzymatically, and stable and measurable indicators that react with superoxide are used. The most widely used method is based on the reduction of cytochrome *c*,[13] nitroblue tetrazolium,[94] autooxidation of epinephrine,[14] or chemiluminescence.[18,95] We describe the method using acetylated cytochrome *c* to avoid the interference with cytochrome *c* reductases and cytochrome *c* oxidases present in tissues.[20,89]

14.5.1.1.2 Tissue preparation. Perfused renal cortex is homogenized at 1:10 (w/v) in a buffer containing 50 m*M* potassium phosphate (pH 7.8), 0.1 m*M* EDTA and 1% (v/v) Triton X-100. The homogenates are centrifuged at 200 × g at 4°C for 10 min, and the supernatants are used for the assay. When individual cells are used, cell suspensions are centrifuged at 14,000 × g at 4°C for 10 to 15 min. The pelleted cells are washed two times with the same phosphate buffer without Triton by centrifugation. Then cells are resuspended in the buffer with 1% (v/v) Triton and sonicated three times for 5 s each time. The samples are centrifuged, and the aliquots of the supernatant are used for the assay.

14.5.1.1.3 Reagents

Buffer for assay at pH 7.8. Potassium phosphate (50 m*M*) containing 0.1 m*M* EDTA (pH 7.8).

Buffer for assay at pH 10.0. Sodium carbonate (50 m*M*, pH 10.0).

All reagents described below are prepared in 50 m*M* potassium phosphate, 0.1 m*M* EDTA, pH 7.8:

Acetylated cytochrome (0.1 m*M*). Cytochrome *c* can be acetylated as described by Azzi et al.[20] At 0°C, 50 mg of cytochrome *c* is dissolved in 5 ml of a 50%-saturated sodium acetate solution. The solution is slowly added with 0.07 ml of acetic anhydride in ice with occasional stirring for 20 to 30 min, and dialyzed at 0°C for 12 h against deionized water. Stock solution is made in 1-ml aliquots in concentrations determined at time of acetylation, usually of about 0.3 m*M* ($E_{550} = 2.1 \times 10^4\ M^{-1}cm^{-1}$).[21]

Xanthine (1 m*M*).

Xanthine oxidase (XO; 25 U/ml) in potassium phosphate buffer. It is diluted at 1:10 (v/v) with phosphate buffer. Use 20 µl of diluted XO per 3-ml cuvette in the assay at pH 7.8.

KCN (300 m*M*). Use 10 µl in a 3-ml cuvette to achieve a final concentration of 1 m*M*.

14.5.1.1.4 Procedure.

Total SOD activity assay.

1. Acetylated cytochrome *c* (0.3 ml), xanthine (0.3 ml), and 2.4 ml of the buffer are placed in a 3-ml cuvette with a light path of 1.0 cm, at 25°C. The reaction is initiated by adding 10 µl of diluted XO solution, and the rate of increase in absorbance at 550 nm is recorded. For this uninhibited reaction condition, the rate of increase in absorbance should be between 0.02 and 0.025 per min at pH 7.8 and near 0.030 at pH 10.0.
2. Another reaction mixture is then prepared in which the sample to be assayed replaces an equal volume (2.4 ml) of the buffer, and the rate of increase in absorbance is again recorded after adding the same amount of diluted XO solution. For the assay at pH 7.8, dilute the supernatant obtained from cortical tissue homogenates 1:10 (v/v) with potassium phosphate buffer containing EDTA to give an amount of protein that produces a 50% reduction of the rate of the uninhibited reaction. Corrections for the reduction of cytochrome *c* not due to SOD should be made by boiling the sample for 30 min and assaying at pH 7.8 and subtracting these units from the total SOD activity. Correction may be as much as 5 to 10%.

Modification of CuZn- and Mn-SOD activity assay

1. At pH 10.0, the CuZn-SOD activity may be increased nine- to tenfold, but the Mn-SOD activity should not be affected. Dilute 1:80 to 1:100 and adjust the protein to achieve 50% inhibition, as described.
2. KCN (1 m*M*) added to the pH 7.8 assay should inhibit 87.5% of the CuZn-SOD activity, but not the Mn-SOD activity.[96] Concentrations of KCN greater than 1 m*M* may affect the rate of the uninhibited reaction. When the SOD activity in the tissue sample is weak, the undiluted sample should be used. Add the undiluted sample, 500 µl of the buffer containing 1 m*M* KCN, and incubate 30 s before the addition of the remaining reagents.
3. Sodium dodecyl sulfate (SDS) inhibits Mn-SOD activity, but not CuZn-SOD activity.[97] The test samples are assayed at pH 7.8 to determine total SOD activity before adding SDS. To determine Mn-SOD activity, dilute test samples 1:10 (v/v), as described. Add 0.2 ml of 10% (w/v) SDS to 0.8 ml of diluted samples to give a final concentration of 2% and incubate at 37°C for at least 30 min. Cool the samples to 4°C and then add 0.1 ml of 3 *M* KCl to precipitate SDS. The sample is then centrifuged at 20,000 × g or higher for 10 min. The supernatant that represents only CuZn-SOD activity is assayed in the same manner as the assay at pH 7.8.

14.5.1.1.5 Definition of unit. One unit SOD is defined as the amount of SOD required to produce 50% inhibition of the rate of cytochrome *c* reduction under the specified conditions. The amount of sample added in 3-ml reaction mixtures that induces a decrease of 50% of the absorbance under uninhibited conditions represents a unit.

14.5.1.1.6 Calculation of data

$$\text{Unit SOD of sample in the assay} = [\Delta A_{\text{sample}}/\Delta A_{\text{uninhibited condition}}]/0.5 \quad (13)$$

SOD activity is expressed as units per gram tissue or milligrams protein.

1. Total SOD activity = (SOD units of sample in the assay – corrected units) at pH 7.8 × assay dilution × dilution rate in the homogenates.
2. CuZn-SOD activity
   a. [(SOD units of sample in the assay – corrected units) at pH 10.0 × assay dilution × dilution rate in homogenates – total SOD activity at pH 7.8]/8.7, calculated by setting up two simultaneous equations that assume that CuZn-SOD activity has a 9.7 times greater activity in the pH 10.0 assay than in the pH 7.8 assay and that Mn-SOD activity has the same activity in both assays.[96]
   b. At pH 7.8, [SOD activity in the absence of KCN – SOD activity in the presence of KCN]/0.875, calculated assuming 1 m*M* KCN inhibits 87.5% of CuZn-SOD activity and produces no inhibition of Mn-SOD activity.[96]
   c. SOD activity after adding SDS at pH 7.8.
3. Mn-SOD activity. Mn-SOD activity = Total SOD activity – CuZn-SOD activity. Thus, Mn-SOD activity is calculated by the data obtained from 1 and 2, or as follows: SOD activity in the absence of SDS–SOD activity after adding SDS at pH 7.8.

14.5.1.1.7 Comments. When the two assays at the two different pH values are used to calculate CuZn-SOD activity instead of using the pH 7.8 assay only with or without KCN, more accurate data can be obtained.[96]

14.5.2 Measurement of catalase

Several methods have been used to measure catalase activity by monitoring the decomposition of hydrogen peroxide or the liberation of oxygen.[30,38] The method to measure catalase activity in tissues spectrophotometrically is described in Section 14.2.2 on measurement of intracellular generation of hydrogen peroxide.

14.5.3 Measurement of glutathione peroxidase (GSH-Px)

There are two types of methods used to determine GSH-Px activity. One is a direct measurement of unconsumed GSH by polarography[98] or by the dithionitrobenzoic acid method.[99] The second method is used to monitor the regeneration of GSH from GSSG by the action of glutathione reductase with NADPH.[100] We present the latter method with modification by Lawrence and Burk.[101]

14.5.3.1 Glutathione peroxidase (GSH-Px) assay

14.5.3.1.1 Principle. Glutathione peroxidases catalyze the reduction of hydroperoxides (ROOH) by glutathione (GSH):

$$\text{ROOH} + 2\,\text{GSH} \rightarrow \text{ROH} + H_2O + \text{GSSG} \quad (14)$$

Assays of glutathione peroxidase (GSH-Px) activity are based on measurement of ROOH or GSH consumption.[98] Alternatively, GSSG production is monitored by coupling to the reaction catalyzed by glutathione reductase:

$$GSSG + NADPH + H^+ \rightarrow 2\,GSH + NADP^+ \quad (15)$$

Oxidation of NADPH is monitored spectrophotometrically or fluorometrically.

There are two major types of GSH-Px — one is selenium-dependent and is active with both organic hydroperoxides and H_2O_2, and the other is selenium-independent and has negligible activity with H_2O_2.[102] Thus, the total GSH-Px activity can be measured with cumene hydroperoxide as a substrate, and selenium-dependent GSH-Px activity can be measured with H_2O_2 as a substrate. The subtraction of selenium-dependent GSH-Px from total activity is used to calculate selenium-independent glutathione peroxidase activity.[103]

14.5.3.1.2 Tissue preparation. To avoid contamination from erythrocyte enzymes, EDTA (final concentration, 1 m*M*) is added to an aliquot of supernatant.

14.5.3.1.3 Total GSH-Px activity assay

Reagents

Potassium phosphate (50 m*M*, pH 7.0) containing 1 m*M* EDTA and 1 m*M* sodium azide (NaN_3) (which inhibits catalase).

The reagents below should be made fresh in potassium phosphate buffer containing EDTA and NaN_3.

NADPH (2 m*M*).
Glutathione reductase (10 U/ml, type IV from yeast).
Reduced glutathione (10 m*M*, GSH).
Cumene hydroperoxide (15 m*M*).

Procedure

Place 0.5 ml of phosphate buffer containing 1 m*M* EDTA and 1 m*M* NaN_3, 0.1 ml of 2 m*M* NADPH, 0.1 ml of 10 U/ml glutathione reductase, and 0.1 ml of 10 m*M* GSH in the test cuvette. Add 0.1 ml of test sample with mixing and incubate the reaction mixture for 5 min at room temperature. Then initiate the reaction by adding 0.1 ml of 15 m*M* cumene hydroperoxide (final concentration, 1.5 m*M*). Record the absorbance at 340 nm for 5 min using a spectrophotometer, and the activity is calculated from the slope of these lines as micromoles NADPH oxidized per minute. It is necessary to adjust the amount of protein in the test sample to give a rate of change in absorbance of approximately 0.1 per minute. As a blank, add the same amount of deionized water (0.1 ml) in the reaction mixture, and the absorbance should be read and subtracted from the absorbance of sample.

14.5.3.1.4 Calculation of data

$$\text{GSH-Px activity (U/mg protein)} = (\Delta A_{340} \times \text{assay dilution} \times \text{dilution factor for homogenate})/(\text{time, min} \times 6.22) \times 1/\text{mg protein} \quad (16)$$

The molar extinction coefficient of NADPH at 340 nm is 6220 $M^{-1}cm^{-1}$.[104] One unit of the enzyme is defined as the amount of enzyme that oxidizes 1 μmol of NADPH per minute.

14.5.3.1.5 Selenium-dependent GSH-Px activity assay. Selenium dependent GSH-Px activity is measured with H_2O_2 as a substrate. Start the reaction by adding 0.1 ml of 2.5 m*M* H_2O_2 (final concentration, 0.25 m*M*) instead of using cumene hydroperoxide. All other reagents and procedures are the same as those for the assay described above.

14.5.3.1.6 Selenium-independent GSH-Px activity. Selenium-independent GSH-Px activity is calculated by the formula:

$$\text{Selenium-independent GSH-Px activity} = \text{Total GSH-Px activity-selenium-dependent GSH-Px activity.} \quad (17)$$

References

1. McCord, J. M., Oxygen-derived free radicals in postischemic tissue injury, *N. Engl. J. Med.*, 312, 159, 1985.
2. Fantone, J. C. and Ward, P. A., Role of oxygen-derived free radicals and metabolites in leukocyte-dependent inflammatory reactions, *Am. J. Pathol.*, 107, 397, 1982.
3. Weiss, S. J., Oxygen, ischemia and inflammation, *Acta Physiol. Scand.*, 126 (Suppl. 548), 9, 1986.
4. Baud, L. and Ardaillou, R., Reactive oxygen species: production and role in the kidney, *Am. J. Physiol.*, 251, F765, 1986.
5. Freeman, B. A. and Crapo, J. D., Free radicals and tissue injury., *Lab. Invest.*, 47, 412, 1982.
6. Cross, C. E., Halliwell, B., Borish, E. T., Pryor, W. A., Ames, B. N., Saul, R. L., McCord, J. M. and Harman, D., Oxygen radicals and human disease, *Ann. Intern. Med.*, 107, 526, 1987.
7. Shah, S. V., Role of reactive oxygen metabolites in experimental glomerular disease, *Kidney Int.*, 35, 1093, 1989.
8. Shah, S. V., Oxidant mechanisms in glomerulonephritis, *Semin. Nephrol.*, 11, 320, 1991.
9. Ueda, N., Walker, P. D., and Shah, S. V., Oxidant stress in acute renal failure, in *Acute Renal Failure: Emerging New Concepts and Therapeutic Strategies,* Goligorsky M. S., Ed., Churchill Livingstone, New York, 1995.
10. Fridovich, I., The biology of oxygen radicals. The superoxide radical is an agent of oxygen toxicity; superoxide dismutases provide an important defense, *Science*, 201, 875, 1978.
11. McCord, J. M. and Fridovich, I., The biology and pathology of oxygen radicals, *Ann. Intern. Med.*, 89, 122, 1978.
12. Halliwell, B. and Gutteridge, J. M. C., Role of free radicals and catalytic metal ions in human disease: an overview, *Methods Enzymol.*, 186, 1, 1990.
13. McCord, J. M. and Fridovich, I., Superoxide dismutase. An enzymic function for erythrocuprein (hemocuprein), *J. Biol. Chem.*, 244, 6049, 1969.
14. Misra, H. P. and Fridovich, I., The role of superoxide anion in the autoxidation of epinephrine and a simple assay for superoxide dismutase, *J. Biol. Chem.*, 247, 3170, 1972.
15. Rosen, G. M., Finkelstein, E., and Rauckman, E. J., A method for the detection of superoxide in biological systems, *Arch. Biochem. Biophys.*, 215, 367, 1982.
16. Rosen, G. M. and Rauckman, E. J., Spin trapping of superoxide and hydroxyl radicals, *Methods Enzymol.*, 105, 198, 1984.
17. Samuni, A., Carmichael, A. J., Russo, A., Mitchell, J. B., and Riesz, P., On the spin trapping and ESR detection of oxygen-derived radicals generated inside cells, *Proc. Natl. Acad. Sci. U.S.A.*, 83, 7593, 1986.
18. Nakano, M., Determination of superoxide radical and singlet oxygen based on chemiluminescence of luciferin analogs, *Methods Enzymol.*, 186, 585, 1990.
19. Johnston, R. B., Jr., Measurement of O_2^- secreted by monocytes and macrophages, *Methods Enzymol.*, 105, 365, 1984.
20. Azzi, A., Montecucco, C., and Richter, C., The use of acetylated ferricytochrome *c* for the detection of superoxide radicals produced in biological membranes, *Biochem. Biophys. Res. Commun.*, 65, 597, 1975.
21. Massey, V., The microestimation of succinate and the extinction coefficient of cytochrome *c*, *Biochim. Biophys. Acta*, 34, 255, 1959.

22. Shah, S. V., Light emission by isolated rat glomeruli in response to phorbol myristate acetate, *J. Lab. Clin. Med.*, 98, 46, 1981.
23. Trush, M. A., Wilson, M. E., and Van Dyke, K., The generation of chemiluminescence (CL) by phagocytic cells, *Methods Enzymol.*, 57, 462, 1978.
24. Cadenas, E. and Sies, H., Low-level chemiluminescence as an indicator of singlet molecular oxygen in biological systems, *Methods Enzymol.*, 105, 221, 1984.
25. Ohara, Y., Peterson, T. E., and Harrison, D. G., Hypercholesterolemia increases endothelial superoxide anion production, *J. Clin. Invest.*, 91, 2546, 1993.
26. Rathakarishnan, C. and Tiku, M. L., Lucigenin-dependent chemiluminescence in articular chondrocytes, *Free Rad. Biol. Med.*, 15, 143, 1993.
27. Faulkner, K. and Fridovich, I., Luminol and lucigenin as detectors for $O_2^{\bar{}}$, *Free Rad. Biol. Med.*, 15, 447, 1993.
28. Ueda, N., Guidet, B., and Shah, S. V., Measurement of intracellular generation of hydrogen peroxide by rat glomeruli *in vitro*, *Kidney Int.*, 45, 788, 1994.
29. Stanley, P. E. and Williams, S. G., Use of the liquid scintillation spectrometer for determining adenosine triphosphate by the luciferase enzyme, *Anal. Biochem.*, 29, 381, 1969.
30. Chance, B., Sies, H., and Boveris, A., Hydroperoxide metabolism in mammalian organs, *Physiol. Rev.*, 59, 527, 1979.
31. Guidet, B. R. and Shah, S. V., In vivo generation of hydrogen peroxide by rat kidney cortex and glomeruli, *Am. J. Physiol.*, 256, F158, 1989.
32. Guidet, B. and Shah, S. V., Enhanced in vivo H_2O_2 generation by rat kidney in glycerol-induced renal failure, *Am. J. Physiol.*, 257, F440, 1989.
33. Yusa, T., Beckman, J. S., Crapo, J. D., and Freeman, B. A., Hyperoxia increases H_2O_2 production by brain *in vivo*, *J. Appl. Physiol.*, 63, 353, 1987.
34. Cohen, G. and Somerson, N. L., Catalase-aminotriazole method for measuring secretion of hydrogen peroxide by microorganisms, *J. Bacteriol.*, 98, 543, 1969.
35. Tephly, T. R., Mannering, G. J., and Parks, Jr., R. E., Studies on the mechanism of inhibition of liver and erythrocyte catalase activity by 3-amino-1,2,4-triazole (AT), *J. Pharmacol. Exp. Ther.*, 134, 77, 1961.
36. Cohen, G., Dembiec, D., and Marcus, J., Measurement of catalase activity in tissue extracts, *Anal. Biochem.*, 34, 30, 1970.
37. Aebi, H., Catalase, in *Methods of Enzymatic Analysis*, Bergmeyer, H. U., Ed., Verlag Chemie International, Deerfield Beach, FL, 1974.
38. Aebi, H., Catalase in vitro, *Methods Enzymol.*, 105, 121, 1984.
39. Keston, A. S. and Brandt, R., The fluorometric analysis of ultramicro quantities of hydrogen peroxide, *Anal. Biochem.*, 11, 1, 1965.
40. Bass, D. A., Parce, J. W., Dechatelet, L. R., Szejda, P., Seeds, M. C., and Thomas, M., Flow cytometric studies of oxidative product formation by neutrophils: a graded response to membrane stimulation, *J. Immunol.*, 130, 1910, 1983.
41. Rosenkranz, A. R., Schmaldienst, S., Stuhlmeier, K. M., Chen, W., Knapp, W., and Zlabinger, G. J., A microplate assay for the detection of oxidative products using 2′,7′-dichlorofluorescin-diacetate, *J. Immunol. Methods*, 156, 39, 1992.
42. Carter, W. O., Narayanan, P. K., and Robinson, J. P., Intracellular hydrogen peroxide and superoxide anion detection in endothelial cells, *J. Leukocyte Biol.*, 55, 253, 1994.
43. Oyama, Y., Hayashi, A., Ueha, T., and Maekawa, K., Characterization of 2′,7′-dichlorofluorescin fluorescence in dissociated mammalian brain neurons: estimation on intracellular content of hydrogen peroxide, *Brain Res.*, 635, 113, 1994.
44. Hockenbery, D. M., Oltvai, Z. N., Yin, X.-M., Milliman, C. L., and Korsmeyer, S. J., Bcl-2 functions in an antioxidant pathway to prevent apoptosis, *Cell*, 75, 241, 1993.
45. Halliwell, B., Grootveld, M., and Gutteridge, J. M.C., Methods for the measurement of hydroxyl radicals in biochemical systems: deoxyribose degradation and aromatic hydroxylation, *Methods Biochem. Anal.*, 33, 59, 1988.
46. Buettner, G. R. and Mason, R. P., Spin-trapping methods for detecting superoxide and hydroxyl free radicals in vitro and in vivo, *Methods Enzymol.*, 186, 127, 1990.
47. Babbs, C. F. and Steiner, M. G., Detection and quantitation of hydroxyl radical using dimethyl sulfoxide as molecular probe, *Methods Enzymol.*, 186, 137, 1990.

48. Kaur, H., Fagerheim, I., Grootveld, M., Puppo, A., and Halliwell, B., Aromatic hydroxylation of phenylalanine as an assay for hydroxyl radicals: application to activated human neutrophils and to the heme protein leghemoglobin, *Anal. Biochem.*, 172, 360, 1988.
49. Kaur, H. and Halliwell, B., Aromatic hydroxylation of phenylalanine as an assay for hydroxyl radicals: measurement of hydroxyl radical formation from ozone and in blood from premature babies using improved HPLC methodology, *Anal. Biochem.*, 220, 11, 1994.
50. Kaur, H. and Halliwell, B., Detection of hydroxyl radicals by aromatic hydroxylation, *Methods Enzymol.*, 233, 67, 1994.
51. Cao, W., Carney, J. M., Duchon, A., Floyd, R. A., and Chevion, M., Oxygen free radical involvement in ischemia and reperfusion injury to brain, *Neurosci. Lett.*, 88, 233, 1988.
52. Ghiselli, A., Laurenti, O., De Mattia, G., Maiani, G., and Ferro-Luzzi, A., Salicylate hydroxylation as an early marker of *in vivo* oxidative stress in diabetic patients, *Free Rad. Biol. Med.*, 13, 621, 1992.
53. Sun, J. Z., Kaur, H., Halliwell, B., Li, X. Y., and Bolli, R., Use of aromatic hydroxylation of phenylalanine to measure production of hydroxyl radicals after myocardial ischemia in vivo: direct evidence for a pathogenic role of the hydroxyl radical in myocardial stunning, *Circ. Res.*, 73, 534, 1993.
54. Aruoma, O. I., Deoxyribose assay for detecting hydroxyl radicals, *Methods Enzymol.*, 233, 57, 1994.
55. Till, G. O., Hatherill, J. R., Tourtellotte, W. W., Luta, M. J., and Ward, P. A., Lipid peroxidation and acute lung injury after thermal trauma to skin. Evidence of a role for hydroxyl radical, *Am. J. Pathol.*, 119, 376, 1985.
56. Ward, P. A., Till, G. O., Hatherill, J. R., Annesley, T. M., and Kunkel, R. G., Systemic complement activation, lung injury, and products of lipid peroxidation, *J. Clin. Invest.*, 76, 517, 1985.
57. Ramsammy, L. S., Josepovitz, C., Ling, K. Y., Lane, B. P., and Kaloyanides, G. J., Effects of diphenyl-phenylenediamine on gentamicin-induced lipid peroxidation and toxicity in rat renal cortex, *J. Pharmacol. Exp. Ther.*, 238, 83, 1985.
58. Paller, M. S., Hoidal, J. R., and Ferris, T. F., Oxygen free radicals in ischemic acute renal failure in the rat, *J. Clin. Invest.*, 74, 1156, 1984.
59. Meister, A., Selective modification of glutathione metabolism, *Science*, 220, 472, 1983.
60. Meister, A., Glutathione metabolism and its selective modification, *J. Biol. Chem.*, 263, 17205, 1988.
61. White, C. W., Mimmack, R. F., and Repine, J. E., Accumulation of lung tissue oxidized glutathione (GSSG) as a marker of oxidant induced lung injury, *Chest*, 89, 111S, 1986.
62. White, C. W., Ghezzi, P., Dinarello, C. A., Caldwell, S. A., McMurtry, I. F., and Repine, J. E., Recombinant tumor necrosis factor/cachectin and interleukin 1 pretreatment decreases lung oxidized glutathione accumulation, lung injury, and mortality in rats exposed to hyperoxia, *J. Clin. Invest.*, 79, 1868, 1987.
63. Dunbar, J. R., DeLucia, A. J., and Bryant, L. R., Glutathione status of isolated rabbit lungs, *Biochem. Pharmacol.*, 33, 1343, 1984.
64. Sies, H. and Akerboom, T. P. M., Glutathione disulfide (GSSG) efflux from cells and tissues, *Methods Enzymol.*, 105, 445, 1984.
65. Scaduto, R. C., Jr., Gattone, V. H., II., Grotyohann, L. W., Wertz, J., and Martin, L. F., Effect of an altered glutathione content on renal ischemic injury, *Am. J. Physiol.*, 255, F911, 1988.
66. Abul-Ezz, S. R., Walker, P. D., and Shah, S. V., Role of glutathione in an animal model of myoglobinuric acute renal failure, *Proc. Natl. Acad. Sci. U.S.A.*, 88, 9833, 1991.
67. Paller, M. S., Renal work, glutathione and susceptibility to free radical-mediated postischemic injury, *Kidney Int.*, 33, 843, 1988.
68. Slater, T. F., Overview of methods used for detecting lipid peroxidation, *Methods Enzymol.*, 105, 283, 1984.
69. Bird, R. P., Hung, S. S. O., Hadley, M., and Draper, H. H., Determination of malonaldehyde in biological materials by high-pressure liquid chromatography, *Anal. Biochem.*, 128, 240, 1983.
70. Esterbauer, H. and Cheeseman, K. H., Determination of aldehydic lipid peroxidation products: malonaldehyde and 4-hydroxynonenal, *Methods Enzymol.*, 186, 407, 1990.
71. Draper, H. H. and Hadley, M., Malondialdehyde determination as index of lipid peroxidation, *Methods Enzymol.*, 186, 421, 1990.

72. Slater, T. F. and Sawyer, B. C., The simulatory effects of carbon tetrachloride and other halogenoalkanes on peroxidative reactions in rat liver fractions *in vitro*, *Biochem. J.*, 123, 805, 1971.
73. Nair, V. and Turner, G. A., The thiobarbituric acid test for lipid peroxidation: structure of the adduct with malondialdehyde, *Lipids*, 19, 804, 1984.
74. Bird, R. P. and Draper, H. H., Comparative studies on different methods of malonaldehyde determination, *Methods Enzymol.*, 105, 299, 1984.
75. Uchiyama, M. and Mihara, M., Determination of malonaldehyde precursor in tissues by thiobarbituric acid test, *Anal. Biochem.*, 86, 271, 1978.
76. Esterbauer, H., Lang, J., Zadravec, S., and Slater, T. F., Detection of malonaldehyde by high-performance liquid chromatography, *Methods Enzymol.*, 105, 319, 1984.
77. Chirico, S., High-performance liquid chromatography based thiobarbituric acid tests, *Methods Enzymol.*, 233, 314, 1994.
78. Recknagel, R. O. and Glende, Jr., E.A., Spectrophotometric detection of lipid conjugated dienes, *Methods Enzymol.*, 105, 331, 1984.
79. Folch, J., Lees, M., and Stanley, G. H. S., A simple method for the isolation and purification of total lipids from animal tissue, *J. Biol. Chem.*, 226, 497, 1957.
80. Corongiu, F. and Banni, S., Detection of conjugated dienes by second derivative ultraviolet spectrophotometry, *Methods Enzymol.*, 233, 303, 1994.
81. Tietze, F., Enzymic method for quantitative determination of nanogram amounts of total and oxidized glutathione: applications to mammalian blood and other tissues, *Anal. Biochem.*, 27, 502, 1969.
82. Meister, A. and Anderson, M. E., Glutathione, *Annu. Rev. Biochem.*, 52, 711, 1983.
83. Griffith, O. W., Determination of glutathione and glutathione disulfide using glutathione reductase and 2-vinylpyridine, *Anal. Biochem.*, 106, 207, 1980.
84. Owens, C. W. I. and Belcher, R. V., A colorimetric micro-method for the determination of glutathione, *Biochem. J.*, 94, 705, 1965.
85. Anderson, M. E., Determination of glutathione and glutathione disulfide in biological samples, *Methods Enzymol.*, 113, 548, 1985.
86. Evans, P. J. and Halliwell, B., Measurement of iron and copper in biological systems: bleomycin and copper-phenanthroline assays, *Methods Enzymol.*, 233, 82, 1994.
87. Gutteridge, J. M. C., Rowley, D. A., and Halliwell, B., Superoxide-dependent formation of hydroxyl radicals in the presence of iron salts. Detection of 'free' iron in biological systems by using bleomycin-dependent degradation of DNA, *Biochem. J.*, 199, 263, 1981.
88. Baliga, R., Ueda, N., and Shah, S. V., Increase in bleomycin-detectable iron in ischaemia/reperfusion injury to rat kidneys, *Biochem. J.*, 291, 901, 1993.
89. Crapo, J. D., McCord, J. M., and Fridovich, I., Preparation and assay of superoxide dismutases, *Methods Enzymol.*, 53, 382, 1978.
90. Ballou, D., Palmer, G., and Massey, V., Direct demonstration of superoxide anion production during the oxidation of reduced flavin and of its catalytic decomposition by erythrocuprein, *Biochem. Biophys. Res. Commun.*, 36, 898, 1969.
91. Klug, D., Rabani, J., and Fridovich, I., A direct demonstration of the catalytic action of superoxide dismutase through the use of pulse radiolysis, *J. Biol. Chem.*, 247, 4839, 1972.
92. Marshall, M. J. and Worsfold, M., Superoxide dismutase: a direct, continuous linear assay using the oxygen electrode, *Anal. Biochem.*, 86, 561, 1978.
93. Flohe, L. and Otting, F., Superoxide dismutase assays, *Methods Enzymol.*, 105, 93, 1984.
94. Beauchamp, C. and Fridovich, I., Superoxide dismutase: improved assays and an assay applicable to acrylamide gel, *Anal. Biochem.*, 44, 276, 1971.
95. Corbisier, P., Houbison, A., and Remacle, J., A new technique for highly sensitive detection of superoxide dismutase activity by chemiluminescence, *Anal. Biochem.*, 164, 240, 1987.
96. Sjostrom, K. and Crapo, J. D., Structural and biochemical adaptative changes in rat lung after exposure to hypoxia, *Lab. Invest.*, 48, 68, 1983.
97. Geller, B. L. and Winge, D. R., A method for distinguishing Cu,Zn- and Mn-containing superoxide dismutases, *Anal. Biochem.*, 128, 86, 1983.
98. Flohe, L. and Gunzler, W. A., Assays of glutathione peroxidase, *Methods Enzymol.*, 105, 114, 1984.

99. Wendel, A., Glutathione peroxidase, *Methods Enzymol.*, 77, 325, 1981.
100. Paglia, D. E. and Valentine, W. N., Studies on the quantitative and qualitative characterization of erythrocyte glutathione peroxidase, *J. Lab. Clin. Med.*, 70, 158, 1967.
101. Lawrence, R. A. and Burk, R. F., Glutathione peroxidase activity in selenium-deficient rat liver, *Biochem. Biophys. Res. Commun.*, 71, 952, 1976.
102. Mannervik, B., Glutathione peroxidase, *Methods Enzymol.*, 113, 490, 1985.
103. Lawrence, R. A. and Burk, R. F., Species, tissue and subcellular distribution of non Se-dependent glutathione peroxidase activity, *J. Nutr.*, 108, 211, 1978.
104. Horecker, B. L. and Kornberg, A., The extinction coefficients of the reduced band of pyridine nucleotides, *J. Biol. Chem.*, 175, 385, 1948.

chapter fifteen

Mechanisms of Repair After Renal Injury

Steven B. Miller

15.1 Introduction ... 283
15.2 Growth factor expression in the regenerating kidney ... 286
15.3 Markers of renal regeneration ... 288
15.3.1 Thymidine incorporation ... 288
15.3.2. [^{3}H]thymidine histoautoradiography ... 289
15.3.3 5-Bromo-2′-deoxyuridine (BrdU) incorporation ... 289
15.3.4 Proliferating cell nuclear antigen (PCNA) ... 290
15.4 Markers of differentiation ... 292
15.4.1 Vimentin ... 292
15.4.2 Clusterin ... 292
15.5 Apoptosis ... 293
15.5.1 Electron microscopy ... 293
15.5.2 DNA fragmentation ... 293
15.5.2.1 DNA extraction ... 294
15.5.2.2 3′ End-labeling of DNA ... 295
15.5.2.3 Gel electrophoresis and autoradiography ... 295
References ... 296

15.1 Introduction

Acute renal failure (ARF) is the most costly kidney condition requiring hospitalization.[1] The number of cases is increasing, probably as a result of more complicated surgical procedures on older and sicker patients. Unfortunately, despite the advent of hemodialysis, the mortality rate for patients with ARF has not changed over the last 40 years.[2] At the current time, the standard therapy for ARF is supportive care to permit regeneration of damaged nephron segments. No therapy exists that can accelerate renal recovery. Consequently, the need exists for a new therapeutic approach that can speed regeneration of damaged renal tissue and reduce mortality.

The kidney possesses a remarkable capacity for restoring its structural and functional capacity after an ischemic or toxic injury. The most susceptible region of the nephron to ischemic injury is the distal segment (S_3) of the proximal tubule and the medullary thick ascending limb of the loop of Henle.[3] Following injury, there is loss of the epithelial lining in these segments as necrotic cells are shed into the lumen. An intense regenerative process

0-8493-3341-5/96/$0.00+$.50

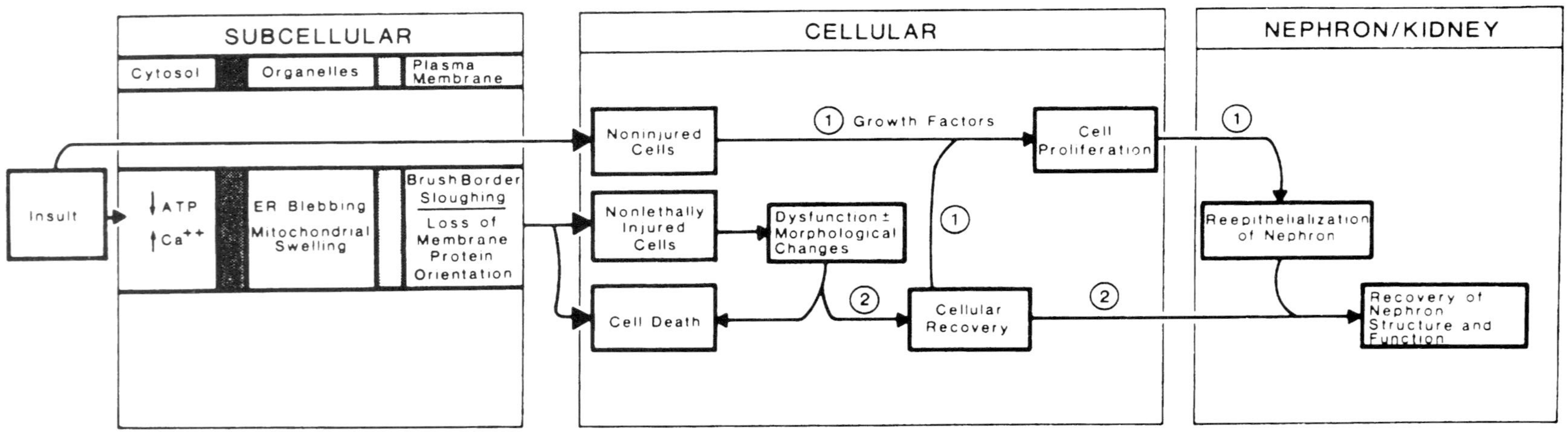

Figure 1 Schematic representing some of the events following a renal insult and epithelial cell repair. Cellular proliferation and reepithelialization by surrounding noninjured cells is indicated by Pathway 1. Recovery of nonlethally injured cells is indicated by Pathway 2. (From Toback, G. R., *Kidney Int.*, 41, 226, 1992. With permission.)

follows. It is theorized that surviving cells situated close to or within the necrotic area dedifferentiate and enter miotic cycles, and then redifferentiate until nephron segment integrity is restored.[4,5] The molecular basis regulating this regenerative process is poorly understood. Figure 1 provides a schematic representation of the renal response to an ischemic or toxic injury.[1]

After an initial renal insult there is a spectrum of cellular damage. Injury can be manifested by subcellular events, which include mitochondrial swelling and blebbing of the endoplasmic reticulum. There is sloughing of the brush border membrane and loss of protein orientation and phospholipid content. The barrier function of the plasma membrane is lost. If the intensity of the insult is limited, the cell becomes dysfunctional but survives. More severe injury results in detachment of the cell from the tubular basement membrane and necrosis. Still other cells have no apparent damage and may proliferate to reepithelialize the damaged nephron segments. Thus, as indicated in Figure 1, several different processes are required to achieve structural and functional integrity of the kidney following a toxic or ischemic insult:[1] (1) noninjured cells must proliferate and reepithelialize damaged nephron segments; (2) nonlethally damaged cells must recover; and (3) some damaged cells may actually die, not as a result of the initial insult, but through a process of programmed cell death known as apoptosis. This chapter reviews some of the methods useful in examining the renal response to injury and the subsequent repair process.

Ischemic or toxic acute renal failure is a reversible form of organ failure. The kidney is unique as a solid organ in its ability to suffer an injury of such magnitude that the organ fails and yet recovers to full function. The injury phase is due to structural damage to renal epithelial cells, predominantly proximal tubule cells. The recovery phase is dependent on the repair and replacement of the injured and necrotic tubule epithelial cells.[6]

At least three growth factors — epidermal growth factor (EGF),[7,8] insulin-like growth factor I (IGF I),[9–10] and hepatocyte growth factor (HGF)[11] — have been shown to be useful as therapeutic agents in rat models of acute renal failure. The rationale for the use of EGF, IGF I, or HGF as therapeutic agents in acute renal failure is as follows: (1) EGF[12] and IGF I[13] bind to specific receptors in the proximal tubule and regulate metabolic and transport processes at this site; (2) EGF,[14] HGF,[15] and to a lesser extent IGF I[11] are mitogens for proximal tubule *in vitro*, and expression of EGF,[16] IGF I,[17] HGF,[18] and the HGF receptor[19] is enhanced in kidneys undergoing compensatory growth; (3) expression of IGF I,[20] HGF,[21] and the HGF receptor[19] in kidney is increased after acute renal injury in rats; and (4) both IGF I[22] and the EGF-like peptide transforming growth factor α (TGF α)[23] are essential for the growth and development of the metanephric kidney *in vitro*, a process that may be recapitulated by tubular regeneration postinjury.

A graphic demonstration of the natural regenerative process that occurs following renal damage is provided by experiments in which growth factors are administered following renal injury.[24] These experiments provide investigators the opportunity to observe the natural regenerative process and compare results obtained after growth factor administration. Figure 2 demonstrates the results obtained from an experiment in which rats received IGF I or vehicle in established ischemic acute renal failure. In this experiment, rats were subjected to bilateral renal artery occlusion for 60 min. Twenty-four hours post-reperfusion, animals were randomized to receive IGF I or vehicle. As evidenced by the serum creatinine, the renal injury was severe. Serum creatinine at the time of randomization, 24 h post-reperfusion was sevenfold over baseline. In animals that received vehicle, renal function continued to worsen, with serum creatinine peaking on day 2. In contrast, rats treated with IGF I beginning 24 h post reperfusion, serum creatinine started to decline toward baseline. Values for creatinine measured between days 1 and 7 were significantly lower in the IGF I-treated than in the vehicle-treated animals, indicating more rapid restoration of normal renal function ($p < 0.05$). Similarly, levels of BUN in IGF I-treated rats were significantly lower than those measured in vehicle-treated animals ($p < 0.02$). Although weights of rats treated with IGF I tended to be higher than weights of vehicle-treated rats during the 7 days postischemia, differences between groups were not significant.

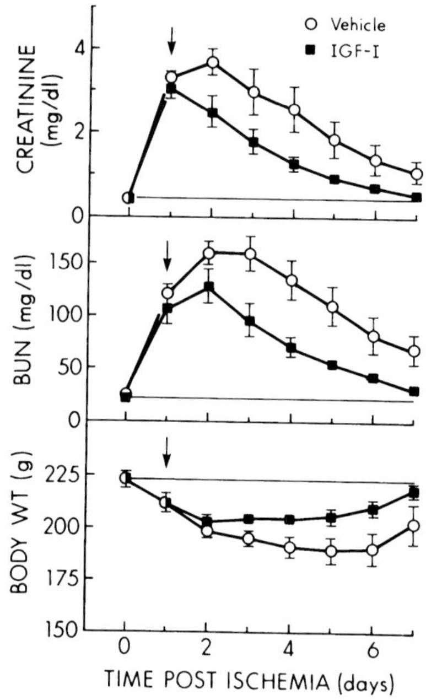

Figure 2 Levels of serum creatinine, blood urea nitrogen (BUN), and weight as function of time in rats treated with vehicle (○) or IGF I (■) beginning 24 h postinduction of ischemic acute renal failure (arrow). Data are means ± SE. (From Miller, S. B., Martin, D. R., Kissane, J., and Hammerman, M. R., *Am. J. Physiol.*, 266, F949, 1994. With permission.)

Regeneration is not only apparent from functional data but also from histologic evidence of structural recovery. Figure 3 is a photomicrograph of a representative histologic section originating from the kidney of an animal in which ischemic acute renal failure was induced 24 h before. As evidenced in the figure there is severe damage to proximal tubular epithelium, with extensive cellular necrosis, sloughing of the brush border, and tubular obstruction.

As previously stated, this is a reversible injury. In animals randomized to either vehicle or IGF I 24 h post-reperfusion, there is substantial improvement in the histologic appearance of the kidneys at the time of sacrifice on day 7 (Figure 4). The kidneys of animals that received vehicle still have evidence of a significant renal injury in that there is dilatation and simplification of the proximal tubules. An ongoing regenerative response is manifested by papillary proliferations within the proximal tubules. The integrity of the tubules is restored and most of the sloughed brush border membranes are no longer evident. The histologic appearance of kidneys from animals that received IGF I have almost recovered to normal. Thus, in both vehicle- and IGF I-treated animals there is histologic evidence of substantial regeneration/proliferation and repair.

15.2 *Growth factor expression in the regenerating kidney*

In several classic reports Cuppage, Tate, and colleagues carefully evaluated renal tubule cell regeneration after mercuric chloride induced acute renal failure in rats.[25-26] This toxin produces necrosis of the proximal tubule cells shortly after administration. Regeneration

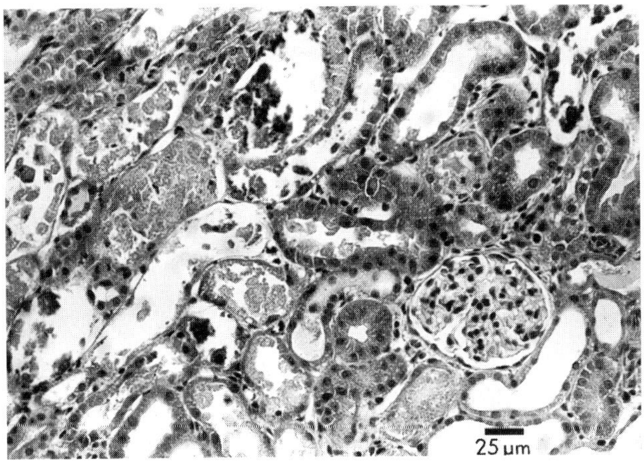

Figure 3 Photomicrograph of histologic section stained with hematoxylin and eosin originating from kidney of rat in which ischemic acute renal failure was induced 24 h before. Section is representative of those originating from five rats. (From Miller, S. B., Martin, D. R., Kissane, J., and Hammerman, M. R., *Am. J. Physiol.*, 266, F949, 1994. With permission.)

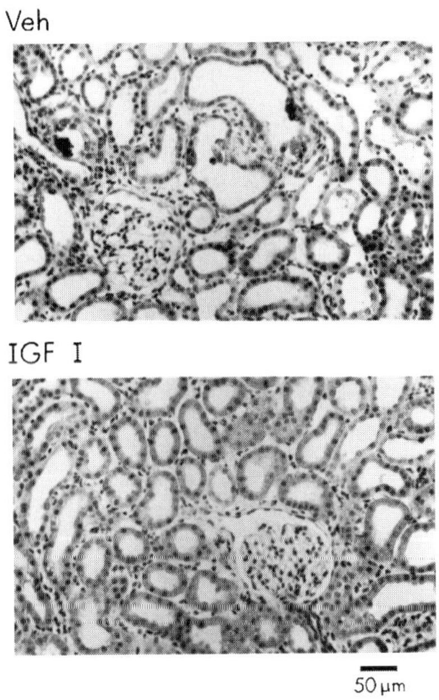

Figure 4 Photomicrographs of histologic sections stained with hematoxylin and eosin originating from kidneys of rats treated with vehicle (top) or IGF I (bottom) beginning 24 h postischemic injury. Sections are representative of those originating from six rats in each group. (From Miller, S. B., Martin, D. R., Kissane, J., and Hammerman, M. R., *Am. J. Physiol.*, 266, F949, 1994. With permission.)

of epithelial cells began within the first 2 days, with immature epithelial cells relining the necrotic area by day 3. Epithelial cells at both ends of the necrotic segments of involved tubules, as well as surviving epithelial cells along the denuded surface of the tubular basement membrane, appear to be responsible for the regenerating cells. Cell doubling time was approximately 14 h so that most tubules were relined with new epithelium by day 5. A time course similar to that observed with mecuric chloride for renal tubule cell regeneration and renal function recovery has also been observed after bilateral renal artery occlusion in rats.[7] These observations suggest that local factors play a significant role in mediating the regenerative process leading to recovery from acute renal failure. The process of regeneration and repair by surviving epithelial cells at the edge of the injured segment is likely dependent on production of local growth factors (Figure 1).[1,27]

Growth factors that are produced in kidney and are known to accelerate recovey following a renal insult may represent logical candidates to study in an attempt to identify the factors associated with the natural regenerative process. We have recently examined the expression of EGF, IGF I, and HGF following an ischemic renal insult. Since the regenerative response starts early after induction of injury, times examined were baseline, 3, 6, 12, and 24 h post-reperfusion. A highly sensitive and specific solution hybridization nuclease protection assay for each growth factor of interest was performed on samples of total RNA.[28] Tissue was obtained from three animals sacrificed at each time point.

The renal expression of mRNA for both EGF and IGF I decreased rapidly following induction of ischemic injury. Verstrepen et al. observed a similar pattern of expression for total kidney mRNA for EGF and IGF I during the course of nephrotoxic acute renal failure.[29] In striking contrast, the expression of renal HGF mRNA after an ischemic insult differs from the pattern observed with EGF and IGF I (Figure 5). HGF expression rapidly increases to a level 3.7-fold above that of the baseline. This is in agreement with observations from other laboratories that report an early increase in expression of HGF message and peptide.[21] This suggests that HGF may participate in the natural regenerative response to acute renal failure.

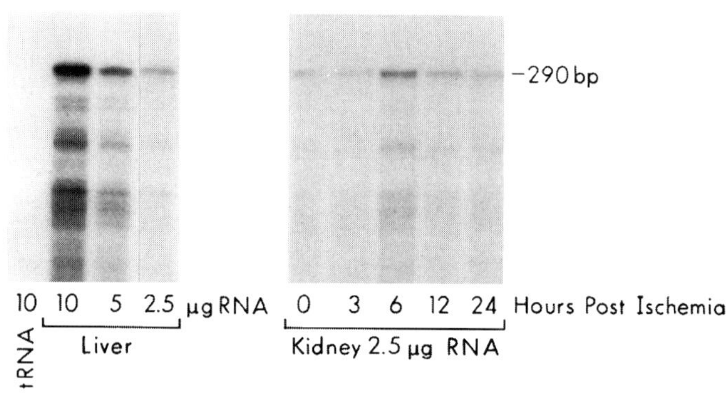

Figure 5 Representative autoradiograph of a solution-hybridization, nuclease protection experiment using total cellular RNA originating from normal rat liver, yeast RNA, or rat kidney at times 0, 3, 6, 12, or 24 post ischemia. A specific 290-nucleotide fragment is protected by the probe for HGF. HGF mRNA expression is significantly increased 6 h postischemia.

15.3 *Markers of renal regeneration*

Investigators have utilized several techniques to examine the regenerative response at the cellular level after an ischemic or toxic renal injury. We review several of these techniques, describe the methodology, and highlight the limitations and advantages of each.

15.3.1 *Thymidine incorporation*

A technique that quantifies regeneration is the incorporation of [^{3}H]thymidine into dividing cells of the tissue to be examined.[7,25,26] The major disadvantages of this technique is the use of [^{3}H], a radioactive material with a long half-life. As with most radioactive agents, [^{3}H] requires special handling of samples and waste, with the associated costs of storage and radioactive waste disposal. In addition, a scintillation counter is required. The advantages of this technique are the relative simplicity and reliability of the method.

The following protocol is recommended for examining regeneration in an intact rat model of either ischemic or toxic acute renal failure.[7,30] Modifications will be required dependent on the animal model utilized, with the major determinant being animal size.

1. One hour prior to sacrifice, the rat receives an intraperitoneal injection of 200 μCi of [methyl-^{3}H]thymidine diluted in 0.25 ml of sterile water.
2. The animal is sacrificed and the kidneys quickly removed. Samples that are not processed immediately should be snap-frozen and stored at –70°C.
3. Tissue is homogenized in ice-cold distilled water (2 ml/100 g tissue) using a tissumizer.
4. DNA content should be determined on 1 ml of the homogenate.
5. Radioactivity is determined in duplicate on 0.5 ml of the sample placed in 2 ml of scintillation solution and counted in a scintillation counter.
6. Counts from the samples are corrected for DNA content.
7. A serum sample should be obtained from each study animal and counted to assure consistent intraperitoneal absorption of the [^{3}H]thymidine.

15.3.2 [^{3}H]thymidine histoautoradiography

While examining homogenized tissue for [^{3}H]thymidine incorporation provides quantitative information concerning regeneration, it does not help in localizing the cells within the tissue that are undergoing proliferation. An extension of the technique that provides localization to the actual proliferating cells is [^{3}H]thymidine histoautoradiography.[7] The major limitation of this technique is, again, the requirement of radioactive material, but, in addition, there is a long exposure time required for visualization of the incorporated [^{3}H]thymidine.

1. One hour prior to sacrifice, the rat receives an intraperitoneal injection of 200 μCi of [methyl-^{3}H]thymidine diluted in 0.25 ml of sterile water.
2. Kidneys are perfused *in vivo* with 2% glutaraldehyde in 0.1 *M* sodium cacodylate buffer (pH 7.2).
3. Tissue sections are placed in 4% formaldehyde, 1% glutaraldehyde, 100 m*M* phosphate buffer (pH 7.2).
4. Specimens are dehydrated and embedded in methacrylate.
5. Tissue sections (4 μm) are dipped in NBT-2 nuclear emulsion (Eastman Kodak Co., Rochester, NY) and stored in the dark at 4°C for three weeks.
6. Sections are developed and counterstained with methylene blue–basic fuchsin.

15.3.3 5-Bromo-2′-deoxyuridine (BrdU) incorporation

A technique that is particularly useful in quantitating or localizing regenerating cells is the incorporation of BrdU.[11] BrdU is an analog of uridine, but is incorporated specifically into DNA in place of thymidine. Cells can be pulse-labeled with BrdU, and those cells that are synthesizing DNA (i.e., in S phase of the cell cycle) will incorporate BrdU into the DNA. Fluorescein-conjugated monoclonal anti-BrdU antibodies can then be used to identify those cells that were undergoing DNA synthesis during exposure to BrdU. The proportion of cells in S phase of the cell cycle can be determined either by fluorescence microscopy or by flow cytometric analysis. Advantages of this technique include ease of use, lack of radioactive materials, and rapid analysis. The major disadvantage is the need for a flow cytometer or fluorescence microscope. The protocol provided below is for fluorescence microscopy. Adjustments must be made depending on animal size and the degree of organ proliferation.

1. One hour prior to sacrifice, the rat receives an intraperitoneal injection of BrdU (50 mg/kg) dissolved in 20% ethanol.
2. The kidneys are perfused *in vivo* with *N*-2-hydroxyethylpiperazine-*N*′-2-ethanesulfonic acid buffer warmed to 37°C.
3. Sections are embedded and sliced at 5 μm on a cryostat. Sections are stored in 70% alcohol at 4°C.
4. Tissue sections are exposed to 0.007 *N* sodium hydroxide for 2 min and then washed in phosphate buffered saline (PBS) three times.
5. Sections are incubated in a humidified chamber for 2 h with monoclonal fluorescein isothiocyanate-conjugated anti-BrdU antibodies (Becton–Dickinson, San Jose, CA) diluted 1:5 with 0.5% Tween 20 in PBS.
6. Sections are washed three times in PBS, air-dried, and cover-slipped.

Figure 6 provides an example of the incorporation of BrdU into renal tissue originating from noninjured normal rats or rats injured 2 days previously that were administered vehicle or the potent renal mitogen HGF.[11] Kidneys originating in noninjured normal rats incorporate relatively little BrdU in cortical tubular epithelia. In contrast, vehicle- and HGF-treated rats incorporate more BrdU than do noninjured animals. Thus this technique allows for both quantification and localization of the proliferative response in the setting of acute renal injury.

15.3.4 Proliferating cell nuclear antigen (PCNA)

Another useful marker of replication is identification of cell-producing PCNA, a DNA polymerase δ-associated protein.[31] This protein is required for synthesis of the leading strand at the replication fork and is necessary for entry of cells from late G_1 into S phase of the cell cycle. PCNA is also expressed during DNA repair. The major advantage of this technique is that no exogenous sustance needs to be administered and incorporated into replicating cells. Thus, variations in the absorption of either [^{3}H]thymidine or BrdU are not an issue. The method described below is a standard streptavidin–biotin method to examine PCNA in Bouin's fixed paraffin-embedded specimens. There are many kits available to simplify this technique. Make sure that the reagents utilized are appropiate for the primary antibody. Several notes of caution should be considered before attempting this method. Formaldhyde is known to induce steric changes in the antigen molecules (intermolecular cross-linking). Excessive formalin fixation can mask antigenic sites and diminish specific staining. Milder fixatives are recommended. Likewise, temperatures in excess of 60°C must be avoided when processing the tissue. Rapid, high-temperature processing destroys antigenicity.

1. Slides should be deparaffinized and rehydrated. This is accomplished by placing the slides in a xylene bath for 5 min and then repeating once. Slides are next placed in absolute ethanol for 3 min × 2 followed by 95% ethanol for 3 min × 2 and finally distiller or deionized water for 30 s.
2. Quench endogenous peroxidase activity by incubating slides for 5 min with 3% hydrogen peroxide. Rinse gently with distilled water.
3. Apply enough mouse anti-rat PCNA antibody (Dako, Carpinteria, CA) to cover the specimen and incubate in a humidified chamber for 30 min. Rinse gently.

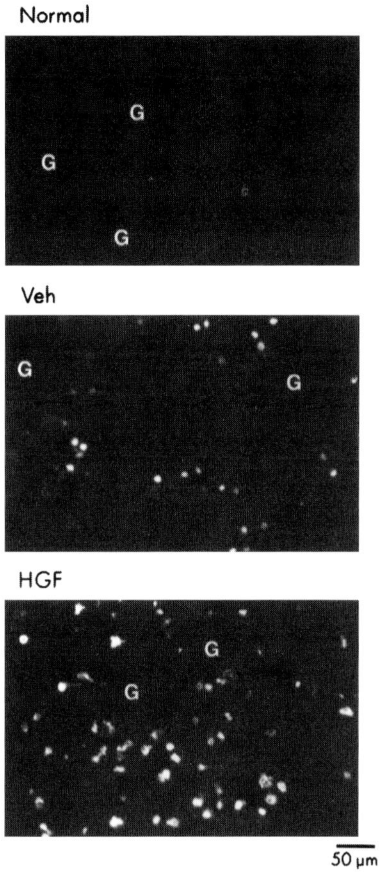

Figure 6 Incorporation of BrdU in renal cortices. Photomicrographs are shown of histologic sections stained with fluorescein-labeled anti-BrdU originating from noninjured normal rats or rats injured 2 days previously administered vehicle or HGF. Sections are representative of those originating from five rats in each group. G = glomeruli. (From Miller, S. B., Martin, D. R., Kissane, J., and Hammerman, M. R., *Am. J. Physiol.*, 266, F129, 1994. With permission.)

4. Apply enough biotinylated anti-mouse secondary antibody to cover the specimen. Incubate in a humidified chamber for 30 min. Rinse gently.
5. Apply enough streptavidin peroxidase to cover the specimen and incubate in a humidified chamber for 30 min. Rinse gently.
6. Add the chromogen, 3% 3-amino-9-ethylcarbazole in *N,N*-dimethylformamide to acetate buffer containing hydrogen peroxide. Cover the specimen and incubate for 10 min. Rinse gently.
7. Counterstain with hematoxylin for 2 to 5 min. Dip in 37 m*M* ammonium hydroxide bath and then place in distilled water for 2 min.
8. Allow to air-dry and then mount. Positive staining is represented by the red reaction product.

Appropriate positive and negative controls must be included because both false-positive and false-negative staining can be seen. The tubular epithelium of kidney may have endogenous avidin-binding activity. Endogenous avidin-binding activity can be suppressed by sequential 20-min incubations, first with 0.1% avidin and then with 0.01% biotin in 0.05 *M* TRIS-HCl buffer, pH 7.2 to 7.6.

15.4 Markers of differentiation

Once the regenerative phase is accomplished, the final repair process is that of differentiation of the regenerative, immature tubule cell into a mature, functional cell. The final differentiation of renal proximal tubule cells requires the development of correct spatial orientation and pattern formation so that the epithelial cells develop polarity within tubule structures.[6] These epithelial cells must be capable of performing the physiologic process of transport along with endocrine and metabolic functions.

Since the kidney is so heterogeneous in structure and function and since the extent of damage to the renal tubule after a toxic or ischemic injury depends upon the location of the tubule within the nephron, knowledge of changes in overall levels of protein or mRNA does not provide much insight into the role a particular protein may play in the recovery process. To better understand the process of differentiation in regenerating renal epithelial cells, it is important to identify which cells are expressing specific differentiation markers.[31] A useful and relatively simple technique is immunohistochemistry for specific differentiation proteins. In this section we review two of the commonly employed markers of differentiation in renal tubular epithelium.[31] Antibodies to these markers are available, and most can be adapted to either immunofluoescence microscopy or immunoperoxidase microscopy.

15.4.1 Vimentin

The intermediate filaments constitute a large multigene family of different proteins whose expression correlates with cell type and phase of cellular differentiation.[32] Within the intermediate filament protein family is the group of cytokeratin filaments.[32] The cytokeratin filaments are predominantly epithelium-specific. Consequently intermediate filament and cytokeratin filament proteins are useful as differentiation markers, especially in the fields of embryogenesis, tumor pathology, and cellular regeneration.

Vimentin is an intermediate filament protein that is expressed in mesenchymal tissue, but not in normal, differentiated kidney epithelial cells. Nephron segments derived from metanephrogenic mesenchyme express vimentin in early stages of development.[31-34] In later stages, vimentin expression is turned off and cytokeratin expression is turned on.[32] In normal adult kidney, tubular epithelial cells do not express vimentin. Vimentin is expressed in renal cell carcinomas, with expression being greatest in those tumors that are most poorly differentiated.[32,33]

Vimentin expression has been demonstrated in regenerating kidney following either an ischemic or toxic insult. Expression is early, during the proliferative phase of regeneration and repair. In fact, following an ischemic insult, expression is greatest in the S_3 segment of the proximal tubule.[31,33] This is the nephron segment that is most suseptible to an ischemic renal insult.

15.4.2 Clusterin

Clusterin is a heterodimeric glycoprotein.[35] Initially isolated from ram rete testis fluid, clusterin is so named for its ability to elicit clustering of Sertoli and red blood cells. Many investigators, working in divergent areas, have isolated or cloned species or tissue homologues, which has resulted in a number of different names for clusterin. Some of these names for clusterin include complement cytolysis inhibitor or CLI, sulfated glycoprotein-2 or SGP-2, testosterone-repressed prostate message-2 or TRMP-s, dimeric acidic glycoprotein or DAG, gp 80, NA1/NA, lipoprotein-associated protein, apolipoprotein J, and glycoprotein III.[35]

Clusterin is induced early during renal injury and is useful as a marker of cellular damage.[31] The role of clusterin remains unknown. The presence of clusterin in developing tubules as well as in cystic renal tissue, immature tubules in hypoplastic/dysplastic kidneys, injured tubules following ischemia or renal toxins, and some renal cancer cells indicates that it is a marker of dedifferentiation.[33]

15.5 Apoptosis

If the extent of cellular hypoxia following an ischemic renal insult is severe, there is extensive cellular necrosis, especially in the S_3 segment of the proximal tubules.[3] The pathologic features of necrosis are due to changes in cellular functions such that there is mitochondrial swelling and loss of plasma membrane integrity, leading to swelling and rupture of cells. Cellular contents are then spilled into the surrounding tissue space provoking an inflammatory response.

Recently, it has been recognized that following an ischemic renal insult, a population of cells undergoes a different form of cell death known as apoptosis.[36-38] This is alluded to in Figure 1 by the pathway in which nonlethally injured cells still proceed to a nonnecrotic cell death.[1] Apoptosis, or programmed cell death, is morphologically and biochemically distinct from necrotic cell death.[39-40] In apoptosis, the appearance of a dying cell is much different. While the mitochondria function normally, the nucleus collapses and chromatin is densely packed around the nuclear envelope.[40] The cell shrinks, losing 20 to 30% of its volume. The plasma membrane ruffles and blebs, but remains intact, and the cell contents are not spilled. Shortly after this process is initiated, the apoptotic cell is recognized and undergoes phagocytosis with no resultant inflammatory response.

Apoptosis is probably an important component of the regeneration/repair process following an ischemic or toxic renal insult. Several studies have demonstrated that during the repair phase there is an initial excess epithelial cell proliferation. Shimizu and Yamanaka confirmed these results and extended the observation.[36] They demonstrated two peaks of apoptosis, occurring on days 3 and 8 following 60 min of bilateral ischemia in rats. They concluded that apoptosis was essential for recovery of normal renal architecture.

There is no absolute marker for apoptosis.[40] Most studies rely on the use of several techniques to confirm the presence of apoptotic cells. In this section we describe several useful techniques that are easy to apply to the study of acute renal injury.

15.5.1 Electron microscopy

While an excellent method by which to identify cells undergoing apopotic death, this technique is labor intensive, expensive, and difficult to obtain on large numbers of samples. In addition, apoptotic cells are rapidly phagocytized and thus exist in tissues for only brief periods of time.[37] This makes it difficult to quantify apoptosis by electron microscopy. This being the case, it is still very useful to establish the presence of apoptotic cells by this method. The collapse of the nucleus is the hallmark of apoptosis and is best studied by electron microscopy.[40] The chromatin forms dense crescent-shaped aggregates lining the nuclear membrane. Complex invaginations develop in the nuclear membrane resulting in segmentation of the nucleus. The plasma membrane also becomes convoluted, and the cell separates into a cluster of membrane-bound segments known as apoptotic bodies. The apoptotic bodies contain morphologically normal mitochondria and other cellular organelles. Figure 7 demonstrates many of these morphological features.

15.5.2 DNA fragmentation

A striking feature of apoptosis is the activation of specific endonucleases that cleave cellular DNA between regularly spaced nucleosomal units.[37,39,40] The apoptotic DNA degradation produces DNA fragments in size multiples of 185 to 200 bp, which can be visualized

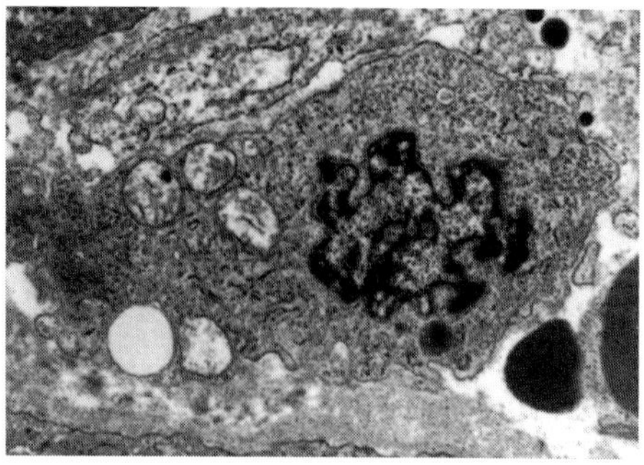

Figure 7 Photoelectronmicrograph of a histologic section originating from kidney of a rat in which ischemic acute renal failure was induced 48 h before. The renal epithelial cell is undergoing morphological changes consistent with apoptotic cell death.

as a distinct ladder of DNA bands following gel electrophoresis and ethidium bromide staining. In the setting of acute toxic or ischemic renal failure, where many of the cells are necrotic, this method is insensitive. Recently, Tilly and Hsueh have described a simple and sensitive autoradiographic method to quantify apopototic DNA fragments.[41]

15.5.2.1 DNA extraction

1. Tissue to be analyzed should be snap-frozen and stored at –70°C to prevent non-specific activation of DNases.
2. Tissue is homogenized in a tissumizer with 2 ml homogenization buffer (0.1 *M* sodium chloride, 0.01 *M* EDTA (pH 8.0), 0.3 *M* TRIS-HCl (pH 8.0), and 0.2 *M* sucrose).
3. Two hundred fifty microliters 10% sodium dodecyl sulfate (SDS) is added to the homogenates, mixed, and incubated at 65°C for 30 min.
4. Three hundred fifty microliters 8 *M* potassium acetate is added to each tube, and the sample is mixed and incubated on ice for 60 min to precipitate proteins.
5. Samples are centrifuged at 5000 × g for 10 min at 4°C to pellet cellular debris. The supernatant is collected and transferred to a clean tube (~ 2.5 ml).
6. The supernatant is extracted with an equal volume of phenol–chloroform–isoamyl alcohol (25:24:1, v:v:v) followed by reextraction with an equal volume of chloroform–isoamyl alcohol (24:1, v:v).
7. The upper aqueous phase is collected and precipitated by addition of 2.5 × volume ice-cold 100% ethanol and incubated at –70°C for a minimum of 60 min.
8. The nucleic acid is collected by centrifugation at 14,000 × g for 30 min at 4°C. The pellets are resuspended in 0.5 ml 1 × TE buffer (10 m*M* TRIS-HCl, 1m*M* EDTA; pH 8.0) and digested by addition of 10 µl DNase-free RNase (500 µg/ml, Boehringer-Mannheim, Indianapolis, IN). Samples are incubated at 37°C for 60 min.
9. Samples are extracted with an equal volume of phenol–chloroform–isoamyl alcohol followed by an equal volume of chloroform–isoamyl alcohol.
10. The supernatant is collected and DNA precipitated by addition of 0.1 × volume 3 *M* sodium acetate and 2.5 volume ice-cold 100% ethanol incubated at –70°C for at least 60 min.
11. DNA is collected by centrifugation at 14,000 × g for 30 min at 4°C, washed in 0.5 ml ice-cold 80% ethanol, and dried under vacuum in a speed vac concentrator. Pellets are resuspended in 50 µl sterile water, quantitated by absorbance at 260 nm, and stored at –20°C.

15.5.2.2 3′ End-labeling of DNA

1. Five hundred nanograms of DNA in 30 µl is placed in a 1.5-ml microcentrifuge tube.
2. Add 10 µl 5 × reaction buffer (1 *M* potassium cacodylate, 0.123 *M* TRIS-HCl, 1.25 mg/ml bovine serum albumin; pH 6.6), 5 µl $CoCl_2$, 5 µl [α^{32}P]-ddATP (17 pmoles; 50 µCi), and 1 µl terminal deoxynucleotidyl transferase enzyme (25 U/µl). Allow the reaction to proceed for 60 min at 37°C.
3. The reaction is terminated by the addition of 5 µl 0.25 *M* EDTA (pH 8.0).
4. Add 50 µg tRNA (2 µl of 25 mg/ml stock) as a carrier. Labeled DNA is separated from unincorporated radionucleotide by addition of 0.2 × volume 10 *M* ammonium acetate and 3 × volume ice-cold 100% ethanol followed by incubation at –70°C for 60 min.
5. The nucleic acid is collected by centrifugation at 14,000 × g for 20 min at 4°C, washed with 0.25 ml ice-cold 80% ethanol, and allowed to air-dry.
6. Samples are resuspended in 25 µl TE buffer and stored at –20°C until electrophoretic gel analysis.

15.5.2.3 Gel electrophoresis and autoradiography

1. Twelve and five-tenths microliters of the labeled sample is loaded onto a 2% agarose gel and separated by electrophoresis for 3.5 h at 50 V using 1× TAE solution (40 m*M* TRIS-acetate, 1 m*M* EDTA) as running buffer.
2. The gel is removed, placed on 3-mm chromatography paper and dried in a slab-gel dryer for 2 h without heat.
3. The dried gel is sealed in plastic wrap and exposed to X-ray film for 2 to 6 h at –70°C. Figure 8 is an example of DNA fragmentation obtained from a normal rat kidney and the kidney of a rat 48 h post-reperfusion. There is no evidence of DNA fragmentation in the sample obtained from the normal rat. The sample obtained from the postischemic rat demonstrates a classic DNA ladder pattern suggestive of apoptosis.

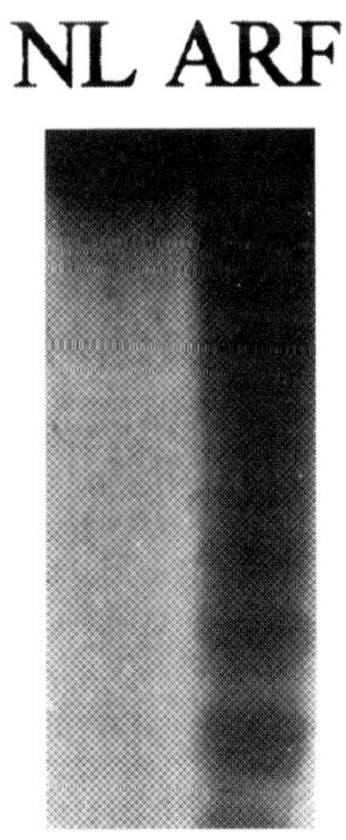

Figure 8 Autoradiograph of apoptotic DNA fragmentation. Cellular DNA was obtained from the kidneys of sham operated normal rats and rats 48 h postischemic injury. The DNA from the normal rat kidney demonstrates minimal fragmentation, while extensive labeling of DNA fragments was observed in the injured kidneys.

References

1. Toback, G.R., Regeneration after acute tubular necrosis, *Kidney Int.*, 41, 226, 1992.
2. Butkus, D.E., Persistent high mortality in acute renal failure, *Arch. Int. Med.*, 143, 209, 1983.
3. Venkatachalam, M.A., Bernard, D.B., Donohoe, J.F., and Levinsky, N.G., Ischemic damage and repair in the rat proximal tubule: differences among the S1, S2, and S3 segments, *Kidney Int.*, 14, 31, 1978.
4. Bacallao, R. and Fine, L.G., Molecular events in the organization of renal tubular epithelium: from nephrogenesis to regeneration, *Am. J. Physiol.*, 257, F913, 1989.
5. Brezis, M. and Heyman, S.N., Diversity of injuries in renal ischemia, *Int. J. Artif. Organs*, 9, 7, 1986.
6. Lake, E.W. and Humes, H.D., Acute renal failure: directed therapy to enhance renal tubular regeneration, *Seminars in Nephrology*, 14, 83, 1994.
7. Humes, D.H., Cieslinski, D.A., Coimbra, T.M., Messana, J.M., and Galvao, C., Epidermal growth factor enhances renal tubule cell regeneration and repair and accelerates the recovery of renal function in postischemic acute renal failure, *J. Clin. Invest.*, 84, 1757, 1989.
8. Norman, J., Tsau, Y-K., Bacay, A., and Fine, L.G., Epidermal growth factor accelerates functional recovery from ischaemic acute tubular necrosis in the rat: role of the epidermal growth factor receptor, *Clin. Sci.*, 78, 445, 1990.
9. Miller, S.B., Martin, D.R., Kissane, J., and Hammerman, M.R., Insulin-like growth factor I accelerates recovery from ischemic acute tubular necrosis in the rat, *Proc. Natl. Acad. Sci. U.S.A.*, 89, 11876, 1992.
10. Ding, H., Kopple, J.D., Cohen, A., and Hirschberg, R., Recombinant human insulin-like growth factor-I accelerates recovery and reduces catabolism in rats with ischemic acute renal failure, *J. Clin. Invest.*, 91, 2281, 1993.
11. Miller, S.B., Martin, D.R., Kissane, J., and Hammerman, M.R., Hepatocyte growth factor accelerates recovery from acute renal ischemic renal injury in rats, *Am. J. Physiol.*, 266, F129, 1994.
12. Breyer, M.D., Redha, R., and Breyer, J.A., Segmental distribution of epidermal growth factor binding sites in rabbit nephron, *Am. J. Physiol.*, 259, F553, 1990.
13. Hammerman, M.R. and Rogers, S.A., Distribution of IGF receptors in the plasma membrane of the proximal tubule cell, *Am. J. Physiol.*, 253, F841, 1987.
14. Norman, J., Badie-Dezfooly, B., and Nord, E.P., EGF-induced mitogenesis in proximal tubule cells: potentiation by angiotensin II, *Am. J. Physiol.*, 253, F299, 1987.
15. Igawa, T., Kanda, S, Kanetake, H., Saitoh, Y., Ichihara, A., Tomita, Y., and Nakamura, T., Hepatocyte growth factor is a potent mitogen for cultured rabbit renal tubular epithelial cells, *Biochem. Biophys. Res. Commun.*, 174, 831, 1991.
16. Miller, S.B., Rogers, S.A., Estes, C.E., and Hammerman, M.R., Increased distal nephron EGF content and altered distribution of peptide in compensatory renal hypertrophy, *Am. J. Physiol.*, 262, F1032, 1992.
17. Lajara, R., Rotwein, P., Bortz, J.C., Hansen, V.A., Sadow, J.L., Betts, C.R., Rogers, S.A., and Hammerman, M.R., Dual regulation of insulin-like growth factor I expression during renal hypertrophy, *Am. J. Physiol.*, 257, F252, 1989.
18. Nagike, M., Hirao, S., Tajima, H., Noji, S., Taniguchi, S., Matsumoto, K., and Nakamura, T., Renotropic functions of hepatocyte growth factor in renal regeneration after unilateral nephrectomy, *J. Biol. Chem.*, 266, 22781, 1991.
19. Ishibshi, K., Sasaki, S., Sakamoto, H., Hoshino, Y., Nakamura, T., and Marumo, F., Expression of receptor gene for hepatocyte growth factor in kidney after unilateral nephrectomy and renal injury, *Biochem. Biophys. Res. Commun.*, 187, 1454, 1992.
20. Matejka, G.L. and Jennische, E., IGF-I and IGF-I mRNA expression in the post-ischemic regenerating rat kidney, *Kidney Int.*, 42, 1113, 1992.
21. Igawa, T., Matsumoto, K., Kanda, S., Saito, Y., and Nakamura, T., Hepatocyte growth factor may function as a renotropic factor for regeneration in rats with acute renal injury, *Am. J. Physiol.*, 265, F61, 1993.
22. Rogers, S.A., Ryan, G., and Hammerman, M.R., Insulin-like growth factor I and II are produced in the metanephros and are required for growth and development in vitro, *J. Cell Biol.*, 113, 1447, 1991.

23. Rogers, S.A., Ryan, G., and Hammerman, M.R., Metanephric transforming growth factor-α is required for renal organogenesis in vitro, *Am. J. Physiol.*, 262, F533, 1992.
24. Miller, S.B., Martin, D.R., Kissane, J., and Hammerman, M.R., Rat models for clinical use of insulin-like growth factor I in acute renal failure, *Am. J. Physiol.*, 266, F949, 1994.
25. Cuppage, F.E., Cunningham, N., and Tate, A., Nucleic acid synthesis in the regenerating nephron following injury with mercuric chloride, *Lab. Invest.*, 21, 449, 1969.
26. Cuppage, F.E., Chiga, M., and Tate, A., Cell cycle in the regenerating rat nephron following injury with mercuric chloride, *Lab. Invest.*, 26, 122, 1972.
27. Bonventre, J.V., Mechanisms of ischemic acute renal failure, *Kidney Int.*, 43, 1160, 1993.
28. Miller, S.B., Rotwein, P., Bortz, J.D., Bechtel, P.J., Hansen, V.A., Rogers, S.A., and Hammerman, M.R., Renal expression of IGF I in hypersomatotropic states, *Am. J. Physiol.*, 259, F251, 1990.
29. Verstrepen, W.A., Nouwen, E.J., Yue, X.S., and De Broe, M.E., Altered growth factor expression during toxic proximal tubular necrosis and regeneration, *Kidney Int.*, 43, 1267, 1993.
30. Coimbra, T.M., Cieslinski, D.A., and Humes, H.D., Epidermal growth factor accelerates renal repair in mercuric chloride nephrotoxicity, *Am. J. Physiol.*, 259, F438, 1990.
31. Witzgall, R., Brown, D., Schwarz, C., and Bonventre, J.V., Localization of proliferating cell nuclear antigen, vimentin, c-Fos, and clusterin in the postischemic kidney, *J. Clin. Invest.*, 93, 2175, 1994.
32. Moll, R., Hage, C., and Thoenes, W., Expression of intermediate filament proteins in fetal and adult human kidney, *Lab. Invest.*, 65, 74, 1991.
33. Ward, J.M., Stevens, J.L., Konishi, N., Kurata, Y., Uno, H., Diwan, B.A., and Ohmori, T., Vimetin metaplasia in renal cortical tubules of preneoplastic, neoplastic, aging, and regenerative lesions of rats and humans, *Am. J. Pathol.*, 141, 955, 1992.
34. Wallin, A., Zhang, G., Jones, T.W., Jaken, S., and Stevens, J.L., Mechanisms of the nephrogenic repair response, *Lab. Invest.*, 66, 474, 1992.
35. Rosenberg, M.E. and Paller, M.S., Differential gene expression in the recovery from ischemic renal injury, *Kidney Int.*, 39, 1156, 1991.
36. Shimizu, A. and Yamanaka, N., Apoptosis and cell desquamation in repair process of ischemic tubular necrosis, *Virchows Arch. B*, 64, 171, 1993.
37. Savill, J., Apoptosis and the kidney, *J. Am. Soc. Nephrol.*, 5, 12, 1994.
38. Schumer, M., Colombel, M.C., Sawczuk, I.S., Gobe, G., Connor, J., O'Toole, K.M., Olsson, C.A., Wise, G.J., and Buttyan, R., Morphologic, biochemical, and molecular evidence of apoptosis during the reperfusion phase after brief periods of renal ischemia, *Am. J. Pathol.*, 140, 831, 1992.
39. Ueda, N. and Shah, S.V., Apoptosis, *J. Lab. Clin. Med.*, 124, 169, 1994.
40. Cohen, J.J., Apoptosis: physiologic cell death, *J. Lab. Clin. Med.*, 124, 761, 1994.
41. Tilly, J.L. and Hsueh, A.J.W., Microscale autoradiographic method for the qualitative and quantitative analysis of apoptotic DNA fragmentation, *J. Cell. Physiol.*, 154, 519, 1993.

chapter sixteen

Mitochondrial Toxicity in Renal Injury

Lawrence H. Lash and Dean P. Jones

16.1 Introduction ... 300
16.2 Biological model systems for assessing mitochondrial function ... 300
16.2.1 Intact renal cells ... 301
16.2.2 Digitonin fractionation of intact cells ... 303
16.2.3 Preparation of mitochondrial suspensions from intact cells by digitonin/nagarse method ... 305
16.2.4 Suspensions of isolated mitochondria ... 305
16.3 Parameters of mitochondrial function ... 306
16.3.1 Respiration ... 306
16.3.2 Membrane integrity ... 308
16.3.3 Mitochondrial energetic and redox status ... 309
16.3.3.1. Membrane potential ... 311
16.3.3.1.1 Measurement of mitochondrial $\Delta\psi$ in intact renal cells with $TPMP^+$ ... 312
16.3.3.1.2 Measurement of mitochondrial $\Delta\psi$ in intact renal cells and isolated mitochondria with rhodamine 123 ... 312
16.3.3.1.3 Measurement of $\Delta\psi$ in isolated renal mitochondria with safranine O ... 313
16.3.3.2 pH Gradient ... 315
16.3.3.3 Adenine and pyridine nucleotides ... 317
16.3.3.3.1 Determination of adenine and oxidized pyridine nucleotides by HPLC ... 317
16.3.3.3.2 Determination of reduced pyridine nucleotides by HPLC ... 318
16.3.3.4 Permeability transition ... 319
16.3.3.5 Thiol/disulfide status ... 320
16.3.3.5.1 Determination of GSH and GSSG with enzymatic recycling and 2-vinylpyridine ... 320
16.3.3.5.2 Determination of GSH and GSSG by reversed-phase, ion-exchange HPLC ... 321
16.3.3.5.3 Determination of mixed disulfides of GSH and cysteine with protein by HPLC ... 322

0-8493-3341-5/96/$0.00+$.50

16.3.4 Calcium ion distribution....322
16.3.4.1 Measurement of Ca^{2+} ion concentrations with fura-2....323
16.3.4.2 Measurement of Ca^{2+} ion concentrations with arsenazo III....323
16.4 Concluding remarks....327
16.5 Acknowledgments....327
References....327

16.1 Introduction

Maintenance of renal function is dependent on a continual source of energy.[1] Energy-requiring processes include active transport of ions and metabolites, including reabsorption and secretion, biosynthesis of macromolecules, and drug metabolism reactions. Renal cellular energy status in cell populations such as those in the proximal tubules is primarily provided by mitochondrial oxidative phosphorylation. Modulation of energy-consuming or energy-generating reactions has been linked to altered susceptibility of the kidneys to chemically or pathologically induced injury.[2-4] Chemically induced renal cellular injury often involves inhibition of mitochondrial function because exogenous chemicals can be actively accumulated within the organelles by the large number of membrane transporters that possess broad substrate specificity and because of the presence of numerous nucleophilic sites that can react with electrophilic metabolites of xenobiotics and drugs. Inhibition of mitochondrial function, leading to decreased energy production (i.e., ATP supply), leads to a cascade of effects, including collapse of ion gradients, decreased membrane potential, decreased biosynthetic reactions, alterations in cytoskeletal structure, and alterations in thiol/disulfide status.

Nephrotoxicants whose mechanism of action likely involves mitochondrial dysfunction include several diverse chemicals, such as the cysteine conjugates *S*-(1,2-dichlorovinyl)-L-cysteine[5,6] and *S*-(1,2,3,4,4-pentachlorobutadienyl)-L-cysteine,[7-9] allyl alcohol and acrolein,[10] cisplatin,[11-13] bromohydroquinone,[14] aminoglycosides,[15] cephalosporin antibiotics,[16] inorganic mercury,[17-19] and cyclosporin A.[20,21] The dissimilar chemical nature of these toxicants implies that mitochondrial toxicity is a common and general mechanism of renal cellular injury. Furthermore, pathological conditions such as hypoxia and ischemia are also associated with mitochondrial dysfunction.[2-4] Understanding of the mechanisms by which mitochondrial dysfunction is produced by various toxicologic and pathologic conditions may thus provide a key to understanding renal cellular injury.

This chapter briefly describes biological preparations derived from renal tissue that can be used to monitor mitochondrial function *in vitro* and specific methods to assess key parameters of mitochondrial function in these systems. Finally, a few examples of chemicals that target renal mitochondria are given to illustrate how mitochondrial dysfunction may be involved in renal pathologies.

16.2 Biological model systems for assessing mitochondrial function

A variety of biological systems can be used *in vitro* to study the role of mitochondrial mechanisms of chemical injury and mitochondrial function. Advantages and disadvantages of each model will be discussed. Since detailed presentations of these methods have been given elsewhere, including in other chapters in this volume, this presentation focuses primarily on the utility of these preparations for study of mitochondrial function, and the reader is referred to other sources for related information.

16.2.1 Intact renal cells

In vitro renal preparations that comprise intact cells, such as suspensions of tubular fragments or isolated cells, have become commonly used systems for study of renal biochemistry and metabolism, metabolite transport, and mechanisms of chemically induced renal cellular injury. Detailed procedures for preparation of rabbit renal proximal tubule fragments are described elsewhere in this volume (Chapter 9). Procedures for preparation of suspensions of isolated renal cortical cells from the rat have been published,[22,23] and methods to separate these cortical cells into separate populations derived from proximal tubular and distal tubular regions using Percoll density gradient centrifugation have been published[24,25] and are described elsewhere in the volume (Chapter 11). It is relatively easy to obtain tubular fragments but is difficult to obtain suspensions of single cells from rabbit kidneys. In contrast, it is relatively easy to obtain suspensions of single cells from rat kidneys. Hence, depending on the animal model being used, different *in vitro* preparations are commonly used.

Important characteristics of these *in vitro* systems are that intact cellular structure is maintained and adequate amounts of biological material are obtained to allow for paired control and treated samples. These are important for screening of potentially nephrotoxic chemicals because they allow for consistency of sampling, rapid detection of toxic effects, and a reduction in the number of animals required to assess chemically induced toxicity. An additional advantage is that cellular effects, including those occurring within specific subcellular organelles such as the mitochondria, can be studied in detail without the complications of treatment effects due to extrarenal processes or those due to changes in renal hemodynamics. Furthermore, mechanisms of chemically induced injury can be studied in detail with these systems because many incubation conditions — such as nutritional status, media composition, media pH, and cellular oxygenation — can be specified to a high degree of accuracy, thereby limiting further the complications due to unknown or unspecified factors.

Certainly, there are cautions or disadvantages that are associated with the use of *in vitro* suspensions of intact renal cells and primary cultures, and these highlight the need to use these systems in conjunction with other biological models. For example, an important consideration in the use of *in vitro* models is the faithfulness with which the systems reflect normal, *in vivo* renal cellular function. In answer to this concern, investigators have characterized in detail the transport and metabolic capabilities of isolated renal tubules, cell suspensions, and primary cultures, and compared properties with those obtained in whole organ and *in vivo* studies. Excellent correlations have been obtained between many properties observed *in vitro* and *in vivo*. However, there remain some limitations due to plasma membrane damage in freshly isolated cells and phenotype changes in primary cultures. With suspensions of renal tubules, not only is intact cellular structure maintained, but renal cellular polarity and cell-to-cell tight junctions are maintained. With suspensions of single cells, however, the ability to distinguish processes that occur on the brush border and basolateral membrane surfaces is limited. This limitation is not critical for many types of investigations, and primary cell cultures can be grown on porous supports so that studies of polarized processes can be conducted. These systems can, therefore, validly provide significant information on many types of processes.

Several approaches can be used with preparations of intact renal cells to investigate mitochondrial function under physiological, toxicological, and pathological conditions. These methods range from measurement of cellular oxygen consumption, which reflects primarily (>90%) that which occurs in the mitochondrial electron transport chain, to measurements of mitochondrial membrane potential and intracellular distribution of ions and metabolites with fluorescent probes and microscopy. An advantage of assessing parameters of mitochondrial function in intact cells is that the integration of these processes with cellular function can be performed. For example, coupling of ATP supply and cellular requirements for ATP can be demonstrated by modulation of (Na^++K^+)-stimulated ATPase activity and measurement of cellular oxygen consumption (Figure 1). Decrease of cellular ATP consumption by inhibition of the (Na^++K^+)-stimulated ATPase with ouabain is coupled to a concomitant decrease in the rate of mitochondrial oxidative phosphorylation, and uncoupling of the (Na^++K^+)-stimulated ATPase by treatment with the monocation ionophore nystatin, which increases ATP consumption, is coupled to an increase in the rate of mitochondrial oxidative phosphorylation.[1] Preincubation of renal epithelial cells with fructose to rapidly consume cellular ATP by phosphorylation of fructose also leads to a modest increase in cellular oxygen consumption. Preincubation of cells with adenosine to provide cells with ATP precursor leads to increased cellular ATP content and also increased rates of oxygen consumption. The increased rates of oxygen consumption due to adenosine may, however, be due to hormonal effects on cellular Ca^{2+} ion homeostasis or on stimulation of purine catabolism. Thus, functionally competent cells can modulate mitochondrial respiration to correlate with cellular ATP consumption.

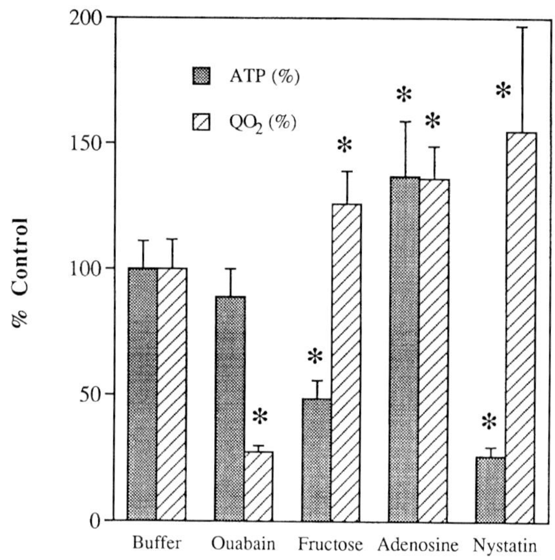

Figure 1 Coupling of mitochondrial respiration with cellular ATP flux in suspensions of renal cortical cells from rat kidney. Isolated renal cortical cells from rat kidney (2.5×10^6 cells/ml) were incubated with either Krebs–Henseleit buffer, 0.1 m*M* ouabain, 10 m*M* fructose, 10 m*M* adenosine, or 1400 U nystatin per milliter for 60 min at 37°C. Cellular concentrations of ATP were measured by a pyridine nucleotide-linked enzymatic assay. Control ATP concentration was 2.7 ± 0.3 nmol/10^6 cells. Rates of cellular oxygen consumption were measured polarographically in the presence of 3.3 m*M* succinate as respiratory substrate. Control rate of oxygen consumption was 44.4 ± 5.2 nmol O_2 consumed per minute per 10^6 cells. Results are the means ± SE of measurements from three separate cell preparations. *Significantly different ($P < 0.05$) from the corresponding control measurement. Statistical analyses were performed on actual data values before transformation to % control. (From Lash, L. H. and Anders, M.W., unpublished data.)

Compartmentation of calcium ions is controlled by several energy-dependent processes involving calcium binding proteins and transport systems on the plasma, microsomal, and mitochondrial membranes. Sequestration of calcium ions in mitochondria of rat renal cortical cells has been measured by dual-wavelength spectroscopy at 654 minus 685 nm with the calcium-sensitive dye arsenazo III.[26] Mitochondrial calcium content can be measured as the carbonyl cyanide *m*-chlorophenylhydrazone (CCCP)-sensitive pool. Treatment of renal cortical cells with the cytotoxic and mitochondrial toxicant conjugate *S*-(1,2-dichlorovinyl)-L-cysteine (DCVC) produces a time-dependent decrease in the ability of mitochondria to retain calcium (Figure 2).[27]

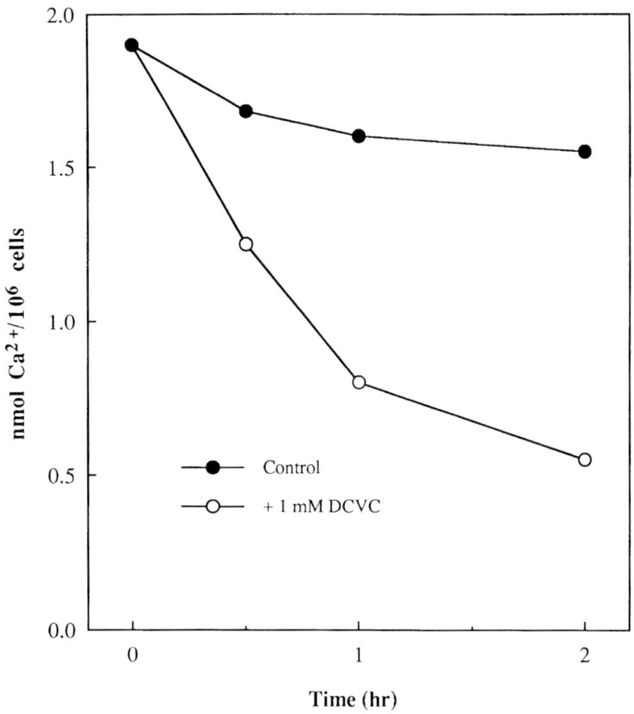

Figure 2 Alterations in mitochondrial sequestration of calcium after treatment of rat renal cortical cells with *S*-(1,2-dichlorovinyl)-L-cysteine (DCVC). Isolated renal cortical cells from rat kidney (4 to 5×10^6 cells/ml) were incubated at 37°C for the indicated times with either buffer (= Control) or 1 m*M* DCVC. Mitochondrial Ca^{2+} content was measured by rapid centrifugation of a 1-ml aliquot of cells through 20% (v/v) Percoll in a Ca^{2+}- and Mg^{2+}-free Hank's buffer. Cells were then resuspended in the modified Hank's buffer and mitochondrial Ca^{2+} content was determined by dual-wavelength spectroscopy (654 minus 685 nm) after addition of 30 μ*M* arsenazo III and 10 μ*M* carbonyl cyanide *p*-trifluoromethoxyphenylhydrazone (FCCP). Results are the means of measurements from four separate cell preparations. (Modified from Lash, L. H. and Anders, M. W., *J. Biol. Chem.*, 261, 13076, 1986.)

16.2.2 Digitonin fractionation of intact cells

Rapid transport processes across mitochondrial inner membranes and collapse of mitochondrial membrane potential during processing of samples can lead to artifactual changes in the subcellular distribution of metabolites. To minimize these artifacts, digitonin fractionation can be used to rapidly separate cytosolic and mitochondrial fractions. By careful selection of digitonin concentration, one can selectively permeabilize cellular plasma membranes, releasing low molecular weight metabolites and proteins but not intracellular organelles. The procedure, which is described in detail by Lash and Sall,[28] involves mixing of cells in polypropylene microcentrifuge tubes with a top layer of digitonin in an aqueous buffer and use of a microcentrifuge to rapidly centrifuge cells through a middle layer of silicone oil–mineral oil into a bottom layer of glycerol or perchloric acid (Figure 3). The oil layer prevents mixing of cytosolic and extracellular media with intracellular organelles, including mitochondria. Glycerol is used when quantitating proteins or enzymatic activities while perchloric acid can be used to measure low molecular weight chemicals. Metabolites or enzyme activities can then be quantitated in the top aqueous layer, which represents material from the extracellular medium and the cytosol, and in the bottom pellet, which represents primarily material from the mitochondria. Separation efficiency is validated by measurement of marker enzymes for cytosolic and mitochondrial fractions (Table 1). In the absence of digitonin in the top layer, material in the supernatant that is obtained by centrifugation through the oil layer gives extracellular media and material in the pellet gives total cellular contents. Under these conditions, less than 15% of the total amount of the cytosolic marker enzyme lactate dehydrogenase (LDH) and less than 5% of the total amount of the mitochondrial marker enzyme glutamate dehydrogenase (GDH) is found in the supernatant, indicating that cellular plasma membranes are largely intact. With digitonin in the top layer, in contrast, more than 80% of LDH activity is recovered in the supernatant while more than 90% of GDH activity is retained in the mitochondrial pellet. This indicates that centrifugation through digitonin yields effective separation of cytosolic and mitochondrial compartments, with the cytosol being found in the supernatant and the mitochondria being found in the pellet.

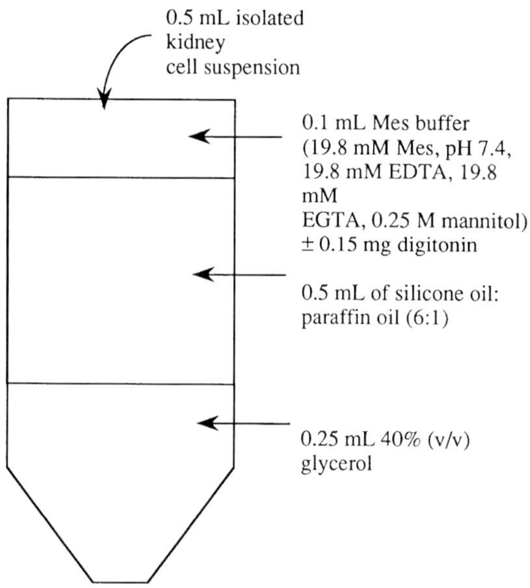

1. Rapidly mix cells with Mes buffer layer in 1.5-mL plastic microcentrifuge tube.
2. Centrifuge 13,000*g* x 3 min.
3. **In absence of digitonin:**
   Supernatant = Extracellular medium
   Pellet = Total cellular contents
   In presence of digitonin:
   Supernatant = Extracellular medium + Cytosol
   Pellet = Mitochondria

Figure 3 Scheme of digitonin fractionation of renal cells for analysis of cytosolic and mitochondrial compartmentation.

By using digitonin fractionation, chemically induced changes in subcellular contents and distributions of intermediary metabolites such as pyruvate, glutathione (GSH), and adenine nucleotides can be evaluated. Additionally, enzymatic activities in cytosol and

Table 1 Distribution of Marker Enzymes in Fractions of Rat Renal Proximal Tubular and Distal Tubular Cells Obtained by Digitonin Treatment

		PT cells		DT cells	
	Digitonin	Supernatant	Glycerol	Supernatant	Glycerol
Lactate Dehydrogenase					
	—	4.05 ± 0.68	70.3 ± 9.0	6.24 ± 1.14	96.7 ± 8.1
	+	65.3 ± 8.2	6.80 ± 1.50	87.0 ± 9.8	10.6 ± 2.0
Glutamate Dehydrogenase					
	—	2.40 ± 0.67	30.9 ± 3.1	2.74 ± 0.29	37.0 ± 3.8
	+	3.70 ± 0.60	30.9 ± 4.6	3.19 ± 0.80	41.2 ± 6.2

Note: Isolated renal PT and DT cells (3 to 5 × 10^6 cells/ml) were fractionated by centrifugation through buffer ± digitonin (1.5 mg/ml). Enzyme activities were measured by pyridine nucleotide-linked spectrophotometric assays. Results are expressed as mU/10^6 cells and are the means ± SE of measurements from six cell preparations for lactate dehydrogenase and ten cell preparations for glutamate dehydrogenase.

mitochondria can be quantitated separately, thereby providing information about the metabolic and drug biotransformation capabilities of renal cortical mitochondria. This knowledge can provide information about the capacity of mitochondria to generate reactive and toxic metabolites.

16.2.3 *Preparation of mitochondrial suspensions from intact cells by digitonin/nagarse method*

Digitonin fractionation of intact renal cells is a useful method for analysis of metabolite and enzyme distributions. Since digitonin acts to selectively permeabilize the plasma membranes, but does not affect cytoskeletal proteins, intracellular organelles cannot be isolated. To enable isolation of mitochondria from suspensions of single hepatocytes, Bai et al.[29] developed a method combining digitonin fractionation with treatment with the protease nagarse and filtration through polycarbonate membranes. With minor modifications, this method has been applied to the isolation of mitochondria from suspensions of renal proximal tubular and distal tubular cells, and is described in detail elsewhere.[28] Nagarse is a nonspecific protease that digests cytoskeletal proteins, thereby releasing organelles, including mitochondria, from digitonin-treated cells. Polycarbonate membranes are used because they are inert toward biological materials. Using the appropriate pore-size filters (2 μm), enriched preparations of mitochondria separated from cytosol and most other subcellular organelles can be obtained. Functional integrity of these mitochondrial preparations is validated by measurements of respiratory control (see below).

Use of the digitonin/nagarse method provides a unique opportunity to study processes in mitochondria derived from distinct populations of renal epithelial cells. Procedures, such as Percoll density gradient centrifugation,[24,25] can be used to obtain enriched preparations of renal cells derived from proximal tubular and distal tubular nephron segments. Application of the digitonin/nagarse procedure can thus enable isolation of proximal tubular and distal tubular mitochondria.[28] This can have important utility for mechanistic toxicology studies because mitochondria are often primary intracellular targets of toxicants and little knowledge is available about the sensitivity of mitochondria from different populations of renal epithelial cells.

16.2.4 *Suspensions of isolated mitochondria*

Suspensions of isolated mitochondria from renal cortical homogenates are a useful model in which to study mitochondrial function separate from processes occurring in cytosol or other cellular organelles. Standard methods using biological buffers and centrifugation methods have been available for many years and have provided significant insight into mitochondrial metabolism and responses to exposures to toxicants. Procedures for differential centrifugation and the appropriate composition of biological buffers to maintain and optimize mitochondrial function have been described elsewhere.[28] Optimal function in suspensions of isolated mitochondria is maintained by using buffers containing an impermeant solute, such as sucrose or mannitol, and salt solutions containing potassium, magnesium, chloride, and phosphate ions.

16.3 Parameters of mitochondrial function

Transport activities, energetics, and redox status are critical components of mitochondrial function. The following four sections describe some examples of specific methodologies to quantitate effects of nephrotoxic chemicals in renal mitochondria. Patterns and rates of oxygen consumption are conveniently measured and provide information on membrane integrity and coupling of metabolism to ATP biosynthesis. Membrane integrity can be assessed directly, and changes can indicate irreversible injury to mitochondria much in the same way that leakage of cytosolic enzymes from intact cells is used to demonstrate irreversible cytotoxicity. Methods to assess several parameters of energetic and redox status, including membrane potential, pH, adenine nucleotides, the permeability transition, and thiol/disulfide status will be described. These procedures can be used to obtain mechanistic information about effects of chemicals on specific target molecules. Finally, maintenance of calcium ion distribution is critical to mitochondrial function. Alterations in mitochondrial calcium ion status, which can result from oxidative stress or ATP depletion, can lead to a variety of pathological changes.

16.3.1 Respiration

Rates of oxygen consumption in intact cells or isolated mitochondria can be measured readily in a thermostat-controlled, jacketed chamber with an attached oxygen-sensitive electrode. A wide variety of isolation and incubation buffers have been used in measurements of respiration. Preparations of intact renal cells typically use media containing balanced salt solutions, such as Krebs–Henseleit buffer with organic buffers — e.g., 4-(2-hydroxyethyl)piperazine-1-(2-ethanesulfonic acid); HEPES — and bicarbonate, or use enriched media such as those used for cell cultures. For suspensions of isolated mitochondria, however, early studies showed that the use of an impermeant molecule such as sucrose or mannitol rather than a balanced salt solution is important for maintenance of function and structural integrity; incubation media typically contain 225 m*M* sucrose or 155 m*M* sucrose + 70 m*M* mannitol. Although many incubation media for isolated mitochondria try to simulate the cytosol, inclusion of only a few cations and anions seems to be critical. These include potassium (30 m*M*), magnesium (5 m*M*), chloride (50 m*M*), and inorganic phosphate (1 to 10 m*M*; 3 m*M* appears to be optimal). Sodium ions should be omitted. An organic buffer (20 m*M*), such as TRIS, triethanolamine, or HEPES, and the divalent cation chelator ethylene glycol bis(β-aminoethyl ether)-*N*,*N*,*N*′,*N*′-tetraacetic acid (EGTA) are also added to provide additional buffering capacity and to remove calcium ions, respectively. Although the pH of media for incubations with intact renal cells is usually 7.4, many investigators use incubation media with the pH adjusted to values closer to that of cytosol (i.e., 6.8 to 7.2) in studies with isolated mitochondria. Aw and Jones[30] have shown that a pH gradient exists in renal proximal tubular cells, with a lower pH existing in the region of mitochondria. The temperature for measurements of respiration in isolated cells or tubules is usually 37°C. For isolated mitochondria, however, measurements are usually done at substantially lower temperatures (20 to 28°C) because processes often occur too rapidly to allow for accurate measurement at higher temperatures and because mitochondrial function is not well maintained at higher temperatures.

Respiratory function in isolated mitochondria is defined by substrate, ADP, and oxygen supply, as first described by Chance and Williams.[31] The following respiratory states were defined:

State 1: mitochondria only (in the presence of inorganic phosphate)
State 2: substrate added, no ADP; respiration rate low
State 3: a limiting amount of ADP added; rapid respiration rate
State 4: all ADP phosphorylated to ATP; respiration rate decreases
State 5: anoxia; no respiration

As substrate and ADP are both present during state 3, this rate of oxygen consumption represents the maximum coupled rate of respiration. If mitochondria are functionally intact, relatively high rates of state 3 and low rates of state 4 respiration are observed, indicating low proton permeability and the ability to carry out oxidative phosphorylation. Many nonspecific injuries to mitochondria lead to an increase in membrane permeability and an uncoupling of oxidative phosphorylation, which is observed as an increase in state 4 relative to state 3 respiration. In other cases, such as the generation of free radicals or other oxidants that lead to specific inactivation of dehydrogenases and other components of the electron transport chain, decreases in state 3 respiration are observed.

The basic procedure to be described is essentially that of Estabrook,[32] and was recently summarized elsewhere.[28] An oxygraph, such as the Gilson Model 5/6H (Gilson Medical Electronics, Middleton, WI), can be used. The sample chamber is a water-jacketed, 1.6-ml glass compartment that has dual ports, one for the oxygen electrode and one, which can be capped, for addition of solutions. The cap contains a long, narrow-bore opening that enables injection of solutions with a syringe but minimizes diffusion of oxygen. The following steps are performed to measure oxygen consumption in renal cells or isolated mitochondria:

1. *Setup and calibration.* A new oxygen-permeable membrane is placed on the electrode tip daily. The oxygraph is calibrated with air-saturated water, which has known concentrations of dissolved oxygen at specified temperatures.[32] The temperature is controlled by a circulating water bath connected to the water jacket ports surrounding the electrode chamber. When a stable, level tracing is obtained, a few grains of sodium dithionite or sodium sulfite are added to consume all the oxygen in the chamber, thereby establishing the zero-oxygen concentration.
2. *Measurement of state 3 and state 4 respiration.* To the 1.6-ml electrode chamber are added 1.0 ml of isolation buffer (Krebs–Henseleit buffer for intact cells or sucrose–mannitol-containing buffer for isolated mitochondria) and 0.5 ml of biological material (isolated cells/tubules or isolated mitochondria; 2 to 5 mg protein per milliliter), and oxygen consumption is measured. After approximately 1 min, respiratory substrate (1 to 5 m*M*) is added and oxygen consumption is measured. When succinate is used as a respiratory substrate, 5 µl of 1.5 m*M* rotenone (dissolved in ethanol; final concentration 5 µ*M*) and 5 µl of 1 *M* succinate (final concentration 3.3 m*M*) are added. After approximately 1 min, 5 µl of 90 m*M* ADP (prepared fresh; final concentration 0.3 m*M*) is added to initiate state 3 respiration. Oxygen consumption is measured for several minutes (2 to 4 min) and should exhibit two phases: a rapid phase (= state 3) and a slower phase (= state 4) that occurs after the added ADP is consumed.

If specific inhibition of components of the mitochondrial electron transport chain is involved in the mechanism of toxicity, respiratory substrates that donate electrons to different coupling sites can be used to help identify targets. For example, substrates that donate electrons to the NADH dehydrogenase (complex I), such as glutamate (4 m*M*) + malate (2 m*M*) or pyruvate (4 m*M*) + malate (2 m*M*), can be used; succinate (3.3 m*M*) is used as a substrate that donates electrons to the succinate dehydrogenase complex (complex II); and ascorbate (1 m*M*) + *N,N,N′,N′*-tetramethyl-*p*-phenylenediamine (TMPD; 0.2 m*M*) are used as substrates that donate electrons directly to cytochrome *c*, thus showing effects occurring at cytochrome oxidase (complex IV, coupling site III).

3. *Calculation of respiratory control ratio.* The respiratory control ratio (RCR) is calculated as the ratio of the state 3 to state 4 respiration by determining slopes of the oxygen concentration vs. time tracings. For renal cortical mitochondria, RCR values of 3.5 to 5 are typical for normal, functionally intact mitochondria. An RCR value of 3.0 is usually set as a lower limit of acceptability for mitochondrial functional integrity.
4. *Calculation of P/O ratio.* The P/O ratio is a measure of the ability of mitochondria to perform oxidative phosphorylation and generate ATP. Assuming that all the added ADP is phosphorylated to ATP, then the P/O ratio is calculated as the ratio of nanomoles of ADP added to nanoatoms of oxygen consumed (i.e., 1/2 O_2); the latter is the amount of oxygen consumed during the state 3 phase of oxygen consumption, which is after addition of substrate and ADP and until all the ADP is consumed and the slower, state 4 phase of oxygen consumption begins.
5. *Assessment of responsiveness of mitochondria to chemicals that alter cellular energetics.* Several approaches that use effects on respiration are available to determine the regulatory competence of renal mitochondria. Correlation of mitochondrial respiratory activity with cellular ATP consumption in intact renal cells was discussed above. In suspensions of isolated mitochondria, a number of uncouplers or metabolic inhibitors can be used as probes of mitochondrial function. As with the chemicals above (i.e., substrates, ADP, etc.), these compounds are added after the addition of ADP to the oxygraph chamber, in small volumes (i.e., < 25 µl) from concentrated stock solutions, by injection with a syringe through the cap in the electrode chamber. Rates of oxygen consumption are recorded to assess effects on state 3 and state 4 respiration. Examples of agents that can be used to modulate mitochondrial respiration in isolated mitochondria and their expected effects are summarized in Table 2. Many of the expected responses, such as increase in state 3 respiration by an ionophore and increase of state 4 respiration by an uncoupler are dependent on the presence of an intact mitochondrial inner membrane and can thus be used as a gauge of functional and structural integrity.

16.3.2 Membrane integrity

Just as release of cytosolic enzymes (such as lactate dehydrogenase) from intact renal cells can be used as a measurement of plasma membrane integrity, and thus of irreversible cellular injury,[23] release of mitochondrial matrix enzymes into the extramitochondrial medium can be used as an assessment of mitochondrial inner membrane integrity and mitochondrial injury. Use of a matrix enzyme that is present at a relatively high activity, such as malate dehydrogenase, is recommended to provide for adequate sensitivity.[6] When investigating chemically induced injury in mitochondria by this method, it is important that the matrix enzyme used as the marker is not inhibited by the chemical under investigation. Otherwise, increased inner membrane permeability will be underestimated.

After incubating suspensions of isolated renal cortical mitochondria for various times at 25°C or 28°C with buffer (= control) or a chemical of interest, aliquots (1 ml) of the

Table 2 Chemicals Used to Modulate Respiratory Function of Isolated Mitochondria from Renal Cortex

	Chemical	Expected effect on respiration
Respiratory chain inhibitors		
	Rotenone	Inhibits state 3 and 4 at complex I; no effect when complex II substrates used
	Cyanide	Inhibits state 3 and 4 by >90%
	Amytal	Inhibits state 3 and 4 at complex I
	Antimycin A	Inhibits state 3 and 4 at complex II
Adenine nucleotide status		
	Bongkrekic acid	Inhibits state 3 rate, ANT
	(Carboxy)atractyloside	Inhibits state 3 rate, ANT
	Oligomycin	Inhibits oxygen consumption; F_0F_1-ATPase inhibitor
Uncouplers/Ionophores		
	2,4-Dinitrophenol	Stimulates state 4; uncouples
	CCCP	Stimulates oxygen consumption; RCR = 1; protonophore

Note: CCCP, carbonyl cyanide *m*-chlorophenylhydrazone; ANT, adenine nucleotide translocase; RCR, respiratory control ratio. Complex I = NADH dehydrogenase; complex II = succinate dehydrogenase; complex III = cytochrome oxidase; coupling site I = NADH–Coenzyme Q; coupling site II = cytochrome b–c_1; coupling site III = cytochrome oxidase.

mitochondrial suspensions are placed in 1.5-ml polypropylene microcentrifuge tubes and are centrifuged for 4 min at 10,000 × g. Protein content and a matrix marker enzyme activity are then measured in the mitochondrial pellet and in the supernatant. Treatment of renal cortical mitochondria with the nephro- and cytotoxic cysteine *S*-conjugate DCVC produces a time-dependent increase in release of malate dehydrogenase (Figure 4), indicating irreversible membrane damage.[6]

Besides measurement of protein leakage from mitochondria, a classic method to assess mitochondrial membrane integrity is to measure swelling of the mitochondria by changes in absorbance. Permeability of the mitochondrial inner membrane can be assessed by determination of the ability of isosmolar solutions of polyethylene glycol (PEG) of different molecular weights to decrease matrix volume.[33,34] Shrinkage is induced by addition of 0.3 ml of 60% (v/v) PEG solutions of M_r = 200, 300, 600, or 1000 to 1 ml of mitochondria (1 mg protein) in the sample cuvette. Sucrose (0.3 ml of 0.25 *M*), which is impermeant to the mitochondrial inner membrane, is added to mitochondria in the sample cuvette. The method, therefore, assesses exclusion of PEG by the mitochondrial inner membrane relative to sucrose. Decreased matrix volume in mitochondria incubated for various times with buffer or toxicants is determined by increases in absorbance at 540 nm. Mitochondria that are functionally and structurally intact are normally impermeable to PEG solutions of $M_r \geq 200$ and thus do not show absorbance changes in such solutions.[34] In contrast, mitochondria incubated with cytotoxic chemicals exhibit time- and concentration-dependent increases in A_{540} with PEG solutions of increasing molecular weight.

16.3.3 Mitochondrial energetic and redox status

As the primary function of mitochondria is to generate ATP for biosynthetic and other ATP-dependent processes such as active transport, methods to assess energetic status are critical to an understanding of chemically induced mitochondrial injury. According to the chemiosmotic hypothesis, which is the generally accepted theory of mitochondrial energy

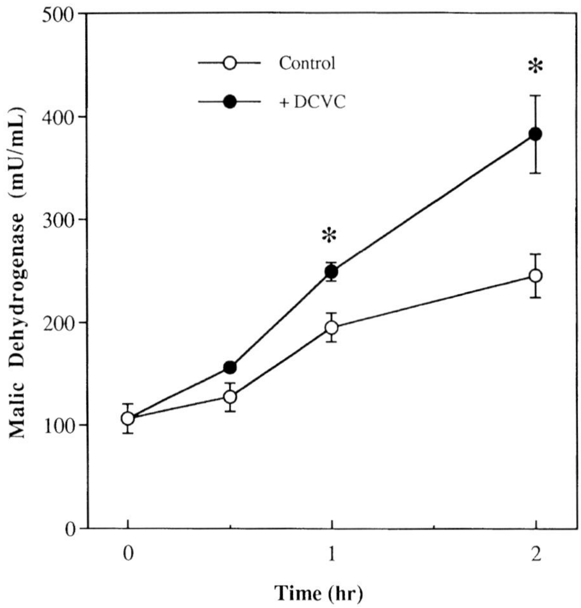

Figure 4 Enzyme release from renal cortical mitochondria incubated with *S*-(1,2-dichlorovinyl)-L-cysteine (DCVC). Suspensions of renal cortical mitochondria (1.5 to 2.0 mg protein per milliliter) were incubated with either buffer or 1 m*M* DCVC at 28°C for up to 2 h. Mitochondria were separated from the extramitochondrial media by centrifugation for 4 min at 10,000 × *g*. Malic dehydrogenase activity in total mitochondrial suspension, in mitochondrial pellet, and in the supernatant was measured by a pyridine nucleotide-linked spectrophotometric assay. Time-zero control activity in the supernatant was 6.0% of activity in the total mitochondrial suspension. Results are the means ± SE of measurements from three separate mitochondrial preparations. *Significantly different ($P < 0.05$) from control at the corresponding incubation time. (Data from Lash, L. H. and Anders, M. W., *Mol. Pharmacol.*, 32, 549, 1987.)

transduction, the common energy pool is the protonmotive force, Δp, which is based on the presence of a proton electrochemical gradient, $\Delta\mu_H+$, which is defined as

$$\Delta\mu_H+ \text{ (kJ mol}^{-1}) = -F\Delta\psi + 2.3RT\ \Delta pH, \quad (1)$$

where F is the Faraday constant (0.0965 kJ mol^{-1} mV^{-1}); $\Delta\psi$ is the membrane potential; R is the gas constant (8.314 J mol^{-1} K^{-1}); T is the absolute temperature in degrees Kelvin (K); and ΔpH is the pH gradient across the inner membrane. The protonmotive force, then, is defined as

$$\Delta p \text{ (mV)} = -(\Delta\mu_H+)/F. \quad (2)$$

Substituting values for R and T at 25°C and the fact that a $\Delta\mu_H+$ of 1 kJ mol^{-1} corresponds to a Δp of 10.4 mV, gives the final equation for protonmotive force as

$$\Delta p \text{ (mV)} = \Delta\psi - 60\Delta pH. \quad (3)$$

Superimposed on the mitochondrial processes that generate the Δp is redox status. Oxidation and reduction of both soluble and membrane-bound components of mitochondria are intrinsic to substrate oxidation and the generation of the $\Delta\mu_H+$. Additionally, numerous enzymes involved in oxidative phosphorylation and ion transport contain critical sulfhydryl groups that are only active in the reduced form. These include dehydrogenases and oxidases as well as the F_0F_1-ATPase. The tripeptide GSH would appear to be a critical protective component of this system because it exists at relatively high concentrations in renal mitochondrial matrix[35] and can undergo reversible oxidation to glutathione disulfide (GSSG). The GSH/GSSG redox couple has a midpoint potential at pH 7 ($E_{m,7}$) of –240 mV, which is between that of physiological reductants such as $NAD(P)^+/NAD(P)H$ [–320 mV] and physiological oxidants such as cytochrome *c* oxidase (Fe^{3+}/Fe^{2+}) [+220 mV] and $O_2/2H_2O$ [+820 mV]. This indicates that GSH can function with thermodynamic efficiency in the maintenance of mitochondrial redox status.

The following selected methods to study these parameters can be employed in either intact renal epithelial cells or in suspensions of isolated renal mitochondria to assess effects on energetics and redox status. The coverage is by no means comprehensive, but is presented to illustrate examples of procedures for quantitation of certain key parameters of mitochondrial bioenergetics.

16.3.3.1 Membrane potential

Since energized mitochondria possess a membrane potential ($\Delta\psi$) and a pH gradient (ΔpH), the distribution of charged species across the inner membrane can be used to calculate the $\Delta\psi$ (negative inside). The Nernst equation is used to correlate the distribution of charged species across a membrane at equilibrium with $\Delta\psi$:

$$\Delta\psi = -[2.3\ RT/mF][\log_{10}([X^{m+}]_B/[X^{m+}]_A)]. \tag{4}$$

Weak acid anions become concentrated in an acidic compartment (A), whereas weak base cations become concentrated in a basic compartment (B). X^{m+} is a charged species with charge *m* in compartments A and B. Since mitochondrial matrix normally has an alkaline pH (typically 7.5 to 7.8) whereas cytosol has a slightly acidic to neutral pH (typically 6.8 to 7.2), weak base cations such as triphenylmethylphosphonium ($TPMP^+$) accumulate in mitochondrial matrix, with the distribution being correlated with the $\Delta\psi$.

Several assumptions and constraints, as described by Lemasters et al.,[36] must be considered in applying membrane-permeant, cationic probes for measurement of $\Delta\psi$. First, the Nernst equation actually uses the logarithm of the ratio of chemical activity in two compartments, rather than chemical concentration. Although the activity and concentration are generally reasonably equivalent, the high protein concentration of mitochondria suggests that this assumption may produce a significant error. Second, since the cationic probes are highly lipophilic, it takes several minutes for them to equilibrate into different intracellular compartments.[37] Therefore, there is a lag in the response time, allowing only relatively slow changes to be measured. Third, it is also assumed that the cationic probe crosses the membrane only in the charged form. These probes can also cross membranes as neutral ion pairs, thus producing an underestimate of $\Delta\psi$. Fourth, since the probes are charged species, they may artifactually alter $\Delta\psi$ or cause osmotic swelling of mitochondria. For this reason, relatively low concentrations of the probes must be used to avoid these artifacts. Fifth, the probes should not bind nonspecifically to proteins or lipids in either the mitochondrial membranes or matrix. Finally, the probes should not interfere with mitochondrial metabolism, as this will artifactually alter $\Delta\psi$. Nonetheless, several probes have become commonly used, and these can provide qualitative information on and reasonable quantitative estimates of $\Delta\psi$. A detailed discussion of the potential problems associated with the measurement of $\Delta\psi$ with these indicators is provided by Rottenberg.[38] For example, tetraphenylphosphonium (TPP^+), a commonly used probe, exhibits a substantial amount of binding to mitochondrial membranes.[38] Another indicator that is discussed below, rhodamine 123, can produce mitochondrial toxicity by inhibiting the F_0F_1-ATPase.[39]

16.3.3.1.1 Measurement of mitochondrial Δψ in intact renal cells with TPMP⁺. To measure Δψ in intact renal epithelial cells with $TPMP^+$, the following steps are taken:

1. Incubate isolated cells (2 to 3×10^6 cells/ml) or tubule fragments (1 to 2 mg protein per milliliter) with 0.5 μCi/ml of [methyl-^{3}H]- or [methyl-^{14}C]-$TPMP^+$ and unlabeled $TPMP^+$ at a final concentration of 2.5 *μM* for 20 min;
2. Fractionate two 0.5-ml aliquots of cells or tubules by digitonin fractionation (one tube + digitonin, one tube without digitonin) as described above;
3. Count radioactivity recovered in supernatant (= extracellular media + cytosol with digitonin; = extracellular media without digitonin) and in pellet (= mitochondria with digitonin; = total intracellular material without digitonin);
4. Subtract nonspecific binding of $TPMP^+$, as determined by use of boiled cells, from total cellular and mitochondrial accumulation of radiolabel. Perform parallel incubations with ^3H_2O and [^{14}C]sucrose or [^{14}C]inulin to determine intracellular volume and trapped extracellular space.[40]
5. Use these values to determine concentrations of $TPMP^+$ relative to those in extracellular media. Calculate the concentration ratio of $TPMP^+$ in mitochondria (C_m) after digitonin fractionation according to equations derived by and Andersson and Jones[41] and Hoek et al.[37] C_m is calculated as the concentration of $TPMP^+$ in the pellet after digitonin fractionation divided by the concentration in the extracellular medium, and the cytosolic/extracellular concentration ratio (C_c) is calculated from Equation 5:

$$C_T\ (\text{mol/l}) = (V_c \times C_c) + (V_m \times C_m), \tag{5}$$

where C_T is the total intracellular concentration of $TPMP^+$ divided by the extracellular concentration of $TPMP^+$, and V_c and V_m are the volumes for the cytosolic and mitochondrial fractions, respectively.

$TPMP^+$ distribution can be used to measure mitochondrial Δψ in intact cells because more than 95% of steady-state intracellular levels of the cation are found in the mitochondrial fraction.[42]

16.3.3.1.2 Measurement of mitochondrial Δψ in intact renal cells and isolated mitochondria with rhodamine 123. Rhodamine 123, similar to $TPMP^+$, is a membrane-permeant cationic probe that distributes into negatively charged intracellular organelles such as mitochondria according to the Δψ. Since rhodamine 123 is also fluorescent, techniques such as confocal microscopy can be used to visually assess Δψ.[36,43] Mitochondria are identified by green fluorescence after excitation with blue light. A simple filter fluorometer or a dual-wavelength spectrometer can be used to quantitate rhodamine 123 accumulation in mitochondria, using suspensions of either isolated cells or isolated mitochondria.

Since rhodamine 123 distributes according to the Nernst equation (also see Equation 4 above)

$$\Delta\psi\ (\text{mV}) = -60 \log (FL_{IN}/FL_{OUT}), \tag{6}$$

where FL = fluorescence intensity and 2.3 RT/mF = 60 (at 37°C, 1 atm of pressure, and with an indicator cation having one positive charge [i.e., m = +1]), a 10:1 mitochondria to cytosol uptake ratio of the probe corresponds to a Δψ of –60 mV. Since energized mitochondria can have Δψ as high as –180 mV, the rhodamine 123 mitochondria to cytosol uptake ratio can be as high as 1000:1. This indicates two important points. First, rhodamine 123 can be used to localize mitochondria and assess intraorganellar distribution within intact cells; second, relatively small amounts of mitochondrial depolarization can produce large changes in rhodamine 123 distribution and, hence, large changes in fluorescence intensity, making the method extremely sensitive. For example, a decrease in $\Delta\psi$ of 60 mV, which readily occurs in mitochondria under both physiological and toxicological conditions, corresponds to a tenfold change in fluorescence intensity.

1. *Protocol for measurements in isolated cell suspensions.* The protocol is essentially that described by Lemasters et al.[36] Isolated cells (10^5 cells/ml) are suspended in a modified Krebs–Ringer–HEPES buffer, containing 115 m*M* NaCl, 5 m*M* KCl, 1 m*M* KH_2PO_4, 2 m*M* $CaCl_2$, 1.2 m*M* $MgSO_4$, 25 m*M* HEPES, 2 mg/ml bovine serum albumin, and 1 μ*M* rhodamine 123, pH 7.4. After various incubation times, 3-ml aliquots are centrifuged at 700 rpm for 2 min in a tabletop centrifuge. After removal of the supernatant, the pellet containing the cells is resuspended in buffer containing 0.1% (v/v) Triton X-100, which lyses the cells, thereby releasing all the rhodamine 123 accumulated. Cells are centrifuged again at 3500 rpm for 2 min to sediment any debris. The rhodamine 123 concentration in the supernatant is then measured by fluorescence, using excitation and emission wavelengths of 490 and 515 nm, respectively. Results are quantified by comparison to rhodamine 123 standards in the same buffer.
2. *Protocol for measurements in isolated mitochondria.* Isolated mitochondria (0.15 to 0.20 mg protein per milliliter) are prepared in a standard buffer, containing 150 m*M* sucrose, 5 m*M* $MgCl_2$, 10 m*M* potassium phosphate, pH 7.4, 20 m*M* HEPES (free acid or potassium salt), respiratory substrate (5 m*M* sodium succinate + 1 μ*M* rotenone or 5 m*M* malate + 5 m*M* pyruvate), and 0.2 μ*M* rhodamine 123. Fluorescence can be measured using wavelengths of 503 and 527 nm for excitation and emission, respectively. Dual-wavelength spectrometry can also be used to measure absorbance change due to rhodamine 123 distribution, using absorbance changes at 516 minus 495 nm.[36] In this case, higher concentrations of rhodamine 123 (0.6 μ*M*) and mitochondria (0.5 mg protein per milliliter) are used to account for differences in sensitivity between fluorescence and absorbance. Results for both methods are calibrated using valinomycin-induced potassium diffusion potentials (see below).

16.3.3.1.3 Measurement of $\Delta\psi$ in isolated renal mitochondria with safranine O. $\Delta\psi$ in suspensions of isolated mitochondria can be determined by measurement of absorbance changes due to the redistribution of a lipophilic cationic probe across the inner membrane as a function of $\Delta\psi$. One such probe is safranine O (3,7-diamino-5-phenylphenazinium chloride; Figure 5),[44] which is freely soluble in both water and alcohol when used as the chloride salt. Aqueous and alcoholic solutions are purplish-red (A_{max} at approximately 530 nm) and have a greenish-yellow fluorescence. The following procedures are used to calibrate and measure $\Delta\psi$ with safranine O:

1. *Calibration of signal with safranine O.*
   a. Add the following to a cuvette (2.9 ml capacity): mitochondria (0.9 ml, 1.2 to 2.0 mg protein per milliliter) in buffer (250 m*M* sucrose, 5 m*M* $MgCl_2$, 20 m*M* triethanolamine/HCl, pH 7.4) + 5 μl of 1 mg rotenone per milliliter ethanol (5 μg/ml final) + 5 μl of 1 mg oligomycin per milliliter ethanol (5 μg/ml final) + 5 μl of 2 m*M* safranine O in water (10 μ*M* final) + 0.1 ml of appropriate KCl solution (0.12 to 20 m*M* final) + 5 μl of 10 μg valinomycin per milliliter ethanol (50 ng/ml final). The final ethanol concentration is 2% (v/v).
   b. Measure absorbance value at 511 minus 533 nm.

c. Add 2 μl of 0.5 m*M* FCCP in ethanol (1 μ*M* final) and 0.1 ml of 0.2 *M* KCl (20 m*M* added) to dissipate the Δψ. Measure absorbance at 511 minus 533 nm again. The signal is the difference in absorbance after addition of valinomycin as compared to that after addition of FCCP and KCl.

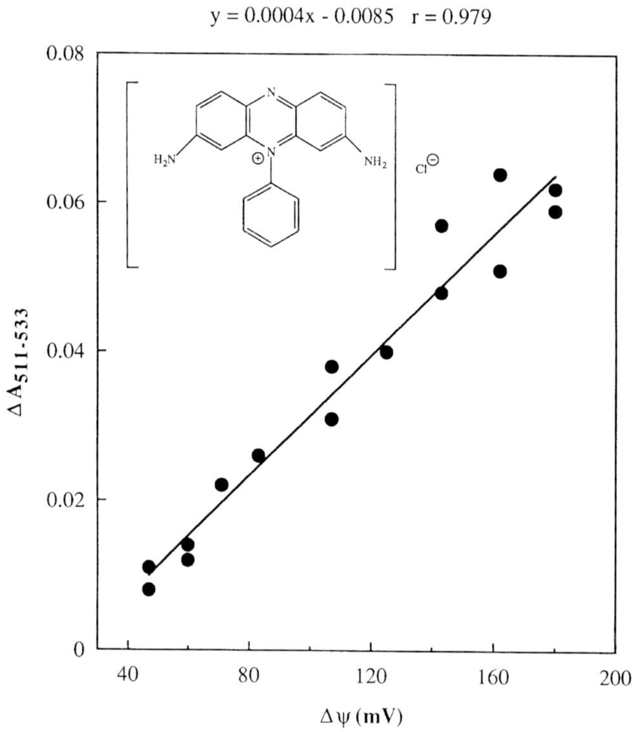

Figure 5 Calibration curve for determination of mitochondrial membrane potential (Δψ) with safranine O. Renal cortical mitochondria (0.9 ml; 1.5 mg protein per milliliter) were mixed with 5 μg/ml rotenone, 5 μg/ml oligomycin, 10 μ*M* safranine O (see inset for chemical structure), 0.1 ml of the appropriately diluted KCl stock solution (see Table 3), and 50 ng/ml valinomycin. After recording $\Delta A_{511-533}$, 1 μ*M* FCCP and 20 m*M* KCl are added. $\Delta A_{511-533}$ is recorded again, and the final value is the difference between the ΔA after addition of valinomycin and that after addition of FCCP and KCl. Δψ was calculated using the Nernst equation, assuming intramitochondrial K^+ ion concentration is 120 m*M* and extramitochondrial K^+ ion concentrations are varied between 0.12 and 20 m*M*. Results are single measurements obtained from two separate mitochondrial preparations.

To prepare a safranine O–Δψ calibration curve, K^+-diffusion potentials are created by varying the extramitochondrial K^+ ion concentration, $[K^+]_{OUT}$, in the presence of valinomycin and applying the Nernst equation (Equation 4) (Table 3). Intramitochondrial K^+ ion concentration, $[K^+]_{IN}$, is assumed to be 120 m*M* whereas normal $[K^+]_{OUT}$ is approximately 20 m*M*. A linear relation (r = 0.979) between a Δψ of 47 mV to 180 mV was obtained (Figure 5), validating the assay method over the range of Δψ values typically observed in mitochondria during different physiological or pathological states. Note that at ΔAbsorbance = 0, a residual Δψ of –21.2 mV is obtained. Inadequacies of available methods make measurements of Δψ values below about –40 mV approximations at best.[38]

2. *Measurement of Δψ in isolated mitochondria with safranine O.* Membrane potential in suspensions of mitochondria incubated with either buffer or a chemical of interest is measured as above except that valinomycin is omitted, 0.2 *M* KCl is used to give

Table 3 Preparation of Calibration Curve for Determination of Mitochondrial Membrane Potential ($\Delta\psi$) with Safranine O

$[KCl]_{OUT}$ (m*M*)	$\Delta\psi$ (mV)[a]	Amount stock added (μl)[b]	Amount buffer added (μl)[c]
20	–47	100	0
12	–60	60	40
8	–71	40	60
5	–83	25	75
2	–107	10	90
1	–125	5	95
0.5	–143	2.5	97.5
0.25	–162	1.25	98.75
0.12	–180	0.6	99.4

Note: For calibration of $\Delta\psi$ (negative inside), cuvettes contain the following (total volume = 1.02 ml): Mitochondria (0.9 ml; 1.5 mg protein/ml), rotenone (5 μl; 1 mg/ml), oligomycin (5 μl; 1 mg/ml), safranine O (5 μl; 2 m*M*), KCl solution (0.1 ml), and valinomycin (5 μl; 10 μg/ml). After recording $\Delta A_{511\text{-}533}$, 2 μl of FCCP (0.5 m*M*) and 0.1 ml of 0.2 *M* KCl are added, and ΔA is recorded. Net signal is difference between two ΔA values.

[a] $\Delta\psi = -60 \log (K^+_{IN}/K^+_{OUT})$, where $[K^+]_{IN}$ assumed to be 120 m*M*.

[b] Stock KCl solution = 0.2 *M* KCl.

[c] Buffer = 250 m*M* sucrose, 5 m*M* $MgCl_2$, 20 m*M* triethanolamine/HCl, pH 7.4.

a final $[K^+]_{OUT}$ of 20 m*M*, and 5 μl of 1 *M* succinate (5 m*M* final concentration) is added to energize the mitochondria.

Control renal cortical mitochondria typically have $\Delta\psi$ = 140 to 180 mV after addition of succinate.[6] Further addition of valinomycin decreases $\Delta\psi$ to 40 to 60 mV; subsequent addition of FCCP decreases $\Delta\psi$ further to 25 to 35 mV; final addition of 20 m*M* KCl decreases $\Delta\psi$ to the residual value of 21 mV. The high concentration of anionic proteins in the mitochondrial matrix provides a significant Donnan potential that is likely responsible for much of the residual $\Delta\psi$ after collapse of ion gradients. Control mitochondria maintain the ability to generate a $\Delta\psi$ of >150 mV during a 2-h incubation. In contrast, renal cortical mitochondria treated with the nephrotoxic cysteine *S*-conjugate DCVC progressively lose the ability to generate a $\Delta\psi$ when energized with succinate in a time- and concentration-dependent manner.[6] For example, renal cortical mitochondria incubated with 1 m*M* DCVC for 2 h only generated a $\Delta\psi$ of 90 mV after addition of succinate, whereas mitochondria incubated with buffer for 2 h generated a $\Delta\psi$ of 150 mV after addition of succinate.

16.3.3.2 pH Gradient

Generation of a pH gradient (ΔpH) by mitochondria is a critical component of the chemiosmotic hypothesis by which substrate oxidation is coupled to ATP synthesis. A decreased ΔpH, therefore, indicates impairment of oxidative phosphorylation capability. In contrast to the use of lipophilic cations that distribute according to membrane potential, measurement of ΔpH depends on the distribution of radiolabeled weak bases that are membrane-permeable only in the non-ionized form (Figure 6). The distribution of A^- + HA or B + BH^+ across the membrane is thus a function of the pK and the pH values on each side of the membrane. As explained above (see Equation 3), the proton electrochemical gradient or protonmotive force (Δp), is composed of both a charge difference (i.e., the $\Delta\psi$) and a proton concentration difference (ΔpH) across the mitochondrial inner membrane. Under physiological conditions, the presence of weak permeant acids (e.g., phosphate, bicarbonate, other organic acids) in biological fluids tends to limit the ΔpH to usually no more than one unit. Consequently, the majority of the Δp is composed of the $\Delta\psi$, with ΔpH accounting for 30% or less of the total energetic driving force.

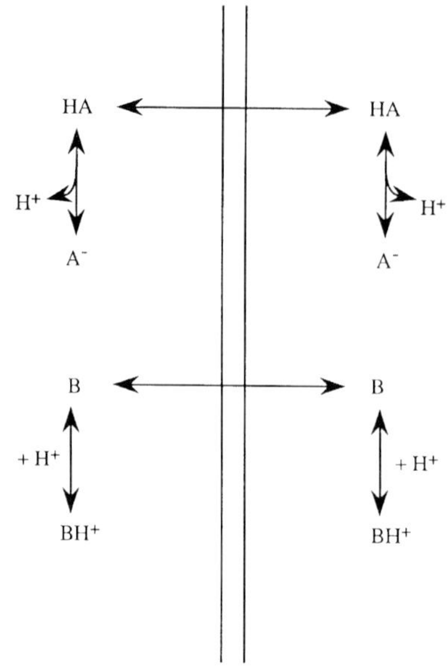

Figure 6 The equilibrium distribution of electroneutrally permeant weak acids and bases as a function of ΔpH. With acids, the concentration of the protonated form (HA) is the same on both sides of the membrane, whereas the deprotonated form (A^-) cannot cross the membrane. With bases, the concentration of the deprotonated form (B) is the same on both sides of the membrane, whereas the protonated form (BH^+) cannot cross the membrane.

Mitochondrial ΔpH can be quantified by use of weak bases such as 5,5-dimethyloxazolidine-2,4-dione (DMO) that distribute into intracellular organelles according to pH by the following procedure,[41] which is analogous to that described above for determination of Δψ with radiolabeled $TPMP^+$:

1. Incubate isolated cells (2 to 3×10^6 cells/ml) or tubule fragments (1 to 2 mg protein/ml) with 0.5 μCi/ml of [2-^{14}C]DMO and unlabeled DMO at a final concentration of 2.5 μ*M* for 20 min.
2. Fractionate two 0.5-ml aliquots of cells or tubules by digitonin fractionation (one tube + digitonin, one tube without digitonin) as described above.
3. Count radioactivity recovered in supernatant (= extracellular media + cytosol with digitonin; = extracellular media without digitonin) and in pellet (= mitochondria with digitonin; = total intracellular material without digitonin).
4. Determine nonspecific binding of DMO by use of boiled cells, and subtract binding from total cellular and mitochondrial accumulation of radiolabel. Perform parallel incubations with ^3H_2O and [^{14}C]sucrose or [^{14}C]inulin to determine intracellular volume and trapped extracellular space.[40] Use these values to determine concentrations of DMO.
5. Quantitate pH values in mitochondria and cytosol from the corrected concentrations of DMO according to Equation 7:

$$pH = \log[C_r(10^{pK + pHout}) - 10^{pK}], \qquad (7)$$

where C_r is the concentration ratio of DMO in each compartment relative to the extracellular concentration and pH_{out} is the extracellular pH. C_r for DMO in each compartment is calculated as described above for $TPMP^+$. A value of 6.13 is used for the pK_a for DMO at 37°C.[37]

16.3.3.3 *Adenine and pyridine nucleotides*

The ability to derive energy from food and nutrients is a fundamental characteristic of all organisms. ATP is the central currency of chemical energy for cells, and the mitochondria are the primary intracellular sites of ATP biosynthesis. Measurement of cellular ATP content is a common method to quantify cellular energetics because maintenance of high intracellular ATP generally means that mitochondria and the ATP-generating mechanisms are functionally intact. The association of maintenance of ATP supply with preservation of cellular and mitochondrial viability or depletion of ATP supply with cellular and mitochondrial injury has been a subject of debate for many years.[45] Reversible changes in ATP content readily occur without loss of cellular viability. Such reversible changes have been investigated extensively in studies of hypoxia and anoxia in which cells deprived of oxygen rapidly lose most (>80%) of their normal ATP content within 10 min but can remain viable for as long as 2 to 3 h,[46] depending on the tissue. Although cellular ATP content always decreases in dead cells, this phenomenon is not always an early occurrence in the progression of events leading to cell death. While necrotic cell death may be associated with an early decrease in the ability of cells to synthesize ATP, cells undergoing apoptosis, or programmed cell death, may retain relatively high concentrations of ATP until relatively late in the progression of events leading to cell death.[47] Therefore, a simple decrease in cellular ATP content may not provide any information regarding time course, mechanism, or target site involved in cellular injury. Additional information on mitochondrial energetic status can be obtained by measurement of both ADP and AMP and calculation of the ATP/ADP ratio and the adenylate energy charge [(ATP + 1/2 ADP)/(ATP + ADP + AMP)].

16.3.3.3.1 *Determination of adenine and oxidized pyridine nucleotides by HPLC.* Adenylates (ATP, ADP, AMP), associated degradation products (IMP, hypoxanthine, xanthine, adenosine), and oxidized pyridine nucleotides (NAD^+, $NADP^+$) can be determined simultaneously by reversed-phase high-performance liquid chromatography (HPLC) using gradient elution according to the method of Jones,[43] with minor modifications. Sample processing and HPLC separation conditions are described below.

1. *Processing of samples.* To a 0.5-ml aliquot of isolated cells or isolated mitochondria is added 0.25 ml of 3 *M* perchloric acid and samples are immediately cooled on ice. Samples can be frozen at this stage and analyzed within 1 to 2 days. The perchloric acid is removed by neutralization with KOH and centrifugation immediately before injection.
2. *HPLC column.* μBondapak C_{18} cartridge (8 mm × 10 cm) (Waters Associates, Milford, MA).
3. *HPLC solvents.* Solvent A: 100 m*M* potassium phosphate, pH 6.0; solvent B: methanol.
4. *General operating conditions.* Flow rate = 1.5 ml/min; recycling time between runs = 10 min; temperature = ambient (20 to 22°C).
5. *HPLC separation conditions.* Seven and one half minutes at 100% A/0% B, 7.5 min linear gradient to 90% A/10% B, 15 min linear gradient to 75% A/25% B, 0.5 min linear gradient back to 100% A/0% B, 10 min reequilibration at initial conditions.
6. *Detection.* Absorbance at 260 nm.

Separation of standard adenine nucleotides and associated metabolites is shown in Figure 7. By simultaneously measuring the seven indicated species, a detailed picture of adenine nucleotide status can be obtained. For example, ischemia or hypoxia is associated with inhibition of mitochondrial respiration and rapid degradation of ATP — initially to ADP and AMP, but then to adenosine and IMP and hypoxanthine and xanthine. By this HPLC method, therefore, formation of these products over time can be followed readily.

In addition to adenine nucleotides and their breakdown products, oxidized pyridine nucleotides can be detected. Although not shown in Figure 7, $NADP^+$ and NAD^+ have retention times of 17.28 min and 23.00 min, respectively.

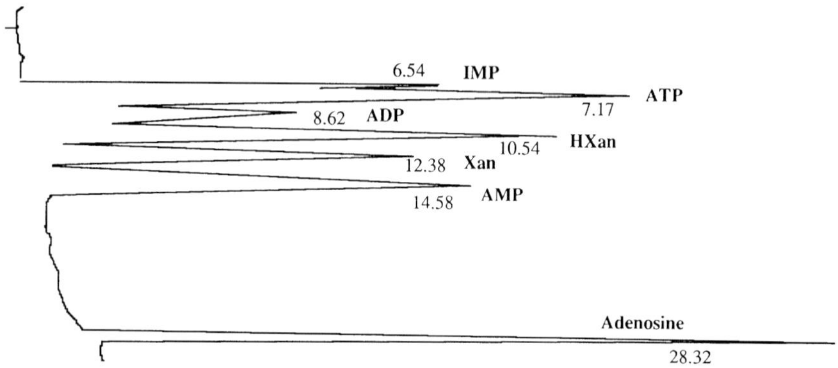

PEAK#	AREA%	RT	AREA
1	7.316	6.54	12733878
2	16.413	7.17	28567317
3	12.648	8.62	22013299
4	16.077	10.54	27982522
5	12.682	12.38	22072717
6	17.561	14.58	30565346
7	17.303	28.32	30116204

Figure 7 Analysis of adenine nucleotides and associated metabolites by HPLC. Standard mixture of 1.5 nmol each of IMP, ATP, ADP, hypoxanthine (HXan), xanthine (Xan), AMP, and adenosine were separated by reversed-phase HPLC on a μBondapak C_{18} column using gradient elution with 100 m*M* potassium phosphate, pH 6.0 (solvent A)–methanol (solvent B) and detection at 260 nm. Separation conditions were as follows: flow rate was 1.5 ml/min; 7.5 min at 100% A/0% B, 7.5 min linear gradient to 95% A/5% B, 15 min linear gradient to 85% A/15% B, 0.5 min linear gradient back to initial conditions.

16.3.3.3.2 Determination of reduced pyridine nucleotides by HPLC. A similar HPLC method is used for detection and quantitation of reduced pyridine nucleotides. Since reduced pyridine nucleotides are unstable in acid, however, sample preparation is modified to quench cellular processes in base.

1. *Processing of samples.* To a 0.5-ml aliquot of isolated cells or isolated mitochondria is added 0.05 ml of 0.5 *M* KOH containing 50% (v/v) ethanol and 35% (w/v) cesium chloride. The KOH–ethanol–CsCl solution should be kept ice-cold. Samples are immediately cooled on ice and then centrifuged to remove insoluble material before injection. Due to the relative instability of the reduced pyridine nucleotides, it is important that samples be analyzed as quickly as possible, usually within 6 h.
2. *HPLC column.* μBondapak C_{18} cartridge (8 mm × 10 cm) (Waters Associates, Milford, MA).
3. *HPLC solvents.* Solvent A: 100 m*M* potassium phosphate, pH 6.0, solvent B: methanol.
4. *General operating conditions.* Flow rate = 1.5 ml/min, recycling time between runs = 10 min, temperature = ambient (20 to 22°C).
5. *HPLC separation conditions.* Five minutes at 95% A/5% B, 10 min linear gradient to 85% A/15% B, 4 min isocratic at 85% A/15% B, 1 min linear gradient back to 95% A/5% B, 7.5 min reequilibration at initial conditions.

6. *Detection.* Absorbance at 340 nm.
7. *Retention times.* NADPH (9.12 min), NADH (16.81 min).

16.3.3.4 Permeability transition

Mitochondria contain a latent mechanism that when activated by certain chemicals produces an increase in permeability of the inner membrane to small ions (<1500 Da), swelling, collapse of the $\Delta\psi$, and uncoupling of oxidative phosphorylation.[49] The process is dependent on the presence of Ca^{2+} ions. Although the precise mechanism by which the transition occurs has not been unequivocally established, a large list of diverse chemical agents have been shown to induce the transition in suspensions of isolated mitochondria from liver, kidney, heart, and other mammalian tissues (Table 4). These agents include lipids and fatty acid derivatives, heavy and transition metals, oxidants, specific mitochondrial inhibitors, and other diverse chemicals.

Table 4 Some Agents That Induce the Mitochondrial Permeability Transition

Fatty acids and lipid metabolites	Reye's syndrome	Sulfhydryl reagents (organic)
Acyl carnitine, long chain	Blood serum from Reye's syndrome patients	Arsenite
Acylcoenzyme A, long chain	Salicylates	Diamide
L-Carnitine	Uncouplers and inhibitors	1,2-Dibromoethane
Lysophospholipids	Indomethacin	Disulfiram
Heavy and transition metals	Rhein	5,5′-Dithiobis(2-nitrobenzoic acid)
Cd^{2+}	Safranine	Iodoacetate
Cu^{2+}	Silymarin	Iodoacetamide
Fe^{2+}	Uncoupler + EGTA	Mersalyl
Hg^{2+} and organic mercurials	Uncoupler + ruthenium red	Phenylarsine oxide
Pb^{2+}	WY 14643 and clofibric acid	Other compounds
Zn^{2+}	Quinones	Allantoin
Metabolites that oxidize NAD(P)H	Benzoquinones	Adriamycin aglycone
Acetoacetate	2,5-Dibromothymoquinone	Cyanide
t-Butylhydroperoxide	Menadione	Dihyroorotate
H_2O_2	Other ions	Dopamine
Oxalacetate	Ca^{2+} only (no inducing agent present)	6-Hydroxydopamine
Adenine nucleotide translocase inhibitors	Phosphate	Nifedipine
Atractyloside	Pyrophosphate	Nitrofurantoin
Carboxyatractyloside		Phosphoenolpyruvate
		Protoporphyrin IX
		Pyridoxal phospate
		Trialkyltin compounds
		Xanthine + xanthine oxidase

Adapted from Gunter, T. E. and Pfeiffer, D. R., *Am. J. Physiol.*, 258, C755, 1990.

The swelling and increased membrane permeability associated with the permeability transition can be measured by the methods described above. A diagnostic for the permeability transition is the ability of the immunosuppressive agent cyclosporin A to inhibit it with very high potency, irrespective of the inducing agent; a cyclosporin A concentration of 0.5 μM is sufficient to completely prevent or reverse the permeability transition. This potency and universality suggest that transition-dependent movements of ions and certain metabolites across the inner membrane of mitochondria occur through a regulated pore as a normal part of mitochondrial function and that the large array of inducing agents ultimately work through a common, final step.

16.3.3.5 *Thiol/disulfide status*

As discussed above, regulation of intramitochondrial thiol/disulfide status, chiefly through GSH-dependent processes, is critical for the maintenance of mitochondrial functional integrity. GSH is the principal nonprotein thiol in mitochondria and can exist in several forms, including GSH, GSSG, and mixed-disulfides with coenzyme A and proteins. Two methods are described to quantify these forms of GSH — an enzymatic assay that allows measurement of GSH and GSSG and an HPLC method that, depending on sample preparation and processing, can be used to measure GSH and GSSG or other disulfide-containing forms of GSH.

16.3.3.5.1 *Determination of GSH and GSSG with enzymatic recycling and 2-vinylpyridine.* GSH and GSSG can be measured by an enzymatic recycling assay[50] involving the use of Ellman's reagent [5,5′-dithiobis(2-nitrobenzoic acid); DTNB], and GSSG reductase, with GSH content correlating with NADPH oxidation (ε_{340} = 6200 $M^{-1}cm^{-1}$) or formation of the *p*-nitrothiophenolate anion (NTP; ε_{412} = 13,600 $M^{-1}cm^{-1}$). The assay occurs in two steps:

$$\textit{nonenzymic}: 2\ \text{GSH} + \text{DTNB} \rightarrow \text{GSSG} + 2\ \text{NTP} \tag{8}$$

$$\textit{GSSG reductase}: \text{GSSG} + \text{NADPH} + \text{H}^+ \rightarrow 2\ \text{GSH} + \text{NADP}^+ \tag{9}$$

As shown above, the assay measures total GSH-equivalents (i.e., GSH + 2 GSSG). The following steps are performed to measure either total GSH-equivalents or GSSG in GSH-equivalents:

1. *Solutions*
   Buffer. 125 m*M* sodium phosphate, 6.3 m*M* EDTA (pH 7.5)
   Triethanolamine base. 25% triethanolamine (v/v)
   Solutions prepared in buffer
   I. 0.3 m*M* NADPH
   II. 6 m*M* DTNB
   III. 50 U GSSG reductase per milliliter
2. *Sample preparation.* Precipitate cellular or mitochondrial protein by adding 0.5 volumes of 10% (w/v) 5-sulfosalicylic acid (SSA): [0.5 ml cells (or mitochondria) + 0.25 ml SSA]; per 100 µl of deproteinized sample, add the following:
   a. For assay of total GSH-equivalents (GSH + 2 GSSG), add 24 µl of 25% (v/v) of triethanolamine base to neutralize;
   b. For assay of GSSG in GSH-equivalents, add 24 µl of 25% (v/v) of triethanolamine base (to neutralize) + 2 µl of 2-vinylpyridine (to bind GSH); incubate at room temperature for 1 h.
3. *Assay procedure.* In a cuvette, add the following: 700 µl of solution I + 100 µl of solution II + 100 µl of neutralized acid extract of sample; mix in cuvette at 30°C and record ΔA_{412} for approximately 5 min; add 10 µl of solution III; and mix and record ΔA_{412}.
4. *Calculations.* Rates of NTB formation are quantitated using the molar absorption coefficient, and NTB is equivalent to GSH-equivalents present. In the absence of 2-vinylpyridine, assay gives total GSH-equivalents (GSH + 2 GSSG); in the presence of 2-vinylpyridine, assay gives GSSG in GSH-equivalents. Content of GSH is calculated by taking total GSH-equivalents minus GSSG in GSH-equivalents. Although this assay

method is commonly used for determination of GSH and GSSG and is completely reliable for determination of total content of glutathione (GSH + 2 GSSG), use of 2-vinylpyridine underestimates the content of GSSG and overestimates the content of GSH because 2-vinylpyridine can react with the GSH that is generated in the assay. Caution should be exercised, therefore, in use of this method to determine GSSG content.

16.3.3.5.2 Determination of GSH and GSSG by reversed-phase, ion-exchange HPLC. The HPLC method is that described by Fariss and Reed,[51] and involves derivatization and separation by reversed-phase, ion-exchange chromatography. Some of the critical features of the assay will be briefly described.

1. *Sample preparation.* Aliquots of cells or mitochondria (0.5 ml) are deproteinated by addition of 0.1 ml of 70% (v/v) perchloric acid (10%, v/v, final concentration). Internal standard (50 µl of 1.5 m*M* L-γ-glutamyl-L-glutamate) and antioxidant to prevent nonenzymic conversion of GSH to GSSG (50 µl of 15 m*M* bathophenanthroline disulfonate) are added. After removal of the perchloric acid-insoluble material, a portion of the extract (0.5 ml) is derivatized and analyzed by HPLC.
2. *Derivatization*
   a. *Reagents.* Iodoacetic acid, 100 m*M* (made fresh); KOH (stock), 10 *M*, dissolved in metal-free water; $KHCO_3$ (stock), 3 *M*, dissolved in metal-free water; KOH (2 *M*)-$KHCO_3$ (2.4 *M*), working solution; 1-fluoro-2,4-dinitrobenzene, 1%, v/v, in ethanol (made fresh).
   b. *Procedure.* To 0.5 ml of acid extract containing the internal standard and antioxidant, add 50 µl of 100 m*M* iodoacetic acid; bring the acidic solution to pH 8 to 9 by the addition of 0.48 ml of KOH (2 *M*)-$KHCO_3$ (2.4 *M*) and allow to incubate in the dark at room temperature for 10 min. Add 1 ml of 1%, v/v, 1-fluoro-2,4-dinitrobenzene, cap reaction mixture, mix with a vortex mixer, and store overnight at 4°C. Centrifuge *S*-carboxymethyl-*N*-dinitrophenyl derivatives and store at 4°C in the dark until analysis; samples are stable for up to two weeks.
3. *HPLC separation*
   a. *Principle.* Dinitrophenyl (DNP) derivatives of acidic amino acids (including thiol-containing compounds) are separated on an amine column by reversed-phase, ion-exchange HPLC. In the mobile phase, methanol is used to elute rapidly the excess 2,4-dinitrophenol and the DNP derivatives of basic and neutral amino acids. The pH of the acetate in the mobile phase maintains the bonded-phase amino groups in the protonated form. By increasing the sodium acetate concentration of the mobile phase, selective elution of the acidic DNP derivatives is accomplished. The eluted DNP derivatives are measured by their absorbance at 365 nm. The internal standard corrects for errors in dilution and alterations in derivatization efficiency, derivatization stability, and chromatographic conditions.
   b. *Reagents and supplies.* Sodium acetate solution (stock), 2.6 *M*, prepared by adding 272 g of sodium acetate and 122 ml of water to 378 ml of glacial acetic acid; stir with low heat until sodium acetate is in solution; cool and then filter with a 4.0- to 5.5-µm polypropylene filter. Mobile phase A: 80% (v/v) methanol. Mobile phase B: 0.5 *M* sodium acetate in 64% (v/v) methanol; prepared by adding 200 ml of the stock sodium acetate solution to 800 ml of 80% (v/v) methanol. HPLC column: µBondapak amine 10-µ cartridge (8 mm × 10 cm) (Waters Assoc., Milford, MA).

c. *Procedure.* An example of separation conditions for a new column is as follows:

Mobile phase is maintained at 80% A, 20% B for 5 min at a flow rate of 1.5 ml/min.

30-min linear gradient to 1% A, 99% B.

Hold mobile phase at 1% A, 99% B until last compound (usually GSSG) has eluted (10 to 15 min).

1-min linear gradient to 80% A, 20% B.

Hold at 80% A, 20% B for 5 min to reequilibrate at initial conditions.

These separation conditions will vary, depending on the efficiency of the column, which decreases with the age of the column. Hence, as resolution decreases, conditions are changed to make the acetate concentration lower and/or the gradient more shallow.

d. *Sensitivity of method.* Sensitivity is based, in part, on the number of amine groups available for chromophore (DNP) derivatization and the sensitivity of the detector. With variable wavelength detectors, disulfides are measured at concentrations as low as 0.5 nmol/ml or 25 pmol/injection and thiols are measured at concentrations as low as 1.0 nmol/ml or 50 pmol/injection. Approximately five- to tenfold greater sensitivities can be achieved with some fixed-wavelength, filter-type detectors. In addition to GSH and GSSG, other relevant compounds that are measurable by this method include glutamate, cystine, cysteine, aspartate, γ-glutamyl-L-cysteine, and the mixed disulfide of GSH and cysteine.

16.3.3.5.3 Determination of mixed disulfides of GSH and cysteine with protein by HPLC. The objective of this procedure is to remove soluble thiols and disulfides rapidly from cellular or mitochondrial protein and then to release covalently bound GSH or cysteine from proteins for analysis.

1. Deproteinate samples by treatment with 10% (v/v) perchloric acid as above.
2. Solubilize protein pellets from 0.5-ml acid extracts by addition of 2 ml of 0.1 *M* NaOH.
3. Add 4 ml of 0.1 *M* sodium phosphate, pH 6.0, containing 5 m*M* dithiothreitol, and incubate 30 min.
4. Add 1.2 ml of 30% (w/v) trichloroacetic acid to deproteinate.
5. Derivatize supernatant with iodoacetic acid and 1-fluoro-2,4-dinitrobenzene and analyze by HPLC as above.

16.3.4 Calcium ion distribution

Regulation of intramitochondrial Ca^{2+} distribution is critical for numerous functions. As described above, high loads of Ca^{2+} induce a permeability transition that leads to alterations in membrane potential and gradients of other ions, thereby inhibiting and/or uncoupling oxidative phosphorylation. These changes occur at concentrations that are orders of magnitude greater than the changes in Ca^{2+} concentration that are involved in regulation of mitochondrial metabolism.[52] Several assays for Ca^{2+} with colorimetric or fluorimetric dyes are based on changes in the absorbance or fluorescence of these dyes on complexation with Ca^{2+} ions. Critical features of the interaction of these dyes with Ca^{2+} are that they occur with a high affinity and a high degree of specificity. In other words, it is important that Ca^{2+} ions remain bound to the dye in proportion to their presence in the biological compartment of interest and that little binding of the dye with other ions, such as Mg^{2+} or other cations, occurs relative to that with Ca^{2+}.

Two dyes that have been used extensively for quantitation of Ca^{2+} ion concentrations in intact cells and in subcellular organelles are fura-2 and arsenazo III. Fura-2 is a fluorescent dye that is used both for direct quantitation of Ca^{2+} ion concentrations and in imaging studies (such as those using confocal microscopy) to determine the intracellular distribution of Ca^{2+} ions. Arsenazo III is a colorimetric dye whose absorbance spectrum changes on binding with Ca^{2+} ions.

16.3.4.1 *Measurement of Ca^{2+} ion concentrations with fura-2*

Isolated renal cells or mitochondria are incubated with 10 μ*M* fura-2-acetoxymethyl ester. The ester form is readily transported across biological membranes by diffusion and is then deesterified within the cell or mitochondria to release fura-2. The method described below for isolated mitochondria is essentially that described by Drewnowska and Schoolwerth.[53]

1. Mitochondria (10 mg protein per milliliter) are loaded with fura-2 in an oxygenated "loading medium" containing (in m*M*): KCl (150), 3-(*N*-morpholino)propanesulfonic acid (MOPS; 20), EGTA (1), ATP (5), $MgCl_2$ (5), pH 7.0, by incubating for 35 min at 25°C.
2. Fura-2-loaded mitochondria are washed by centrifugation and resuspended in "wash medium," containing (in m*M*): KCl (130), HEPES (20), EGTA (1), ATP (5), $MgCl_2$ (5), KH_2PO_4 (5), and NaCl (5), pH 7.0. Loaded and washed mitochondria are stored on ice until used for measurements of Ca^{2+} concentration.
3. Fifty microliters of the mitochondrial suspension are placed in a cuvette maintained at 25°C containing 1.95 ml of "assay buffer," containing (in m*M*): KCl (150), MOPS (20), EGTA (7.5), KH_2PO_4 (5), and NaCl (5), pH 7.0. With a dilution of 1:40, the final Mg^{2+} ion concentration is 125 μ*M*. The fluorescence ratios are obtained from excitation wavelengths of 340 and 380 nm with 510 nm emission. Autofluorescence of mitochondria that are not loaded with fura-2 are also measured at 340 and 380 nm, and these values are subtracted from those of the loaded mitochondria.
4. The ratio (R) of emission intensities obtained by excitation at 340 and 380 nm are then used to calculate the matrix Ca^{2+} concentration, $[Ca^{2+}]_m$, according to the following equation:

$$[Ca^{2+}]_m \text{ (mol/l)} = K_d \times [(R - R_{min})/(R_{max} - R)] \times S_f/S_b, \tag{10}$$

   where K_d is the apparent dissociation constant of Ca^{2+}, R_{max} is the ratio R when all the dye is bound with Ca^{2+}, R_{min} is the ratio when all the dye is in the unbound form, and S_f and S_b are the fluorescence of the free dye and the Ca^{2+}-bound dye, respectively, at 380 nm.
5. Calibration is performed using the brominated form of A23187 (3 μ*M*) and nigericin (5 μ*M*) to permeabilize the mitochondrial membrane to Ca^{2+}, K^+, and H^+ to enable calculation of the K_d for the intramitochondrial dye for Ca^{2+} ions. K_d for Ca^{2+} binding to fura-2 calculated by Drewnowska and Schoolwerth[47] was 323 n*M*. K_d was independent of pH over the range of pH = 7.0 to 7.4.

An illustration of an application of this methodology to the measurement of intramitochondrial Ca^{2+} ion concentration in renal cortical mitochondria is shown in Figure 8.

16.3.4.2 *Measurement of Ca^{2+} ion concentrations with arsenazo III*

Arsenazo III (*o*-1,8-dihydroxy-3,6-disulfo-naphthalene-2,7-bisazo-bisbenzenearsonic acid) is a water-soluble dye that exhibits no detectable binding to cellular membranes and exists as a purple dye in the absence of Ca^{2+} ions (l_{max} < 550 nm) and as a blue violet dye in the Ca^{2+}-bound form (l_{max} = 595 and 658 nm). The Ca^{2+}-bound dye has a molar absorption

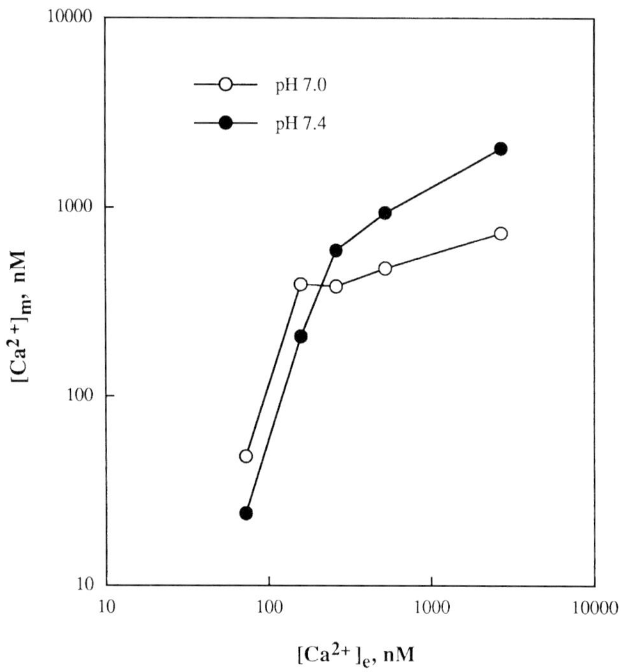

Figure 8 Correlation between extramitochondrial calcium ion concentration, $[Ca^{2+}]_e$, and intramitochondrial calcium ion concentration, $[Ca^{2+}]_m$, in renal cortical mitochondria incubated at pH 7.0 and 7.4. Isolated renal cortical mitochondria from Sprague–Dawley rats were loaded with fura 2-acetoxymethyl ester for measurement of $[Ca^{2+}]_m$ at different $[Ca^{2+}]_e$ at pH 7.0 and 7.4 by fluorescence (excitation ratio at 340 and 380 nm, emission at 510 nm). Results are plotted on log scales. Each data point is the mean of 27 to 49 determinations at each pH value and are obtained from Drewnowska and Schoolwerth.[53] (Adapted from Drewnowska, K. and Schoolwerth, A. C., *Am. J. Physiol.*, 267, F153, 1994.)

coefficient ($\Delta\varepsilon_{654-685}$) of 21,500 M^{-1}cm^{-1}, indicating a high sensitivity. Arsenazo III can be used to determine the distribution of Ca^{2+} ions in different subcellular fractions of intact renal epithelial cells, as described above, using selective release of mitochondrial Ca^{2+} ions with the protonophore FCCP and subsequent release of remaining Ca^{2+} ion, which is predominantly microsomal, with the Ca^{2+}-ionophore A23187.[5] Arsenazo III can also be used in suspensions of isolated renal cortical mitochondria to assess the ability of mitochondria to sequester and retain Ca^{2+} ions.[6]

1. *Treatment of glassware.* All glassware and columns used in experiments with arsenazo III are prewashed with 1 m*M* EGTA and then thoroughly rinsed with deionized water.
2. *Purification of arsenazo III.* Arsenazo III that is obtained commercially (e.g., Sigma Chemical Co., St. Louis, MO) must be purified first to remove any bound cations. The procedure involves passage through two successive columns, takes about 5 to 7 days, and is based on the procedure described by Kendrick.[54]
   a. Wash a 2.5 × 41-cm preparative column of DEAE-cellulose with 800 ml of *n*-butanol–pyridine–acetic acid–water (3:1:1:3) (BPAW) solvent for 24 h at 0.6 ml/min.
   b. Apply 0.5 g of arsenazo III (dissolved in 2 ml of water and 3 ml of BPAW) to the column top. Any residue remaining in the arsenazo III vessel is dissolved in 2 ml of BPAW and is applied to the column. This is followed by three 2-ml rinses,

which are also applied to the column. Arsenazo III is eluted from the column with BPAW at a flow rate of 14 ml/h. Approximately two hundred fifty 7-ml fractions are collected.

c. Gross color differences in eluate fractions should be seen: fractions 1 to 25 (brownish), fractions 26 to 49 (amber), fractions 50 to 75 (rose), fractions 76 to 93 (light rose), fractions 94 to 210 (dark purple).

d. Fractions 118 to 232 (805 ml) are pooled and taken to dryness under vacuum using a rotary evaporator. Water is added several times to the residue and it is reevaporated to eliminate the pyridine odor. Approximately 300 mg of product is obtained from the DEAE column.

e. Product from the DEAE column is dissolved in 150 ml of water and is passed over a 2.5 × 10-cm Chelex-100 (Na^+ form) column.

f. Eluate from the Chelex column is reduced in volume under vacuum and is then lyophilized to yield approximately 335 mg of dry product, which is purified arsenazo III.

3. *Ca^{2+} ion standard curve*

a. *Solutions*

Ca^{2+}- and Mg^{2+}-free Hank's buffer. Prepare as a 2× stock containing the following (final concentration in m*M*): NaCl (137), KCl (5.4), KH_2PO_4 (0.44), $NaHCO_3$ (4.2), Na_2HPO_4 (0.33), and HEPES (20). For use, the stock is diluted 1:1 with deionized water, is bubbled with 95% O_2/5% CO_2 for 30 min, and the pH is adjusted to 7.4.

$CaCl_2$ standard solution, 0.5 m*M*.

EGTA, 10 m*M* in 0.9% (w/v) NaCl.

Arsenazo III stock, 5 mg/ml of 0.9% (w/v) NaCl (= 6.44 m*M*).

b. To prepare a standard curve, the following additions are made to a cuvette: 1 ml Ca^{2+}- and Mg^{2+}-free Hank's buffer, 0 to 30 μl of 0.5 m*M* $CaCl_2$ stock (= 0 to 15 nmol), and 4.65 μl arsenazo III stock (final concentration = 30 μ*M*). Absorbance is measured by dual-wavelength spectrometry at 654 minus 685 nm. A standard curve is shown in Figure 9.

c. From these data and Equation 11, the parameters for the interaction of Ca^{2+} ions with arsenazo III can be derived:

$$K_d = [Ca^{2+}]_{Free}[AsIII]_{Total}/[Ca^{2+}\text{-}AsIII] = 11.3\ \mu M, \quad (11)$$

where $[Ca^{2+}\text{-}AsIII]$ is determined by adding excess EGTA and $[AsIII]_{Total}$ is determined by adding excess Ca^{2+} ions.

4. *Procedure for measurement of calcium sequestration by isolated renal cells*

a. Isolated kidney cells (4 to 6 × 10^6 cells/ml) are separated from the Ca^{2+}-containing Krebs–Henseleit medium by rapid centrifugation through 20% (v/v) Percoll in Ca^{2+}- and Mg^{2+}-free Hank's buffer (see above). Cells are resuspended in 1.5 ml of the modified Hank's medium and are recentrifuged. Cells are resuspended in a final volume of 1.2 ml of the modified Hank's medium.

b. In a cuvette (2.9-ml capacity) is added 1 ml of cells, 4.65 μl of arsenazo III stock (30 μ*M* final concentration), and 2 μl of 5 m*M* FCCP (in absolute ethanol; 10 μ*M* final concentration). Record $\Delta A_{654-685}$ until reading is stable. This gives the mitochondrial Ca^{2+} pool.

c. Two microliters of 7.5 m*M* A23187 (15 μ*M* final concentration) is added and $\Delta A_{654\text{-}685}$ is recorded until a stable reading is obtained. The remainder of the intracellular Ca^{2+} that is released is derived primarily from the microsomal pool.

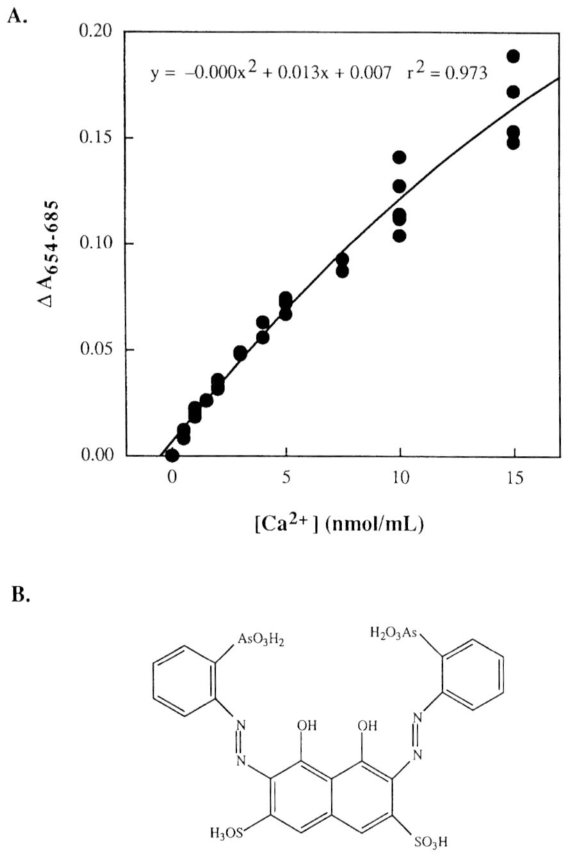

Figure 9 Standard curve for determination of Ca^{2+} ion concentration with arsenazo III. (A) Ca^{2+}- and Mg^{2+}-free Hank's buffer (1 ml) was mixed with 0 to 15 nmol of $CaCl_2$ and 30 μ*M* arsenazo III in a cuvette. Absorbance at 654 minus 685 nm was determined. Each data point represents a single determination. The regression curve was a second-order polynomial. (B) Structure of arsenazo III.

5. *Procedure for measurement of calcium sequestration by renal cortical mitochondria.* Although the microsomes have the primary function in the cell in sequestering Ca^{2+} to maintain low cytosolic Ca^{2+} concentration, mitochondria have several energy-dependent systems that take up and retain Ca^{2+} ions. Suspensions of isolated renal cortical mitochondria can be loaded with Ca^{2+} and the ability of these mitochondria to retain Ca^{2+} after exposure to a chemical toxicant can then be assessed to determine toxic effects on mitochondrial function.[6]
   a. Mitochondria (1 mg protein per milliliter) are suspended in 240 m*M* sucrose, 10 m*M* potassium phosphate, pH 7.4, 20 m*M* triethanolamine/HCl, and 20 m*M* KCl.
   b. Before exposure to a putative mitochondrial toxicant, incubate mitochondria with 50 μ*M* $CaCl_2$ for 5 min.
   c. At specified times, add 40 μ*M* arsenazo III and measure $\Delta A_{654-685}$ to determine the content of Ca^{2+} ions released from the mitochondria.

   Control mitochondria incubated with buffer released only 4.6 and 7.0 nmol Ca^{2+} per milliliter during a 1-h and 2-h incubation, respectively. In contrast, mitochondria incubated with 1 m*M* DCVC released 14.6 and 23.6 nmol Ca^{2+} per milliliter during a 1-h and 2-h incubation, indicating a decreased ability of renal cortical mitochondria to retain Ca^{2+} ions.[6]

16.4 Concluding remarks

This chapter reviews several *in vitro* systems that can be used to determine toxic effects on renal mitochondria and methods to determine several key parameters of mitochondrial function in those systems. Although there has been much argument about the role of mitochondrial dysfunction in the mechanism by which chemicals produce cellular injury, it is clear that assessments of mitochondrial function after exposure to chemicals can provide critical diagnostic information concerning the advent of cellular injury. Alterations in mitochondrial respiration, membrane structural integrity, $\Delta\psi$, ΔpH, adenine and pyridine nucleotides contents, GSH status, or Ca^{2+} ion distribution typically occur at early time points after exposure of renal cells to cytotoxic chemicals. Whether these effects are primary cytotoxic responses or consequences of changes in other cellular processes is not always clear. However, examination of the status of these parameters can provide early information on the potential cytotoxicity of many chemicals and provide a sensitive indicator of their effects on cellular energy metabolism.

16.5 Acknowledgments

Research from the author's laboratory was supported by a grant from the National Institute of Diabetes and Digestive and Kidney Diseases (Grant R01-DK40725). L.H.L. is a recipient of a Research Career Development Award from the National Institute of Diabetes and Digestive and Kidney Diseases (Grant K04-DK02090).

References

1. Soltoff, S. P., ATP and the regulation of renal cell function, *Annu. Rev. Physiol.*, 48, 9, 1986.
2. Brezis, M., Rosen, S., Spokes, K., Silva, P., and Epstein, F. H., Transport-dependent anoxic injury in the isolated perfused rat kidney, *Am. J. Pathol.*, 116, 327, 1984.
3. Epstein, F. H., Silva, P., Spokes, K., Brezis, M., and Rosen, S., Renal medullary Na-K-ATPase and hypoxic injury in perfused rat kidney, *Kidney Int.*, 36, 768, 1989.
4. Shanley, P. F., Brezis, M., Spokes, K., Silva, P., Epstein, F. H., and Rosen, S., Transport-dependent cell injury in the S_3 segment of the proximal tubule, *Kidney Int.*, 29, 1033, 1986.
5. Lash, L. H. and Anders, M. W., Cytotoxicity of *S*-(1,2-dichlorovinyl)glutathione and *S*-(1,2-dichlorovinyl)-L-cysteine in isolated rat kidney cells, *J. Biol. Chem.*, 261, 13076, 1986.
6. Lash, L. H. and Anders, M. W., Mechanism of *S*-(1,2-dichlorovinyl)-L-cysteine- and *S*-(1,2-dichlorovinyl)-L-homocysteine-induced renal mitochondrial toxicity, *Mol. Pharmacol.*, 32, 549, 1987.
7. Wallin, A., Jones, T. W., Vercesi, A. E., Cotgreave, I., Ormstad, K., and Orrenius, S., Toxicity of *S*-pentachlorobutadienyl-L-cysteine studied with isolated rat renal cortical mitochondria, *Arch. Biochem. Biophys.*, 258, 365, 1987.
8. Schnellmann, R. G., Lock, E. A., and Mandel, L. J., A mechanism of *S*- (1,2,3,4,4-pentachloro-1,3-butadienyl)-L-cysteine toxicity to rabbit renal proximal tubules, *Toxicol. Appl. Pharmacol.*, 90, 513, 1987.
9. Schnellmann, R. G., Cross, T. J., and Lock, E. A., Pentachlorobutadienyl-L-cysteine uncouples oxidative phosphorylation by dissipating the proton gradient, *Toxicol. Appl. Pharmacol.*, 100, 498, 1989.
10. Ohno, Y., Jones, T. W., and Ormstad, K., Allyl alcohol toxicity in isolated renal epithelial cells: Protective effects of low molecular weight thiols, *Chem. Biol. Interact.*, 52, 289, 1985.
11. Brady, H. R., Kone, B. C., Stromski, M. E., Zeidel, M. L., Giebisch, G., and Gullans, S. R., Mitochondrial injury: an early event in cisplatin toxicity to renal proximal tubules, *Am. J. Physiol.*, 258, F1181, 1990.
12. Zhang, J.-G. and Lindup, W. E., Role of mitochondria in cisplatin-induced oxidative damage exhibited by rat renal cortical slices, *Biochem. Pharmacol.*, 45, 2215, 1993.

13. Zhang, J.-G. and Lindup, W. E., Cisplatin nephrotoxicity: decreases in mitochondrial protein sulfhydryl concentration and calcium uptake by mitochondria from rat renal cortical slices, *Biochem. Pharmacol.*, 47, 1127, 1994.
14. Schnellmann, R. G., Ewell, F. P. Q., Sgambati, M., and Mandel, L. J., Mitochondrial toxicity of 2-bromohydroquinone in rabbit renal proximal tubules, *Toxicol. Appl. Pharmacol.*, 90, 420, 1987.
15. Mela-Riker, L. M., Widener, L. L., Houghton, D. C., and Bennett, W. M., Renal mitochondrial integrity during continuous gentamicin treatment, *Biochem. Pharmacol.*, 35, 979, 1986.
16. Lash, L. H., Tokarz, J. J., and Woods, E. B., Renal cell type specificity of cephalosporin-induced cytotoxicity in suspensions of isolated proximal tubular and distal tubular cells, *Toxicology*, 94, 97, 1994.
17. Weinberg, J. M., Harding, P. G., and Humes, H. D., Mitochondrial bioenergetics during initiation of mercuric chloride-induced renal injury. I. Direct effects of *in vitro* mercuric chloride on renal cortical mitochondrial function, *J. Biol. Chem.*, 257, 60, 1982.
18. Weinberg, J. M., Harding, P. G., and Humes, H. D., Mitochondrial bioenergetics during initiation of mercuric chloride-induced renal injury. II. Functional alterations of renal cortical mitochondria isolated after mercuric chloride treatment, *J. Biol. Chem.*, 257, 68, 1982.
19. Lund, B.-O., Miller, D. M., and Woods, J. S., Studies on Hg(II)-induced H_2O_2 formation and oxidative stress *in vivo* and *in vitro* in rat kidney mitochondria, *Biochem. Pharmacol.*, 45, 2017, 1993.
20. Jung, K. and Pergande, M., Influence of cyclosporin A on the respiration of isolated rat kidney mitochondria, *FEBS Lett.*, 183, 167, 1985.
21. Strzelecki, T., Kumar, S., Khauli, R., and Menon, M., Impairment by cyclosporin A of membrane-mediated functions in kidney mitochondria, *Kidney Int.*, 34, 234, 1988.
22. Jones, D. P., Sundby, G.-B., Ormstad, K., and Orrenius, S., Use of isolated kidney cells for the study of drug metabolism, *Biochem. Pharmacol.*, 28, 929, 1979.
23. Lash, L. H., Isolated kidney cells in the study of chemical toxicity, in *In Vitro Toxicology: Model Systems and Methods*, McQueen, C. A., Ed., Telford Press, Caldwell, NJ, 1989, 231.
24. Lash, L. H. and Tokarz, J. J., Isolation of two distinct populations of kidney cells from rat kidney cortex and their use in the study of chemical-induced toxicity, *Anal. Biochem.*, 182, 271, 1989.
25. Lash, L. H., Purification of renal cortical cell populations by Percoll density-gradient centrifugation, in *In Vitro Biological Systems: Preparation and Maintenance, Methods in Toxicology*, Vol. 1A, Tyson, C. A. and Frazier, J. M., Eds., Academic Press, San Diego, 1993, 397.
26. Di Monte, D., Bellomo, G., Thor, H., Nicotera, P., and Orrenius, S., Alterations in intracellular thiol homeostasis during metabolism of menadione by isolated rat hepatocytes, *Arch. Biochem. Biophys.*, 235, 343, 1984.
27. Lash, L. H. and Anders, M. W., Cytotoxicity of *S*-(1,2-dichlorovinyl)glutathione and *S*-(1,2-dichlorovinyl)-L-cysteine in isolated rat kidney cells, *J. Biol. Chem.*, 261, 13076, 1986.
28. Lash, L. H. and Sall, J. M., Mitochondrial isolation from liver and kidney: strategy, techniques, and criteria for purity, in *Mitochondrial Dysfunction, Methods in Toxicology*, Vol. 2, Lash, L. H. and Jones, D. P., Eds., Academic Press, San Diego, 1993, 8.
29. Bai, C., Slife, C. W., Aw, T. Y., and Jones, D. P., Fractionation and analysis of mitochondria with polycarbonate membrane filters, *Anal. Biochem.*, 179, 114, 1989.
30. Aw, T. Y. and Jones, D. P., Heterogeneity of pH in the aqueous cytoplasm of renal proximal tubular cells, *FASEB J.*, 3, 52, 1989.
31. Chance, B. and Williams, G. R., The respiratory chain and oxidative phosphorylation, *Adv. Enzymol.*, 17, 65, 1956.
32. Estabrook, R. W., Mitochondrial respiratory control and the polarographic measurement of ADP:O ratios, *Methods Enzymol.*, 10, 41, 1967.
33. Haworth, R. A. and Hunter, D. R., The Ca^{2+}-induced membrane transition in mitochondria. II. Nature of the Ca^{2+} trigger site, *Arch. Biochem. Biophys.*, 195, 460, 1979.
34. Mittnacht, S., Jr. and Farber, J. L., Reversal of ischemic mitochondrial dysfunction, *J. Biol. Chem.*, 256, 3199, 1981.
35. Schnellmann, R. G., Gilchrist, S. M., and Mandel, L. J., Intracellular distribution and depletion of glutathione in rabbit renal proximal tubules, *Kidney Int.*, 34, 229, 1988.

36. Lemasters, J. J., Nieminen, A.-L., Chacon, E., Imberti, R., Gores, G. J., Reece, J. M., and Herman, B., Use of fluorescent probes to monitor mitochondrial membrane potential in isolated mitochondria, cell suspensions, and cultured cells, in *Mitochondrial Dysfunction, Methods in Toxicology,* Vol. 2, Lash, L. H. and Jones, D. P., Eds., Academic Press, San Diego, 1993, 404.
37. Hoek, J. B., Nicholls, D. G., and Williamson, J. R., Determination of the mitochondrial protonmotive force in isolated hepatocytes, *J. Biol. Chem.*, 255, 1458, 1980.
38. Rottenberg, H., The measurement of membrane potential and ΔpH in cells, organelles, and vesicles, *Methods Enzymol.*, 55, 547, 1979.
39. Modica-Napolitano, J. S. and Aprille, J. R., Basis for selective cytotoxicity of rhodamine 123, *Cancer Res.*, 47, 4361, 1987.
40. Palmieri, F. and Klingenberg, M., Direct methods for measuring metabolite transport and distribution in mitochondria, *Methods Enzymol.*, 56, 279, 1979.
41. Andersson, B. S. and Jones, D. P., Use of digitonin fractionation to determine mitochondrial transmembrane ion distribution in cells during anoxia, *Anal. Biochem.*, 146, 164, 1985.
42. Berry, M. N., Gregory, R. B., Grivell, A. R., Henly, D. C., Nobles, C. D., Phillips, J. W., and Wallace, P. G., Intracellular mitochondrial membrane potential as an indicator of hepatocyte energy metabolism: further evidence for thermodynamic control of metabolism, *Biochim. Biophys. Acta*, 936, 294, 1988.
43. Lemasters, J. J., Nieminen, A.-L., Chacon, E., Bond, J. M., Harper, I., Reece, J. M., and Herman, B., Single-cell microscopic techniques for studying toxic injury, in *In Vitro Toxicity Indicators, Methods in Toxicology,* Vol. 1B, Tyson, C. A. and Frazier, J. M., Eds., Academic Press, San Diego, 1994, 438.
44. Zanotti, A. and Azzone, G. F., Safranine as membrane potential probe in rat liver mitochondria, *Arch. Biochem. Biophys.*, 201, 255, 1980.
45. Farber, E., ATP and cell integrity, *Fed. Proc. Fed. Am. Soc. Exp. Biol.*, 32, 1534, 1973.
46. Andersson, B. S., Aw, T. Y., and Jones, D. P., Mitochondrial transmembrane potential and pH gradient during anoxia, *Am. J. Physiol.*, 252, C349, 1987.
47. Park, Y., Aw, T. Y., and Jones, D. P., ATP and other energetic parameters as indicators of cell injury, in *In Vitro Toxicity Indicators, Methods in Toxicology,* Vol. 1B, Tyson, C. A. and Frazier, J. M., Eds., Academic Press, San Diego, 1994, 140.
48. Jones, D. P., Determination of pyridine dinucleotides in cell extracts by high-performance liquid chromatography, *J. Chromatogr.*, 225, 446, 1981.
49. Gunter, T. E. and Pfeiffer, D. R., Mechanisms by which mitochondria transport calcium, *Am. J. Physiol.*, 258, C755, 1990.
50. Griffith, O. W., Determination of glutathione and glutathione disulfide using glutathione reductase and 2-vinylpyridine, *Anal. Biochem.*, 106, 207, 1980.
51. Fariss, M. W. and Reed, D. J., High-performance liquid chromatography of thiols and disulfides: dinitrophenyl derivatives, *Methods Enzymol.*, 143, 101, 1987.
52. McCormack, J. G. and Denton, R. M., The role of intramitochondrial Ca^{2+} in the regulation of oxidative phosphorylation in mammalian tissues, *Biochem. Soc. Trans.*, 21, 793, 1993.
53. Drewnowska, K. and Schoolwerth, A. C., Stimulatory effect of calcium on metabolism and its sensitivity to pH in kidney mitochondria, *Am. J. Physiol.*, 267, F153, 1994.
54. Kendrick, N. C., Purification of arsenazo III, a Ca^{2+}-sensitive dye, *Anal. Biochem.*, 76, 487, 1976.

chapter seventeen

Biotransformation and Membrane Transport in Nephrotoxicity

Peter J. Harvison and Gary O. Rankin

17.1 Introduction to renal metabolism ... 331
17.2 Techniques to study renal metabolism ... 335
17.2.1 Subcellular fractions ... 335
17.2.1.1 Tissue homogenization ... 337
17.2.1.2 Centrifugation ... 337
17.2.1.3 Storage of subcellular fractions ... 337
17.2.1.4 Incubation conditions ... 337
17.2.2 Isolated cells ... 339
17.2.2.1 Isolation techniques ... 340
17.2.2.2 Incubation conditions ... 340
17.3 Methods for study of renal metabolism ... 340
17.3.1 Preparation of renal microsomes and cytosol ... 341
17.3.2 Bradford protein assay ... 341
17.3.3 UDP-glucuronosyltransferase assay ... 342
17.3.4 Glutathione *S*-transferase assay ... 343
17.3.5 Cysteine conjugate β-lyase assay ... 344
17.4 Membrane transport ... 344
17.4.1 General description ... 344
17.4.2 Renal cortical slices ... 345
17.4.3 Membrane vesicles ... 346
References ... 348

17.1 Introduction to renal metabolism

The kidney is a target organ for toxicity due in part to its capabilities for xenobiotic biotransformation and membrane transport. In general, most of the hepatic enzymes that are involved in xenobiotic metabolism are also present in the kidney (for a review see Tarloff et al.[1]). Many of the methods used to study metabolism in other organs (subcellular fractions, isolated cells, etc.) can be used with renal preparations. However, the kidney presents some special difficulties that must be taken into consideration when experiments are being planned and conducted. These are described in more detail below and in the subsequent sections.

0-8493-3341-5/96/$0.00+$.50

Although cytochrome P450 (P450) is found in the renal proximal convoluted tubules, the concentration is lower than that in the liver.[1] Furthermore, the P450 isozyme profiles in these two organs are not identical. Complex species- and sex-dependent differences in renal P450 induction and inhibition also exist. For example, pretreatment of rats with phenobarbital (PB; Table 1), an inducer of hepatic P450, does not enhance renal P450 activity in rats since the 2B isozymes are absent in the kidney of this species.[1,2] In contrast, P450 is inducible by PB in the rabbit and hamster kidney.[2,3] Polycyclic aromatic hydrocarbons, such as β-naphthoflavone (β-NF) and 3-methylcholanthrene (3-MC), are effective inducers of renal P450s in several species, including rats (Table 1).[2-5] Renal, but not hepatic, P450 2E1 activity is androgen-dependent in mice.[6] On the other hand, pyrazole and 4-methylpyrazole induce both the hepatic and renal forms of 2E1 in rats.[7] The choice of which P450 inhibitors to use in renal metabolism experiments must also be made carefully. Metyrapone, for example, inhibits hepatic P450 but has no effect on renal P450 in the rat.[2] Other inhibitors, such as α-naphthoflavone (α-NF)[2] or 1-aminobenzotriazole (ABT)[8] may be useful alternatives (Table 2).

Table 1 Recommended Protocols for the Induction of Renal Xenobiotic Metabolizing Enzymes *in Vivo*

Enzyme	Inducer	Typical pretreatment regimen	Comments	Ref.
P450	PB	80 mg/kg for 4 days, i.p. in saline	Ineffective in rodents and guinea pigs	2, 3
	β-NF	80 mg/kg for 4 days, i.p. in corn oil	Multiple forms induced in rats	2
	3-MC	25 mg/kg for 3 days, i.p. in corn oil	Multiple forms induced in rats and mice	4, 5
	Pyrazole	200 mg/kg for 2 days, i.p. in saline	2E1 isozyme induced in rat liver and kidney	7
UDPGT	PB	100 mg/kg for 4 days, i.p. in saline	Ineffective in rats	10
	β-NF	100 mg/kg for 4 days, i.p. in corn oil	Multiple forms induced in rats	10
	3-MC	20 mg/kg for 4 days, i.p. in corn oil	Ineffective in rats	10
	Salicylic acid	5 mmol/kg for 3 days, intragastric	Renal UDPGT selectively induced in rats	11
GST	PB	80 mg/kg for 6 days, i.p. in saline	Ineffective in rats	13
	3-MC	40 mg/kg for 6 days, i.p. in olive oil	Ineffective in rats	13
	Ethoxyquin	200 mg/kg for 3 days, i.p. in olive oil	Multiple hepatic and renal forms induced	13

Note: P450, cytochrome P-450; PB, phenobarbital; β-NF, β-naphthoflavone; 3-MC, 3-methylcholanthrene; UDPGT, UDP-glucuronosyltransferance; GST, glutathione *S*-transferase.

Phase II enzymes, such as UDP-glucuronosyltransferase (UDPGT), sulfotransferase (ST), and glutathione *S*-transferase (GST), are also found in the kidney. However, the activities tend to be lower than their hepatic counterparts.[1,9] UDPGT is localized in the proximal and distal tubules. Although isozymes are known to exist for rat renal UDPGT, this enzyme is resistant to induction by PB or 3-MC.[10,11] Salicylic acid reportedly induces renal, but not hepatic, UDPGT in rats.[11] Although relatively little is known about the capacity of the kidney to form sulfate conjugates, ST activity is highest in the cortex. As

Table 2 Recommended Protocols for the Inhibition of Renal Xenobiotic Metabolizing Enzymes *in Vitro*

Enzyme	Inhibitor	Typical concentration	Comments	Ref.
P450	Metyrapone	0.1 m*M*	Ineffective in rodent kidney microsomes	2
	α-NF	0.001 m*M*	Selective for β-NF-induced microsomes	2
	ABT	1.0 m*M*	Nonselective suicide substrate	8
PHS	Aspirin	1.0 m*M*	Irreversible cyclooxygenase inhibitor	16
	Indomethacin	0.2 m*M*	Cyclooxygenase inhibitor	16
	Methimazole/ propylthiouracil	0.05 m*M*	Nonspecific hydroperoxidase inhibitors	17
GGT	AT-125 (acivicin)	0.25 m*M*	Irreversible inhibitor	19
	Serine-borate	20 m*M*	Reversible inhibitor	20
CysGly dipeptidase	Phenylalanylglycine	10 m*M*	Competitive inhibitor	20
Aminopeptidase M	1,10-phenanthroline	0.4 m*M*	Metal chelator	21
Cys conjugate β-lyase	AOAA	0.1 m*M*	Mitochondrial form more sensitive than cytosolic form	22, 23

Note: P450, cytochrome P-450; α- and β-NF, α- and β-naphthoflavone; ABT, 1-aminobenzotriazole; AOAA, aminooxyacetic acid.

seen with UDPGT, renal ST is unaffected by pretreatment of rats with 3-MC.[12] Formation of glutathione (GSH) conjugates in the kidney also occurs primarily in the cortex. The effect of common hepatic enzyme inducers, such as PB or 3-MC, on renal GST activity is highly substrate- and sex-dependent.[1] Ethoxyquin is an effective inducer of GSH conjugation for several substrates in kidneys of male Sprague–Dawley rats.[13]

In addition to the common phase I and phase II metabolic pathways, the kidney has other enzymes that may be involved in biotransformation of xenobiotics. Prostaglandin H synthase (PHS) activity, although absent in the liver, is relatively high in the renal inner medulla.[14] This membrane-bound, heme-containing enzyme consists of two closely related activities, cyclooxygenase and hydroperoxidase (Figure 1). The latter activity has been implicated in renal metabolic activation of a number of compounds that can serve as cosubstrates.[15] A fatty acid such as arachidonic acid is essential for the cyclooxygenase component, whereas many peroxides, including prostaglandin G_2 and hydrogen peroxide, can support the hydroperoxidase activity. The appropriate choice of cofactor can therefore be used to distinguish between these enzymatic activities (i.e., H_2O_2 can be used to skip the cyclooxygenase-mediated step entirely). Inhibitors can also be used to effectively differentiate between the two activities present in PHS. Aspirin and indomethacin are selective inhibitors of cyclooxygenase,[16] whereas methimazole or propylthiouracil inhibit the hydroperoxidase activity nonspecifically (Table 2).[17]

The kidney also contains enzymes, such as γ-glutamyltranspeptidase (GGT), various dipeptidases, and cysteine conjugate β-lyase, that are involved in the further metabolism of glutathione (GSH) conjugates (Figure 2).[18] Activities of these three enzymes are either absent in the liver or are much lower than in the kidney. GGT is located along the brush border of the proximal tubules and converts GSH conjugates into the corresponding cysteinylglycine conjugates.[19] Several different brush border enzymes, such as cysteinylglycine dipeptidase and aminopeptidase M, can then remove the glycyl residue to produce

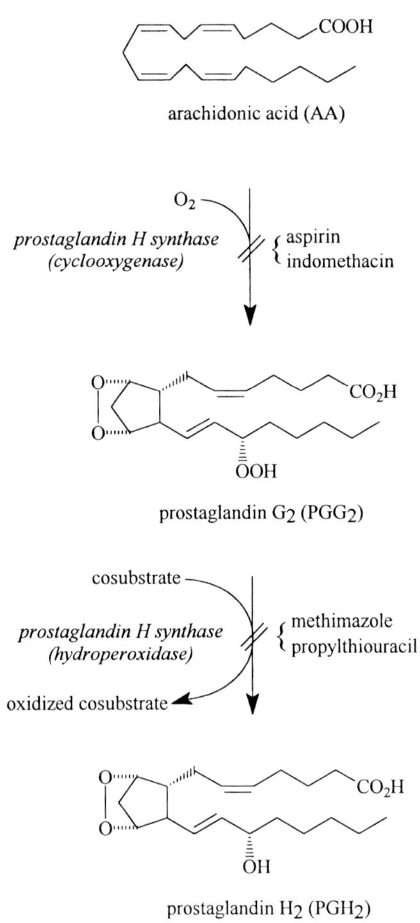

Figure 1 Metabolism of arachidonic acid by prostaglandin H synthase.

the corresponding cysteine conjugate.[20,21] The final step in the process is catalyzed by the pyridoxal-5′-phosphate-dependent enzyme cysteine conjugate β-lyase. This enzyme, which is present both in the cytosol and the mitochondria, converts the cysteine conjugate to a thiol, ammonia, and pyruvate.[22] Inhibitors are available that can block each step in this process (Figure 2 and Table 2). For example, GGT activity is selectively and potently inhibited by AT-125 (acivicin).[19] Serine–borate and glutathione disulfide (GSSG) have also been used to inhibit GGT activity in isolated renal cells.[20] Cysteinylglycine dipeptidase and aminopeptidase M can be inhibited by phenylalanylglycine or 1,10-phenanthroline, respectively.[20,21] Although aminooxyacetic acid (AOAA) is commonly used to inhibit cysteine conjugate β-lyase,[22] the mitochondrial form of this enzyme is considerably more sensitive to this compound than the cytosolic form.[23]

An example of the unique role of the kidney in processing GSH conjugates can be seen by comparing the metabolism of acetaminophen (paracetamol, APAP) in isolated cells from rat liver and kidney. In rat hepatocytes, the acetaminophen–GSH conjugate (GS-APAP) predominates over the cysteine conjugate.[24] When APAP was incubated with rat renal tubular epithelial cells, however, GS-APAP was not detected.[12] Metabolites derived from the GSH conjugate (i.e., cysteine and *N*-acetylcysteine conjugates) were found instead. Furthermore, GS-APAP was directly converted to APAP-cysteinylglycine and APAP-cysteine conjugates by isolated rat kidney cells.[20] These differences may be less important in other species, such as the guinea pig, where renal and hepatic levels of these enzymes are similar.[25]

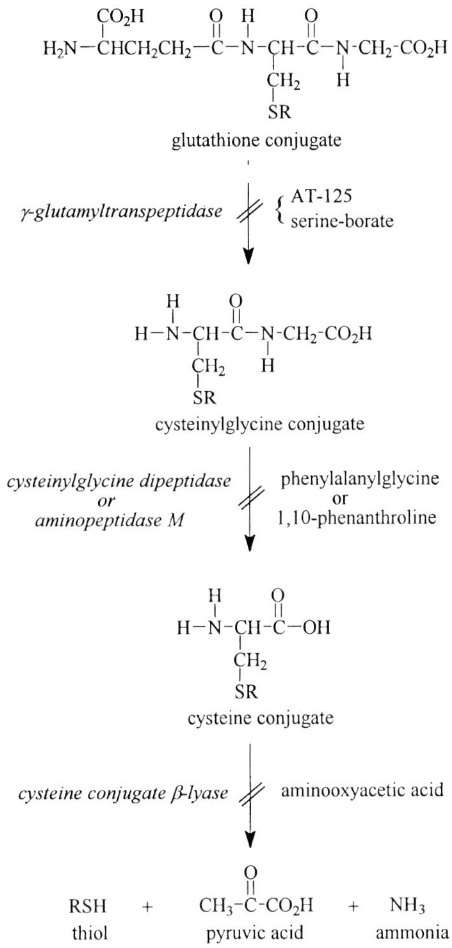

Figure 2 Renal processing of glutathione conjugates.

17.2 Techniques to study renal metabolism

Although a number of systems are available to study renal xenobiotic biotransformation, this section focuses on two *in vitro* approaches, subcellular fractions and isolated cells. Details on the preparation and use of these systems in metabolism experiments are provided below. The advantages and disadvantages of each technique are also described.

Induction and inhibition experiments can provide useful information in metabolism studies. Enzyme inducers must be admininstered *in vivo* (see Table 1 for recommended dosing schedules) prior to preparation of the subcellular fractions or cells. Suggested inhibitor concentrations for use in *in vitro* incubations are summarized in Table 2.

17.2.1 Subcellular fractions

Subcellular fractions (microsomes, cytosol, and mitochondria) are commonly used in metabolism studies and can be prepared by differential centrifugation.[2,26] This process separates the organelles based on their densities and is summarized in Figure 3 (see below for detailed procedure). Mitochondria can be further fractionated by digitonin treatment.[27] If mitochondria are not being prepared, the initial centrifugation step (600 × g) can be omitted. The tissue must be kept cold during all steps to prevent enzyme inactivation.

Preparation of microsomes and cytosol requires about 3 to 4 h; these fractions can then be used immediately or may be frozen for later use (see below).

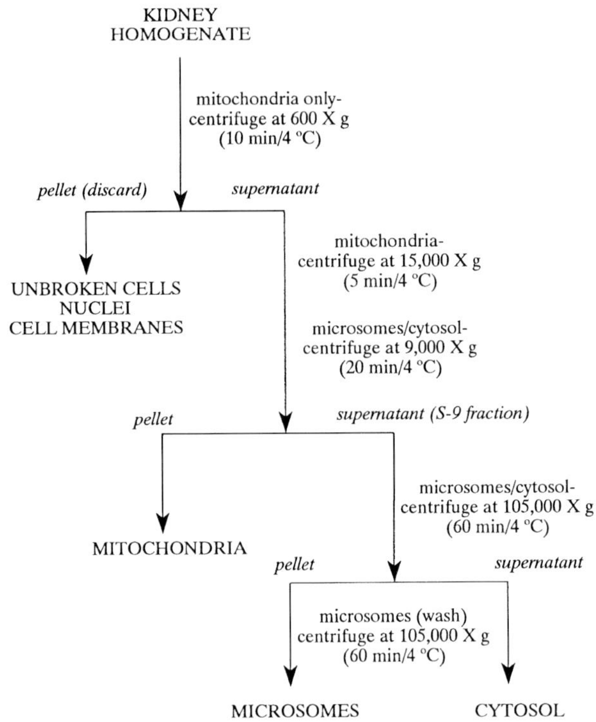

Figure 3 Preparation of kidney subcellular fractions by differential centrifugation.

One major advantage of this approach is its simplicity. However, this system also suffers from several disadvantages, including sensitivity to method of preparation, loss of enzyme activity on storage, and lack of correlation with *in vivo* metabolism studies. In addition, enzyme cofactors are lost during preparation of the subcellular fractions and must therefore be replenished in the incubations.

As in other tissues, most renal phase I enzymes are microsomal, whereas phase II activities (with the important exception of UDPGT) are primarily cytosolic. The S-9 fraction (see Figure 3) can be used to monitor phase I and II metabolism in the same incubation; however, enzyme activity will be lower than that in microsomes and cytosol. Other membrane-bound enzymes that may be important in renal metabolism and nephrotoxicity are PHS and GGT. Cysteine conjugate β-lyase is found in the cytosolic and mitochondrial fractions, but these forms are not identical.[23]

There are several special considerations that must be taken into account when preparing subcellular fractions from the kidney. One of the most important of these is related to the heterogeneity of the organ, because renal xenobiotic metabolic enzymes are differentially distributed throughout the organ and along the nephron.[1] For example, P450 is located primarily in renal cortical proximal tubules, whereas PHS is found mainly in the inner medulla.[1] Thus, it may be essential to dissect these regions apart prior to tissue homogenization, depending on the activity that one wants to measure. Because the specific activities of renal enzymes are often lower than their hepatic counterparts,[1] increasing the protein concentration during incubations may be necessary to achieve detectable levels of metabolism.

The results of experiments employing subcellular fractions are usually normalized to a unit protein concentration (i.e., amount of product formed per milligram protein).

17.2.1.1 Tissue homogenization

The initial step in the preparation of subcellular fractions involves homogenization of the organ. A soft organ like the kidney can be readily homogenized using a Teflon® (Registered Trademark of E. I. Du Pont de Nemours and Company, Inc., Wilmington, DE) pestle/glass vessel (Potter-Elvehjem) tissue grinder. Sizes B or C (30- and 55-ml chamber volumes, respectively) work well for pooled rat or mouse kidneys.

After sacrifice (preferably by cervical dislocation or decapitation, to avoid altering enzyme activities) the kidneys should be removed from the animal and carefully dissected into the medullary and cortical regions. With small animals such as rodents, kidneys from several animals will have to be pooled in order to obtain a sufficient amount of tissue. The dissected tissue should then be weighed and minced in ice-cold homogenizing buffer (3 ml of buffer per gram tissue). While either isotonic sucrose (0.25 M) or phosphate–KCl (100 m*M* phosphate containing 1.15%, w/v, KCl, pH 7.4) can be used for the tissue homogenization, KCl is reportedly beneficial in removing residual hemoglobin that may interfere with later measurements of cytochrome P450 content.[28] The presence of sucrose in the homogenizing buffer may be important for assessing UDPGT activity (see below). Ethylenediamine tetraacetic acid (EDTA, 1 to 5 m*M*) can be added to the homogenizing media to minimize lipid peroxidation.[29] A protease inhibitor, such as phenylmethylsulfonyl fluoride (PMSF, 0.1 m*M*), is sometimes also added to subcellular fractions prepared from extrahepatic tissues.[29] To help remove excess blood from the tissue, the buffer should be decanted and replaced several times. The grinding vessel should not be filled more than one third to one half with the minced tissue preparation. Although the pestle can be driven by a motor mounted on a ring stand, an electric drill also works well. Usually three to four strokes of the pestle are sufficient to completely disrupt the cells. Immersion of the homogenizer in an ice bath throughout this process will keep the tissue cold, and the ice bath helps prevent injury if the grinding vessel shatters.

17.2.1.2 Centrifugation

Virtually all refrigerated, high-speed centrifuges and ultracentrifuges will suffice. Actual revolutions per minute will depend on the rotor, and the total spin time should be adjusted to account for acceleration and braking. To ensure that the microsomal fraction is not contaminated by cytosolic enzymes, a second spin at 105,000 × g is recommended (Figure 3). After the final centrifugation step, microsomes can be resuspended in an appropriate buffer (usually one third the volume that was originally employed during homogenization) and then diluted for use in incubations. Protein concentrations can be measured by the method of Lowry et al.[30] or the Bradford assay[31] (see below for procedure).

17.2.1.3 Storage of subcellular fractions

Ideally, the subcellular fractions should be used as soon as possible after preparation to prevent unpredictable loss of enzyme activity. Although the preparations can be stored at ≤ –78°C for several months, careful consideration must be given to the fact that the activities of different enzymes (and even different isozymes of a single enzyme) may decline with time.[28] If microsomes are to be frozen, glycerol (20%, v/v) should be added to the buffer. Furthermore, the glycerol must be removed from the tissue fractions (by centrifugation at 105,000 × g) before they are used in incubations.

17.2.1.4 Incubation conditions

Incubations with renal subcellular fractions are typically performed under air at 37°C in pH 7.4 buffer unless otherwise noted below. The incubation vessel should be chosen to insure that an adequate surface area for oxygenation (essential for monooxygenase activities) is maintained; small Erlenmeyer flasks (about 25 ml) or glass scintillation vials (20 ml) work well. Reactions should be agitated throughout the experiment with a shaking incubator. Any of the common buffers can be used. However, TRIS is an amine and may react with certain substrates. For example, we have found that TRIS forms adducts with *N*-(3,5-dichlorophenyl)succinimide and related compounds (unpublished). Buffer pH should be adjusted at the incubation temperature since the pH of certain buffers, notably TRIS, are highly sensitive to temperature.[32]

The substrate or inhibitors can be added in buffer (preferable) or in an organic solvent. Some caution should be used in the choice of organic solvent to prevent interference with the reaction that is under investigation (see below). Furthermore, the amount of solvent added should not exceed 0.5 to 1% of the total incubation volume. The use of appropriate controls can eliminate problems with data interpretation that may arise from solvent effects.

To optimize the incubation conditions, preliminary experiments may be performed in which substrate or protein concentration or incubation time are varied. To confirm that enzymatic reactions are being measured, control experiments can be conducted in which the protein is either omitted or boiled for 5 to 10 min prior to addition to the incubations. Depending on the activity being measured, omission of the appropriate cofactor may also provide useful information. Reactions can be terminated by adding an acid (such as trichloroacetic acid) or an organic solvent, followed by centrifugation to remove the precipitated proteins. Additional recommendations (protein concentration, cofactor requirements, etc.) for using renal subcellular fractions to monitor activity of specific enzymes are described below. All concentrations are suggestions only and may need to be modified.

P450 activity can be monitored in either microsomes or the S-9 fraction. P450 levels in the preparation should be measured by carbon monoxide difference spectra by the method of Omura and Sato, using a molar absorptivity value of 91 mM^{-1} cm^{-1}.[33] Renal microsomal P450 content is typically about 0.1 nmol/mg protein or approximately one tenth the concentration in the liver.[1] To compensate for this, it may be necessary to increase the protein concentration in incubations with renal microsomes (i.e., 2 to 5 mg/ml) to obtain measurable P450 activity. Although the cofactor NADPH can be added directly to the incubations, an NADPH-generating system is frequently used instead. One formulation of an NADPH-generating system can be prepared as follows: 8 mg of $NADP^+$ (sodium salt), 80 mg of glucose 6-phosphate (G6P, disodium salt/monohydrate), and 20 U of glucose 6-phosphate dehydrogenase (G6PDH, type VII) are dissolved in 5 ml of buffer (pH 7.4, 37°C) to which 0.2 ml of 1.0 *M* $MgCl_2$ is added. If 0.5 ml of this is used in 1-ml incubations (total volume), the following concentrations are obtained: G6P (25 m*M*), G6PDH (2 U), $NADP^+$ (1.0 m*M*), and $MgCl_2$ (20 m*M*). The stock solution must be used on the day of preparation. Some caution should be used in adding substrates or inhibitors in alcohols, since these compounds are type I substrates of P450.[34] As mentioned above, metyrapone does not inhibit rat renal P450. However, other inhibitors, such as metyrapone or ABT, are available (see Table 2 for concentrations).[2,8] Since ABT is a suicide substrate for P450, a short preincubation (5 to 10 min) prior to addition of substrate is necessary for inhibitory activity to occur. There are a number of assays that can be used to monitor P450 activity, such as dealkylation of ethoxyresorufin or pentoxyresorufin. These are described elsewhere in this volume.

Microsomal preparations can also be used to monitor glucuronidation. However, Rush and Hook found that renal UDPGT activity may be sensitive to the method of preparation.[10] For example, glucuronidation of 1-naphthol by rat renal microsomes was enhanced twofold when the microsomes were prepared in buffer containing 0.25 *M* sucrose rather than in buffer alone. This difference was not apparent in hepatic tissue. UDPGT activity can be difficult to measure, even in hepatic microsomes or S-9 fraction, since this enzyme is very tightly membrane-bound. To release the latent enzyme activity, the microsomes can be preincubated for approximately 30 min at 5°C with a biochemical detergent, such as Triton X-100, Brij 58, or deoxycholic acid (0.05%, v/v) prior to addition of substrate.[10] With substrates such as acetaminophen or 1-naphthol, protein concentrations of 2 to 4 mg renal microsomal protein per milliliter of buffer have typically been used.[9,10] The cofactor uridine 5′-diphosphoglucuronic acid (UDPGA, 5 to 10 m*M*) and $MgCl_2$ (10 m*M*) must also be included.[9,10] UDPGT activity can be spectrophotometrically assessed by monitoring the glucuronidation of *p*-nitrophenol (see below for procedure).[8,35]

Sulfate conjugates of acetaminophen or isoprenaline were produced in the presence of renal cytosol (2 to 10 mg protein per milliliter) and the cofactor adenosine 3′-phosphate 5′-phosphosulfate (PAPS, 0.1 m*M*).[9,36] Sulfotransferase activity is reportedly sensitive to thawing, and the cytosol should not be stored longer than one week.[36] β-Mercaptoethanol or dithiothreitol (0.5 to 3 m*M*) is often added to the incubations to stabilize the enzyme activity.[37] Since renal ST activity is generally lower than that in the liver, the use of [^{35}S]-PAPS or radiolabeled substrate can greatly enhance assay sensitivity.[38]

In the liver, cytosolic and microsomal forms of GST are known. In the kidney, however, this enzyme is found exclusively in the cytosol.[1] When reactions were conducted with 1-chloro-2,4-dinitrobenzene (CDNB) as substrate, 25 to 75 mg of cytosolic protein were used per incubation (2 ml volume).[8,9] Although no cofactor is required, GSH (5 m*M*) is usually added to the incubations.[8,9] A detailed procedure for monitoring GST activity using CDNB as substrate is presented below.[39]

PHS activity can be measured in microsomes or homogenates prepared from renal medulla or papilla. This enzyme has two distinct activities with different substrate requirements (Figure 2).[15] Many easily oxidized substances, such as phenols and aromatic amines, can serve as cosubstrates for the hydroperoxidase-mediated step. Protein concentrations of 0.4 to 2.5 mg/ml are used with acetaminophen and benzidine as cosubstrates, respectively.[16,17] Arachidonic acid (0.025 to 0.08 m*M*) may be added to the incubations to support the complete reaction pathway.[16,17] Alternatively, the first step in the reaction can be bypassed by using H_2O_2 (0.2 m*M*) as a cofactor instead.[17] Inhibitors can be used to selectively suppress the cyclooxygenase or hydroperoxidase components (see Table 2 for suggested concentrations).

Cysteine conjugate β-lyase can be measured in renal cytosolic or mitochondrial preparations, although these forms differ in their substrate and inhibitor specificity (Table 2).[23] Activity of this enzyme is frequently assayed using *S*-(2-benzothiazolyl)-L-cysteine (BTC) as the substrate.[40] Incubations are conducted at pH 8.6 with protein concentrations of 0.17 to 1.2 mg/ml.

17.2.2 Isolated cells

Freshly isolated renal tubular epithelial cells are less commonly used than subcellular fractions in renal biotransformation studies. This may be due in part to the fact that isolation of the cells is technically more demanding than the preparation of subcellular fractions. Nevertheless, this technique has been used to investigate metabolism of xenobiotics such as acetaminophen (APAP),[12,20] benzo[*a*]pyrene,[41] 2-acetylaminofluorene,[41] and *N*-(3,5-dichlorophenyl)succinimide (NDPS).[42] Unlike isolated rat hepatocytes, isolated rat renal tubular epithelial cells do not normally accumulate GSH conjugates in incubations with GSH and electrophilic substrates.[20] As mentioned above, this is due to the high levels of enzymes, such as GGT and cysteinylglycine dipeptidase, in the rat kidney as compared with the rat liver.

One advantage of this system is that all metabolic pathways are present in the isolated cells. Indeed, with the exception of NDPS, all of the compounds listed above are converted into both phase I and phase II metabolites. Furthermore, the relation between biotransformation and cytotoxicity can be explored in the same incubations. In fact, isolated renal cells have been employed in elucidating the role of the kidney in metabolic activation of nephrotoxic glutathione and cysteine conjugates.[43] Another advantage over subcellular fractions is that enzyme cofactors do not have to be added to the incubations since the isolated cells are metabolically competent. Preparation of the isolated cells (without separation of the proximal and distal tubular cells) typically requires 60 to 90 min.

Primary cultures of renal cortical cells have also been used in some metabolism and cytotoxicity studies. One benefit of this system over freshly isolated cells is that the apical and basolateral polarity of the cells is retained. In one study, P450-, GST-, and β-lyase-dependent activities could be detected in cultured cells isolated from rat renal cortex.[44] Unfortunately, as is seen with other cell culture systems, enzyme activities are not maintained uniformly in the cultured renal cells. For example, although GST activity remained relatively constant over 5 days (albeit at a much lower level than that present in freshly isolated cells), P450 could not be detected after only 24 h in culture.[44] This system shows promise for use in metabolism and cytotoxicity studies if the problems with loss of enzyme activity can be solved.

The results of studies utilizing isolated cells are typically presented on the basis of a unit cell concentration (i.e., amount of product formed per 10^6 cells).

17.2.2.1 *Isolation techniques*

Renal cells can be isolated by perfusion of the kidneys with a collagenase-containing, modified Hank's buffer.[12] Detailed procedures are provided elsewhere in this volume. All solutions must be adequately oxygenated (95% O_2/5% CO_2) and humidified throughout the procedure. Since the medulla does not usually digest as well as the cortex, this method produces a mixed population consisting primarily of proximal and distal tubular cells.[45] Most of the enzymes involved in xenobiotic metabolism are found in the proximal tubular cells. If desired, the cortical cells can be separated into proximal and distal tubular cell populations by centrifugation through a Percoll gradient.[46] Cell viability can be assessed by measuring trypan blue exclusion or lactate dehydrogenase release.[47] In general, only cell preparations with viabilities $\geq$ 80% should be used in metabolism experiments.

17.2.2.2 *Incubation conditions*

Incubations with isolated kidney cells are typically performed at 37°C in oxygenated (95% O_2/5% CO_2) Krebs–Henseleit buffer (pH 7.4). Reactions may be run in small Erlenmeyer flasks (25 ml); the use of polypropylene flasks or siliconized glassware may help prevent cell aggregation.[45] As with subcellular fractions, preliminary experiments can be run to optimize the incubation conditions. However, to ensure that cells are adequately oxygenated and nourished, the cell concentration should generally not exceed 2×10^6 cells/ml.[45] The cells should be gently agitated throughout the incubations, and the use of a gyratory incubator may help avoid the cell damage that could occur with a shaking incubator. The agitation speed should not exceed 100 cpm.[45] Due to loss of cell viability, incubation times are typically limited to no more than 4 h. Control experiments should also be conducted to determine if cell viability is adversely affected by any additions (solvent, substrate, inhibitors, etc.) that are made to the incubations.

The spectrally determined P450 content in renal cortical cells isolated from control rats is approximately 0.068 nmol/10^6 cells, or about one fourth the value reported in rat hepatocytes (0.23 ± 0.05 nmol/10^6 cells).[20,47] Unfortunately, there are very few examples in the literature where cytochrome P450 inhibitors have been used in conjunction with renal cells. In one study, 1 m*M* ABT successfully reversed chloroform-induced cytotoxicity to isolated rat kidney cells, but did not significantly affect cell viability on its own.[42]

17.3 *Methods for study of renal metabolism*

This section provides detailed procedures for assessing the activities of several of the enzymes mentioned above. Methods that are specific to P450 (i.e., CO-difference spectra, ethoxyresorufin *O*-deethylation, etc.) or isolated kidney cells (viability measurements, etc.) are described in other chapters.

17.3.1 Preparation of renal microsomes and cytosol

This procedure is taken from Rush et al.[2] and is suitable for most of the xenobiotic metabolizing enzymes in the kidney. The KCl-containing buffers are preferred if P450 levels will be determined in microsomes. However, if renal UDPGT activity is to be measured, the sucrose–phosphate buffer should be used in steps 3 to 8.[10]

Buffers

1. 100 m*M* sodium phosphate–154 m*M* KCl buffer: dissolve 11.5 g of KCl in 1 l of 100 m*M* sodium phosphate buffer, pH 7.4.
2. 100 m*M* sodium phosphate–154 m*M* KCl buffer–1 m*M* EDTA: dissolve 11.5 g of KCl and 0.372 g of EDTA in 1 l of 100 m*M* sodium phosphate buffer, pH 7.4.
3. 0.25 *M* sucrose buffer: dissolve 42.79 g of sucrose in 500 ml of 100 m*M* sodium phosphate buffer, pH 7.4.
4. Also needed: 1.15% (w/v) KCl.

Procedure

1. Sacrifice animals by cervical dislocation or decapitation. Remove the kidneys and place them in ice-cold 1.15% (w/v) KCl.
2. Dissect the cortex and the medulla apart; save the appropriate region, depending on the enzyme activity that is being measured.
3. Weigh the tissue and mince it in 3 volumes of ice-cold sodium phosphate–KCl buffer. Wash the tissue with buffer three times.
4. Homogenize the tissue in 3 volumes of sodium phosphate–KCl–EDTA buffer (pH 7.4) with a Potter–Elvehjem homogenizer.
5. Centrifuge at $9000 \times g$ for 30 min at 4°C.
6. Remove the supernatant (S-9 fraction) and centrifuge at $105{,}000 \times g$ for 60 min at 4°C.
7. Remove the supernatant (cytosol) and set it aside, if desired.
8. Suspend the microsomes in 3 volumes of sodium phosphate–KCl–EDTA buffer and centrifuge them at $105{,}000 \times g$ for 60 min at 4°C.
9. Resuspend the microsomes in 0.5 volumes of buffer.
10. Measure the protein concentration of the microsomes and the cytosol with the Lowry or Bradford assay (see below).

17.3.2 Bradford protein assay

This assay measures the shift in absorbance maximum (from 464 to 595 nm) that occurs when the dye Coomassie brilliant blue G-250 binds to protein.[31] The procedure is simple to use and is less prone to interference than the Lowry assay. Protein concentrations are determined by comparison to a standard curve derived using bovine serum albumin (BSA).

Reagents. Dye reagent: dilute 20 ml of Coomassie blue dye with 80 ml of H_2O (prepare fresh daily). If necessary, filter diluted reagent by gravity to remove any precipitate.

BSA standard curve

1. Prepare a 1 mg/ml BSA stock solution by dissolving 5 mg of BSA in 5 ml of H_2O (prepare fresh daily).

2. Dilute the BSA stock solution as follows:

BSA stock solution (ml)	H_2O (ml)	Protein concentration (mg/ml)
0.2	0.8	0.2
0.4	0.6	0.4
0.6	0.4	0.6
0.8	0.2	0.8
1.0	0.0	1.0

3. Assay as described below.

Assay procedure

1. Dilute 0.2 ml of tissue samples with 9.8 ml of H_2O (50:1 dilution).
2. Place 0.1 ml of diluted tissue samples and BSA standards in test tubes (all samples should be run in duplicate). Also prepare a blank that contains 0.1 ml of H_2O in place of the protein.
3. Add 5 ml of the diluted Coomassie dye to each tube and vortex gently.
4. Read the absorbance of each tube at 595 nm against the H_2O blank. The color is stable for up to 60 min.
5. Determine the protein concentration in tissue samples by comparison with the BSA standard curve.
6. If the tissue samples are out of range of the standard curve, a further dilution should be used.

17.3.3 *UDP-glucuronosyltransferase assay*

This spectrophotometric assay monitors the disappearance of *p*-nitrophenol (PNP) from the incubations.[8] PNP has an absorbance maximum at 400 nm whereas the product of the reaction (PNP-glucuronide) absorbs at 312 nm.

Reagents and buffers

1. 2.5 m*M* PNP: dissolve 34.78 mg of PNP in 100 ml of H_2O (prepare fresh daily).
2. 9.8 m*M* UDPGA: dissolve 5.69 mg of UDPGA in 1 ml of H_2O (prepare fresh daily).
3. 200 m*M* glycine buffer: dissolve 1.5 g of Gly in 100 ml of H_2O and adjust pH to 10.4 with NaOH.
4. Also needed: 0.15 *M* phosphate buffer (pH 7.4), 50 m*M* $MgCl_2$, 10% (w/v) trichloroacetic acid (TCA), 1 *M* NaOH.

PNP standard curve

1. Prepare a 0.25 m*M* PNP stock solution by diluting 1 ml of 2.5 m*M* PNP with 9 ml of H_2O.
2. Dilute 0.25 m*M* PNP stock solution as follows:

0.25 m*M* PNP (µl)	H_2O (µl)	Final concentration (pmol/ml)
0	1000	0
50	950	5
100	900	10
250	750	25
500	500	50
750	250	75
1000	0	100

3. Add 1 ml of 1 *M* NaOH and 1 ml of glycine buffer, and read the absorbance at 400 nm.

Assay procedure

1. Mix the following reagents together for each incubation:

   100 μl of 9.8 m*M* UDPGA
   100 μl of 50 m*M* $MgCl_2$
   4 μl of Triton X-100 (1%, v/v, solution)
   100 μl of microsomes (equivalent to 0.4 to 0.5 mg protein)
   300 μl of 0.15 *M* phosphate buffer, pH 7.4.

2. Add 100 ml of 2.5 m*M* PNP solution to each reaction mixture and incubate at 37°C for 30 min in a shaking incubator bath. Run a control incubation by using boiled microsomes.
3. Terminate reactions by adding 0.5 ml of 10% (w/v) TCA, then add 0.5 ml of glycine buffer.
4. Vortex well and centrifuge.
5. Remove 1.0 ml of the supernatant and add 2 ml of 1 *M* NaOH to this aliquot.
6. Vortex and read absorbance at 400 nm.
7. Determine the PNP concentration in samples by comparison with the standard curve.
8. Calculate the protein concentration of an aliquot of microsomes using the Lowry or Bradford protein assay.
9. Calculate the amount of PNP-glucuronide formed (in nanomoles per milligram protein per minute) from the following equation:

$$\frac{\left[\text{conc. PNP (blank)} - \text{conc. PNP (sample)}\right] \text{(in nmol/ml)} \times 2.7 \text{ ml}}{\text{protein conc. (in mg/ml)} \times \text{vol. microsomes (in ml)} \times 30 \text{ min}}$$

17.3.4 Glutathione S-transferase assay

The GST-catalyzed conjugation of GSH with 1-chloro-2,4-dinitrobenzene (CDNB) is measured spectrophotometrically at 340 nm.[39]

Reagents and buffers

1. 100 m*M* GSH: dissolve 614.6 mg of GSH in 20 ml of buffer (prepare fresh daily).
2. 1 m*M* CDNB: dissolve 20.25 mg of CDNB in 100 ml of 95% (v/v) ethanol.
3. Also needed: 100 m*M* sodium phosphate buffer, pH 6.5.

Assay procedure

1. Dilute the cytosol 1:5 with buffer. Measure the protein concentration using the Lowry or Bradford assay.
2. Mix together the following reagents:

   1.86 ml of 100 m*M* phosphate buffer, pH 6.5
   0.1 ml of 100 m*M* GSH
   0.02 ml of 1 m*M* CDNB

3. Initiate reaction by adding 0.02 ml of the diluted cytosol.
4. Read the absorbance on a spectrophotometer (340 nm) at time-zero and at 30-s intervals for 3 min against a blank containing all the reagents except CDNB. Calculate the change in absorbance per minute (A_{340}/min).

5. Determine the nonenzymatic conjugation rate (A_{340}/min) by measuring the absorbance at time-zero and 1 min later of a reaction mixture in which the cytosol is omitted. Subtract the nonenzymatic rate (no cytosol present) from the enzyme-catalyzed rate (cytosol present).
6. Calculate the amount of CDNB-GSH conjugate formed (in micromoles per milligram protein per minute) using a molar absorptivity of 8.5 mM^{-1} cm^{-1} as follows:

$$\frac{A_{340}/\text{min} \times 1000}{\text{protein (mg/ml)} \times 8.5}$$

17.3.5 *Cysteine conjugate β-lyase assay*

Formation of 2-mercaptobenzothiazole from *S*-(2-benzothiazolyl)-L-cysteine (BTC) can be monitored spectrophotometrically at 321 nm.[40] BTC is synthesized from 2-chlorobenzothiazole, L-cysteine, and sodium metal in liquid ammonia.[40]

Reagents and buffers

1. BTC has limited solubility in aqueous buffers in the pH range 7 to 10. A 4-m*M* stock solution of BTC (20 ml) can be prepared as follows:
   a. Suspend 20.3 mg of BTC in 8 ml of H_2O.
   b. Add a sufficient amount (0.5 ml/20 ml final volume) of 1 *M* KOH to dissolve the solid rapidly.
   c. After dissolution is complete, immediately add 10 ml of 0.2 *M* boric acid.
   d. Adjust the pH to 8.6 with 1 *M* KOH.
   e. Adjust the volume to 20 ml with H_2O.
2. Also needed: 0.1 *M* potassium borate buffer (pH 8.6) and 10% (w/v) TCA.

Assay procedure

1. Preincubate 1.5 ml of 4 m*M* BTC with 1.3 ml of 0.1 *M* borate buffer (pH 8.6) for 4 min at 37°C in a shaking water bath.
2. Add 0.2 ml of enzyme sample and incubate at 37°C for 2.5 min.
3. Terminate the reaction by adding 0.6 ml of 10% (w/v) TCA.
4. Centrifuge to remove protein.
5. Measure the absorbance in samples at 321 nm.
6. Calculate the amount of product formed (in nanomoles per minute per milliliter) from the following equation (the product of the reaction has a molar absorptivity coefficient of 21,600 M^{-1} cm^{-1}):

$$\frac{\Delta A_{321}\ \text{min}^{-1} \times 10^6\ \text{nmol}}{21.6\ \text{mmol}^{-1}\ \text{liter} \times 10^3 \text{ml liter}^{-1} \times \text{mmol}} \times 18$$

17.4 *Membrane transport*

17.4.1 *General description*

One important characteristic of renal tubular epithelial cells (especially those lining the segments of the proximal tubule) is their ability to transport a wide variety of endogenous compounds and xenobiotics from blood into luminal fluid (secretion) and from luminal fluid into blood (reabsorption). The transport systems involved in secretion and reabsorption processes are primarily membrane-bound protein carriers, but toxicants can also cross renal membranes via passive diffusion (e.g., chloroform), via membrane processing (e.g., GSH conjugates), or by endocytosis (e.g., cadmium–metallothionein complexes). A number of reviews detail the specific mechanisms by which toxicants and endogenous compounds are transported, secreted, and/or reabsorbed in the kidney.[48-52] While these systems function primarily to promote the excretion of xenobiotics and reabsorption of filtered endogenous compounds, one consequence of transporting toxicants across renal plasma membranes is that these toxicants can accumulate in renal cells to levels much higher than those found in plasma or other organs. Thus, the transport ability of the kidney can ultimately lead to toxic effects from transported substrates.

There are several ways in which one can take advantage of a knowledge of renal transport systems to answer questions relevant to toxicology. Many transport systems, such as the basolateral organic anion or organic cation transport systems found in proximal tubular cells, require cellular energy to promote transport. If a compound is a proximal tubular toxicant, it should alter accumulation of transport substrates in renal cortical tissue or cells. Thus, diminished accumulation of transported substrates can be used as one measure of renal function. In addition, an examination of the effects of a compound on transport by renal plasma membrane vesicles (basolateral or luminal) will allow for the detection of direct membrane toxicity.

The model renal systems used to monitor toxicant transport or the toxic potential of a chemical, with changes in transport of a prototypic substrate used as a marker for nephrotoxicity, are the same model systems used for most renal studies. Renal cortical slices,[53,54] the isolated perfused kidney,[55] isolated renal epithelial cells,[56] isolated renal tubular segments,[57] isolated perfused tubular segments,[58] cell cultures,[59,60] and membrane vesicles[61,62] have all been used for these purposes.

Perhaps one of the more common models that uses changes in organic ion transport for monitoring the development of nephrotoxicity *in vivo* or *in vitro* is the renal cortical slice model. Methodology for the use of membrane transport in this model system is described in the next section. The methodology used with renal cortical slices is also easily adapted for use in several other *in vitro* renal model systems (isolated tubular segments, isolated renal epithelial cells, and primary cell cultures).

Markers of membrane transport are also important in the use of basolateral or luminal membrane vesicles as a toxicological model. In this model, transport can be determined at each membrane surface independent of cellular metabolism, storage within organelles, or binding to cytosolic components. In addition, the direct effects of a toxicant on each membrane can be determined by monitoring accumulation of transport substrates. This model is discussed below.

17.4.2 Renal cortical slices

Organic ions are secreted by distinct transport systems for organic anions (weakly acidic compounds) or organic cations (weakly basic and quaternary ammonium compounds) in the kidney. These transporters are located in the proximal tubule and demonstrate axial heterogeneity. Studies in rabbit with *p*-aminohippurate (PAH), the prototypical substrate for the organic anion transporter, have demonstrated that the decreasing order of secretory activity by proximal tubular segments is $S_2 > S_1 = S_3$.[63] For secretion of organic cations, such as tetraethylammonium (TEA), the order of activity of secretion rates is $S_1 > S_2 > S_3$ for superficial nephrons and $S_1 = S_2 > S_3$ for juxtamedullary nephrons.[64] Thus, renal cortical slices will contain the majority of proximal tubular cells and both organic ion transport systems.

Renal cortical slices can be used to detect toxicity following *in vivo*[53] or *in vitro*[54] exposure to a nephrotoxicant. Decreased accumulation of organic anions (e.g., PAH) or organic cations (e.g., TEA) is a sensitive indicator of proximal tubular toxicity, and changes in the accumulation of the transported substrates frequently occur before other parameters of renal function are altered.[65]

To utilize membrane transport by renal cortical slices as a measure of *in vivo* nephrotoxicity for a compound, the following procedure can be used:[53]

1. Treat the test animal with the compound to be evaluated.
2. At a specified time, one or both kidneys are removed and rapidly placed in ice-cold Krebs–Ringer buffer containing 5.0 m*M* potassium phosphate.
3. Renal cortical slices are prepared either freehand, with a razor blade, or with a tissue slicer (e.g., Stadie–Riggs, McIlwain, or Krumdieck).[66,67] Slices should be approximately 0.2 to 0.5 mm in thickness to allow for proper oxygenation.
4. Incubate approximately 100 mg of slices in 3 ml of the Krebs–Ringer buffer/5.0 m*M* potassium phosphate in a shaking water bath under a 100% oxygen atmosphere at 25°C for 15 min. Then add [^{14}C]-PAH or [^{14}C]-TEA and continue the incubations for 1.5 h. Sufficient radioactive PAH or TEA is added to yield about 0.02 μCi/ml of incubation medium and enough unlabeled material is added to yield a final concentration of 7×10^{-5} *M* for PAH and 1×10^{-5} *M* for TEA. To determine lactate-stimulated PAH accumulation, lactate (10 m*M*) should be present in the incubation medium.
5. At the end of the incubation period, the tissue is removed from the medium, blotted dry, weighed, and placed in a vial containing 4.0 ml of distilled water. The tissue is then homogenized and a 500-μl aliquot is added to 4.5 ml of scintillant for counting. In a separate counting vial, a 250-μl aliquot of medium is added to 4.75 ml of scintillant for counting.
6. Accumulation of PAH and TEA by the renal cortical slices is expressed as the slice-to-medium (S/M) ratio, where S equals the radioactivity (disintegrations per minute) per gram of tissue and M equals the radioactivity (disintegrations per minute) per milliliter of incubation medium. A decrease in the S/M ratio for PAH and/or TEA is indicative of toxicity to the proximal tubules.

Nonradiolabeled PAH alone can also be used in these experiments,[68] but the S/M ratios tend to be higher. With radiolabeled PAH and TEA, common S/M ratios are as follows: basal PAH = 3.0 to 5.0; lactate-stimulated PAH = 8.0 to 11.0; and TEA = 15 to 20. Values using nonradiolabeled PAH are about two times larger than those reported for [^{14}C]-PAH. Decreased food intake can also reduce PAH accumulation, so pair-fed controls should always be used to account for this potential variable. TEA accumulation does not appear to be altered by changes in food intake.

This same basic procedure can also be used for *in vitro* studies. In general, kidneys are removed from untreated animals, and renal cortical tissues slices are prepared and preincubated for about 15 min. The test compound is then added, and after incubating the slices for 0.5 h with the test compound, [^{14}C]-PAH or [^{14}C]-TEA is added as above and the incubations are continued for 1.0 to 1.5 h. S/M ratios are then determined as described above. Some investigators remove the tissue slices from the medium containing the test compound and add the slices to fresh medium containing PAH or TEA.[68] This method allows for the accumulation of the organic ions without the possibility that the test compound is competing with PAH or TEA for transport.

17.4.3 *Membrane vesicles*

Membrane vesicles can be used to determine the direct toxic effects of a compound on the basolateral or luminal (brush border) membrane.[62,69,70] Membrane vesicles can also be

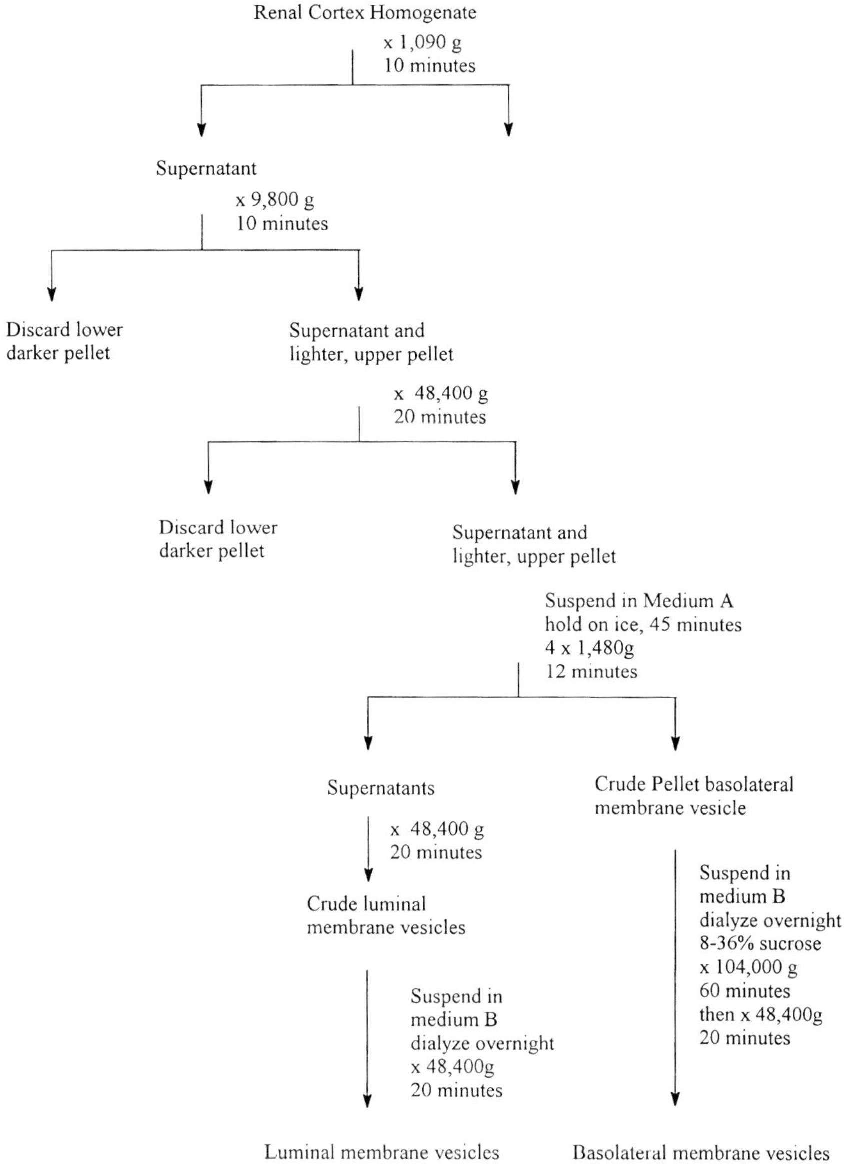

Figure 4 Preparation of basolateral and luminal membrane vesicles from rabbit kidney cortex. (Modified from Wright, S. H. and Wunz, T. M., *Am. J. Physiol.*, 253, F432, 1987.)

used to determine how compounds are transported at each membrane.[71,72] Preparation of separate pools of basolateral and luminal membrane vesicles generally starts with a renal cortical homogenate that is subjected to differential centrifugation with divalent cation precipitation and density gradient centrifugation techniques.

An example of the methodology for preparing rabbit renal basolateral and luminal membrane vesicles can be taken from the work of Wright and Wunz,[71] and is shown in Figure 4. Following injection of the rabbit with a lethal dose of pentobarbital, the kidneys are perfused with 50 ml each of 250 m*M* sucrose and 10 m*M* *N*-2-hydroxyethylpiperazine-*N*′-2-ethanesulfonic acid (HEPES) that has been buffered to pH 7.0 with tris(hydroxymethyl)aminomethane (TRIS). The kidneys are then removed, the cortices are excised and minced, and the tissue from two rabbits is pooled for the isolation procedures. The two media used for the isolation of the membrane vesicles in Figure 4 are medium A: 100 m*M* mannitol, 5 m*M* $MgCl_2$, 5 m*M* $CaCl_2$, 25 m*M* HEPES–TRIS, pH 7.0; and medium B: 100 m*M* mannitol, 25 m*M* HEPES–TRIS, pH 7.0. Once the crude membrane vesicles are obtained, they are dialyzed against 2 l of medium B. Centrifugation alone yields the luminal membrane vesicles, but basolateral membrane vesicles must undergo discontinuous sucrose gradient centrifugation (8 to 36% sucrose gradient, centrifuged at 104,000 × g for 60 min) prior to a final centrifugation step. Although the procedure in Figure 4 was developed for rabbit renal membrane vesicles, similar procedures are available for other species, including the rat[69,70] and dog.[73]

Identity and purity of the membrane vesicles can be determined by monitoring enzymatic activities and transport characteristics in the vesicle preparations.[71,73] For example, alkaline phosphatase, trehalase, and γ-glutamyltransferase activity and glucose transport are much greater in luminal membrane vesicles than in basolateral membrane vesicles, while PAH transport and (Na^+ + K^+)-stimulated ATPase activity are higher in basolateral membrane vesicles than in luminal membrane vesicles.

Although membrane vesicles have been widely used to examine transport of prototypical transport substrates, it is somewhat surprising that more studies have not taken advantage of the unique features of this *in vitro* model. Since cellular metabolism or other intracellular events do not interfere with the effects of the test compound directly at the membrane level, the contributions of direct and indirect cellular effects of a compound can easily be discerned and complement results from other *in vitro* models.

In the few studies that have been conducted, effects at the basolateral membrane are monitored by assessing a decrease in the transport of radiolabeled PAH, while luminal membrane effects can be monitored by determining changes in radiolabeled glucose transport. For example, Ansari et al.[69] found that mercuric chloride (100 n*M*) altered PAH transport in rat basolateral membrane vesicles, but glucose transport was not altered in luminal membrane vesicles. In a study of the effect of aminoglycosides on luminal membrane function, Takahashi et al.[70] noted a decrease of glucose transport into rat renal luminal membrane vesicles by gentamicin. Thus, the use of renal cortical membrane vesicles can help identify targets for toxicants and can complement results from other *in vitro* models and from histological studies.

References

1. Tarloff, J. B., Goldstein, R. S., and Hook, J. B., Xenobiotic biotransformation by the kidney: pharmacological and toxicological aspects, in *Progress in Drug Metabolism*, Vol. 12, Gibson, G. G., Ed., Taylor & Francis, London, 1990, chap. 1.
2. Rush, G. F., Wilson, D. M., and Hook, J. B., Selective induction and inhibition of renal mixed function oxidases in the rat and rabbit, *Fundam. Appl. Toxicol.*, 3, 161, 1983.
3. Smith, J. H., Rush, G. F., and Hook, J. B., Induction of renal and hepatic mixed function oxidases in the hamster and guinea pig, *Toxicology*, 38, 209, 1986.
4. Lake, B. G., Hopkins, R., Chakraborty, J., Bridges, J. W., and Parke, D. V. W., The influence of some hepatic enzyme inducers and inhibitors on extrahepatic drug metabolism, *Drug Metab. Dispos.*, 1, 342, 1973.
5. Kluwe, W. M., McCormack, K. M., and Hook, J. B., Selective modification of the renal and hepatic toxicities of chloroform by induction of drug-metabolizing enzyme systems in kidney and liver, *J. Pharmacol. Exp. Ther.*, 207, 566, 1978.
6. Henderson, C. J., Scott, A. R., Yang, C. S., and Wolf, C. R., Testosterone-mediated regulation of mouse renal cytochrome P450 isoenzymes, *Biochem. J.*, 266, 675, 1990.
7. Wu, D. and Cederbaum, A. I., Characterization of pyrazole and 4-methylpyrazole induction of cytochrome P4502E1 in rat kidney, *J. Pharmacol. Exp. Ther.*, 270, 407, 1994.

8. Mugford, C. A., Mortillo, M., Mico, B. A., and Tarloff, J. B., 1-Aminobenzotriazole-induced destruction of hepatic and renal cytochromes P450 in male Sprague–Dawley rats, *Fundam. Appl. Toxicol.*, 19, 43, 1992.
9. Tarloff, J. B., Goldstein, R. S., Sozio, R. S., and Hook, J. B., Hepatic and renal conjugation (phase II) enzyme activities in young adult, middle-aged, and senescent male Sprague–Dawley rats, *Proc. Soc. Exp. Biol. Med.*, 197, 297, 1991.
10. Rush, G. F. and Hook, J. B., Characteristics of renal UDP-glucuronosyltransferase, *Life Sci.*, 35, 145, 1984.
11. Hanninen, O. and Aitio, A., Enhanced glucuronide formation in different tissues following drug administration, *Biochem. Pharmacol.*, 17, 2307, 1968.
12. Jones, D. P., Sundby, G.-B., Ormstad, K., and Orrenius, S., Use of isolated kidney cells for study of drug metabolism, *Biochem. Pharmacol.*, 28, 929, 1979.
13. Derbel, M., Igarashi, T., and Satoh, T., Differential induction of glutathione *S*-transferase subunits by phenobarbital, 3-methylcholanthrene and ethoxyquin in rat liver and kidney, *Biochim. Biophys. Acta*, 1158, 175, 1993.
14. Zenser, T. V., Levitt, M. J., and Davis, B. B., Effect of oxygen and solute on PGE and PGF production by rat kidney slices, *Prostaglandins*, 13, 143, 1977.
15. Eling, T. E. and Curtis, J. F., Xenobiotic metabolism by prostaglandin H synthase, *Pharmacol. Ther.*, 53, 261, 1992.
16. Mohandas, J., Duggin, G. G., Horvath, J. S., and Tiller D. J., Metabolic oxidation of acetaminophen (paracetamol) mediated by cytochrome P450 mixed-function oxidase and prostaglandin endoperoxide synthetase in rabbit kidney, *Toxicol. Appl. Pharmacol.*, 61, 252, 1981.
17. Zenser, T. V., Mattammal, M. B., Wise, R. W., Rice, J. R., and Davis, B. B., Prostaglandin H synthase-catalyzed activation of benzidine: a model to assess pharmacologic intervention of the initiation of chemical carcinogenesis, *J. Pharmacol. Exp. Ther.*, 227, 545, 1983.
18. Elfarra, A. A. and Anders, M. W., Renal processing of glutathione conjugates. Role in nephrotoxicity, *Biochem. Pharmacol.*, 33, 3729, 1984.
19. Tate, S. S. and Meister, A., γ-Glutamyl transpeptidase from kidney, *Methods Enzymol.*, 113, 400, 1985.
20. Jones, D. P., Moldéus, P., Stead, A. H., Ormstad, K., Jörnvall, H., and Orrenius, S., Metabolism of glutathione and a glutathione conjugate by isolated kidney cells, *J. Biol. Chem.*, 254, 2787, 1979.
21. McIntyre, T. and Curthoys, N. P., Renal catabolism of glutathione. Characterization of a particulate rat renal dipeptidase that catalyzes the hydrolysis of cysteinylglycine, *J. Biol. Chem.*, 257, 11915, 1982.
22. Stevens, J. L., Robbins, J. D., and Byrd, R. A., A purified cysteine conjugate β-lyase from rat kidney cytosol. Requirement for an α-keto acid or an amino acid oxidase for activity and identity with soluble glutamine transaminase K, *J. Biol. Chem.*, 261, 15529, 1986.
23. Lash, L. H., Elfarra, A. A., and Anders, M. W., Renal cysteine conjugate β-lyase. Bioactivation of nephrotoxic cysteine *S*-conjugates in mitochondrial outer membrane, *J. Biol. Chem.*, 261, 5930, 1986.
24. Moldéus, P., Paracetamol metabolism and toxicity in isolated hepatocytes from rat and mouse, *Biochem. Pharmacol.*, 27, 2859, 1978.
25. Hinchman, C. A. and Ballatori, N., Glutathione-degrading capacities of liver and kidney in different species, *Biochem. Pharmacol.*, 40, 1131, 1990.
26. Johnson, D. and Lardy, H., Isolation of liver or kidney mitochondria, *Methods Enzymol.*, 10, 94, 1967.
27. Schnaitman, C. and Greenawalt, J. W., Enzymatic properties of the inner and outer membranes of rat liver mitochondria, *J. Cell Biol.*, 38, 158, 1968.
28. Lake, B. G., Preparation and characterisation of microsomal fractions for studies on xenobiotic metabolism, in *Biochemical Toxicology. A Practical Approach*, Snell, K. and Mullock, B., Eds., IRL Press, Oxford, 1987, chap. 8.
29. Guengerich, F. P., Microsomal enzymes involved in toxicology — analysis and separation, in *Principles and Methods of Toxicology*, student ed., Hayes, A. W., Ed., Raven Press, New York, 1984, chap. 20.

30. Lowry, O. H., Rosebrough, N. J., Farr, A. L., and Randall, R. J., Protein measurement with the Folin phenol reagent, *J. Biol. Chem.*, 193, 265, 1951.
31. Bradford, M. M., A rapid and sensitive method for the quantitation of microgram quantities of protein utilizing the principle of protein-dye binding, *Anal. Biochem.*, 72, 248, 1976.
32. Cooper, T. G., *The Tools of Biochemistry*, John Wiley & Sons, New York, 1977, chap. 1.
33. Omura, T. and Sato, R., The carbon monoxide-binding pigment of liver microsomes. I. Evidence for its hemoprotein nature, *J. Biol. Chem.*, 239, 2370, 1964.
34. Jefcoate, C. R., Measurement of substrate and inhibitor binding to microsomal cytochrome P450 by optical-difference spectroscopy, *Methods Enzymol.*, 52, 258, 1978.
35. Temple, A. R., Done, A. K., and Clement, M. S., Studies of glucuronidation. III. The measurement of *p*-nitrophenyl glucuronide, *J. Lab. Clin. Med.*, 77, 1015, 1971.
36. Wong, K. P., Sulphate conjugation of isoprenaline by lung, small intestine and other organs, *Biochem. Pharmacol.*, 31, 59, 1982.
37. Sekura, R. D. and Jakoby, W. B., Phenol sulfotransferases, *J. Biol. Chem.*, 254, 5658, 1979.
38. Sekura, R. D., Marcus, C. J., Lyon, E. S., and Jakoby, W. B., Assay of sulfotransferases, *Anal. Biochem.*, 95, 82, 1979.
39. Habig, W. H., Pabst, M. J., and Jakoby, W. B., Glutathione *S*-transferases. The first enzymatic step in mercapturic acid formation, *J. Biol. Chem.*, 249, 7130, 1974.
40. Dohn, D. R. and Anders, M. W., Assay of cysteine conjugate β-lyase activity with *S*-(2-benzothiazolyl)cysteine as the substrate, *Anal. Biochem.*,120, 379, 1982.
41. Rudo, K. M., Dauterman, W. C., and Langenbach, R., Human and rat kidney cell metabolism of 2-acetylaminofluorene and benzo[a]pyrene, *Cancer Res.*, 49, 1187, 1989.
42. Henesey, C. M. and Harvison, P. J., Potential metabolism and cytotoxicity of *N*-(3,5-dichlorophenyl)succinimide and its hepatic metabolites in isolated rat renal cortical tubule cells, *Toxicology*, 104, 9, 1995.
43. Lash, L. H. and Anders, M. W., Cytotoxicity of *S*-(1,2-dichlorovinyl)glutathione and *S*-(1,2-dichlorovinyl)-L-cysteine in isolated rat kidney cells, *J. Biol. Chem.*, 261, 13076, 1986.
44. Bruggeman, I. M., Mertens, J. J. W. M., Temmink, J. H. M., Lans, M. C., Vos, R. M. E., and van Bladeren, P. J., Use of monolayers of primary rat kidney cortex cells for nephrotoxicity studies, *Toxicol. In Vitro*, 3, 261, 1989.
45. Lash, L. H., Isolated kidney cells in the study of chemical toxicity, in *In Vitro Toxicology: Model Systems and Methods*, McQueen, C. A., Ed., Telford Press, Caldwell, NJ, 1989, chap. 8.
46. Lash, L. H. and Tokarz, J. J., Isolation of two distinct populations of cells from rat kidney cortex and their use in the study of chemical-induced toxicity, *Anal. Biochem.*, 182, 271, 1989.
47. Moldéus, P., Högberg, J., and Orrenius, S., Isolation and use of liver cells, *Methods Enzymol.*, 52, 60, 1978.
48. Grantham, J. J., Studies of organic anion and cation transport in isolated segments of proximal tubules, *Kidney Int.*, 22, 519, 1982.
49. Giacomini, K. M., Hsyu, P.-H., and Gisclon, L. G., Renal transport of drugs: an overview of methodology with application to cimetidine, *Pharm. Res.*, 5, 465, 1988.
50. Guggino, W. B. and Guggino, S. E., Renal anion transport, *Kidney Int.*, 36, 385, 1989.
51. Pritchard, J. B. and Miller, D. S., Comparative insights into the mechanisms or renal organic anion and cation secretion, *Am. J. Physiol.*, 261, R1329, 1991.
52. Ullrich, K. J. and Rumrich, G., Renal transport mechanisms for xenobiotics: chemicals and drugs, *Clin. Invest.*, 71, 843, 1993.
53. Rankin, G. O., Shih, H.-C., Yang, D. J., Richmond, C. D., Teets, V. J., and Brown, P. I., *Toxicol. Appl. Pharmacol.*, 96, 405, 1988.
54. Wolfgang, G. H., Gandolfi, A. J., Stevens, J. L., Brendel, K., *N*-Acetyl *S*-(1,2-dichlorovinyl)-L-cysteine produces a similar toxicity to *S*-(1,2-dichlorovinyl)-L-cysteine in rabbit renal slices: differential transport and metabolism, *Toxicol. Appl. Pharmacol.*, 101, 205, 1989.
55. Sumpio, B. E., Chaudry, I. H., and Baue, A. E., Reduction of the drug-induced nephrotoxicity by ATP-$MgCl_2$. I. Effects on the cis-diamminedichloroplatinum-treated isolated perfused kidneys, *J. Surgical Res.*, 38, 429, 1985.
56. Lash, L. H. and Anders, M. W., Uptake of nephrotoxic *S*-conjugates by isolated rat renal proximal tubular cells, *J. Pharmacol. Exp. Ther.*, 248, 531, 1989.

57. Hassall, C. D., Gandolfi, A. J., Duhamel, R. C., and Brendel, K., The formation and biotransformation of cysteine conjugates of halogenated ethylenes by rabbit renal tubules, *Chem. Biol. Interact.* 49, 283, 1984.
58. Zalups, R. K. and Barfuss, D. W., Transport and toxicity of methylmercury along the proximal tubule of the rabbit, *Toxicol. Appl. Pharmacol.*, 121, 176, 1993.
59. Boogaard, P. J., Zoeteweij, J. P., vanBerkle, T. J. C., van'tNoordende, J. M., Mulder, G. J., and Nagelkerke, J. F., Primary culture of proximal tubular cells from normal rat kidney as an *in vitro* model to study mechanisms of nephrotoxicity: toxicity of nephrotoxicants at low concentrations during prolonged exposure, *Biochem. Pharmacol.*, 39, 1335, 1990.
60. Aleo, M. D., Taub, M. L., and Kostyniak, P. J., Primary cultures of rabbit renal proximal tubule cells. III. Comparative cytotoxicity of inorganic and organic mercury, *Toxicol. Appl. Pharmacol.*, 112, 310, 1992.
61. Charkrabardi, S., Vu, D. D., and Cote, M. G., Effects of cysteine derivatives of styrene on the transport of *p*-aminohippurate ion in renal plasma membrane vesicles, *Arch. Toxicol.*, 65, 366, 1991.
62. Ansari, R. A., Thakran, R. S., and Berndt, W. O., Effects of mercuric chloride on renal plasma function after depletion or elevation of renal glutathione, *Toxicol. Appl. Pharmacol.*, 111, 364, 1991.
63. Woodhall, P. B., Tisher, C. C., Simonton, C. A., and Robinson, R. R., Relationship between *p*-aminohippurate secretion and cellular morphology in rabbit proximal tubules, *J. Clin. Invest.*, 51, 1320, 1978.
64. McKinney, T. D., Heterogeneity of organic base secretion by proximal tubules, *Am. J. Physiol.*, 243, F404, 1982.
65. Rankin, G. O., Cressey-Veneziano, K., and Brown, P. I., Onset of and recovery from acute *N*-(3,5-dichlorophenyl)succinimide-induced nephrotoxicity in Sprague–Dawley rats, *Toxicology*, 30, 205, 1984.
66. Berndt, W. O., Use of the tissue slice technique for evaluation of renal transport processes, *Environ. Health Perspect.*, 15, 73, 1976.
67. McGuinness, S., Gandolfi, A. J., and Brendel, K., Use of renal slices and renal tubule suspensions for *in vitro* studies, *In Vitro Toxicol.*, 6, 1, 1993.
68. Smith, J. H., The use of renal cortical slices from the Fischer 344 rat as an *in vitro* model to evaluate nephrotoxicity, *Fundam. Appl. Toxicol.*, 11, 132, 1988.
69. Ansari, R. A., Thakran, R. S., and Berndt, W. O., The effects of mercuric chloride on transport by brush border and basolateral membrane vesicles isolated from rat kidney, *Toxicol. Appl. Pharmacol.*, 106, 145, 1990.
70. Takahashi, M., Aramaki, Y., Inaba, A., and Tsuchiya, S., Inhibition of alkaline phosphatase activity and D-glucose uptake in rat renal brush-border membrane vesicles by aminoglycosides, *Biochim. Biophys. Acta*, 903, 31, 1987.
71. Wright, S. H. and Wunz, T. M., Succinate and citrate transport in renal basolateral and brush-border membranes, *Am. J. Physiol.*, 253, F432, 1987.
72. Wright, S. H. and Wunz, T. M., Transport of tetraethylammonium by rabbit renal brush-border and basolateral membrane vesicles, *Am. J. Physiol.*, 253, F1040, 1987.
73. Kinsella, J. L., Holohan, P. D., Pessah, N. I., and Ross, C. R., Isolation of luminal and antiluminal membranes from dog kidney cortex, *Biochim. Biophys. Acta*, 552, 468, 1979.

chapter eighteen

Methods to Evaluate Renal Cytochrome P450 as a Bioactivation System for Nephrotoxicants

Kimberley J. Woodcroft, Richard C. Zangar, and Raymond F. Novak

18.1 Introduction ... 354
18.2 Localization of P450 expression in renal tissue ... 355
18.3 Isozymes present in renal tissue ... 356
18.3.1 1A subfamily ... 357
18.3.2 2A subfamily ... 357
18.3.3 2B subfamily ... 357
18.3.4 2C subfamily ... 358
18.3.5 2E subfamily ... 358
18.3.6 3A subfamily ... 359
18.3.7 4A subfamily ... 360
18.4 Methods to quantitate and modulate P450 activities ... 360
18.4.1 Preparation of renal microsomes ... 361
18.4.2 Measurement of P450 content ... 361
18.4.3 Enhancement of P450 expression ... 361
18.4.4 Inhibition of P450 activity ... 362
18.4.5 Monitoring of P450 activity ... 362
18.4.5.1 CYP1A1 and CYP2B: ethoxy- and pentoxyresorufin *O*-dealkylation assays ... 363
18.4.5.2 *Cyp2a-4/5* and CYP2C11: testosterone hydroxylation assay ... 363
18.4.5.3 CYP2E1: *N*-nitrosodimethylamine *N*-demethylation assay ... 363
18.4.5.4 CYP3A: erythromycin *N*-demethylation ... 364
18.4.5.5 CYP4A: lauric acid ω-hydroxylation ... 364
18.4.5.6 P450-dependent arachidonic acid oxidation ... 365
18.4.6 Immunochemical detection of P450 ... 365
18.4.7 Reverse transcriptase–polymerase chain reaction (RT-PCR) for detection of P450 mRNA ... 367
18.4.8 Immunohistochemical localization of P450 ... 367
18.4.9 *In situ* hybridization of P450 mRNA ... 368
References ... 369

0-8493-3341-5/96/$0.00+$.50

18.1 Introduction

This chapter is intended as a methodological guide for those wishing to pursue research on renal cytochrome P450 expression and the role of this family of enzymes in the metabolism of exogenous and endogenous (e.g., fatty acids and eicosanoids) substrates, some of which may be associated with renal toxicity. Since the chapter is designed for investigators who may not be completely familiar with P450, the nomenclature, as well as current knowledge of P450 localization, isozyme complement, and expression in renal tissue, is included in addition to the methodological approaches and techniques for examining expression and metabolism.

While a large number of nephrotoxic xenobiotics are bioactivated by the cytochromes P450, not all of these agents are bioactivated by renal P450s. In several cases, the toxic metabolite(s) are produced in the liver and are subsequently transported to the kidneys. Thus, determination of the role of renal P450s in the bioactivation of nephrotoxicants is essential for understanding the mechanism(s) by which xenobiotics may mediate renal toxicity.

The following section provides a descriptive approach of the pursuit of such studies, including various techniques that may be used to address the problem. Subsequent sections address the localization, isozyme complement, and experimental techniques in greater detail.

There are several approaches to determine whether xenobiotic activation is catalyzed by renal P450s, and these involve both *in vivo* and *in vitro* techniques. The correlation of the location of renal damage or lesions with the intranephron localization of P450 may suggest the involvement of renal P450s in the production of such damage.[1,2] The correlation of renal P450 levels, isozyme composition, or P450-dependent metabolism with susceptibility to nephrotoxicity — where gender, strain, or species differences in these parameters exist — may also be used to infer renal P450 involvement.[3-7] Likewise, changes in the degree of nephrotoxicity under *in vivo* conditions of enhanced P450 expression or of inhibition of P450 activation may be used to implicate P450-mediated metabolism.[8-10] Because many alterations in P450 expression produced by drugs administered *in vivo* simultaneously affect both renal and hepatic P450 expression, additional approaches using *in vitro* systems are required to establish the primary role and/or identity of renal P450s in metabolism and toxicity.

In vitro systems include renal tissue slices, microsomes, isolated cultured renal cells, purified P450s in a reconstituted system, and heterologously expressed P450s. The use of kidney slices removes the complicating factor of hepatic P450 metabolism while allowing the measurement of functional indices of toxicity, such as organic ion accumulation and other transport properties.[11]

The dependence of xenobiotic metabolism on the presence of oxygen and the cofactor NADPH implicates P450 in the catalytic mechanism. P450-dependent biotransformation of a xenobiotic may be decreased by inhibitors, including inhibitory antibodies, and may be increased by using tissue or microsomes from animals that have been pretreated with agents known to enhance P450 expression, such as those listed in Table 1.

Once renal P450 has been implicated in the bioactivation of a xenobiotic, it is necessary to determine whether specific isozymes are responsible. The participation of specific P450 isoforms in xenobiotic metabolism may be assessed *in vitro* through the use of isozyme-selective mechanism-based and/or competitive inhibitors, inhibitory antibodies, heterologously expressed single isozymes, or isozyme-selective metabolic assays. Xenobiotic metabolism catalyzed by P450 should be decreased substantially (>80 to 90%), if not completely inhibited, in the presence of an isozyme-selective P450 inhibitor, or an isozyme- or P450 subfamily-selective inhibitory antibody. The degree of inhibition should increase with increasing concentration of the inhibitor or level of antibody. Many isozyme-selective,

Table 1 Protocols for Enhancing P450 Expression in Rat Renal Tissues

P450	Compound	Route of administration and treatment regimen	Ref.
CYP1A1	3MC	i.p. 25 mg/kg per day for 3 days	41
	3MC	i.p. 80 mg/kg 2 days prior to death	42
	TCDD	oral 25 μg/kg 3 days prior to death	40
CYP2B	PB	i.p. 100 mg/kg per day for 3 days	41
CYP2E1	DMSO	i.p. 2250 mg/kg twice per day for 3 days	64
	Pyridine	i.p. 200 mg/kg per day for 3 days	65
	Ciprofibrate	i.p. 20 mg/kg per day for 1 to 3 days	67
	Acetone	oral 0.1% (v/v) in drinking water for 7 days	59
	Ethanol	oral 10% (v/v) in drinking water for 14 days	59
	Imidazole	i.p. 200 mg/kg, 20 hr and 12 hr prior to death	59
CYP4A	Clofibrate	i.p. 500 mg/kg 24 hr prior to death	59
		i.p. 400 mg/kg per day for 3 days	70, 74
	Ciprofibrate	i.p. 20 mg/kg per day for 1 to 3 days	67

Note: 3MC, 3-methylcholanthrene; TCDD, 2,3,7,8-tetrachlorodibenzo-*p*-dioxin; PB, phenobarbital; DMSO, dimethylsulfoxide.

mechanism-based P450 inhibitors may also be administered *in vivo* to determine isozyme-specific effects on xenobiotic metabolism and/or nephrotoxicity. However, complications associated with the pharmacodynamics of such agents (e.g., distribution times, tissue levels), and inhibition of hepatic enzymes, require thorough consideration.

Metabolism of xenobiotics by specific isoforms of P450 can be examined with the technique of cDNA-directed heterologous expression using a variety of systems, including yeast,[12] COS cells,[13] vaccinia virus,[14] and baculovirus.[15] However, it must be noted that the ability of an isozyme of P450 to metabolize a chemical in an expression system does not guarantee that the same activity will occur in renal tissue *in vivo*.

An alternative method is to test for inhibition of isozyme-selective metabolic activities in the presence of the xenobiotic to be studied. The xenobiotic should competitively inhibit the metabolism of those substrates that are metabolized by the same P450 isozyme. This method is particularly useful if the metabolism of the xenobiotic itself cannot be measured.

The measurement of indices of renal toxicity (e.g., blood urea nitrogen, proteinuria, urine osmolality, organic ion accumulation and transport) are described elsewhere in this volume, as is the preparation of kidney slices. This chapter focuses on current concepts and methodologies relating to renal P450 expression and the P450-catalyzed metabolism of exogenous and endogenous substrates.

18.2 *Localization of P450 expression in renal tissue*

The physiological effects of metabolites of endogenous substrates, such as fatty acids and eicosanoids, as well as the toxicity of xenobiotics that are bioactivated by P450 in the kidney, appear to correlate with the pattern of P450 isozyme expression and distribution in the nephron.

The localization of P450 within the kidney has been based on both activity measurements as well as immunolocalization studies. The largest P450 content is found in the renal cortex in the proximal tubules (Figure 1). P450 has been reported to be located primarily in the proximal tubule,[16-20] with the greatest levels appearing in the S_2 segment.[16] P450 is also present, albeit to a lesser extent, in the distal convoluted tubule[18-20] and the cortical collecting duct.[21,22]

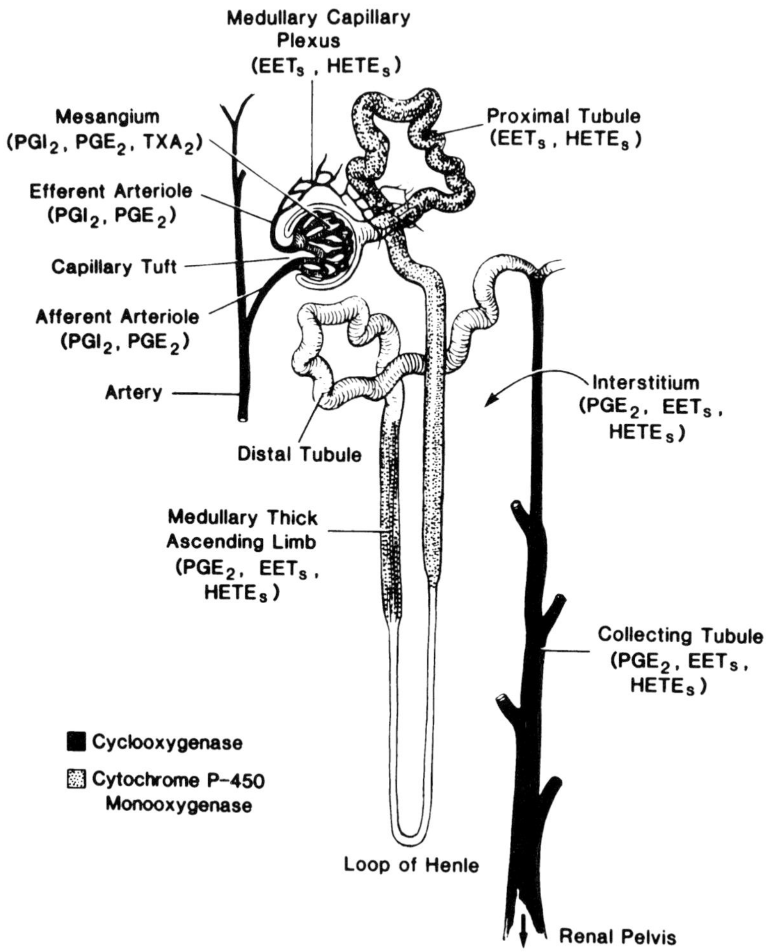

Figure 1 Distribution of renal drug metabolizing enzymes. (From Murray, M. D. and Brater, D. C., *Annu. Rev. Pharmacol. Toxicol.*, 32, 435, 1993. With permission.)

Evidence has also been presented that suggests that P450 expression occurs in the renal medulla. The proximal straight tubule (the S_3 segment; pars recta), located in the outer medulla, was reported to have the highest P450-dependent arachidonic acid (AA) ω- and (ω-1)-fatty acid hydroxylase, and AA epoxygenase activities in rat.[19,23] Arachidonic acid epoxygenase activity has also been reported in the medullary collecting duct.[19] The presence of P450 isozymes catalyzing the metabolism of AA has also been shown in isolated cells from the medullary thick ascending limb of the loop of Henle in rabbits,[24,25] and AA epoxygenase and (ω-1)-hydroxylase activities have been demonstrated to occur in the rat thick ascending limb.[19]

18.3 *Isozymes present in renal tissue*

Cytochrome P450 has been reported to be present in the kidney of rats,[26-28] rabbits,[16,29,30] mice,[28,31] guinea pigs,[32] hamsters,[32] pigs,[33,34] and humans.[35-38]

A number of P450 isozymes have been identified in renal tissue. Evidence for the presence of these P450s has included the detection of P450 protein and mRNA as well as catalytic activities. Some forms have been detected only at the mRNA level. Much of this difficulty is associated with the heterogenous nature of cell types and regions in renal tissue and hence the "dilutional" effect associated with preparation of whole organ homogenates for use in conventional immunoblot or Northern blot analysis. The absence of an isozyme from this presentation should not be interpreted to imply that it is not expressed in the kidney. Rather, the expression of some isozymes has not been examined, while others may be present at levels below the limits of detection of conventional assays for metabolic activity, protein, or mRNA.

The cytochrome P450 superfamily has been categorized into gene families and subfamilies based on amino acid sequence similarity and named according to the nomenclature system of Nelson et al.[39] P450 proteins with ≥40% sequence similarity are grouped in the same family (with some exceptions), while sequences within the same subfamily are >55% identical. The nomenclature includes the root symbol "CYP" ("Cyp" for mouse), which is italicized for the gene and cDNA and not italicized for the protein and mRNA. The root symbol is followed by an Arabic number denoting the family, a capital letter representing the subfamily, and an Arabic number for the individual gene. The correspondence between the different nomenclatures used prior to this system is also provided in Nelson et al.[39]

18.3.1 1A subfamily

CYP1A1 protein has been reported to be constitutively present at very low levels in rat kidney.[40,41] On the other hand, Sesardic et al.[42] found that 1A1 protein was below the limits of detection in untreated rat kidney. CYP1A1 mRNA was reported in trace amounts in untreated fetal and neonatal rat kidney, but was not detectable in kidneys of 46-day-old rats using reverse transcriptase–polymerase chain reaction (RT-PCR).[43] Kim et al.,[44] however, using the same technique, detected constitutive expression of 1A1 mRNA in adult rat kidney.

Treatment of rats with typical CYP1A subfamily inducers, such as 3-methylcholanthrene (3MC), or 2,3,7,8-tetrachlorodibenzo-*p*-dioxin (TCDD), elevated both CYP1A1 mRNA[43,44] and protein[40-42,45] in the kidneys of treated, as compared with untreated, animals.

CYP1A2 protein was reported at low levels in kidney of untreated rat and was increased three-fold by the administration of TCDD.[40] Because of the large increase in CYP1A1 produced by this agent, however, the percentage of total P450 that 1A2 constituted did not change.[40] Kim et al.[44] have recently found that CYP1A2 mRNA, while below the limit of detection using RT-PCR in untreated rat renal tissue, increased in response to treatment with either 3MC or pyridine.

18.3.2 2A subfamily

Two forms of *Cyp2a* — *Cyp2a-4* and *Cyp2a-5* — have been reported to be present in mouse kidney.[46] These forms catalyze the 15α-hydroxylation of testosterone and share approximately 98% amino acid identity. *Cyp2a-4* (testosterone 15α-hydroxylase Type I) mRNA was found to be the predominant form of *Cyp2a* mRNA in male mouse kidney, whereas *Cyp2a-5* (testosterone 15α-hydroxylase Type II) mRNA was the predominant form in female mouse kidney.[46] This pattern of gender specificity was also observed at the protein level in mouse kidney.[47] The male-specific expression was reported to be dependent on the presence of testosterone,[46,47] but not growth hormone.[47]

18.3.3 2B subfamily

Using oligonucleotide probes specific for CYP2B1 and 2B2 mRNAs, Omiecinski[48] and Srivastava et al.[49] were unable to detect either of these mRNA species in kidney of untreated or phenobarbital (PB)-treated rats. However, Srivastava et al.,[49] using a cDNA probe complementary to the mRNAs of 2B1/2B2, were able to detect a single mRNA species, at extremely low levels, in untreated kidney, and the amount of this message was increased following administration of PB and increased to an even greater extent following treatment with the mechanism-based P450 inhibitor, 2-allyl-2-isopropylacetamide. Christou et al.[41] reported that CYP2B1 and 2B2 protein were below the limits of detection in untreated kidney, but were increased to detectable levels in 50% of the kidneys examined following treatment with PB. In contrast, Imaoka et al.[50] were unable to detect 2B1/2B2 protein in kidney of either untreated or phenobarbital-treated rats. Immunodetectable levels of a CYP2B-immunoreactive protein have been reported in rat kidney following cyclosporine treatment.[51] Male mice have been reported to express CYP2B, or an immunologically related form, in renal tissue. This form was not detectable in females. Its expression was not enhanced in response to PB, but was enhanced in both male and female mice in response to dexamethasone treatment.[47]

18.3.4 2C subfamily

The CYP2C subfamily is also represented in the kidney. The presence of testosterone 2α- and 16α-hydroxylase, CYP2C11, was reported in the kidneys of mature, but not immature, male rats,[52] suggesting that 2C11 expression may be developmentally regulated in the kidney. Although CYP2C11 has been reported to be present in hepatic tissue of adult male, but not female, rats,[53] it is unclear whether renal 2C11 expression is also male-specific in the rat.

The arachidonic acid epoxygenases 2CAA (closely related to CYP2C2) in rabbit[54] and 2C23 in rat[55] have also been reported in kidney. Two additional arachidonic acid epoxygenases have been reported in rat kidney that are members of the CYP2C family, one that was demonstrated to be expressed constitutively and was immunochemically related to rat liver CYP2C11 and human liver 2C10,[56] and another that was present following dietary salt loading.[56]

18.3.5 2E subfamily

CYP2E1 mRNA and protein have been reported in kidney of rats,[57] rabbits,[58,59] mice,[60] hamsters,[61,62] and humans.[63] Expression of this protein in the kidney is enhanced in response to administration of a number of xenobiotics, including ethanol,[58,59] acetone,[59] imidazole,[59] dimethylsulfoxide,[64] pyridine,[65] and pyrazole.[66] Ethanol, acetone, imidazole, dimethylsulfoxide, and pyrazole were reported not to increase 2E1 mRNA,[59,64,66] whereas pyridine treatment enhanced both protein and mRNA levels (Figures 2 and 3).[65] Ciprofibrate treatment also increased CYP2E1 mRNA and protein levels in rat renal tissue.[67] Under conditions such as fasting[59,60] and olive oil treatment,[60] 2E1 mRNA and protein levels were reportedly increased in kidney.

Interestingly, 2E1 mRNA and protein levels were reported to be significantly lower in kidney of female compared with male mice. This gender-specific expression was not apparent in the liver. This difference in renal 2E1 expression could be overcome, however, by administration of testosterone to female mice.[60,68] The testosterone-dependent regulation of 2E1 expression in the kidney of male mice has been reported to be dependent on the presence of functional androgen receptors.[68,69] In accordance with these gender-related differences in CYP2E1 expression, male mice are reportedly more susceptible to renal toxicity by CYP2E1-bioactivated compounds, such as acetaminophen,[6] chloroform,[4,5] and 1,1-dichloroethene,[7] than are female mice. In contrast to gender-dependent CYP2E1 expression in mouse kidney, no gender-related difference was reported in rat kidney,[57] and testosterone treatment has been shown to decrease renal CYP2E1 expression in hypophysectomized rats.[70]

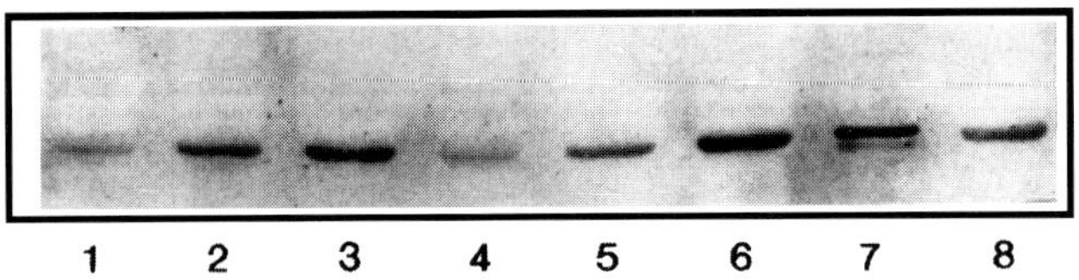

Figure 2 Western blot analysis of time- and dose-dependent increases in renal CYP2E1 after pyridine or pyridine *N*-oxide treatment. Lanes 1 through 6 and 8 contain 20 μg of renal microsomal protein from rats; lane 7 contains purified CYP2E1 protein. The protein band represents the level of immunochemically detectable CYP2E1 protein monitored in untreated animals, (lanes 1 and 4) or in animals treated with either 100 mg pyridine/kg/day for 1 or 3 days (lanes 2 or 3, respectively), 200 mg pyridine/kg/day for 1 or 3 days (lanes 5 or 6, respectively), or 200 mg *N*-oxide/kg/day for 3 days (lane 8). (From Kim, H., Kim, S. G., Lee, M.-Y., and Novak, R. F., *Biochem. Biophys. Res. Commun.*, 186, 846, 1992. With permission.)

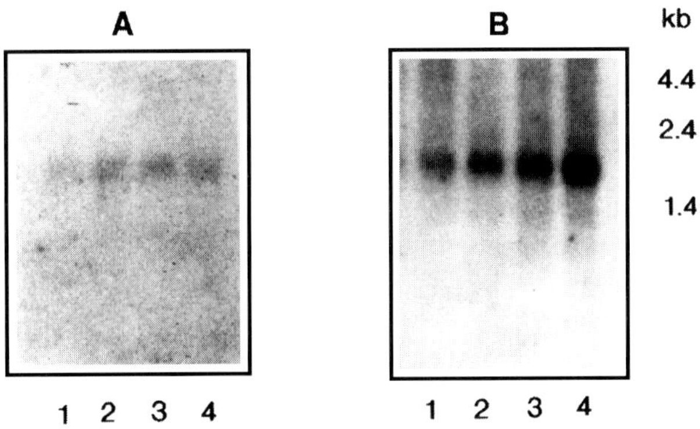

Figure 3 Northern blot analysis of renal CYP2E1 poly(A)$^+$ RNA: Time dependence. Panel A: Poly(A)$^+$ RNA (1 μg/lane) isolated from untreated rat kidney (lane 1) and from rat kidney following treatment with 100 mg pyridine/kg/day, i.p., for 1, 2, or 3 days (lanes 2, 3, or 4, respectively). Panel B: Poly(A)$^+$ RNA (1 μg/lane) isolated from untreated rat kidney (lane 1) and from rat kidney following treatment with 200 mg pyridine/kg/day, i.p., for 1, 2, or 3 days (lanes 2, 3, or 4, respectively). (From Kim, H., Kim, S. G., Lee, M.-Y., and Novak, R. F., *Biochem. Biophys. Res. Commun.*, 186, 846, 1992. With permission.)

18.3.6 3A subfamily

Members of the CYP3A subfamily have been detected in the kidney using immunoblot analysis. CYP3A1 was detected in rat kidney, while 3A3/4 and 3A5 were detected in human renal tissue.[22] These human isozymes apparently exhibited polymorphic expression, with only one in seven adult human kidneys expressing CYP3A3/4, while all human kidney samples examined contained CYP3A5.[22] de Waziers et al.,[63] using immunoblot analysis and erythromycin *N*-demethylase activity, also reported CYP3A4 protein in human kidney.

Schuetz et al.[22] examined an epithelial cell line derived from toad kidney (A6 cells) and detected the CYP3A-catalyzed corticosterone 6β-hydroxylase activity, which was steroid inducible. Immunochemical studies detected a microsomal protein that cross-reacted with CYP3A antibodies, while Northern blot analysis detected an mRNA that cross-hybridized with a CYP3A cDNA. These results suggest that the presence of a steroid-inducible CYP3A in renal tissue may be highly conserved across species.

18.3.7 4A subfamily

Members of the CYP4A subfamily are present in kidney of several species, including rat,[70-72] rabbit,[73,74] mouse,[47] and human.[38] Although these enzymes have not been shown to have a major role in the bioactivation of xenobiotics, they have been shown to catalyze the ω- and (ω-1)-hydroxylation of fatty acids and eicosanoids that may have significant physiological and/or functional effects. This may also represent a rate-limiting step in fatty acid degradation, since the ω-hydroxylated fatty acids are rapidly converted to the di-acids, which can then undergo peroxisomal β-oxidation.

CYP4A2 mRNA was reported to be constitutively expressed at relatively high levels in the renal tissue of male rats,[70,71] but was below the limits of detection using conventional techniques in the renal tissue of female rats, suggesting that testosterone acts as a positive regulator of 4A2 expression in the kidney.[70] CYP4A1 mRNA was reported to be constitutively expressed at relatively low levels in male rat kidney,[71] whereas CYP4A3 mRNA has been reported in renal tissue of male[70,71] and female[70] rats. The expression of these rat renal CYP4A species (4A1, 4A2, 4A3) may be elevated in response to the peroxisome proliferator, clofibrate, although the degree of induction of CYP4A2, which is constitutively expressed at relatively high levels, is substantially less than that of either 4A1 or 4A3.[71,75] CYP4A8 mRNA has also been reported to be constitutively expressed at relatively high levels in rat renal tissue.[76]

P450s 4A5, 4A6, and 4A7 are the major constitutive forms of rabbit renal P450 identified to date,[73,74,77,78] and their expression may be enhanced by treatment with clofibrate or other peroxisome proliferators.[77,79] Expression of CYP4A5 has also been reported to be increased in response to cyclosporine treatment.[77] CYP4A5 and 4A7 were reported to be constitutively expressed at relatively high levels, and their expression was not substantially increased in response to peroxisome proliferators.[74,79] In contrast, CYP4A6 was constitutively expressed at very low levels and its expression was elevated significantly by peroxisome proliferators.[74,79] CYP4A4 mRNA levels, which are normally below the limit of detection in rabbit kidney, have been reported to be increased to detectable levels in renal tissue during pregnancy.[79]

To date, only limited information exists on CYP4A subfamily expression in human renal tissue. CYP4A11 is the only 4A isozyme to have been isolated and purified from human kidney.[38,80]

Given the changes in expression of CYP4A subfamily isozymes in response to peroxisome proliferators and pregnancy, and the role of this subfamily in the metabolism of endogenous lipids and eicosanoids, it has been suggested that altered CYP4A isozyme expression may result in important physiological changes in renal and cardiovascular function, presumably as a result of changes in the levels of bioactive lipids and eicosanoids.[23,81] For example, when placed on a high salt diet, Dahl salt-sensitive rats develop hypertension resulting from abnormal renal function.[82] Development of hypertension appears to be related to low levels of medullary ω-hydroxylation of arachidonic acid to the bioactive 20-hydroxyeicosatetraenoic acid.[83] Treatment with the CYP4A inducer, clofibrate, however, prevented the onset of hypertension in this predisposed strain,[83] suggesting a potentially significant role for CYP4A-mediated metabolism in the development of hypertension. In contrast to the Dahl salt-sensitive rats, renal levels of CYP4A2 are elevated in spontaneously hypertensive rats compared to the parent strain of normotensive rats.[72] Further discussion of the physiological significance of P450-mediated eicosanoid metabolism can be found later in this chapter.

18.4 Methods to quantitate and modulate P450 activities

This section provides a summary of methodologies for use in studies of P450 expression and P450-catalyzed metabolism.

18.4.1 Preparation of renal microsomes

Kidneys are quickly removed from the animal following sacrifice and placed into ice-cold 0.1 *M* sodium (or potassium) phosphate buffer, pH 7.4, containing 1.15% (w/v) KCl.[8] Kidneys can be processed individually, as pairs from an individual animal, or as pools of organs from a number of identically treated animals, depending on the size of the animal and the amount of microsomal protein required for subsequent assays. Moreover, microsomes can be made from either the whole kidney or from cortex and medulla separately by dissecting these sections apart. The tissue is minced and homogenized, on ice, in three volumes of buffer using a Potter–Elvehjem homogenizer with a Teflon® pestle (Registered Trademark of E. I. Du Pont de Nemours and Co., Inc., Wilmington, DE). The homogenate is centrifuged at 9000 × g for 30 min to remove cellular debris, nuclei, and mitochondrial fractions, and the supernatant is centrifuged at 105,000 × g for 60 min. The resulting supernatant is the cytosolic fraction. The pellet (microsomal fraction) is resuspended in the same buffer and is centrifuged at 105,000 × g for 60 min. The final microsomal pellet is resuspended in 0.1 *M* sodium (or potassium) phosphate buffer, pH 7.4, to a final concentration of 10 to 20 mg protein per milliliter.

18.4.2 Measurement of P450 content

Specific P450 content is determined from the carbon monoxide difference spectrum of sodium dithionite-reduced microsomes.[84] Microsomes are suspended in 0.1 *M* potassium phosphate buffer, pH 7.4, to a concentration of 1 to 1.5 mg/ml in a spectrophotometer cuvette. The microsomal suspension is then saturated with carbon monoxide by bubbling for 1 to 2 min, and a baseline spectrum from 500 to 400 nm is recorded. The microsomal suspension is then reduced by the addition of a small amount (1 to 2 mg) of sodium dithionite, and the sample is rescanned to record the difference spectrum. The specific P450 content is calculated using a molar extinction coefficient of 104 $mM^{-1}cm^{-1}$ for $OD_{450\ nm}$ minus $OD_{490\ nm}$.

Orrenius et al.[85] reported that renal microsomes can be significantly contaminated by mitochondrial cytochrome oxidase depending on the severity of the conditions used to prepare the microsomes. If present in substantial amounts, this cytochrome oxidase may interfere with the spectral analysis of renal P450 content by conventional methods. If contamination by mitochondrial enzymes is suspected, the following method may be used to remove or limit interference in determination of P450 content. Mitochondrial cytochrome oxidase exists primarily in the oxidized form, and hence, it is necessary to reduce it prior to assaying the P450 content. Following the addition of 10 m*M* succinate to renal microsomes (1 to 3 mg protein per milliliter) suspended in 50 m*M* TRIS-Cl buffer, pH 7.5, the microsomal suspension is bubbled with carbon monoxide for 2 min. After incubation at room temperature for 5 min (to ensure complete reduction of cytochrome oxidase), a baseline spectrum is recorded from 500 to 400 nm. The P450 in the microsomal suspension is then reduced by the addition of a few milligrams of sodium dithionite, and the difference spectrum of reduced-CO bound P450 minus oxidized P450 is recorded over the same wavelengths.[85] The specific P450 content is calculated using a molar extinction coefficient of 102 $mM^{-1}cm^{-1}$ for $OD_{450\ nm}$ minus $OD_{490\ nm}$.[86]

18.4.3 Enhancement of P450 expression

Levels of renal P450 subfamily members have been shown to increase following treatment with certain xenobiotics. In some cases, these inducing agents may act primarily to enhance a single P450 enzyme or subfamily, although less pronounced effects on other P450 forms and drug metabolizing enzymes, including those involved in phase II metabolism, may also occur. Although these xenobiotics may produce similar changes in P450 expression in both renal and hepatic tissues, as is the case for the compounds listed in Table 1, the mechanisms governing expression as well as the extent and duration of elevated expression may differ. Thus, optimal dosing regimens and times may need to be established.

18.4.4 Inhibition of P450 activity

Mechanism-based P450 inhibitors are substrates that are converted to reactive intermediates through P450 catalysis, with subsequent modification of the enzyme by the reactive metabolite(s), leading to inactivation of the P450.[87] Because of the need for metabolic activation, these agents are generally administered *in vivo* from 1 to 6 h prior to administration of the nephrotoxicant or prior to sacrifice. If used in a microsomal or purified reconstituted system, preincubation periods of 5 to 30 min, in a mixture including the P450 cofactor NADPH, are required prior to addition of the xenobiotic.

Some mechanism-based inhibitors of P450 that have been utilized in studies of renal P450 metabolism include SKF 525A,[88] piperonyl butoxide,[10] methoxsalen,[9] and 17-octadecynoic acid.[89]

Carbon monoxide inhibition of xenobiotic metabolism can be used *in vitro* to determine the overall contribution of P450 to metabolism. The active site of P450 binds carbon monoxide with greater affinity than oxygen, rendering the enzyme catalytically nonfunctional. Incubations are carried out in an atmosphere of $CO–O_2$ (80:20) instead of air or 100% O_2.[90]

Competitive inhibitors are P450 substrates that compete with the xenobiotic for the active site of the enzyme. Competitive inhibitors do not alter the K_m of a substrate, but do result in a decreased V_{max}. Several substrates for specific P450 isoforms are described below. Since competitive inhibitors, by definition, do not require metabolic activation by P450 to cause their inhibitory effects, they can be added to an incubation mixture simultaneously with the xenobiotic in question.

Antibodies raised against a specific P450 can be used to inhibit the catalytic activity of that P450.[37,52] Likewise, antibodies against NADPH–cytochrome P450 reductase can be used to generally inhibit P450 metabolism.[37] Parallel assays are performed using preimmune antisera or IgG to insure that inhibition is the result of the specific antibody, rather than other factors present in the serum or IgG. The antibody, antisera, or IgG, is usually added to the microsomal reaction mixture from 10 to 30 min prior to initiation of metabolism by addition of NADPH or substrate. The inhibition of P450 metabolism by antibodies should occur in a concentration-dependent manner. Cross-reactivity of antibodies with other P450s, especially with closely related forms in a subfamily, needs to be considered when interpreting the results of antibody-inhibition studies.

18.4.5 Monitoring of P450 activity

Several enzymatic assays that are routinely used to determine the catalytic activity of the various P450 forms identified to date in renal tissue are described below. While this is not a comprehensive description of all the assays available, we feel that those listed provide the greatest ease in analysis of metabolic activity, combined with a reasonable degree of selectivity for particular isozymes or subfamilies.

Microsomal incubations to determine metabolic activity are generally performed in 0.1 *M* potassium (or sodium) phosphate or TRIS buffer, pH 7.4, in the presence of 10 m*M* $MgCl_2$ and 1 m*M* NADPH (often supplemented with an NADPH-generating system) at 37°C with constant mixing or shaking to ensure adequate aeration. Although standard protein and substrate concentrations and incubation times are given below, these parameters should be optimized in each case, because enzymatic activities vary with tissue, gender, strain, and age and among different laboratories.

18.4.5.1 CYP1A1 and CYP2B: ethoxy- and pentoxyresorufin O-dealkylation assays

The ethoxyresorufin and pentoxyresorufin *O*-dealkylase activities provide information on the relative levels of rat CYP1A and CYP2B subfamilies, respectively.[91-93] These assays are dynamic fluorometric assays, performed in a 37°C heated fluorometer cuvette in a pH 7.6 potassium phosphate buffer, with 2.5 μ*M* of the appropriate alkoxyresorufin substrate and microsomal protein concentrations of 0.1 to 1 mg/ml. The reactions, initiated by the addition of 1 m*M* NADPH, are generally allowed to proceed for 2 to 10 min. The reaction rate is determined from the slope of product (resorufin) formation, as determined with excitation and emission wavelengths of 530 and 585 nm, respectively. Since the degree of quenching will vary between samples, 10 to 100 pmol of resorufin is added to the cuvette at the end of each assay as an internal standard, and the resulting increase in fluorescence is used to calculate the amount of product formed.

The substrates and product for the alkoxyresorufin assays are susceptible to photohydrolysis, and thus 1 m*M* stock solutions in dimethylsulfoxide are generally stored as aliquots at –20°C or below and are protected from light. Aliquots of substrate and product are added in volumes ≤ 5 μl of dimethylsulfoxide per milliliter of reaction volume to limit possible solvent effects.

18.4.5.2 Cyp2a-4/5 *and CYP2C11: testosterone hydroxylation assay*

The testosterone hydroxylation assay constitutes the most widely accepted assay for these forms. CYP2C11 catalyzes the 16α- and 2α-hydroxylation of testosterone in addition to the conversion of testosterone to androstenedione.[94] The latter conversion, however, may also be catalyzed by 17β-hydroxysteroid oxidoreductase, which is not a P450 enzyme. The *Cyp2a* forms catalyze the 15α-hydroxylation of testosterone.[46] The assay is performed using 50 μ*M* steroid substrate and 0.05 to 0.1 mg of microsomal protein per milliliter. The reaction is initiated by the addition of 1 m*M* NADPH and is allowed to proceed for up to 20 min.[95] Following extraction into organic solvent, the testosterone metabolites are typically separated by thin-layer chromatography[95] or reversed-phase high-performance liquid chromatography (HPLC),[96] with detection at 254 nm and/or by radiometric analysis, with comparison to synthetic standards. Several other P450 forms identified in the kidney also have significant testosterone hydroxylase activity. CYP3A hydroxylates testosterone at the 6β position, while CYP2B hydroxylates the 16β position.[94] Thus, this assay may be used to assess simultaneously the activity or presence of *Cyp2a*, CYP2C11, CYP3A, and CYP2B.

18.4.5.3 CYP2E1: N*-nitrosodimethylamine* N*-demethylation assay*

CYP2E1 associated *N*-nitrosodimethylamine *N*-demethylase (NDMAd) activity has been reported to be increased in hamster kidney by fasting[97] and in rat kidney following isoniazid treatment.[98] Levin et al.[99] examined the conversion of NDMA to formaldehyde by 11 purified hepatic P450s and found that CYP2E1 was at least 15-fold more active in catalyzing the metabolism of 5 m*M* NDMA than any of the other P450 forms examined. Even greater specificity for CYP2E1 activity was obtained when 0.5 m*M* NDMA was tested, although absolute activity rates decreased for all enzymes tested. Similar results have been reported for P450s isolated from rabbit liver.[100]

Inhibition of NDMAd activity by numerous low-molecular-weight organic compounds (e.g., glycerol, semicarbazide, and dithiothreitol) has been reported,[101] and levels of these compounds should be kept at a minimum. When addition of these compounds is unavoidable, such as when microsomes suspended in 20% (v/v) glycerol are used, then care must be taken to ensure that concentrations of these reagents are identical in all sample, standard, and control incubations, in order to control for any inhibitory effects. Since CYP2E1 levels are low in renal microsomes, it may be necessary to use 5 m*M* NDMA to detect basal activity.

Enzymatic assays are performed with microsomal protein concentrations of 0.2 to 2 mg/ml and substrate concentrations of 0.05 to 5 m*M*. The reaction is initiated by addition of 1 m*M* NADPH and is continued for 10 to 20 min. Formaldehyde formation can be determined colorimetrically by the method of Nash[102] or radiometrically by direct scintillation counting of generated [^{14}C]formaldehyde,[99] with comparison to standard amounts of formaldehyde. The Nash procedure is relatively simple and does not require the use of radioactivity, but it is not as sensitive as the radiometric assay. In order to minimize background when utilizing the Nash procedure, only fresh, uncolored acetylacetone should be used.

An alternative, more sensitive, method for the measurement of CYP2E1-dependent catalytic activity is the 6-hydroxylation of chlorzoxazone.[103] This assay has been used to detect CYP2E1 activity in mouse and rat renal microsomes.[7] Chlorzoxazone (0.4 to 1 m*M*) is incubated with microsomal protein (0.4 to 1 mg/ml) and 1 m*M* NADPH for 0 to 30 min, followed by acidification with phosphoric acid and extraction into organic solvent. The 6-hydroxy metabolite is detected by reversed-phase HPLC with detection at 287 nm and quantitation by comparison with standard curves of 6-hydroxychlorzoxazone.[104] Although CYP1A1 has also been reported to catalyze this reaction, it does so with a much higher K_m value and hence should contribute minimally to this activity.[104]

18.4.5.4 *CYP3A: erythromycin* N-*demethylation*

Several reasonably specific assays for CYP3A exist, including testosterone 6β-hydroxylation,[94] triacetyloleandomycin complex formation,[105] and erythromycin *N*-demethylation.[105] Of these three assays, the erythromycin *N*-demethylation analysis is the least complicated. This assay is conducted under conditions similar to those of the NDMAd assay described above, except that 0.4 m*M* erythromycin is used as the substrate. Formation of formaldehyde can be measured spectrophotometrically by the method of Nash.[102]

18.4.5.5 *CYP4A: lauric acid ω-hydroxylation*

The CYP4A-catalyzed ω-hydroxylation of lauric acid appears to be highly conserved in mammalian species. However, the ω-hydroxylation of lauric acid is catalyzed by most members of the CYP4A subfamily, including 4A1,[106] 4A2,[72] 4A5, 4A6, and 4A7.[107] Therefore, this assay is not indicative of the activity of any one specific member of this subfamily. P450-mediated (ω-1)-hydroxylation of fatty acids also occurs and appears to be mediated by several forms of P450. In human liver, (ω-1)-hydroxylase activity is highly correlated with chlorzoxazone 6-hydroxylation, a CYP2E1-catalyzed reaction, and hence does not appear to be associated with CYP4A.[108] In rat liver, treatment with isoniazid,[108] a CYP2E1 inducer, or phenobarbital,[109] which does not increase CYP2E1 or CYP4A, has been reported to increase (ω-1)-hydroxylase activity. However, rabbit 4A isozymes have been shown to exhibit fatty acid (ω-1)-hydroxylase activity.[77,79,107] It therefore appears highly likely that (ω-1)-hydroxylase activity may be catalyzed by more than one P450 subfamily in some species.

The P450-catalyzed ω- and (ω-1)-hydroxylation of lauric acid can be monitored by reverse-phase HPLC separation of 11- and 12-hydroxylaurate.[110] The reaction is carried out using 0.5 mg of microsomal protein per milliliter and 20 to 100 μ*M* lauric acid as substrate. The reaction is initiated by the addition of 1 m*M* NADPH and, following a 5- to 10-min incubation, is stopped by acidification with HCl, followed by extraction of the products into ethyl acetate[111] or diethyl ether.[108,109] This assay has traditionally been performed with ^{14}C-laurate as the substrate with the HPLC-separated products being detected by radiochromatography.[110] However, Dirven et al.[112] recently described derivatization and fluorometric detection of the HPLC-fractionated products.

It is recommended that glassware used for this assay be siliconized to prevent adsorption of the fatty acids to the glass.[111]

18.4.5.6 P450-dependent arachidonic acid oxidation

P450-dependent AA metabolism is thought to play a role in homeostatic control of renal function and blood pressure, as well as in the pathophysiology of hypertension. Several P450-dependent AA metabolites are bioactive, with wide-ranging effects on renal and vascular function. These effects include alterations in transport of Na^+ and K^+ in cortical collecting tubules[113] and loop of Henle[114] and of Na^+ in proximal tubules;[115] inhibition of vasopressin-stimulated water reabsorption;[21,116] renal vasoconstriction;[117,118] stimulation[119] or inhibition[25] of renal $Na^+ - K^+$ ATPase activity; inhibition of renal renin secretion;[120] and potentiation of the tubuloglomerular feedback response.[121] For a more detailed discussion of the biological effects of P450-generated AA metabolites, see Fitzpatrick and Murphy,[122] McGiff,[81] and Omata et al.[23]

Renal P450s metabolize AA to several oxygenated metabolites. Epoxygenase activity results in the formation of four possible regioisomeric epoxyeicosatrienoic acids (EETs) at the 5–6, 8–9, 11–12, and 14–15 positions,[81] which are formed in a regio- and enantioselective manner.[123] These products can then be hydrolyzed by epoxide hydrolase, which is also present in the kidney,[63] to the corresponding dihydroxyeicosatrienoic acids (DHETs).[29,124] Arachidonic acid can also be oxidized at the 5-, 8-, 9-, 11-, 12-, and 15-positions to six regioisomeric *cis–trans* conjugated monohydroxyeicosatetraenoic acids (HETEs).[81] ω/(ω-1)-Hydroxylase activity leads to the formation of 20- and 19-hydroxyeicosatetraenoic acid (20- and 19-HETE), respectively, which can be further metabolized to the 1,20-dioic acid (20-COOH-AA) and to 19 keto-AA.[29,125]

EETs have been detected as endogenous eicosanoids in human kidney[36,37] and urine,[126,127] and 19- and 20-HETEs have also been found in human kidney.[37] 20-HETE has been detected in rat urine, and the concentration was found to be almost twofold higher in the urine of seven-week-old hypertensive rats as compared to normotensive rats.[128]

The P450-dependent metabolism of AA is generally studied *in vitro* through the separation of [1-^{14}C]AA metabolites by HPLC, with identification and quantitation by radiochemical detection.[19,89,129] This assay can be performed with microsomes prepared from whole kidney,[56] renal cortex,[89] or renal medulla or in isolated nephron segments[19] and isolated[17] and cultured[115] renal epithelial cells.

The tissue preparation of choice is incubated for 5 to 20 min in a reaction mixture containing 0.5 mg of microsomal protein per milliliter, 1 to 100 μ*M* [1-^{14}C]AA, and 1 m*M* NADPH. The reaction is terminated by acidification or addition of an organic solvent, and the metabolites are extracted into diethyl ether. Metabolites are separated by reverse-phase HPLC with radiochemical detection (Figure 4).[129] The regioisomeric composition of the generated metabolites can be determined in greater detail by normal-phase HPLC of the pooled ω/ω-1 alcohols, HETEs, or EETs fraction.[129] The enantiomeric composition of the EET regioisomers can be analyzed by HPLC separation of the derivatized regioisomers as described by Capdevila et al.[123]

Endogenous P450 AA metabolites in urine, plasma, or tissues can be determined by gas–liquid chromatography with mass spectrometry (GC/MS), as described by Capdevila et al.[56,123] and Schwartzman et al.[128]

18.4.6 Immunochemical detection of P450

The isolation of microsomes from the whole kidney effectively dilutes out the relatively high level of P450 forms expressed in certain regions or cell types of the kidney. For this reason, sensitive procedures for immunoblot analysis are typically required. While conditions for immunoblot assays are dependent on the affinities of the primary and secondary antibodies used, we have found that the general protocol described below allows detection of the more abundant forms of P450 as well as phase II enzymes.

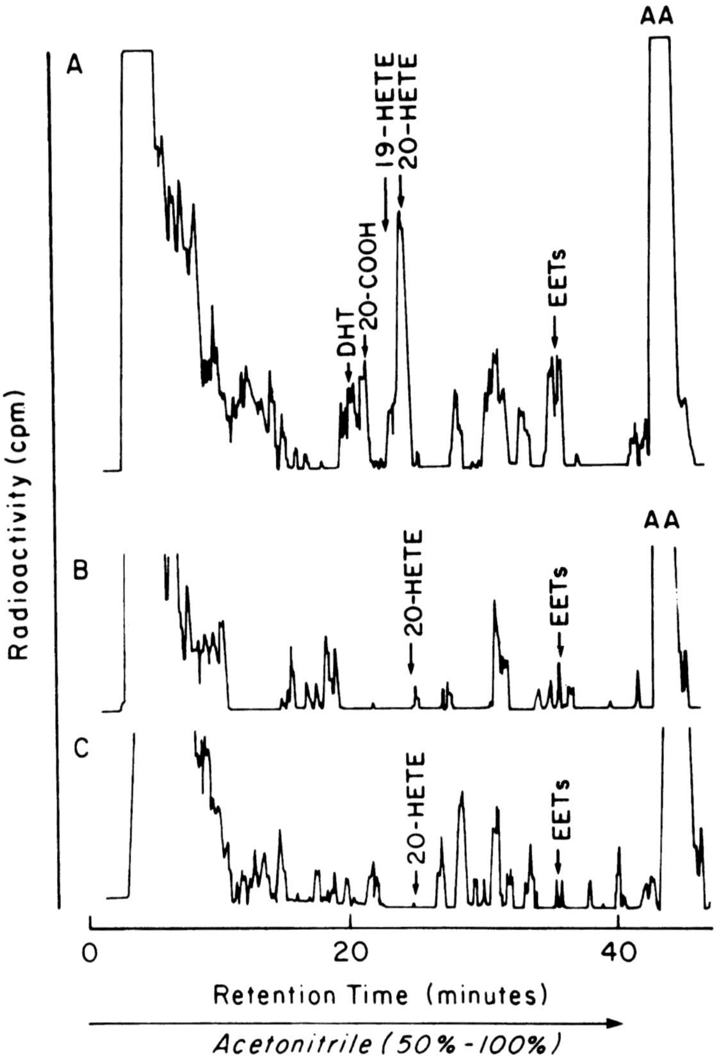

Figure 4 Representative high-performance liquid chromatographic separation of arachidonate metabolites. Arachidonate metabolites were formed by S_2 segments of proximal convoluted tubules incubated with [^{14}C] arachidonate (0.2 μCi, 76 μ*M*), and NADPH (2 m*M*) for 90 min at 37°C (A), in the absence of tubular segments (B), and in the absence of NADPH (C). DHT, diol; 20-COOH, 1,20-dioic acid; HETE, hydroxyeicosatetraenoic acid; EETs, epoxyeicosatrienoic acids; cpm, counts per minute. (From Omata, K., Abraham, N. G., and Schwartzman, M. L., *Am. J. Physiol.*, 262, F591, 1992. With permission.)

Antibody specificity and background interference can be improved by the use of more dilute antibody solutions in combination with longer incubation times. Typically, blots are incubated overnight with highly dilute primary antibody. Incubation conditions should be sterile, if possible, to prevent bacterial growth and antibody degradation. The use of highly sensitive detection systems, such as enhanced chemiluminescence (ECL®; registered trademark of Amersham International plc, Buckinghamshire, England), allows for the use of more dilute antibody solutions and also for the economical use of commercially available antibodies. Our laboratory has found that primary antibodies can often be used at concentrations that are 100-fold more dilute than those suggested by the manufacturer when chemiluminescence detection is employed.

Microsomal proteins are separated using sodium dodecyl sulfate–polyacrylamide gel electrophoresis (SDS-PAGE) and are then electrophoretically transferred to a nitrocellulose membrane.[130] The membrane can be stained using 4 μ*M* amido black, to determine whether uniform transfer has occurred. The following steps are performed at room temperature and with gentle mixing. The blotted membrane is blocked with a 5% (w/v) solution of nonfat powdered milk in phosphate buffered saline (PBS) containing Tween-20 (PBS-T: 10 m*M* sodium phosphate, 154 m*M* NaCl, pH 7.4, 0.05%, v/v, Tween-20). The membrane is washed with PBS-T, then covered with PBS-T containing 0.1% (w/v) bovine serum albumin and 0.01% (v/v) thimerosal. Thimerosal is added to inhibit bacterial growth. Sodium azide is not used because it may inhibit peroxidase activity. Primary antibody is added, and the blot is incubated overnight. The blot is washed with PBS-T, and the secondary antibody is added in 5% (w/v) milk powder in PBS-T and incubated for 3 to 6 h. The membrane is then washed in PBS-T, and film is exposed by chemiluminescent procedures as recommended by the manufacturer. We have found that these procedures are linear over at least a tenfold range of antigen concentrations.[131]

A generalized dark background over the entire blot suggests that primary and/or secondary antibody concentrations are too high. If dark bands are readily detectable in 15 s or less, more dilute antibody solutions should be employed in order to avoid substrate depletion prior to placing the membrane on the film (this procedure takes about 1 min). If "nonspecific" bands (e.g., those not of the expected molecular weight) are detected, repeat the procedure without the primary antibody to determine if the secondary antibody is the source of the problem. If the primary antibody appears to be the source of the problem, occasionally the use of more dilute antibody solutions will disproportionately decrease nonspecific binding.

18.4.7 *Reverse transcriptase–polymerase chain reaction (RT-PCR) for detection of P450 mRNA*

RT-PCR is a highly sensitive method for detection of very low levels of mRNA. Cellular total RNA or poly(A^+) RNA is transcribed to single-stranded cDNA using reverse transcriptase, dNTPs, and random DNA hexamers as primers. The single stranded cDNAs serve as a template in repeated cycles of DNA synthesis using *Taq* DNA polymerase, dNTPS, and sense and antisense oligomers as primers specific for the target P450 cDNA. By carefully selecting the oligomers, annealing temperatures, and Mg^{2+} concentrations, only the region of the target DNA between the selected primers should be amplified. In theory, the target DNA can be amplified 100 million-fold or more, resulting in quantities of DNA that can be detected on an agarose gel by staining with ethidium bromide (Figure 5). The correct size of the product can be confirmed by comparing the migration of the PCR band with that of a DNA ladder and additional confirmation accomplished through restriction analysis and cloning/sequence analysis.

Shown in Table 2 are PCR primers that have been used successfully with RNA that has been isolated from rat kidney to obtain P450 cDNA fragments using RT-PCR.

18.4.8 *Immunohistochemical localization of P450*

The various P450 enzymes are localized in the kidney to specific regions and cell types. Immunohistochemical localization of specific P450 protein(s) to regions or cells in renal tissue may be accomplished using immunohistochemical approaches. Kidneys are fixed in 10% (v/v) formalin, embedded in paraffin, sectioned, and mounted on poly-L-lysine-coated slides. Kidney sections are then deparaffinized in xylene and dehydrated through a series of ethanol baths.[20] The sections are then incubated with primary antibody and immunostained with biotinylated secondary antibody, peroxidase-conjugated avidin, and

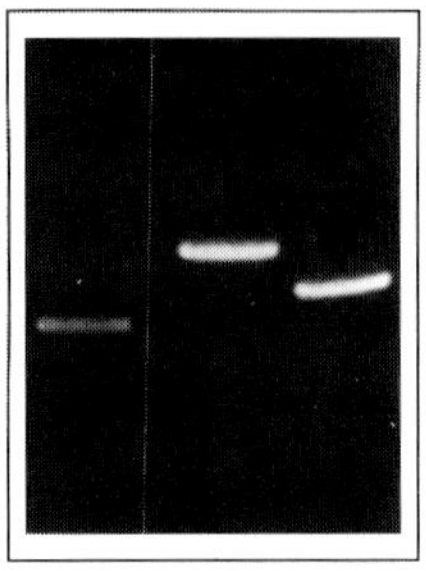

Figure 5 RT-PCR products of renal CYP1A1, 1A2, and 2E1. Rat renal 1A1, 1A2 and 2E1 RT-PCR products were obtained from poly(A)$^+$ RNA isolated from pyridine-treated animals at 24 h following treatment (lane 1) or untreated animals (lanes 2 and 3). (From Kim, H., Reddy, S., and Novak, R. F., 3-Methylcholanthrene and pyridine effects on CYP1A1 and 1A2 expression in rat renal tissue, *Drug Metab. Dispos.*, 23, 818. With permission.)

Table 2 PCR Primers and Product Sizes for CYP1A1, 1A2, and 2E1 Isozymes in Rat

P450	Primer sequence	Product size	Ref.
CYP1A1	5′-CCATGACCAGGAACTATGGG-3′ 5′-TCTGGTGAGCATCCAGGACA-3′	341 bp	43
CYP1A1	5′-TGACCTCTTTGGAGCT-3′ 5′-TTGAGCCTCAGCAGAT-3′	1050 bp	44
CYP1A2	5′-TGACCTCTTTGGAGCT-3′ 5′-GACGTCTTCACAGGTT-3′	600 bp	44
CYP2E1	5′-TCTGAGGCTCATGAGT-3′ 5′-GACAGGAGCAGAAACA-3′	770 bp	44

peroxidase substrate, as described previously (Figure 6).[18,20] Alternatively, the bound antibody can be visualized with alkaline phosphatase-conjugated secondary antibody and phosphatase substrate.[2] The parallel analysis of samples using pre-immune sera, or IgG, is essential to demonstrate specific binding of the primary antibody. To examine whether enhanced expression occurred in response to treatment, a dilutional analysis of staining density should be accomplished in concert with the pre-immune sera or IgG controls.

18.4.9 In situ *hybridization of P450 mRNA*

In situ hybridization of mRNA, like immunohistochemical localization of a P450 protein, can be used to examine the intraorgan distribution and cellular localization of P450 mRNA expression. However, in cases where there are several highly related forms expressed in the kidney, such as with the CYP4A subfamily, *in situ* hybridization may be more selective for a particular P450 form than immunohistochemical localization, because of the potentially greater specificity of the probe.[76]

Kidneys are embedded in Tissue Tek O.C.T.® compound (registered trademark of Miles Laboratories Inc., Naperville, IL), frozen on dry ice, and sectioned onto poly-L-lysine-coated slides. Sections are fixed in 4% (v/v) paraformaldehyde in PBS, washed with ethanol, treated with 0.2 *M* HCl and washed with PBS. The slides are then incubated with 0.25% (v/v) acetic anhydride, washed with PBS, and dehydrated with ethanol.[76,132] Sections are then hybridized with a specific cDNA or oligomeric probe that has been radiolabeled.[76,132] Localization of the probe in the renal slice is then visualized by direct exposure of the sample to film.

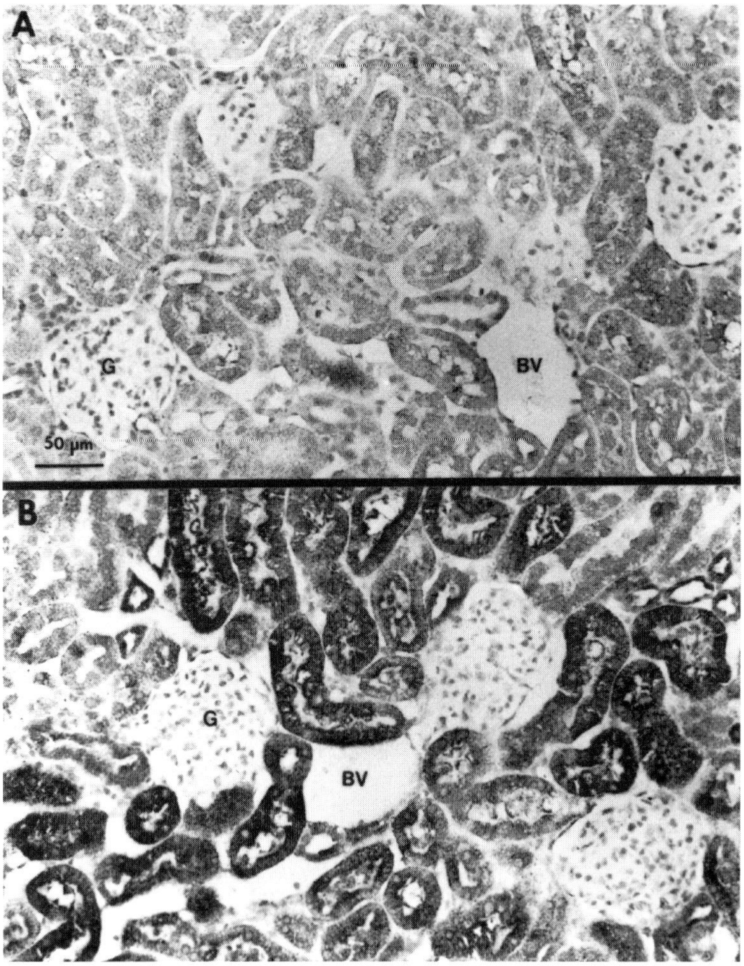

Figure 6 Light photomicrographs of kidney sections from rats intraperitoneally injected with saline once (A) or with 200 mg/kg pyridine/day for 3 days. The tissue sections were immunohistochemically stained to detect CYP2E1. G, glomerulus; BV, blood vessel. (From Hotchkiss, J. A., Kim, H., Hahn, F. F., Novak, R. F., and Dahl, A. R., *Toxicol. Lett.*, 78, 1, 1995.)

References

1. Liehr, J. G., Hall, E. R., Avitts, T. A., Randerath, E., and Randerath, K., Localization of estrogen-induced DNA adducts and cytochrome P-450 activity at the site of renal carcinogenesis in the hamster kidney, *Cancer Res.*, 47, 2156, 1987.
2. Emeigh Hart, S. G., Cartun, R. W., Wyand, D. S., Khairallah, E. A., and Cohen, S. D., Immunohistochemical localization of acetaminophen in target tissues of the CD-1 mouse: correspondence of covalent binding with toxicity, *Fundam. Appl. Toxicol.*, 24, 260, 1995.
3. Newton, J. F., Yoshimoto, M., Bernstein, J., Rush, G. F., and Hook, J. B., Acetaminophen nephrotoxicity in the rat. I. Strain differences in nephrotoxicity and metabolism, *Toxicol. Appl. Pharmacol.*, 69, 291, 1983.
4. Smith, J. H., Maita, K., Sleight, S. D., and Hook, J. B., Mechanism of chloroform nephrotoxicity. I. Time course of chloroform toxicity in male and female mice, *Toxicol. Appl. Pharmacol.*, 70, 467, 1983.
5. Smith, J. H., Maita, K., Sleight, S. D., and Hook, J. B., Effect of sex hormone status on chloroform nephrotoxicity and renal mixed function oxidases in mice, *Toxicology*, 30, 305, 1984.

6. Hu, J. J., Lee, M.-J., Vapiwala, M., Reuhl, K., Thomas, P. E., and Yang, C. S., Sex-related differences in mouse renal metabolism and toxicity of acetaminophen, *Toxicol. Appl. Pharmacol.*, 122, 16, 1993.
7. Speerschneider, P. and Dekant, W., Renal tumorigenicity of 1,1-dichloroethene in mice: the role of male-specific expression of cytochrome P450 2E1 in the renal bioactivation of 1,1-dichloroethene, *Toxicol. Appl. Pharmacol.*, 130, 48, 1995.
8. Bailie, M. B., Smith, J. H., Newton, J. F., and Hook, J. B., Mechanism of chloroform nephrotoxicity. IV. Phenobarbital potentiation of *in vitro* chloroform metabolism and toxicity in rabbit kidneys, *Toxicol. Appl. Pharmacol.*, 74, 285, 1984.
9. Letteron, P., Degott, C., Labbe, G., Larrey, D., Descatoire, V., Tinel, M., and Pessayre, D., Methoxsalen decreases the metabolic activation and prevents the hepatotoxicity and nephrotoxicity of chloroform in mice, *Toxicol. Appl. Pharmacol.*, 91, 266, 1987.
10. Valentovic, M. A., Ball, J. G., Anestis, D., and Madan, E., Modification of P450 activity and its effect on 1,2-dichlorobenzene toxicity in Fischer 344 rats, *Toxicology*, 79, 169, 1993.
11. Smith, J. H. and Hook, J. B., Mechanism of chloroform nephrotoxicity. II. *In vitro* evidence for renal metabolism of chloroform in mice, *Toxicol. Appl. Pharmacol.*, 70, 480, 1983.
12. Guengerich, F. P., Brian, W. R., Sari, M-A., and Ross, J. T., Expression of mammalian cytochrome P450 enzymes using yeast-based vectors, *Methods Enzymol.*, 206, 130, 1991.
13. Clark, B. J. and Waterman, M. R., Heterologous expression of mammalian P450 in COS cells, *Methods Enzymol.*, 206, 100, 1991.
14. Gonzalez, F. J., Aoyama, T., and Gelboin, H. V., Expression of mammalian cytochrome P450 using vaccinia virus, *Methods Enzymol.*, 206, 85, 1991.
15. Gonzalez, F. J., Kimura, S., Tamura, S., and Gelboin, H. V., Expression of mammalian cytochrome P450 using baculovirus, *Methods Enzymol.*, 206, 93, 1991.
16. Endou, H., Cytochrome P450 monooxygenase system in the rabbit kidney: its intranephron localization and its induction, *Jpn. J. Pharmacol.*, 33, 423, 1983.
17. Koop, D., Morrison, A., and Douglas, J., Co-expression of cytochrome P450 and metabolism of arachidonic acid to novel products by early proximal tubular epithelial cells, *Kidney Int.*, 33, 162, 1988.
18. Hu, J. J., Rhoten, W. B., and Yang, C. S., Mouse renal cytochrome P450IIE1: immunocytochemical localization, sex-related difference and regulation by testosterone, *Biochem. Pharmacol.*, 40, 2597, 1990.
19. Omata, K., Abraham, N. G., and Schwartzman, M. L., Renal cytochrome P450-arachidonic acid metabolism: localization and hormonal regulation in SHR, *Am. J. Physiol.*, 262, F591, 1992.
20. Hotchkiss, J. A., Kim, H., Hahn, F. F., Novak, R. F., and Dahl, A. R., Pyridine induction of Sprague–Dawley rat renal cytochrome P4502E1: immunohistochemical localization and quantitation, *Toxicol. Lett.*, 78, 1, 1995.
21. Hirt, D. L., Capdevila, J., Falck, J. R., Breyer, M. D., and Jacobson, H. R., Cytochrome P450 metabolites of arachidonic acid are potent inhibitors of vasopressin action on rabbit cortical collecting duct, *J. Clin. Invest.*, 84, 1805, 1989.
22. Schuetz, E. G., Schuetz, J. D., Grogan, W. M., Naray-Fejes-Toth, A., Fejes-Toth, G., Raucy, J., Guzelian, P., Gionela, K., and Watlington, C. O., Expression of cytochrome P450 3A in amphibian, rat, and human kidney, *Arch. Biochem. Biophys.*, 294, 206, 1992.
23. Omata, K., Abe, K., Sheu, H.-L., Yoshida, K., Tsutsumi, E., Yoshinaga, K., Abraham, N. G., and Schwartzman, M. L., Roles of renal cytochrome P450-dependent arachidonic acid metabolites in hypertension, *Tohoku J. Exp. Med.*, 166, 93, 1992.
24. Schwartzman, M., Carroll, M. A., Abraham, N. G., Ferreri, N. R., Songu-Mize, E., and McGiff, J. C., Renal arachidonic acid metabolism: the third pathway, *Hypertension*, 7, I-136, 1985.
25. Schwartzman, M., Ferreri, N. R., Carroll, M. A., Songu-Mize, E., and McGiff, J. C., Renal cytochrome P450-related arachidonate metabolite inhibits (Na^+-K^+)ATPase, *Nature*, 314, 620, 1985.
26. Jakobsson, S., Thor, H., and Orrenuis, S., Fatty-acid inducible cytochrome P450 of rat kidney cortex microsomes, *Biochem. Biophys. Res. Commun.*, 39, 1073, 1970.
27. Ellin, A., Jakobsson, S. V., Schenkman, J. B., and Orrenius, S., Cytochrome $P450_K$ of rat kidney cortex microsomes: its involvement in fatty acid ω- and (ω-1)-hydroxylation, *Arch. Biochem. Biophys.*, 150, 64, 1972.

28. Hook, J. B., Elcombe, C. R., Rose, M. S., and Lock, E. A., Characterization of the effects of known hepatic monooxygenase inducers on male and female rat and mouse kidneys, *Life Sci.*, 31, 1077, 1982.
29. Oliw, E. H., Lawson, J. A., Brash, A. R., and Oates, J. A., Arachidonic acid metabolism in rabbit renal cortex: formation of two novel dihydroxyeicosatrienoic acids, *J. Biol. Chem.*, 256, 9924, 1981.
30. Dees, J. H., Masters, B. S. S., Muller-Eberhard, U., and Johnson, E. F., Effect of 2,3,7,8-tetrachlorodibenzo-*p*-dioxin and phenobarbital on the occurrence and distribution of four cytochrome P450 isozymes in rabbit kidney, lung and liver, *Cancer Res.*, 42, 1423, 1982.
31. Hawke, R. L. and Welch, R. M., Major differences in the specificity and regulation of mouse renal cytochrome P450-dependent monooxygenases: a comparison of xenobiotic and endogenous substrates, *Mol. Pharmacol.*, 27, 283, 1985.
32. Smith, J. H., Rush, G. F., and Hook, J. B., Induction of renal and hepatic mixed function oxidases in the hamster and guinea pig, *Toxicology*, 38, 209, 1986.
33. Masters, B. S. S., Parkhill, L. K., Yasukochi, Y., Okita, R. T., Theoharides, A. D., and Kupfer, D., Pig liver and kidney microsomal cytochromes P450: specificities for drugs, fatty acids, and prostaglandins in reconstituted systems, in *Biochemistry, Biophysics, and Regulation of Cytochrome P450*, Gustafsson, J. A., Carlstedt-Duke, J., Mode, A., and Rafter, J., Eds., Elsevier/North-Holland, Amsterdam, 1980, 101.
34. Okita, R. T., Parkhill, L. K., Yasukochi, Y., Masters, B. S. S., Theoharides, A. D., and Kupfer, D., The ω-and (ω-1)-hydroxylase activities of prostaglandins A_1 and E_1 and lauric acid by pig kidney microsomes and a purified kidney cytochrome P450, *J. Biol. Chem.*, 256, 5961, 1981.
35. Jakobsson, S. W. and Cinti, D. L., Studies on the cytochrome P450-containing monooxygenase system in human kidney cortex microsomes, *J. Pharmacol. Exp. Ther.*, 185, 226, 1973.
36. Karara, A., Dishman, E., Jacobson, H., Falck, J. R., and Capdevila, J. H., Arachidonic acid epoxygenase: stereochemical analysis of the endogenous epoxyeicosatrienoic acids of human kidney cortex, *FEBS Lett.*, 268, 227, 1990.
37. Schwartzman, M. L., Martasek, P., Rios, A. R., Levere, R. D., Solangi, K., Goodman, A. I., and Abraham, N. G., Cytochrome P450-dependent arachidonic acid metabolism in human kidney, *Kidney Int.*, 37, 94, 1990.
38. Kawashima, H., Kusunose, E., Kubota, I., Maekawa, M., and Kusunose, M., Purification and NH_2-terminal amino acid sequences of human and rat kidney fatty acid ω-hydroxylases, *Biochim. Biophys. Acta*, 1123, 156, 1992.
39. Nelson, D. R., Kamataki, T., Waxman, D. J., Guengerich, F. P., Estabrook, R. W., Feyereisen, R., Gonzalez, F. J., Coon, M. J., Gunsalus, I. C., Gotoh, O., Okuda, K., and Nebert, D. W., The P450 superfamily: update on new sequences, gene mapping, accession numbers, early trivial names of enzymes, and nomenclature, *DNA Cell Biol.*, 12, 1, 1993.
40. Goldstein, J. A. and Linko, P., Differential induction of two 2,3,7,8-tetrachlorodibenzo-*p*-dioxin-inducible forms of cytochrome P450 in extrahepatic vs. hepatic tissues, *Mol. Pharmacol.*, 25, 185, 1984.
41. Christou, M., Wilson, N. M., and Jefcoate, C. R., Expression and function of three cytochrome P-450 isozymes in rat extrahepatic tissues, *Arch. Biochem. Biophys.*, 258, 519, 1987.
42. Sesardic, D., Cole, K. J., Edwards, R. J., Davies, D. S., Thomas, P. E., Levin, W., and Boobis, A. R., The inducibility and catalytic activity of cytochromes P450c (P4501A1) and P450d (P4501A2) in rat tissues, *Biochem. Pharmacol.*, 39, 499, 1990.
43. Omiecinski, C. J., Redlich, C. A., and Costa, P., Induction and developmental expression of cytochrome P450IA1 messenger RNA in rat and human tissues: detection by the polymerase chain reaction, *Cancer Res.*, 50, 4315, 1990.
44. Kim, H., Reddy, S., and Novak, R. F., 3-Methylcholanthrene and pyridine effects on CYP1A1 and 1A2 expression in rat renal tissue, *Drug Metab. Dispos.*, 23, 818, 1995.
45. Ogita, K., Kusunose, E., Ichihara, K., and Kusunose, M., Multiple forms of cytochrome P450 in kidney cortex microsomes of rabbits treated with 3-methylcholanthrene, *J. Biochem.*, 92, 921, 1982.
46. Squires, E. J. and Negishi, M., Reciprocal regulation of sex-dependent expression of testosterone 15α-hydroxylase ($P450_{15\alpha}$) in liver and kidney of male mice by androgen: evidence for a single gene, *J. Biol. Chem.*, 263, 4166, 1988.

47. Henderson, C. J., Scott, A. R., Yang, C. S., and Wolf, C. R., Testosterone-mediated regulation of mouse renal cytochrome P-450 isoenzymes, *Biochem. J.*, 266, 675, 1990.
48. Omiecinski, C. J., Tissue-specific expression of rat mRNAs homologous to cytochromes P-450b and P-450e, *Nucleic Acids Res.*, 14, 1525, 1986.
49. Srivastava, G., Bawden, M. J., Anderson, A., and May, B. K., Drug induction of P450IIB1/IIB2 and 5-aminolevulinate synthase mRNAs in rat tissues, *Biochem. Biophys. Acta*, 1007, 192, 1989.
50. Imaoka, S., Terano, Y., and Funae, Y., Expression of four phenobarbital-inducible cytochrome P450s in liver, kidney, and lung of rats, *J. Biochem.*, 105, 939, 1989.
51. Yoshimura, R., Yoshimura, N., Kusunose, E., Matsui, S., Hamashima, T., Kishimoto, T., Oka, T., Kusnose, M., and Maekawa, M., Role of kidney cytochrome P-450 in cyclosporin induced nephropathy, *Transplant. Proc.*, 21, 934, 1989.
52. Sonderfan, A. J., Arlotto, M. P., and Parkinson, A., Identification of the cytochrome P-450 isozymes responsible for testosterone oxidation in rat lung, kidney, and testis: evidence that cytochrome P-450a (P450IIA1) is the physiologically important testosterone 7α-hydroxylase in rat testis, *Endocrinology*, 125, 857, 1989.
53. Yoshioka, H., Morohashi, K.-I., Sogawa, K., Miyata, T., Kawajiri, K., Hirose, T., Inayama, S., Fujii-Kuriyama, Y., and Omura, T., Structural analysis and specific expression of microsomal cytochrome P-450(M-1) mRNA in male rat livers, *J. Biol. Chem.*, 262, 1706, 1987.
54. Laethem, R. M., Laethem, C. L., and Koop, D. R., Purification and properties of a cytochrome P450 arachidonic acid epoxygenase from rabbit renal cortex, *J. Biol. Chem.*, 267, 5552, 1992.
55. Imaoka, S., Wedlund, P. J., Ogawa, H., Kimura, S., Gonzalez, F. J., and Kim, H.-Y., Identification of CYP2C23 expressed in rat kidney as an arachidonic acid epoxygenase, *J. Pharmacol. Exp. Ther.*, 267, 1012, 1993.
56. Capdevila, J. H., Wei, S., Yan, J., Karara, A., Jacobson, H. R., Falck, J. R., Guengerich, F. P., and DuBois, R. N., Cytochrome P450 arachidonic acid epoxygenase: regulatory control of the renal epoxygenase by dietary salt loading, *J. Biol. Chem.*, 267, 21720, 1992.
57. Hong, J.-Y., Pan, J., Dong, Z., Ning, S. M., and Yang, C. S., Regulation of *N*-nitrosodimethylamine demethylase in rat liver and kidney, *Cancer Res.*, 47, 5948, 1987.
58. Ding, X., Koop, D. R., Crump, B. L., and Coon, M. J., Immunochemical identification of cytochrome P450 isozyme 3a (P-450_{ALC}) in rat nasal and kidney microsomes and evidence for differential induction by alcohol, *Mol. Pharmacol.*, 30, 370, 1986.
59. Porter, T. D., Khani, S. C., and Coon, M. J., Induction and tissue-specific expression of rabbit cytochrome P450IIE1 and IIE2 genes, *Mol. Pharmacol.*, 36, 61, 1989.
60. Hong, J.-Y., Pan, J., Ning, S. M., and Yang, C. S., Molecular basis for the sex-related difference in renal *N*-nitrosodimethylamine demethylase in C3H/HeJ mice, *Cancer Res.*, 49, 2973, 1989.
61. Menicagli, S., Puccini, P., Longo, V., and Gervasi, P. G., Effect of acetone administration on renal, pulmonary and hepatic monooxygenase activities in hamster, *Toxicology*, 64, 141, 1990.
62. Ueng, T-H., Tsai, J-N., Ju, J-M., Ueng, Y-F., Iwasaki, M., and Guengerich, F. P., Effects of acetone administration on cytochrome P450-dependent monooxygenases in hamster liver, kidney, and lung, *Arch. Toxicol.*, 65, 45, 1991.
63. de Waziers, I., Cugnenc, P. H., Yang, C. S., Leroux, J-P., and Beaune, P. H., Cytochrome P450 isoenzymes, epoxide hydrolase and glutathione transferases in rat and human hepatic and extrahepatic tissues, *J. Pharmacol. Exp. Ther.*, 253, 387, 1990.
64. Zangar, R. C. and Novak, R. F., Enhanced expression of renal cytochrome P450 2E1 (CYP2E1) following treatment with dimethylsulfoxide (DMSO), *Toxicologist*, 14, 119, 1994.
65. Kim, H., Kim, S. G., Lee, M.-Y., and Novak, R. F., Evidence for elevation of cytochrome P4502E1 (alcohol-inducible form) mRNA levels in rat kidney following pyridine administration, *Biochem. Biophys. Res. Commun.*, 186, 846, 1992.
66. Wu, D. and Cederbaum, A. I., Characterization of pyrazole and 4-methylpyrazole induction of cytochrome P4502E1 in rat kidney, *J. Pharmacol. Exp. Ther.*, 270, 407, 1994.
67. Zangar, R. C., Woodcroft, K. J., and Novak, R. F., Enhancement of cytochrome P450 2E1 (CYP2E1) in rat kidney by ciprofibrate, *Toxicologist*, 15, 3, 1995.
68. Davis, J. F. and Felder, M. R., Mouse ethanol-inducible cytochrome P-450 (P450IIE1): characterization of cDNA clones and testosterone induction in kidney tissue, *J. Biol. Chem.*, 268, 16584, 1993.

69. Pan, J., Hong, J.-Y., and Yang, C. S., Post-transcriptional regulation of mouse renal cytochrome P450 2E1 by testosterone, *Arch. Biochem. Biophys.*, 299, 110, 1992.
70. Sundseth, S. S. and Waxman, D. J., Sex-dependent expression and clofibrate inducibility of cytochrome P450 4A fatty acid ω-hydroxylases: male specificity of liver and kidney CYP4A2 mRNA and tissue-specific regulation by growth hormone and testosterone, *J. Biol. Chem.*, 267, 3915, 1992.
71. Kimura, S., Hardwick, J. P., Kozak, C. A., and Gonzalez, F. J., The rat clofibrate-inducible *CYP4A* subfamily. II. cDNA sequence of IVA3, mapping of the *Cyp4A* locus to mouse chromosome 4, and coordinate and tissue-specific regulation of the *CYP4A* genes, *DNA*, 8, 517, 1989.
72. Imaoka, S. and Funae, Y., Hepatic and renal cytochrome P-450s in spontaneously hypertensive rats, *Biochem. Biophys. Acta*, 1074, 209, 1991.
73. Kusunose, E., Sawamura, A., Kawashima, H., Kubota, I., and Kusunose, M., Isolation of a new form of cytochrome P450 with prostaglandin A and fatty acid ω-hydroxylase activities from rabbit kidney cortex microsomes, *J. Biochem.*, 106, 194, 1989.
74. Yokotani, N., Bernhardt, R., Sogawa, K., Kusunose, E., Gotoh, O., Kusunose, M., and Fujii-Kuriyama, Y., Two forms of ω-hydroxylase toward prostaglandin A and laurate: cDNA cloning and their expression, *J. Biol. Chem.*, 264, 21665, 1989.
75. Sharma, R. K., Lake, B. G., Makowski, R., Bradshaw, T., Earnshaw, D., Dale, J. W., and Gibson, G. G., Differential induction of peroxisomal and microsomal fatty-acid-oxidising enzymes by peroxisome proliferators in rat liver and kidney: characterisation of a renal cytochrome P450 and implications for peroxisome proliferation, *Eur. J. Biochem.*, 184, 69, 1989.
76. Stromstedt, M., Hayashi, S-I., Zaphiropoulos, P. G., and Gustafsson, J-A., Cloning and characterization of a novel member of the cytrochrome P450 subfamily IVA in rat prostate, *DNA Cell Biol.*, 9, 569, 1990.
77. Yokotani, N., Kusunose, E., Sogawa, K., Kawashima, H., Kinosaki, M., Kusunose, M., and Fujii-Kuriyama, Y., cDNA cloning and expression of the mRNA for cytochrome $P\text{-}450_{kd}$ which shows a fatty acid ω-hydroxylating activity, *Eur. J. Biochem.*, 196, 531, 1991.
78. Kusunose, M., Kikuta, Y., Kusunose, E., Matsubara, S., Yokotani, N., Kubota, I., Sogawa, K., and Fujii-Kuriyama, Y., Prostaglandin ω-hydroxylase and related cytochrome P450, in *Advances in Prostaglandin, Thromboxane, and Leukotriene Research*, Vol. 19, Samuelsson, B., Wong, P. Y-K., and Sun, F. F., Eds., Raven Press, New York, 1989, 343.
79. Roman, L. J., Palmer, C. N. A., Clark, J. E., Muerhoff, A. S., Griffin, K. J., Johnson, E. F., and Masters, B. S. S., Expression of rabbit cytochromes P4504A which catalyze the ω-hydroxylation of arachidonic acid, fatty acids, and prostaglandins, *Arch. Biochem. Biophys.*, 307, 57, 1993.
80. Imaoka, S., Ogawa, H., Kimura, S., and Gonzalez, F. J., Complete cDNA sequence and cDNA-directed expression of CYP4A11, a fatty acid omega-hydroxylase expressed in human kidney, *DNA Cell Biol.*, 12, 893, 1993.
81. McGiff, J. C., Cytochrome P450 metabolism of arachidonic acid, *Annu. Rev. Pharmacol. Toxicol.*, 31, 339, 1991.
82. Dahl, L. K. and Heine, M., Primary role of renal homografts in setting chronic blood pressure levels in rats, *Circ. Res.*, 36, 692, 1975.
83. Roman, R. J., Ma, Y.-H., Frohlich, B., and Markham, B., Clofibrate prevents the development of hypertension in Dahl salt-sensitive rats, *Hypertension*, 21, 985, 1993.
84. Matsubara, T., Koike, M., Touchi, A., Tochino, Y., and Sugeno, K., Quantitative determination of cytochrome P450 in rat liver homogenate, *Anal. Biochem.*, 75, 596, 1976.
85. Orrenius, S., Ellin, A., Jakobsson, S. V., Thor, H., Cinti, D. L., Schenkman, J. B., and Estabrook, R. W., The cytochrome P450-containing mono-oxygenase system of rat kidney cortex microsomes, *Drug Metab. Dispos.*, 1, 350, 1973.
86. Jones, D. P., Sundby, G.-B., Ormstad, K., and Orrenius, S., Use of isolated kidney cells for study of drug metabolism, *Biochem. Pharmacol.*, 28, 929, 1979.
87. Rando, R. R., Mechanism-based enzyme inactivators, *Pharmacol. Rev.*, 36, 111, 1984.
88. Geneve, J., Larrey, D., Letteron, P., Descatoire, V., Tinel, M., Amouyal, G., and Pessayre, D., Metabolic activation of the tricyclic antidepressant amineptine. I. Cytochrome P450-mediated *in vitro* covalent binding, *Biochem. Pharmacol.*, 36, 323, 1987.

89. Zou, A.-P., Ma, Y.-H., Sui, Z.-H., Ortiz de Montellano, P. R., Clark, J. E., Masters, B. S., and Roman, R. J., Effects of 17-octadecynoic acid, a suicide-substrate inhibitor of cytochrome P450 fatty acid ω-hydroxylase, on renal function in rats, *J. Pharmacol. Exp. Ther.*, 268, 474, 1994.
90. Smith, J. H. and Hook, J. B., Mechanism of chloroform nephrotoxicity. III. Renal and hepatic microsomal metabolism of chloroform in mice, *Toxicol. Appl. Pharmacol.*, 73, 511, 1984.
91. Burke, M. D. and Mayer, R. T., Ethoxyresorufin: direct fluorimetric assay of a microsomal *O*-dealkylation which is preferentially inducible by 3-methylcholanthrene, *Drug Metab. Dispos.*, 2, 583, 1974.
92. Burke, M. D., Thompson, S., Elcombe, C. R., Halpert, J., Haaparanta, T., and Mayer, R. T., Ethoxy-, pentoxy- and benzyloxyphenoxazones and homologues: a series of substrates to distinguish between different induced cytochromes P-450, *Biochem. Pharmacol.*, 34, 3337, 1985.
93. Lubet, R. A., Mayer, R. T., Cameron, J. W., Nims, R. W., Burke, M. D., Wolff, T., and Guengerich, F. P., Dealkylation of pentoxyresorufin: a rapid and sensitive assay for measuring induction of cytochrome(s) P-450 by phenobarbital and other xenobiotics in the rat, *Arch. Biochem. Biophys.*, 238, 43, 1985.
94. Waxman, D. J., Interactions of hepatic cytochromes P-450 with steroid hormones: regioselectivity and stereospecificity of steroid metabolism and hormonal regulation of rat P450 enzyme expression, *Biochem. Pharmacol.*, 37, 71, 1988.
95. Waxman, D. J., P450-catalyzed steroid hydroxylation: assay and product identification by thin-layer chromatography, *Methods Enzymol.*, 206, 462, 1991.
96. Arlotto, M. P., Trant, J. M., and Estabrook, R. W., Measurement of steroid hydroxylation reactions by high-performance liquid chromatography as indicator of P450 identity and function, *Methods Enzymol.*, 206, 454, 1991.
97. Ueng, T.-H., Ueng, Y.-F., Chen, T.-L., Park, S. S., Iwasaki, M., and Guengerich, F. P., Induction of cytochrome P450-dependent monoxygenases in hamster tissues by fasting, *Toxicol. Appl. Pharmacol.*, 116, 66, 1993.
98. Thomas, P. E., Bandiera, S., Maines, S. L., Ryan, D. E., and Levin, W., Regulation of cytochrome P-450j, a high-affinity *N*-nitrosodimethylamine demethylase, in rat hepatic microsomes, *Biochemistry*, 26, 2280, 1987.
99. Levin, W., Thomas, P. E., Oldfield, N., and Ryan, D. E., *N*-demethylation of *N*-nitrosodimethylamine catalyzed by purified rat hepatic microsomal cytochrome P-450: isozyme specificity and role of cytochrome b_5, *Arch. Biochem. Biophys.*, 248, 158, 1986.
100. Yang, C. S., Tu, Y. Y., Koop, D. R., and Coon, M. J., Metabolism of nitrosamines by purified rabbit liver cytochrome P-450 isozymes, *Cancer Res.*, 45, 1140, 1985.
101. Yoo, J.-S. H., Cheung, R. J., Patten, C. J., Wade, D., and Yang, C. S., Nature of *N*-nitrosodimethylamine demethylase and its inhibitors, *Cancer Res.*, 47, 3378, 1987.
102. Nash, T., The colorimetric estimation of formaldehyde by means of the Hantzsch reaction, *Biochemistry*, 55, 416, 1953.
103. Peter, R., Bocker, R., Beaune, P. H., Iwasaki, M., Guengerich, F. P., and Yang, C. S., Hydroxylation of chlorzoxazone as a specific probe for human liver cytochrome P450IIE1, *Chem. Res. Toxicol.*, 3, 566, 1990.
104. Carriere, V., Goasduff, T., Ratanasavanh, D., Morel, F., Gautier, J-C., Guillouzo, A., Beaune, P., and Berthou, F., Both cytochromes P450 2E1 and 1A1 are involved in the metabolism of chlorzoxazone, *Chem. Res. Toxicol.*, 6, 852, 1993.
105. Wrighton, S. A., Maurel, P., Schuetz, E. G., Watkins, P. B., Young, B., and Guzelian, P. S., Identification of the cytochrome P-450 induced by macrolide antibiotics in rat liver as the glucocorticoid responsive cytochrome P-450p, *Biochemistry*, 24, 2171, 1985.
106. Gibson, G. G., Orton, T. C., and Tamburini, P. P., Cytochrome P450 induction by clofibrate: Purification and properties of a hepatic cytochrome P450 relatively specific for the 12- and 11-hydroxylation of dodecanoic acid (lauric acid), *Biochem. J.*, 203, 161, 1982.
107. Johnson, E. F., Walker, D. L., Griffin, K. J., Clark, J. E., Okita, R. T., Muerhoff, A. S., and Masters, B. S. S., Cloning and expression of three rabbit kidney cDNAs encoding lauric acid ω-hydroxylases, *Biochemistry*, 29, 873, 1990.
108. Clarke, S. E., Baldwin, S. J., Bloomer, J. C., Ayrton, A. D., Sozio, R. S., and Chenery, R. J., Lauric acid as a model substrate for the simultaneous determination of cytochrome P450 2E1 and 4A in hepatic microsomes, *Chem. Res. Toxicol.*, 7, 836, 1994.

109. Okita, R. T. and Masters, B. S. S., Effect of phenobarbital treatment and cytochrome P450 inhibitors on the laurate ω- and (ω-1)-hydroxylase activities of rat liver microsomes, *Drug Metab. Dispos.*, 8, 147, 1980.
110. Fan, L. L., Masters, B. S. S., and Prough, R. A., Microsomal lauric acid 11- and 12-hydroxylation: a new assay method utilizing high pressure liquid chromatography, *Anal. Biochem.*, 71, 265, 1976.
111. Okita, R. T., Clark, J. E., Okita, J. R., and Masters, B. S. S., ω- and (ω-1)-Hydroxylation of eicosanoids and fatty acids by high-performance liquid chromatography, *Methods Enzymol.*, 206, 432, 1991.
112. Dirven, H. A. A. M., de Bruijn, A. A. G. M., Sessink, P. J. M., and Jongeneelen, F. J., Determination of the cytochrome P-450 IV marker, ω-hydroxylauric acid, by high-performance liquid chromatography and fluorimetric detection, *J. Chromatogr.*, 564, 266, 1991.
113. Jacobson, H. R., Corona, S., Capdevila, J., Chacos, N., Manna, S., Womack, A., and Falck, J. R., Effects of epoxyeicosatrienoic acid on ion transport in the rabbit cortical collecting tubule, in *Prostaglandins and Membrane Ion Transport*, Braquet, P., Garay, R. P., Frolich, J. C., and Nicosia, S., Eds., Raven Press, New York, 1984, 311.
114. Escalante, B., Erlij, D., Falck, J. R., and McGiff, J. C., Effect of cytochrome 450 arachidonate metabolites on ion transport in rabbit kidney loop of Henle, *Science*, 251, 799, 1991.
115. Romero, M. D., Madhum, Z. D., Hopfer, U., and Douglas, J. G., An epoxygenase metabolite of arachidonic acid mediates angiotensin-induced natriuresis in proximal tubular epithelium, in *Advances in Prostaglandin, Thromboxane, and Leukotriene Research*, Vol. 21A, Samuelsson, B., Ramwell, P. W., Paoletti, R., Folco, G., and Granstrom, E., Eds., Raven Press, New York, 1991, 205.
116. Schlondorff, D., Petty, E., Oates, J. A., Jacoby, M., and Levine, S. D., Epoxygenase metabolites of arachidonic acid inhibit vasopressin response in toad bladder, *Am. J. Physiol.*, 253, F464, 1987.
117. Katoh, T., Takahashi, K., Capdevila, J., Karara, A., Falck, J. R., Jacobson, H. R., and Badr, K. F., Glomerular stereospecific synthesis and hemodynamic actions of 8,9-epoxyeicosatrienoic acid in rat kidney, *Am. J. Physiol.*, 261, F578, 1991.
118. Kauser, K., Clark, J. E., Masters, B. S., Ortiz de Montellano, P. R., Ma, Y.-H., Harder, D. R., and Roman, R. J., Inhibitors of cytochrome P450 attenuate the myogenic response of dog renal arcuate arteries, *Circ. Res.*, 68, 1154, 1991.
119. Escalante, B., Falck, J. R., Yadagiri, P., Sun, L., and Schwartzman, M. L., 19(S)-Hydroxyeicosatetraenoic acid is a potent stimulator of renal Na^+-K^+-ATPase, *Biochem. Biophys. Res. Commun.*, 152, 1269, 1988.
120. Henrich, W. L., Falck, J. R., and Campbell, W. B., Inhibition of renin release by 14,15-epoxyeicosatrienoic acid in renal cortical slices, *Am. J. Physiol.*, 258, E269, 1990.
121. Zou, A.-P., Imig, J. D., Ortiz de Montellano, P. R., Sui, Z., Falck, J. R., and Roman, R. J., Effect of P-450 ω-hydroxylase metabolites of arachidonic acid on tubuloglomerular feedback, *Am. J. Physiol.*, 266, F934, 1994
122. Fitzpatrick, F. A. and Murphy, R. C., Cytochrome P450 metabolism of arachidonic acid: formation and biological actions of epoxygenase-derived eicosanoids, *Pharmacol. Rev.*, 40, 229, 1988.
123. Capdevila, J. H., Dishman, E., Karara, A., and Falck, J. R., Cytochrome P450 arachidonic acid epoxygenase: stereochemical characterization of epoxyeicosatrienoic acids, *Methods Enzymol.*, 206, 441, 1991.
124. Winokur, T. S. and Morrison, A. R., Regional synthesis of monohydroxy eicosanoids by the kidney, *J. Biol. Chem.*, 256, 10221, 1981.
125. Morrison, A. R. and Pascoe, N., Metabolism of arachidonate through NADPH-dependent oxygenase of renal cortex, *Proc. Natl. Acad. Sci. U.S.A.*, 78, 7375, 1981.
126. Toto, R., Siddhanta, A., Manna, S., Pramanik, B., Falck, J. R., and Capdevila, J., Arachidonic acid epoxygenase: detection of epoxyeicosatrienoic acids in human urine, *Biochim. Biophys. Acta*, 919, 132, 1987.
127. Catella, F., Lawson, J. A., Fitzgerald, D. J., and Fitzgerald, G. A., Endogenous biosynthesis of arachidonic acid epoxides in humans: increased formation in pregnancy-induced hypertension, *Proc. Natl. Acad. Sci. U.S.A.*, 87, 5893, 1990.

128. Schwartzman, M. L., Omata, K., Lin, F., Bhatt, R. K., Falck, J. R., and Abraham, N. G., Detection of 20-hydroxyeicosatetraenoic acid in rat urine, *Biochem. Biophys. Res. Comm.*, 180, 445, 1991.
129. Capdevila, J. H., Falck, J. R., Dishman, E., and Karara, A., Cytochrome P-450 arachidonate oxygenase, *Methods Enzymol.*, 187, 385, 1990.
130. Laemmli, U. K., Cleavage of structural protein during the assembly of the head of bacteriophage T4, *Nature*, 227, 680, 1970.
131. Zangar, R. C., Springer, D. L., and Buhler, D. R., Alterations in cytochrome P-450 levels in adult rats following neonatal exposure to xenobiotics, *J. Toxicol. Environ. Health*, 38, 43, 1993.
132. Hardwick, J. P., *CYP4A* subfamily: functional analysis by immunohistochemistry and *in situ* hybridization, *Methods Enzymol.*, 206, 273, 1991.

chapter nineteen

Molecular Methods in Renal Toxicology

Jim Koropatnick

19.1 Introduction 378
19.1.1 Gene expression in eukaryotes 378
19.1.2 Deregulation of gene expression 380
19.1.2.1 Gain-of-function events 380
19.1.2.2 Loss-of-function events 380
19.2 Measuring genetic changes in response to nephrotoxicants 380
19.2.1 Transcription rate 380
19.2.1.1 Preparation of nuclei 381
19.2.1.2 Transcription in isolated nuclei 381
19.2.1.3 Detection of specific radiolabeled transcripts 382
19.2.2 Accumulation of specific mRNAs 383
19.2.2.1 RNA isolation 383
19.2.2.2 Northern blot analysis 387
19.2.2.3 Slot and dot blot analysis 389
19.2.2.4 Probe selection and labeling 389
19.2.2.5 Standardization and quantitation 390
19.2.2.6 Reverse transcription–polymerase chain reaction (RT-PCR) analysis 391
19.2.2.7 Ribonuclease protection and primer extension analysis 395
19.2.2.8 *In situ* hybridization 396
19.2.2.9 Interpretation of mRNA measurements 397
19.3 Intervention in gene expression 398
19.3.1 Transfection of structural genes 398
19.3.1.1 Stable transfection 398
19.3.1.2 Transient transfection 399
19.3.2 Gene inactivation 400
19.3.2.1 Transgenic mouse mutation assays 400
19.3.2.2 Site-directed insertional inactivation 401
19.3.3 Antisense nucleic acids 402
19.4 Cellular responses to intervention in gene expression 402
19.4.1 Gain-of-function events 402
19.4.2 Loss-of-function events 403
19.5 Summary 404
19.6 Acknowledgment 404
References 404

0-8493-3341-5/96/$0.00+$.50

19.1 Introduction

Toxicity results from impairment of normal functions and is caused by extracellular agents. Because there are many such functions, it is necessarily an aggregate event encompassing a broad range of specific changes in cells in culture and in tissues. A sufficiently high level of most, if not all, physical and chemical agents can induce toxicity. However, toxic agents do not impair normal cellular functions at all doses. Depending on the level of toxicant and the degree of susceptibility, a broad range of responses can be elicited from cells.

Low level exposure induces changes in cell behavior without nonphysiological chemical alteration of cellular molecules (including lipids, proteins, or nucleic acids). These changes generally include detection, by cells, of agents that are normally present in physiological environments or that mimic physiological constituents normally found within and surrounding cells and tissues.

Medium level exposure induces changes in cell behavior accompanied by (and, perhaps, resulting from) nonphysiological modification of cellular structures by exogenous agents. Again, these agents may arise as a result of normal physiological events (free radical species in mitochondria, for example), or they may not (environmental mercury and cadmium). Damage of this sort can be reversible. Cells may then survive, although not always without long-term consequences that may be deleterious to the host organism, including mutation and cancer. Alternatively, cells may undergo gene-dependent self-autonomous death, or apoptosis.

High level exposure induces changes in cell structures without requiring the action of specific genes within cells (gene-independent cell death). These changes are incompatible with continued survival. Cells undergoing meiotic or mitotic division may die at the next division event or (if toxic events are drastic enough) in nondividing cells in interphase. However, gene-mediated events are irrelevant to the process of death.

In the jargon of genetic toxicology, the use of "molecular" methods to study damage to living things no longer simply means that damage at the level of molecules is studied, however logical such an inference is. Rather, the term means specifically that genes and their direct product (RNA) are studied through manipulation and measurement of nucleic acids within cells. Differences in gene activity — either as a preexisting condition in a heterogeneous population of cells (either the association of cells that compose a single multicelled organism or a heterogeneous group of independent organisms) or as a result of heterogeneous responses among cells to normal physiological signals and toxic events — are critical in predicting whether cells will (1) avoid toxic events and changes in cell behavior, (2) avoid permanent toxic events but alter cell behavior to do so, (3) suffer toxic events but survive (perhaps with long-term consequences for behavior), or (4) suffer toxic events and die, either by gene-dependent processes (programmed cell death, or apoptosis) or independent of gene-mediated events.

A description of the specific genes important in toxic events or resistance to toxicity is beyond the scope of this review. Instead, this chapter addresses techniques that are particularly relevant to assessing toxicity and resistance to toxicity in mammalian cells and organs in general and that may be applied to the study of renal toxicity in particular. Molecular techniques to detect and manipulate gene expression in prokaryotes and plants have been addressed in excellent reviews elsewhere[1-3] and will not be addressed here. To make the discussion more meaningful, however, familiarity with the mechanisms by which cells normally control gene expression is required.

19.1.1 Gene expression in eukaryotes

Some genes (the so-called housekeeping genes) are expressed in all cells, regardless of tissue origin, in order to sustain life. Examples include those encoding major structural proteins of chromosomes (such as histones), structural cytoskeleton proteins (actins, for example), and enzymes catalyzing basic metabolic processes common to all cells (glyceraldehyde-3-phosphate dehydrogenase, for example, a critical enzyme in glycolysis). It is important to note that housekeeping genes, although expressed in all cells, are not expressed at the same level at all times. They may be cell cycle-dependent or vary in activity according to cellular metabolic rates. Nevertheless, their rates of expression are commonly used as standards against which to measure the expression of inducible genes that respond to signals of extracellular origin. These genes direct production of RNAs required in some, but not all, cells or in response to changes in cellular environment. The process by which cells inform themselves of these environmental changes is termed signal transduction.[4,5] Signal transduction involves the following processes:

1. Stimulation of cells by hormones and other signalling molecules on membrane receptors (ion channel-linked, G protein-linked, and enzyme-linked[6]) directly induces, or leads to induction of, an intracellular signal.
2. Stimulated receptors act on protein kinases to induce a cascade of phosphorylation events involving transfer of phosphate groups to serine, threonine, and tyrosine groups on proteins. Phosphorylated proteins relay signals from the cell surface to the nucleus, where production and/or activity of transcription factors is affected.
3. Transcription factors are gene regulatory proteins that increase or decrease production of RNA from specific genes by their recognizing and binding to short DNA regions within or surrounding those genes.[7,8]
4. Higher level chromatin structure (including nucleosomes) may cooperate with transcription factors in controlling transcription.[9,10]

Control at the level of transcription is the predominant factor in mediating expression of most genes. However, posttranscriptional controls are critical in some cases. These include:

1. Attenuation, or premature termination of transcription (present in bacteria).
2. Alternative RNA splicing. Intron sequences, which are present within immature nuclear RNA, do not code for part of a functional protein and are enzymatically removed (RNA splicing) as part of the normal process of eukaryotic RNA maturation. Higher eukaryotic RNA, however, can be spliced in multiple ways to produce different proteins. Alternative splicing can be regulated to produce mRNAs coding for functional or nonfunctional proteins, depending on the needs of the organism.[11]
3. Regulated export of mRNA from the nucleus to cytoplasm for translation into protein.[12,13]
4. Localization of mRNA in cytoplasm at sites permissive for translation and regulated initiation of translation. For example, translation of mRNA encoding the intracellular iron storage protein ferritin is repressed by its binding to the translation repressor protein aconitase.[14]
5. Regulated control of RNA degradation. Eukaryotic mRNAs vary in stability: half-lives range from minutes to 10 h or more. A sequence rich in A and U nucleotides confers instability on some mRNAs by stimulating loss of the poly-A tail on the 3′ end of most eukaryotic mRNAs. In addition, stability of specific mRNA can change in response to extracellular signals. For example, increased intracellular iron induces decreased transferrin receptor mRNA stability, resulting in lower transferrin receptor production overall and diminished iron transport into cells.[15]
6. Regulation of availability of mRNA for translation. "Masking" of mRNA by its binding to a regulatory protein[16] or mRNA association with proteins that enhance

translation[17] have been reported. Association of "antisense" RNA sequences may also regulate mRNA availability in prokaryotes.[18]

These multiple levels of regulation of gene expression at the nucleic acid level are only part of the regulation story: cells and organisms use multiple strategies to regulate the activity and availability of proteins, too. Therefore, any single measure of "gene expression" (i.e., techniques to measure gene transcription rate and mRNA accumulation) outlined below must necessarily be interpreted cautiously. Physiological changes within the same cells and organs must be assessed and interpreted as part of the gene expression story.

19.1.2 Deregulation of gene expression

Deregulation of genes means, in molecular terms, altering normal physiological control of gene expression by deliberately manipulating the genome such that normal signal transduction and gene expression pathways are circumvented. In this way, specific genes can be induced or suppressed without first inducing constitutive genes and relying on cellular response. The advantage is that changes can be focused specifically to genes of interest and do not involve multiple genes that may respond to signals of extracellular origin. The consequences of specific genetic changes for cellular response to toxic or subtoxic agents, or a combination of toxic agents and changes in physiological status (differentiation, proliferation, etc.), can then be assessed. Strategies aimed at this level include the following events.

19.1.2.1 Gain-of-function events

When functioning foreign genes are inserted into cultured cells and whole organisms, increased expression of those genes in the absence of normal signalling can be achieved.

19.1.2.2 Loss-of-function events

Normal gene expression can be disrupted by random, induced mutation events, by site-directed mutation ("gene knockout"), or by insertion of antisense nucleic acids into cultured cells or whole organisms. Gene knockout or exposure to specific antisense nucleic acids are, therefore, methods to inhibit expression of selected genes. Loss of gene expression by mutation events can be used as a marker of genetic damage and is discussed below.

Molecular genetic techniques can be used first to generate gain- or loss-of-function events and then to measure changes in gene expression at the levels of gene transcription and mRNA accumulation. Techniques to measure toxicant-induced changes in gene expression are fundamental and are addressed first.

19.2 Measuring genetic changes in response to nephrotoxicants

Agents or conditions toxic to renal or other cells can induce changes in the activity of specific genes. These changes include the rate at which RNA molecules are synthesized from single-stranded DNA templates (the transcription rate) and the level of accumulation of specific mRNAs. Techniques to measure the translation of mRNA into protein; the enzymatic modification of proteins to alter their activity (by phosphorylation, acetylation, proteolytic cleavage, dimerization, and other events); and cellular localization are described elsewhere in this volume.

19.2.1 Transcription rate

Gene transcription involves several events, including initiation (interaction of a complex of associated transcription proteins with DNA to begin production of a new mRNA molecule), elongation (the generation of an increasingly lengthy nascent RNA molecule), and termination (the release of immature heteronuclear RNA [hnRNA] for further processing and export to cytoplasm). Nascent hnRNA molecules undergoing elongation in isolated nuclei over a short, defined time period (usually 30 to 45 min) can be measured by incorporation of ^{32}P-labeled RNA precursors. ^{32}P-labeled RNA can then be purified and used to detect specific RNA transcripts by physical association (hybridization) to DNA of unique sequence immobilized on membranes. The process is termed nuclear run-on transcription (N-ROT), and the degree of hybridization measured is proportional to the overall transcription rate. N-ROT can be especially useful in determining whether increased accumulation of specific mRNAs in response to signalling is due to a change in RNA synthesis or a change in mRNA degradation or transport from the nucleus to the cytoplasm. The technique has been used to measure transcription of kidney genes *in vivo*, including genes for HSP32 (heme oxygenase–1),[19] and metallothionein.[20]

19.2.1.1 *Preparation of nuclei*

Isolated cell nuclei, not intact cells, are required for N-ROT. This is a critical advantage when using whole tissues, where preparation of nuclei does not generally pose a problem. Detailed protocols are available.[21-25] Since labile ribonucleic acids (RNAs) are handled in this procedure, utmost cleanliness and sterility are required (see Section 19.2.2.1 for details). Briefly, whole organisms, organs cultured *ex vivo*, or cells *in vitro* are exposed to conditions that may induce altered gene expression. Tissues are excised using ice-cold, sterile instruments and rinsed with ice-cold phosphate-buffered saline (pH 7). Aliquots are removed for assays other than N-ROT (mRNA and DNA isolation and analysis, histology, immunohistochemistry, etc.), and a portion is reserved for N-ROT. Typically, nuclei from 5×10^7 cells is sufficient for a single assay, although a minimum of 5×10^6 nuclei may be used under some circumstances. Nuclei are then isolated from excised tissues by a variety of methods, including Teflon-glass homogenization[26,27] or Dounce homogenization:[28] it is this step that is the most critical in the assay. If nuclei are damaged during isolation, or contain excessive amounts of cytoplasmic and membrane contaminants, the result will be poor incorporation of ^{32}P-labeled uridine triphosphate (UTP) into RNA and failure to detect and measure specific radiolabeled transcripts. Methods for cultured cells, lymphocytes,[28] and cells in tissues[23] have been reviewed. A modification of the methods of Kikuchi et al.[26] and Almendral et al.[29] works well for renal cells.[20] Tissue fragments are homogenized in a motor-driven Teflon-glass homogenizer in 2 volumes of added ice-cold buffer I (0.32 *M* sucrose, 3 m*M* $CaCl_2$, 2 m*M* $Mg(OAc)_2$, 0.1 m*M* EDTA, 1 m*M* dithiothreitol, 10 m*M* TRIS-HCl, pH 8) and centrifugation through a 10 ml cushion of Buffer C (2 *M* sucrose, 5 m*M* magnesium acetate, 0.1 m*M* EDTA, 10 m*M* TRIS-HCl, pH 8) at 30,000 × g for 45 min at 4°C. The pellet of nuclei at the bottom of the tube is then resuspended in nuclei storage buffer (NSB)(40% glycerol, 5 m*M* $MgCl_2$, 50 m*M* TRIS-HCl [pH 8], 0.1 m*M* EDTA) at a concentration of 1.5 to 3.8×10^8 nuclei per milliliter and inspected in a hemocytometer with a phase-contrast microscope to ensure that cells are lysed and nuclei are free of cytoplasmic material. Aliquots containing 2×10^7 nuclei are immediately frozen in liquid nitrogen for future use.[30,31] Although nuclei isolated from healthy, unstressed cells are usable more than a year later, those isolated from cells treated with toxicants may have a considerably shorter usable life. For example, storage of mouse liver cell nuclei isolated from animals exposed to toxic cadmium salts for longer than two weeks leads to a marked decrease in transcription efficiency.[25]

19.2.1.2 *Transcription in isolated nuclei*

Cell nuclei (2×10^7) are thawed, transferred to a disposable 15-ml tube, and made up to 80 µl with NSB. Thirty microliters of 10× Reaction Buffer (RB) (700 m*M* KCl, 50 m*M* $MgCl_2$, 50 m*M* TRIS-HCl [pH 8], 25 m*M* dithiothreitol, 1 m*M* EDTA) is immediately added, followed (in order) by 15 µl each of ATP, CTP, and GTP (each 4 m*M*), 16 µl sterile distilled water, and 250 μCi [α-^{32}P]UTP (specific activity = 3000 Ci/mmol, approximately 0.08 nmoles in 25 μl, from a 10 μCi/μl stock). Radioactive UTP is incorporated into RNA during a 30-min run-on transcription at 30°C, and the reaction is stopped by addition of the chaotropic agent guanidinium isothiocyanate (GITC) followed by isolation of RNA by GITC/phenol extraction in a fume hood (see Section 19.2.2.1 for details). Increasing the amount of radioactive UTP or the length of time of elongation beyond 30 min is generally ineffective in enhancing radiolabel incorporation into RNA, although increasing the number of nuclei to 5×10^7 can be useful.[24] Extreme caution should be used in this process, because radiolabeled RNA and precursors will contaminate all items they contact. Before the final ethanol precipitation of RNA, remove unincorporated radiolabeled UTP by passing isolated RNA through a Sephadex® G-50 column (the Pharmacia Biotech Nick™ Column works well). Ethanol-precipitated RNA is then resuspended in 2× TESS buffer (10 m*M* TES [*N*-tris(hydroxymethyl)methyl-2-aminoethanesulfonic acid], pH 7.4, 300 m*M* sodium chloride, 10 m*M* EDTA, 0.2% sodium dodecyl sulfate [SDS], 100 μg/ml of yeast tRNA) at a concentration of 2×10^6 cpm/ml. Isolated radiolabeled RNA will be a mixture of messenger RNAs (mRNAs), transfer RNAs (tRNAs), and ribosomal RNAs (rRNAs): recovery of total labeled RNA should be between 30 and 50% of applied radiolabeled UTP. An advantage of the method is that because radiolabel is incorporated into all transcribed mRNAs, measurement of transcription from many different genes in a single experiment is possible.

19.2.1.3 *Detection of specific radiolabeled transcripts*

Radiolabeled RNA in solution is hybridized to separate nylon membrane strips on which nonradioactive cDNA (complementary DNAs) or single-stranded nonradioactive oligonucleotides[20] (2 μg per slot or dot) have been immobilized by dot or slot blotting (see Section 19.2.2.3). These unlabeled "driver" nucleic acids are in much higher quantity than the complementary radiolabeled mRNA and will force a relatively high proportion of available mRNA molecules to bind. The use of chemically synthesized oligonucleotides as unlabeled probe has added flexibility to N-ROT assays in that transcription of DNA directing production of "artificial" RNAs (including antisense RNA) is possible at the same time and in the same nuclei that transcription of natural mRNAs is measured (Figure 1 and DeMoor et al., manuscript submitted) (see Section 19.3.3 for details). Thus, transcription of both artificial and naturally occurring DNA templates is possible. Two × 10^6 cpm of radiolabeled RNA in 1 ml of 2× TESS buffer is incubated with driver DNA on filters for 48 h at 65°C under standard hybridization buffer conditions (see Section 19.2.2.2). Filters are then washed in 2× TESS buffer without radiolabel at 65° for 30 min, incubated with 20 μg/ml RNase A for 20 min to digest unhybridized RNA, incubated with 200 μg/ml proteinase K for 15 min to remove RNase A, and washed in 2× TESS buffer for 20 min at 65°C to remove unhybridized residual radiolabel. Washing steps remove radiolabeled RNA nonspecifically associated with filters. The amount of remaining radioactivity associated with each "dot" of unlabeled driver nucleic acid is then measured by autoradiography or (more sensitively and accurately) by storage phosphor technology and a laser–optical imager (phosphorimagery) (Figure 1) or liquid scintillation.[20,25] Bound radioactivity indicates the activity of the gene in the cells from which the nuclei were isolated.

Raw data from these analyses can be expressed as counts per minute hybridized per total counts per minute in radiolabeled RNA. However, only a small proportion (typically less than 5%) of radiolabeled RNAs are mRNAs. Variations in the amount of mRNA comprising radiolabeled total RNA can lead to false estimates of increases or decreases in transcription rate measured in this way. In most cases, therefore, it is essential that the radiolabeled RNA transcribed from both the gene of interest and a control gene be measured in the same hybridization bag, preferably on the same piece of nylon membrane. The inclusion of such a control (important for both N-ROT and Northern blot analysis of mRNA level [Section 19.2.2.2]) allows a measure of relative transcription rate (transcription rate of the gene of interest relative to a gene that is presumably unaffected by test conditions). Appropriate control RNAs may include those for such housekeeping genes as glyceraldehyde phosphate dehydrogenase (GAPDH)[32] or β actin[20,25] (Figure 1).

Measuring specific mRNA hybridization at only one level of added total radioactive RNA may be sufficient for some genes[32] (Figure 1). For other mRNAs, this may be inaccurate under some circumstances since the level of nonspecific background radioactivity bound to filters can vary (Figure 2).[20,25] To minimize error, the level of hybridized radiolabeled RNA can be measured in two hybridization bags: one with twice the amount of total radiolabeled RNA exposed to the nylon filter as in the first bag. The slope of "cpm hybridized" for target and control genes will allow assessment of the absolute rate of transcription (in parts per million) of each gene against minimal background variation (Figure 2).[20,25,33] The "slope method" has the added advantage that — assuming that hybridization efficiency (the proportion of radiolabeled transcripts capable of binding to immobilized DNA that actually do bind) in each chamber is equal — 100% hybridization efficiency is not required. In practice, only approximately 50% efficiency is achievable.

Information provided by measurement of N-ROT can be complex. At the same time that transcription of a specific target gene is increased, there may be increased transcription of multiple genes involved in cellular metabolism (including housekeeping genes whose transcription rate is measured as a reference point). Thus, test conditions may enhance cellular metabolic activity overall rather than selectively induce specific target genes or a small subset of target genes.[20] Measurement of target gene transcription rate relative to more than one control, housekeeping gene transcription rate may be informative in this situation.

Nuclear run-on transcription assays can be used to measure the activity of genes in response to inducing signals, toxic or otherwise. However, the next step in gene expression — increased mRNA level — must be achieved if increased transcription is to be effective. The following section describes measurement of mRNA levels in cells and tissues.

19.2.2 *Accumulation of specific mRNAs*

The most common methods to infer altered gene expression at the molecular level — Northern blot analysis, reverse transcription–polymerase chain reaction (RT-PCR) analysis, dot and slot blot analysis, and others — to infer altered gene expression at the molecular level depend upon measurement of changes in accumulation of specific mRNA molecules. However, gene expression can be controlled at multiple points (see above). This makes it essential that measurements focused on RNA alone not be accepted as a reliable indication of altered protein accumulation, activity, or phenotype change. mRNA accumulation measurements should be used as only one of several indicators of response to signals affecting gene expression. In this section, several methods to detect and quantitate mRNAs transcribed from specific genes are discussed, with emphasis on the applications of each method and inherent advantages and disadvantages.

19.2.2.1 RNA isolation

Virtually all mRNA measurement assays (other than *in situ* hybridization in cells and tissues) require partial or complete isolation of cellular or tissue RNA. Isolation methods vary in their capacity to produce RNA in high yield and in the purity of the final RNA product (i.e., the amount of contamination with lipid, protein, ribonucleoside phosphates, or chemical used in the purification process): a detailed description of these methods has been compiled.[34,35] RNA purification can be costly and time-consuming, so procedures should be chosen according to the application for which the RNA is required. For example,

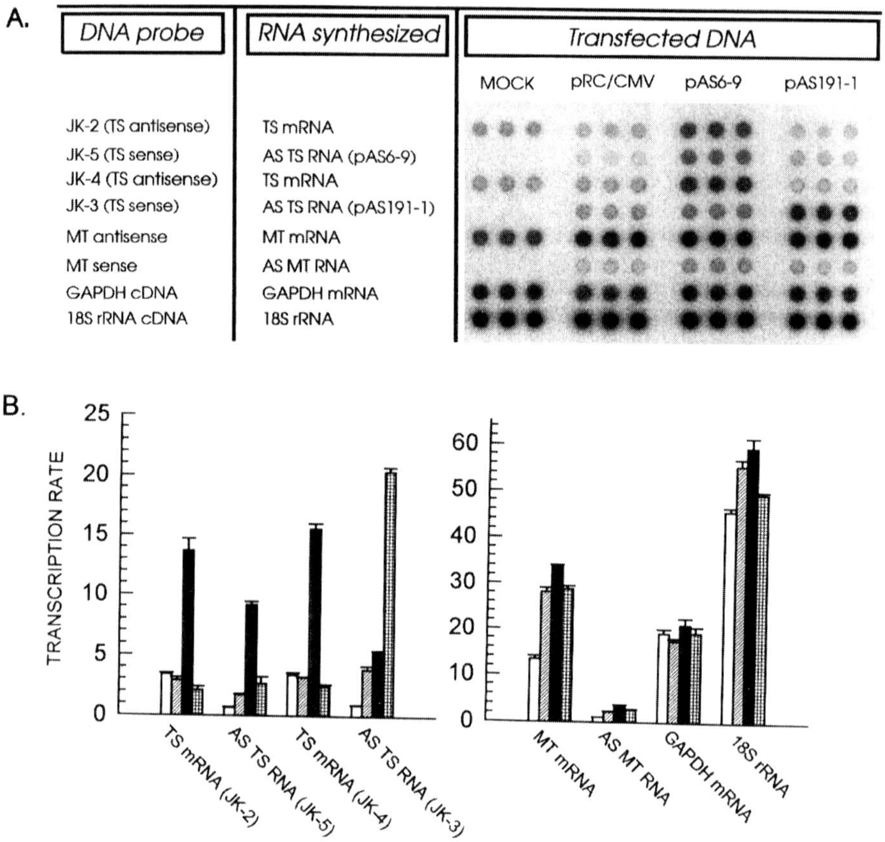

Northern blot analysis requires more highly purified RNA than that required for reverse transcription–polymerase chain reaction measurement of mRNA level. Spectrophotometric methods to monitor RNA concentration and purity, based on relative UV absorbance at 260 nm and 280 nm, have been described.[34]

RNA transcripts are present in both the nucleus (in immature, heteronuclear RNA [hnRNA] form) and cytoplasm (in mature mRNA form) in cells. It is possible to preferentially purify mature cytoplasmic mRNA from cultured eukaryotic cells *in vitro*,[36] but this is rarely practical for cells from solid tissues. In most cases where tissue samples will be analyzed, total tissue RNA (not cytoplasmic RNA) will be isolated.

RNA, even more than DNA, is extremely susceptible to enzymatic cleavage. A major concern during RNA isolation is the possibility of degradation due to the presence of nucleolytic ribonucleases (RNases). The enzymes are heat stable, do not require cofactors for activity, and are ubiquitous. Some tissues contain high levels (pancreas and spleen, for example), while others have relatively low amounts or contain naturally occurring inhibitors of RNases (liver and placenta, for example).[37] Use of sterile gloves, treatment of buffer solutions with diethylpyrocarbonate (DEPC), and autoclaving are essential precautions to avoid RNase contamination. DEPC should not be used with TRIS buffers, however, as TRIS inactivates DEPC. Cells and tissues from which RNA is to be isolated should be snap-frozen in liquid nitrogen and maintained at –70°C or colder temperatures. Although a variety of protocols exist for isolating RNA (some requiring lengthy gradient sedimentation), a single-step RNA isolation procedure of value for whole tissues, especially after treatment with potentially toxic agents or conditions, has been described by Chomczynski and Sacchi.[38] It begins with disruption of cells and tissues in the presence of a chaotropic agent (4 *M* guanidinium isothiocyanate, pH 4, is the agent of choice) that simultaneously lyses cells and denatures and inactivates proteolytic enzymes. Phenol and chloroform are included in the mixture to form separate phases: protein, lipid, and small DNA fragments are found in the phenol/chloroform layer, and larger DNA fragments (greater than 10 kb) remain in the interphase. RNA is in solution in the aqueous phase, from which it is precipitated in the presence of isopropanol. Even simpler methods designed for processing large numbers of samples have been described by Birnboim.[39] Kits for simultaneous RNA, DNA, and protein isolation from the same tissue sample, based on the phenol/GITC method (TRIzol™ reagent, Life Technologies, for example), and kits that depend upon

---

Figure 1 (opposite) Nuclear run-on transcription (N-ROT) of constitutive genes, and transfected expression vectors, in cultured human MCF-7 breast cancer cells. **(A)** Phosphorimager visualization of specific radiolabeled RNAs transcribed over a 30-min period from constitutive genes (thymidylate synthase [TS] mRNA; metallothionein-2 [MT-2] mRNA; glyceraldehyde phosphate dehydrogenase [GAPDH] mRNA; 18S rRNA), or from transiently transfected foreign DNA vectors (antisense thymidylate synthase [AS TS] RNA; antisense metallothionein-2 [AS MT] RNA). "DNA probe" indicates the unlabeled driver DNA immobilized, in three identical dots, on filters: the probe bound RNA radiolabeled during the 30-min transcription period. JK-2 and JK-4 are different probes that specifically bound RNA antisense to thymidylate synthase, but not thymidylate synthase mRNA. JK-3 and JK-5 are different probes that specifically bound thymidylate synthase mRNA, but not antisense TS RNA. Similarly, the MT antisense probe detected MT-2 mRNA, and the MT sense probe detected antisense MT-2 RNA. cDNA probes for "housekeeping" genes (GAPDH, 18S rRNA) are capable of binding to both antisense RNA and mRNA: in this case, only mRNAs were detected. "RNA synthesized" indicates the RNA whose transcription is being detected by each DNA probe. Bracketed names (pAS6-9, for example) refer to transfected vectors from which foreign RNA is transcribed, where such vectors were used. "Mock" refers to MCF-7 cells that undergo vector transfection conditions using cationic liposomes, except that no foreign DNA was included in the transfection mixture. "pRC/CMV" refers to cells transfected with parent vector alone without antisense RNA-expressing sequences. "pAS6-9" and "pAS191–1" refer to cells transfected with two different pRC/CMV-based vectors transcribing short (30 bases long) RNAs antisense to different regions of human thymidylate synthase mRNA. Radiolabeled RNA (2×10^6 cpm) synthesized from cells harboring each of these vectors was hybridized, in four separate bags (2 ml of hybridization solution per bag), as described in the text. The darkness of the phosphorimage indicates the amount of radiolabel and is directly proportional to the level of transcription of each constitutive gene or transfected foreign DNA. **(B)** Graphic representation of N-ROT for each assessed gene. "Transcription rate" (on the Y-axis) is the darkness of the phosphorimage (assessed by computer densitometry, the mean of 3 dots ± standard error) per 2×10^6 cpm of total radiolabeled cellular RNA. The X-axis labels denote the RNA (messenger or antisense) detected: the bracketed name indicates the immobilized driver DNA used to bind and detect the synthesized RNA. The right panel indicates that MT and GAPDH mRNA, and 18S rRNA, are transcribed at roughly the same rate irrespective of the presence of antisense RNA expression vector (except for MT-2 genes, which were transcribed at a higher rate in the presence of foreign DNA of any kind). As expected, antisense MT RNA was not transcribed: no antisense MT RNA was present. The left panel shows that foreign antisense TS genes were transcribed at a high rate in cells transfected with antisense TS expression vectors producing antisense RNA that bound to probes JK-5 or JK-3. However, cells expressing antisense TS RNA from vector pAS6-9 (complementary to the TS mRNA translation start site) had elevated transcription from constitutive TS genes (detected by increased binding to driver DNAs JK-2 and JK-4). Cells harboring and transcribing vector pAS191–1, on the other hand, did not transcribe constitutive TS genes at a higher rate (indicated by low level binding to JK-2 and JK-4). Therefore, antisense RNA directed at the thymidylate synthase mRNA translation start site, but not another region of TS mRNA, stimulated transcription of constitutive TS genes. □, Mock-transfected cells (no foreign DNA); ▨, control vector-transfected cells (no antisense RNA sequences); ■, cells transfected with pAS6-9 and expressing RNA antisense to the translation start site of TS mRNA; ▦, cells transfected with pAS191-1 and expressing RNA antisense to a sequence 156 bases downstream (in the 3′ direction) of the translation start site. This analysis illustrates the potential for measuring, by N-ROT, both the expression of specific genes and the effect of antisense RNA on transcription of those genes. (From DeMoor et al., manuscript submitted).

minicolumn chromatography and eliminate the requirement for handling toxic isolation reagents (phenol, for example) are available (RNeasy™ columns, Qiagen, Inc.).

The yield of RNA depends upon the tissue. For whole kidney and kidney tissue fractions (cortex, outer stripe, inner stripe plus papilla), between 300 and 1300 μg total

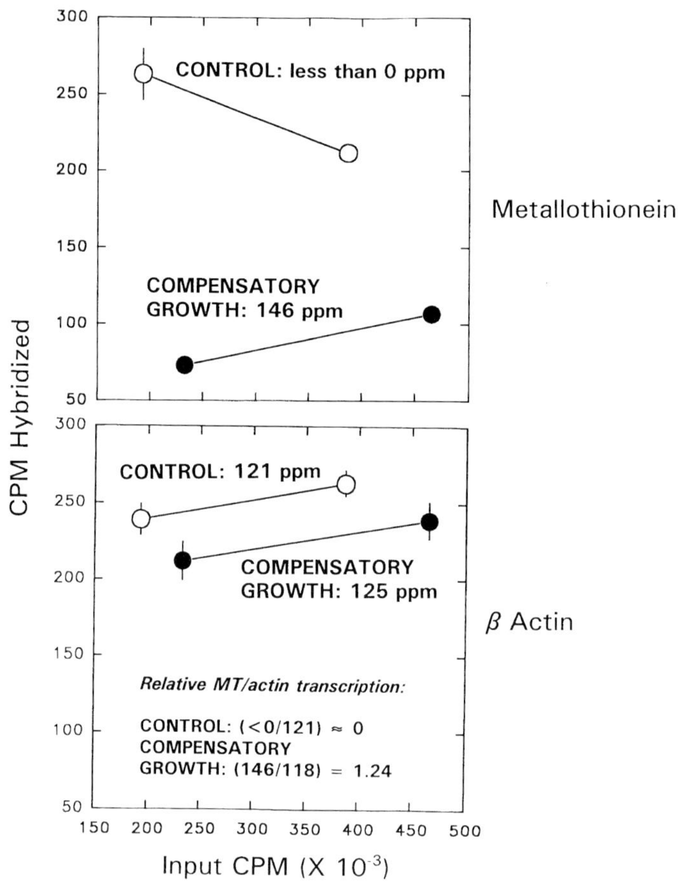

Figure 2 Nuclear run-on transcription (N-ROT) of metallothionein-1 and metallothionein-2 (MT-1 + MT-2) genes, and β actin genes, in rat kidney. In this experiment, the effect of removal of one kidney on MT gene transcription in the remaining kidney was determined. "COMPENSATORY GROWTH" (uninephrectomized) refers to adult male Sprague–Dawley rats whose right kidney was removed 15 days prior to N-ROT. "CONTROL" (sham-operated) refers to animals subjected to identical surgical trauma, but with both kidneys left intact. Nuclei were isolated from the remaining kidney 15 days after surgery, and N-ROT performed as described,[20] similar to the method outlined in the text. However, radiolabeled RNA generated during the 30-min N-ROT period was hybridized to unlabeled immobilized driver DNA (MT-1 + MT-2 oligonucleotides, and β actin cDNA, each immobilized separately on four separate nitrocellulose discs) in two separate hybridization bags: the second bag contained twice the concentration of radiolabeled RNA as the first. Two blank nitrocellulose discs were included to allow measurement of background binding of radiolabeled RNA. The slope of a graph of "input count/min (cpm)" (a measure of total cellular transcription) vs. "cpm hybridized" for the MT and β actin genes allowed assessment of the relative rate of transcription of MT–1 and MT-2 genes against minimal variation in background hybridization.[20,25] Data represent the mean of measurements from four discs ± SE for MT and actin genes. These data indicate that the compensatory hypertrophy undergone in the remaining kidney after uninephrectomy was accompanied by enhanced MT-1 + MT-2 gene transcription. "Housekeeping" β actin gene transcription remained relatively unaffected. (Data from Reference 20.)

RNA per gram wet tissue is typical.[20] This is less than half that isolated side by side from equivalent wet weights of liver and kidney.[20,40]

This method produces total tissue RNAs, the majority of which are ribosomal and transfer RNAs, which do not act as templates for protein production. Mature cytoplasmic mRNA constitutes only about 3% of total RNA.[41] In addition, the majority of eukaryotic mRNAs contain a string of adenosine ribonucleoside residues at the 3′ end: they are polyadenylated and constitute the poly(A)$^+$ RNA pool. Messenger RNAs present at low levels (less than 0.001% of the mRNA population) are generally difficult to detect. It may be necessary to enrich isolated RNA for the polyadenylated fraction by binding to cellulose conjugated with oligo(dT) or poly(U) Sephadex,[42] washing away unbound poly(A)$^-$ RNA, and eluting poly(A)$^+$ mRNA under low salt conditions.[43] Messenger RNA fractions isolated in this way are appropriate to detect low-abundance, specific mRNAs.

19.2.2.2 *Northern blot analysis*

Both the amount and approximate molecular weight of individual mRNA species are most commonly determined by Northern blot analysis. Protocols for this procedure have been described extensively elsewhere.[34,44] Briefly, total tissue or cellular RNA (usually about 10 μg, although up to 40 μg may be used to enhance sensitivity) or poly(A)$^+$ RNA (usually about 3 μg) is separated in an agarose gel under the influence of an electric field in the presence of formaldehyde, glyoxal, or dimethyl sulfoxide to discourage formation of intrastrand RNA hydrogen bonding (which produces anomalous migration). Agarose–formaldehyde gels are, arguably, the most reliable method. RNAs migrate according to molecular weight and are transferred to a solid nylon or nitrocellulose membrane support where they are detected by specific hybridization to radiolabeled cDNA or oligonucleotide probes (Figure 3). Nylon membranes have greater tensile strength and capacity to bind and retain RNA, but are subject to higher nonspecific background radioactivity binding. Hybridization may be carried out using high salt/high temperature (65°) or formamide (low temperature) hybridization buffers.[34] Radiolabeled probes are (1) single-stranded DNA molecules, (2) denatured, double-stranded DNA, or (3) RNA molecules. Each type has advantages and disadvantages (see below). Generally, ^{32}P is the isotope of choice as a tracer because of its high β particle energy and specific activity (suitable for detection by autoradiography and phosphorimagery) and reasonably short half-life (approximately 14 days). A wide range of methods (end-labeling of single-stranded DNA, riboprobe synthesis of single-stranded RNAs, and nick translation or random-primed labeling of double-stranded DNAs) are available. End-labeling techniques provide probes with lower specific activity than other methods, but is the only practical method for single-stranded DNA. Single-stranded DNA and RNA probes can be made to be bind exclusively to cellular RNA or genomic DNA sequences and can be used to distinguish between mRNA and antisense RNA. Double-stranded DNA probes (which contain sequences complementary to genomic DNA, mRNA, and antisense RNA) do not have that capability. In every case, probes used for Northern blot analysis have a nucleotide sequence complementary to the specific mRNA of interest. However, they may bind to the mRNA of more than one member of a related gene family (see below). If mRNAs from different gene family members differ in size, then hybridization of probe to bands of appropriate molecular weight serves as a check for specificity. The size of the mRNA can be interpolated by reference to internal rRNA bands visualized by ethidium bromide staining and/or hybridization to probes specific for rRNA species. 28S rRNA (4718 nucleotides) and 18S rRNA (1874 nucleotides) are the two most prominent bands visualized by ethidium bromide staining of agarose gels after electrophoresis of total tissue RNA (Figure 3).

Because all RNAs expressed in cells are present, a single blot may be reused several times to assess the presence and quantity of multiple transcripts. To avoid interference, however, bound probe from previous hybridizations should, in most cases, be removed

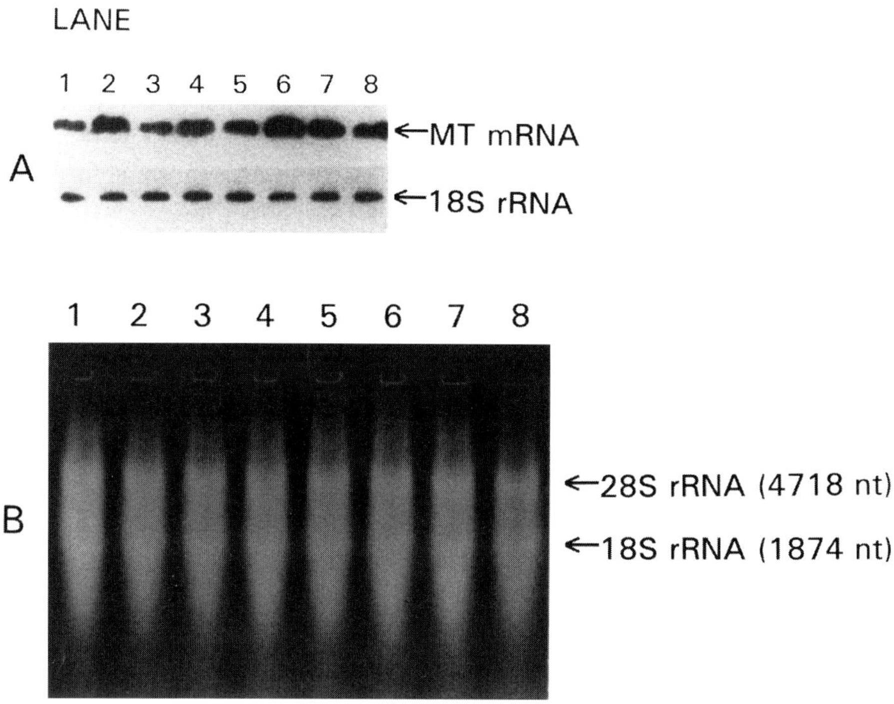

Figure 3 Northern blot measurement of specific mRNAs in kidney tissues. (A): MT-1 + MT-2 mRNA level (assessed by hybridization to a radiolabeled DNA probe containing sequences complementary to both MT-1 and MT-2) and 18S rRNA level (assessed by hybridization to a specific radiolabeled cDNA probe) in rat kidney tissues from animals treated as described in the legend to Figure 2. These data demonstrate altered accumulation, in whole kidney and in subregions with specialized renal cell function, of MT mRNA (but not 18S rRNA) accompanying compensatory renal growth.[20] (Lane 1) CONTROL rat whole kidney from CONTROL rat; (Lane 2) COMPENSATORY GROWTH rat whole kidney; (Lane 3) CONTROL rat renal cortex; (Lane 4) COMPENSATORY GROWTH rat renal cortex; (Lane 5) CONTROL rat renal outer stripe of outer medulla; (Lane 6) COMPENSATORY GROWTH rat renal outer stripe of outer medulla; (Lane 7) CONTROL rat inner stripe of outer medulla plus papilla; (Lane 8) COMPENSATORY GROWTH rat inner stripe of outer medulla plus papilla. Hybridized MT-1 + MT-2 probe was stripped from the blot before rehybridization to the 18S rRNA probe. Hybridization was visualized by autoradiography. (B) Total mouse kidney tissue RNA, including the constitutive 28S (4718 bases) and 18S (1874 bases) RNA apparent in the RNA followed electrophoretic separation through a denaturing formaldehyde/0.8% agarose gel, and prior to transfer to nitrocellulose paper and hybridization to probe. Lanes 1 to 4 contain RNA (10 μg per lane) isolated from control animals untreated with toxic compounds. Lane 5 contains kidney RNA from a mouse treated with $CdSO_2$ (1.0 mg Cd per kilogram mouse, in saline, administered intraperitoneally 3 h prior to tissue sampling). Lanes 6 to 8 contain RNA from mice treated with increasing concentration of cadmium associated with rat MT-2 (CdMT, 0.15 to 0.45 mg Cd per kilogram mouse, administered intraperitoneally 3 h prior to tissue sampling).[40]

by washing at high stringency before hybridization to new probes. Standard procedures have been described.[34,44] Nylon rather than nitrocellulose filter supports stand up best to multiple probing because of their higher tensile strength and more tenacious binding of RNA.

Northern blot detection of hybridization to a single radiolabeled probe is appropriate for *qualitative* detection of specific mRNAs. Quantitation (measurement of relative amounts of specific mRNAs in cells under conditions that induce gene expression, or between different cell types) requires careful use of appropriate controls and is subject to limited interpretation. Relevant considerations are discussed below.

19.2.2.3 Slot and dot blot analysis

These methods detect and measure specific mRNA levels in total tissue RNA applied directly to nitrocellulose or nylon membranes. Blotting manifolds (available commercially from a variety of sources) generate uniform dots (Figure 4) or slots that differ only in the shape of the area to which RNA is applied: otherwise, all methods pertaining to hybridization of probes are identical. Advantages of slot and dot blots over Northern blotting include the ability to process larger numbers of samples, enhanced retention of RNA due to omission of relatively inefficient and variable transfer from agarose gels to nylon or nitrocellulose filters, and the ability to apply larger amounts of RNA per unit area on filters. Detailed protocols for this procedure have been described[34,44] and have been used extensively.[25,40,45] Some special considerations and limitations apply to slot and dot blot analysis. Because no information on the molecular weight of hybridized species is provided by the technique, specificity of hybridization is not assured: it is wise to first ensure that probes hybridize to an RNA molecule of appropriate molecular weight on a Northern blot before proceeding to dot or slot blots.

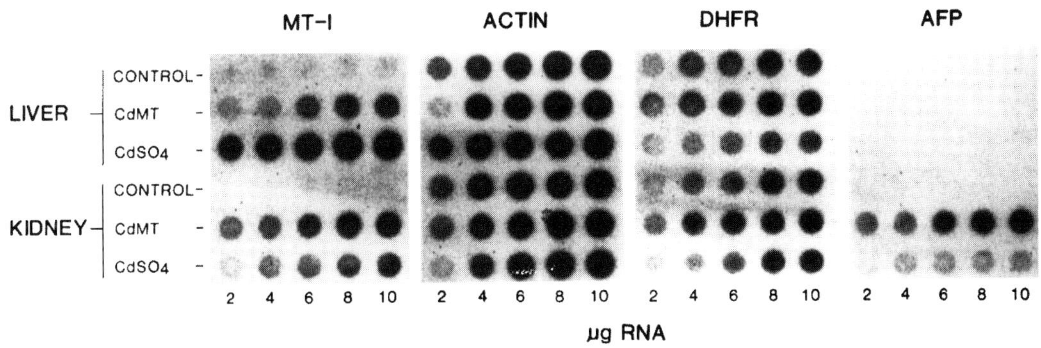

Figure 4 RNA dot blot measurement of specific mRNAs in mouse liver and kidney tissue. Total cellular RNA was isolated from mouse liver and kidney 3 h after saline (CONTROL), CdMT, or $CdSO_4$ treatment (0.3 mg Cd per kilogram mouse in each case; see legend to Figure 3) and quantitated by absorbance at A_{260}. RNA, 2 to 10 µg, was immobilized in five separate dots on nitrocellulose filters and hybridized to radiolabeled cDNA probes for mouse MT-1, β actin, dihydrofolate reductase (dhfr), or alfafetoprotein (AFP) mRNA. Hybridization was visualized by autoradiography. These data indicate that both cadmium (both as an inorganic salt [$CdSO_4$], and bound to rat MT-2 [CdMT]) effectively induce hepatic MT-1. MT-bound cadmium also induced renal AFP mRNA accumulation, while inorganic cadmium salt treatment did so only weakly. AFP mRNA was not induced in liver by either inorganic Cd or CdMT.

19.2.2.4 Probe selection and labeling

Probes to detect specific mRNA are of three types. Double-stranded complementary DNAs (cDNAs) are synthesized from the mRNA transcribed from the gene of interest, and are generally produced in quantity by insertion into a bacterial shuttle vector. For best results on Northern blots, cDNA sequences should be isolated from bacterial sequences by restriction endonuclease cleavage and gel electrophoresis before radiolabeling and hybridization. This minimizes nonspecific binding of bacterial DNA sequences to RNA. DNA oligonucleotides are single-stranded DNAs produced by automated DNA synthesizers via the phosphite triester method[46] and may be of virtually any sequence. Single-stranded oligonucleotides can be end-labeled with T4 polynucleotide kinase:[34] specific activity is limited by the ability to label only terminal nucleotides. For higher specific activity, RNA probes ("riboprobes") transcribed from cDNAs (or synthesized oligonucleotides) inserted into *in vitro* transcription vectors containing viral SP6 or T7 promoters can be used. Like

DNA oligonucleotides, they can be antisense and complementary to the mRNA of interest or sense and complementary to only one of the DNA strands of the gene of interest, depending on the direction of transcription and the RNA polymerase (SP6 or T7) used in the reaction.[34,36]

Radiolabeled probes must bind to the mRNA of interest with high specificity in order to preclude false positive signals. False positive signals can be caused by nonspecific binding to sequences similar to the target sequence, but found in RNA molecules other than the target mRNA. Smaller probes such as synthetic oligonucleotides (20 to 40 bases long) are at greater risk of binding inappropriately because of the increasing likelihood of random complementarity with decreasing length of defined sequence. Complementary DNA probes, on the other hand, are usually longer (greater than 400 base pairs) and, consequently, tend to bind more specifically, assuming that sequences complementary to non-unique RNAs are not embedded in the longer probe.

Synthetic oligonucleotide probes may also be used. Their sequence is chosen to be complementary to published mRNA sequences. However, researchers may, unwittingly, synthesize oligonucleotides complementary to nonrelevant nucleic acids. To minimize this, it is important to scan the known array of RNA sequences for complementarity to the planned oligonucleotide sequence beforehand. Several databases (European Molecular Biology Laboratory, Heidelberg, Germany [EMBL]; GenBank (sponsored by the U.S. National Institutes of Health [NIH]); and the DNA Data Bank of Japan [DDBJ], for example) contain known DNA, RNA, and protein sequences and are available through electronic mail (E-mail) or the Internet to researchers with personal computers with appropriate software.[47] It is important to realize, though, that gene databases contain only known DNA and RNA sequences. Synthesized probes may just as easily bind to nonrelevant nucleic acids not yet described in the literature, and a trial-and-error process is necessary to exclude this possibility.

Genomic DNA sequences are not generally recommended for use as probes for RNA. They contain untranslated sequences not represented in mature cytoplasmic mRNA that may contain repetitive sequences, leading to nonspecific binding. However, some mRNAs may be appropriately detected with genomic DNA probes provided appropriate controls are included.[20,48]

Kits and enzymes for the production of probes are available from a number of manufacturers.

19.2.2.5 *Standardization and quantitation*

Radiolabeled probes bound to Northern blots, dot blots, or N-ROT filters can be visualized by X-ray film autoradiography (Figure 3) or phosphor screen technology (Figure 1). The amount of hybridization is measured by densitometry. Quantitation of densitometric analysis of X-ray film darkening can be complicated by the nonlinear response of autoradiographic film to radioactivity. Phosphor screens release energy at a rate that is proportional to the amount of radioactivity over a greater dynamic range than is possible for X-ray films used with or without intensifying screens.[49] Therefore, phosphor imagery of hybridized probes is rapidly becoming the method of choice for quantitation of mRNA levels from Northern blots.

Interpretation of measurement of the level of hybridization to specific bands in Northern blots is heavily dependent upon standards and controls. The simplest method of standardization is to load equal amounts of total RNA — tissue, cellular, or poly(A)$^+$ — and visualize that loading through enhanced fluorescence after staining with ethidium bromide[34] (Figure 3). This method is inaccurate due to error-prone absorbance spectroscopy quantitation of RNA and low sensitivity of ethidium bromide staining. In addition, most enhanced fluorescence in the presence of total tissue or cellular RNA — approximately

97%[41] is due to RNA that does not code for specific proteins (transfer RNAs, ribosomal RNAs) or is immature coding RNA (heteronuclear RNA). Relatively large changes in the amount of mature cytoplasmic mRNA are not likely to induce detectable changes in fluorescence, but would nevertheless be important in estimating relative changes in specific mRNA levels. Therefore, better controls against which hybridization to the probe of interest can be compared are necessary to provide a measure of relative mRNA levels.

Most investigators rely on an internal standard RNA such as 18S rRNA (an RNA component of the small ribosomal subunit, without protein-coding information) or specific mRNAs for β actin, GAPDH, 18S rRNA or other housekeeping genes as indicators of equal loading of mRNA per lane (Figure 3).[42,43] Radiolabeled probes for such standards are hybridized to the same blot to which the probe for the gene of interest has been hybridized. An intervening "stripping" step removes the first probe without much loss of RNA bound to the membrane (see Section 19.2.2.2 for details). The quantity of mRNA from the gene of interest can be expressed as a fraction of the level of the chosen standard RNA. This provides only a relative measure of specific mRNA level. Therefore, measurement of changes in mRNA accumulation are most reliable when assessed in cells of closely related type or from the same tissue. Comparisons between fundamentally different cell types are more difficult and may require assessment of absolute mRNA levels (i.e., measures of specific mRNA molecules per cell) by solution hybridization.[50]

The use of housekeeping genes as standards against which to measure inducible gene expression depends critically on the assumption that these mRNAs are common and necessary to all cell types and are invariable within one cell type. However, the amount of mRNA from housekeeping genes may vary with tissue type, cell lineage, growth conditions, or cell cycle. Treatment of the cells *in vitro* with drugs, hormones, or growth factors can alter the expression of genes generally regarded as housekeeping.[51,52] The level of ribosomal RNA (e.g., 18S rRNA) as an indicator of the amount of mRNA can also be deceptive. Since mature cytoplasmic mRNA makes up only a small proportion of total cellular RNA, a major change in the amount of mRNA would have only a small effect on the level of rRNA in that sample. Increased overall cellular gene activity (that enhanced all mRNA levels nonspecifically, for example) might appear to be specific expression of the gene of interest when compared to 18S rRNA levels.[20] Measurement of expression of more than one internal standard mRNA and/or rRNA, therefore, can aid in interpreting relative quantitation of induced gene expression.

There are other strategies to address the problem of relative mRNA levels. Variation in gene expression can be evaluated statistically, using a multigene slot blot analysis of a large number of cell or tissue samples.[52] Alternatively, hybridization can be expressed on an average-per-cell basis by normalizing to levels of DNA isolated from the same tissues[25,40] or added radiolabeled cellular RNA with incorporated radiolabeled ribonucleosides.[53] The entire pool of poly(A)$^+$ RNA can also be detected and measured using a radiolabeled oligo(dT) probe.[54] The fraction of this pool provided by mRNA from the gene of interest is a useful comparator for specific mRNAs.

19.2.2.6 *Reverse transcription–polymerase chain reaction (RT-PCR) analysis*

The sensitivity of Northern blot analysis and the loss of material in the isolation of RNA limit the amount of specific mRNAs that can be detected in tissues. The polymerase chain reaction (PCR) has enormously enhanced the ability to detect rare DNA sequences.[55] If the sensitivity of PCR is harnessed for the quantitation of mRNA, smaller sample sizes and less sample preparation is necessary for measurement of gene expression. However, PCR works only on DNA. Therefore, it is necessary to copy mRNA into complementary DNA (cDNA) before the method can be applied. A combined RT-PCR technique to measure the level of specific mRNAs was first reported by Veres et al.[56] and has been described in detail for any mRNA sequence.[57] RT-PCR is approximately 1000 times more sensitive than dot blots or solution hybridization.[58,59] The method does not require highly purified RNA, so RNA loss during processing is minimized. RT-PCR is semiautomated so that large numbers of samples can be processed at one time. Briefly, 0.1 to 1 μg of total tissue RNA (isolated as described above) is used as a template to synthesize a heterogeneous library of cDNAs using a viral reverse transcriptase (RT) enzyme[34]. RT is an RNA-dependent DNA polymerase that uses single-stranded RNA or DNA as a template to synthesize the complementary DNA strand in the presence of dCTP, dGTP, dATP, and dTTP and appropriate primer sequences. The latter are included because production of cDNAs must first be "primed" by initial hybridization of short synthetic single-stranded oligonucleotides to the RNA: reverse transcriptase initiates cDNA synthesis where primers associate with RNA by complementary base-pairing. Primer oligonucleotides may be oligo(dT) designed to bind only to poly(A)$^+$ tails (and therefore prime most, but not all mRNAs), or they may be constructed to bind only to sequences unique to the gene of interest. Generally, however, random primers of heterogeneous sequence, capable of initiating cDNA production from virtually all RNA sequences present, are preferred: the resulting cDNA library will be of value in assessing the level of virtually any mRNA present in the cells. Unique primers restrict the technique to measurement of the mRNA of initial interest alone.[60] Several companies supply kits for this purpose (for example, the AMV reverse transcriptase system from Life Technologies, Inc., Gaithersburg, MD, or the first strand cDNA synthesis kit from Boehringer Mannheim GmbH). When a kit is used (for example, that supplied by Life Technologies), a reaction mixture of 50 m*M* TRIS-HCl (pH 8.3), 75 m*M* KCl, 10 m*M* dithiothreitol, 3 m*M* $MgCl_2$, 500 μ*M* of each dNTP (deoxyribonucleotides: dCTP, dATP, dGTP, and dTTP), 0.5 μg oligo(dT_{18}) or random primers, 0.1 to 1.0 μg of total or poly(A)$^+$ RNA isolated from cells or tissue, and 50 units of reverse transcriptase in a 50-μl reaction volume is prepared and incubated at 37°C for 60 min. Ten microliters is removed for use in a subsequent PCR reaction, and the remainder is stored at –70°C.

The cDNAs produced by the RT reaction are then amplified by PCR using oligonucleotides that prime only the synthesis of the cDNA of interest by multiple rounds of activity of thermostable *Taq* polymerase. To do so, 20 μl of the RT reaction mix is placed in a sterile polypropylene 0.5-ml PCR reaction tube, and to this is added appropriate volumes of 10× PCR reaction buffer, stock $MgCl_2$, mixed dNTPs, sterile water, oligonucleotide primers, and *Taq* DNA polymerase. The final volume is between 50 and 100 μl, depending on the choice of kit (for example, PCR Reagent System from Life Technologies, Inc.). Because of the extremely sensitive nature of the PCR reaction, control tubes should be included that contain either no cDNA, or RNA that has not undergone the RT reaction, to test for false-positive results. In addition, tubes containing known quantities of control DNA template and appropriate primers to amplify that template (both usually supplied by the manufacturer) should also be included as positive controls to quantitate and validate the system and thermal cycler performance. The mixture is overlaid with sterile mineral oil to prevent evaporation and maintain stable reagent concentrations, and the tube inserted into the heating block of a *thermal cycler*. This apparatus sequentially heats samples to 95°C for 5 min to denature nucleic acids, cools them to 55°C for 2 min to allow primers to associate in a sequence-specific manner, and finally heats them to 72°C for 3 min to allow *Taq* polymerase to synthesize a new DNA strand from the primers. This heating/cooling sequence is repeated from 20 to 40 times to allow multiple rounds of replication and high final concentrations of specific DNA product, which are visualized and measured as described below.

In PCR, unique primers that allow amplification of the DNA of interest, and that DNA only, are employed. This is critical, because accurate measurement of mRNA levels depends absolutely on the efficiency and specificity of primer binding to cDNA. Important considerations in the design of such primers have been discussed,[57,61] and a host of primers designed to specifically associate with human and other DNAs of interest to toxicologists are commercially available (Stratagene Cloning Systems, Inc., CA; Clontech Laboratories, Inc., CA, and others). Even so, inappropriate amplification of nontarget cDNAs can occur, and it may be necessary to confirm the identity of RT-PCR products by hybridization to a radiolabeled probe by Southern hybridization.[34] In cases where nonspecific amplification is a problem, "nested" cDNA primers have been used to increase specificity.[62] Although primers that bind by complementary base-pairing with virtually any chosen sequences within target cDNAs is possible, primers should

1. Have noncomplementary ends to prevent primer–dimer formation.
2. Be derived from separate exons to make it simple to identify products arising from contaminating genomic DNA. Genomic DNA contains the same sequences as cDNA and can give rise to false-positive amplification products by binding to primers intended to associate specifically with cDNA. If the sequences with which primers associate are chosen to span an intron, however, genomic DNA products are identifiable by slower migration on the final agarose gel electrophoresis step in RT-PCR.
3. Have similar composition of guanine and cytosine (50 to 60%) to ensure comparable melting temperatures.
4. Avoid runs of guanines and cytosines, which promote nonspecific priming.
5. Be at least 18 to 28 nucleotides in length to maximize specificity.[63]

These factors control the association of primers and targeted DNA sequences. The number of amplification steps (cycles) in the PCR reaction affects the yield of PCR product in a manner that depends critically on the starting number of cDNA (and initial mRNA) molecules. If the number of cycles or starting cDNA concentration is too low, the final concentration of DNA product will also be low, and visualization following electrophoresis will be difficult. On the other hand, accumulation of more than 1 pmol of product results in a "plateau effect." In this case, the concentration of primers and dNTPs and the activity of *Taq* polymerase becomes limiting, and the exponential rate of product accumulation is attenuated. This can lead to inaccurate estimates of starting mRNA levels along with an increase in nonspecific background products.[63] Optimization of the number of cycles and/or the starting amount of cDNA is required to avoid this problem.

RT-PCR increases the sensitivity of mRNA detection by several orders of magnitude. Rare mRNA sequences have been accurately measured in a few thousand cells compared to the 10^6 to 10^7 cells needed for Northern analysis.[64] The high inherent sensitivity of PCR, however, means that all reactants (especially $MgCl_2$ concentrations) must be optimized if target sequences (and not nontarget sequences) are to be maximally amplified. This has been a problem in quantitating mRNA: small differences in the variables that control reaction rate have extreme effects on the yield of PCR product.[57,61] Between-tube error can comprise up to 15% of the yield for identical samples and must be minimized to allow reliable interpretation. An internal control provides two important pieces of information: quantitation of relative expression of a target gene for each sample, and an indication of the purity and integrity of RNA in the samples.[65] The addition of modified synthetic sequences, which are co-amplified with the target gene cDNA, is an internal control for the PCR portion of the RT-PCR reaction.[59] However, this does not provide information about RNA quality. To obtain a reliable measure of relative mRNA level, internal standards that control for variables that affect both the reverse transcription and PCR steps are required. Three approaches have been used to address this problem:

1. Co-amplification of cDNA from an mRNA for a housekeeping protein, including β actin, α actin, HPRT, GAPDH, dihydrofolate reductase, and/or β_2-microglobulin:[65,66] many of these primers are commercially available
2. Quantitation against a synthetic internal standard DNA with priming sites that allow amplification using 12 or more different sets of primers, each specific for a different DNA sequence:[67] this internal standard can be used to measure the efficiency of amplification of a range of different nucleic acids
3. Quantitation against a competitive template that uses the same primers as the target cDNA, but can be distinguished from the target cDNA after co-amplification.

The standard can be identical to the cDNA of interest except for the presence of a mutated restriction site or the inclusion of a small intervening sequence (present in the standard DNA, but not in the mRNA being measured) to increase its size and decrease its rate of migration in an agarose gel.[57,58] The intervening sequence should be small enough to leave the amplification rate unaffected. Competitive templates can be used as controls for both the reverse transcriptase and PCR steps, since synthetic RNA molecules (generated by cloning DNA into an RNA expression vector) can be added to the RNA sample prior to cDNA synthesis. However, such "RNA doping" techniques provide no information about the integrity of mRNA.

A good way to address this problem is to co-amplify a housekeeping gene product — β_2-microglobulin (β_2m) cDNA, for example — using a separate pair of primers in each tube in which the gene of interest is being amplified (Figure 5). The β_2m cDNA must be synthesized by reverse transcription of endogenous β_2m mRNA by random primers in the cells being assessed.[66,68] This method serves simultaneously to measure expression of a housekeeping gene and to control for the integrity of cellular mRNA and the efficiencies of both the reverse transcription and PCR steps.

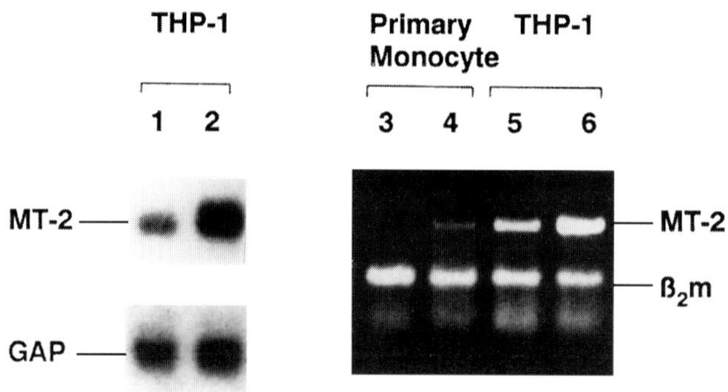

Figure 5 Comparison of Northern blotting and reverse transcription–polymerase chain reaction (RT-PCR) to measure relative metallothionein mRNA expression. Lanes 1 and 2 are autoradiographs of Northern blots of total cellular RNA isolated from a human monocytic leukemia cell line (THP-1) untreated with metals (lane 1), or treated with 1 μ*M* cadmium sulfate to induce MT expression (lane 2). The blot was hybridized, in sequence, to radiolabeled probes detecting human MT-2 and GAPDH mRNA, with an intervening stripping step to remove bound MT-2 probe. The ethidium bromide-stained bands in lanes 3 to 6 represent the abundance of MT-2 and $\beta_2$microglobulin cDNA following RT-PCR of primary human monocyte or THP-1 mRNA. Cadmium sulfate (Cd, 1 μ*M*) was used to induce MT expression. Bacterial lipopolysaccharide (LPS, 10 μg/ml) was used to stimulate a respiratory burst in human monocytes. (Lane 1) – Cd; (Lane 2) + Cd; (Lane 3) – LPS; (Lane 4) + LPS; (Lane 5) – Cd; (Lane 6) + Cd. These data indicate that both Northern blot and RT-PCR analysis detect increased MT-2 mRNA in human monocytes treated with cadmium and undergoing a respiratory burst after LPS induction. (From Leibbrandt, M. E. I. and Koropatnick, J., *Toxicol. Appl. Pharmacol.*, 124, 72, 1994. With permission.)

The amplified products can be identified by size on an ethidium bromide-stained agarose gel (Figure 5) and quantitated by a densitometer scan of a Southern blot hybridization.[66] Alternatively, radioactive DNA precursors can be incorporated during PCR amplification and the resulting products visualized directly by autoradiography or phosphorimagery.[65] Caution should be exercised if this approach is used, since the omission of hybridization to a specific probe does not allow a check for specificity of amplification.

RT-PCR is becoming an increasingly attractive technique to measure mRNA levels where small amounts of available tissue and/or very low level expression precludes measurement by Northern blot analysis. Cytokine gene mRNA levels (interleukin-4 (IL-4),[69] IL-1, IL-3, IL-5, IL-6, interferon-γ[70]) and accumulation of glucagon receptor,[71] renin,[72] nitric oxide synthase,[73] transforming growth factor β1,[74] C-type natriuretic peptide,[75] Na^+/K^+-ATPase α and β subunit[76,77] mRNAs (to name only a few) have been measured. In some cases, microlocalization and quantitation of mRNAs in kidney cellular subpopulations has been possible.[73,75-77] Human adrenal cortex mRNAs (for endothelin A and B) have also been measured in small tissue samples obtained from patients.[78] As a note of caution, however, quantitative RT-PCR measurements are not as reliable, in most cases, as Northern blot or primer extension analysis. RT-PCR is most useful as a qualitative and relative measure of mRNA level, and accurate measurement of mRNAs by this technique depends critically on the use of positive and negative controls as well as measurement in replicate samples to accurately assess experimental error.

19.2.2.7 *Ribonuclease protection and primer extension analysis*

Where mRNA transcripts are rare (between 0.001% and 0.01% of total tissue RNA), modifications of Northern blot analysis have been developed to enhance sensitivity and provide additional information. The ribonuclease protection assay[79] depends upon production of sequence-specific RNA hybridization probes of high specific activity. These probes are complementary to specific mRNAs and are produced by *in vitro* transcription of DNA templates inserted adjacent to bacteriophage promoters (SP6 or T7) in the presence of radiolabeled ribonucleotide triphosphate precursors.[80] The bacteriophage RNA polymerases responsible for producing RNA from these promoters polymerize RNA approximately ten times faster than *Escherichia coli* polymerases and faster than DNA polymerases.[81] Resulting radiolabeled RNA is purified by digestion with deoxyribonuclease (to remove transcription template DNA), phase separation purification with phenol/chloroform (to remove proteins of the transcription complex), and precipitation in ethanol in the presence of 2 *M* ammonium acetate (to remove unincorporated radiolabeled precursors). Hybridization of the complementary radiolabeled RNA probe to mRNA is then carried out in solution — unlike Northern blot analysis, not to RNA immobilized on a membrane. Unhybridized probe is digested with ribonuclease. Radiolabeled probe annealed to specific target mRNA is, however, left intact. Annealed probe/mRNA is purified by ethanol precipitation and analyzed by electrophoresis through a denaturing polyacrylamide/urea gel. The amount of radioactivity associated with the mRNA protected from ribonuclease protection, and present in a characteristic band visualized by gel electrophoresis, is a measure of the amount of that mRNA in total tissue RNA and can be measured by autoradiography or phosphorimagery.

The primer extension assay[82,83] is an alternative to the ribonucleotide protection assay. However, rather than using an RNA probe synthesized apart from the target mRNA, the enzyme reverse transcriptase (RT) is used to synthesize a DNA strand complementary to the mRNA of interest (Figure 6). Just as for the RT-PCR reaction described above, RT requires a short DNA oligonucleotide to anneal to an interior region of the target mRNA to prime synthesis of a complementary strand: the oligonucleotide should be 20 to 40 nucleotides long with a sequence chosen to minimize cross-hybridization to nontarget mRNAs. It should also bind to a sequence situated no more than 100 nucleotides from the 5′ end of the mRNA to reduce the likelihood of premature termination of DNA synthesis (Figure 6). The synthesized DNA strand is assessed for quantity and nucleotide length by autoradiograph or phosphorimager analysis on a denaturing polyacrylamide/urea gel.

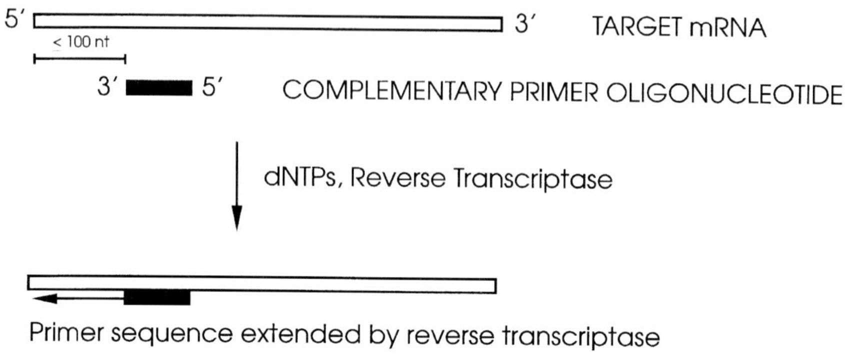

Figure 6 Primer extension to measure specific mRNA transcripts.

Both nuclease protection and primer extension assays assess specific mRNA quantity. Because the lengths of the radiolabeled products critically depend on the length of the target mRNA, they can also (unlike Northern, RT-PCR, or slot and dot blot analyses) map the 5′ terminus of the mature transcript. In practice, primer extension assays are used most often for the latter purpose (i.e., mapping transcription start sites).[84] However, nuclease protection assays have been extensively used to measure kidney mRNAs, including those for growth hormone receptor,[85,86] α2-adrenergic receptor subtypes,[87] natriuretic peptide receptor subtypes,[88] and Ah receptor.[89]

19.2.2.8 In situ *hybridization*

Techniques described above to measure specific mRNA transcripts provide an estimate of the average transcription rate or mRNA level among pooled cells. Assessment of gene expression in individual cells is not practical unless *in situ* methods to measure mRNA or resulting protein levels are used. A description of *in situ* protein measurement protocols is beyond the scope of this chapter, but has been extensively reviewed elsewhere.[90]

Although *in situ* nucleic acid hybridization was first described as a technique to detect specific DNA sequences within cells,[91] it has since been modified to detect specific mRNA transcripts in tissue sections. Detailed protocols for a variety of tissues from different organisms are available.[92-97] Briefly, highly vascularized tissues in test animals (including kidney) are perfused with phosphate-buffered saline (PBS) *in situ* through the left ventricle of the heart. Once the animal's blood has been exchanged for saline, the saline is then exchanged with freshly prepared ice-cold (4°C) 4% paraformaldehyde (PFA) fixative. It is absolutely essential for success that perfusion be complete and speedy: unless blood-rich organs (liver, spleen, and kidney) are seen to turn greyish-white, further steps in the procedure will be a waste of time. Fresh, and not commercially available, PFA stock solutions must be used. Following perfusion, organs are removed to glass vials containing 4% PFA fixative and stored at 4°C until embedded in paraffin and sectioned on a microtome. Alternatively, tissues may be frozen and sectioned in a cryostat.[98] Sections are dewaxed, single cells hydrated, and the sections treated to denature and remove some of the proteins to improve the accessibility of RNA transcripts to radiolabeled hybridizing probe. Probes are usually antisense riboprobes (described in Section 19.2.2.4) with a sequence complementary to target mRNA. They are radiolabeled with ^{32}P-uridine triphosphate (UTP) and are incubated with sections for up to 4 h. Unhybridized probe is removed afterward by digestion with RNase (as described in Section 19.2.2.7). Radiolabeled probe can be visualized by exposure to autoradiograph film (Du Pont Cronex Video Imaging Film [MRF 34 Clear], or Kodak XRP–1) or by coating slides with autoradiographic emulsion (Kodak NTB-2 autoradiographic emulsion for use in emulsion autoradiography).[96]

Some critical precautions to consider[95] for *in situ* hybridization are

1. Sections from tissues known (from Northern blots, slot or dot blots, or RNase protection or primer extension assays) to express the target mRNA at a high level should be included as a positive control.
2. Because over- or underfixation impedes good hybridization, use two different fixation time points that provide tissues that section well.
3. Hybridize for different lengths of time (30 min, 1 h, 2 h, 4 h) to optimize the signal-to-noise ratio.

Critical controls that must be done are

1. Hybridize the first set of sections to an antisense riboprobe to detect target mRNA transcripts and a second set of sections to a complementary sense riboprobe, under exactly the same conditions, to establish nonspecific background. The complementary sense riboprobe can be synthesized from the same template DNA, but transcribed in the opposite direction.
2. Prior to hybridization to the antisense probe, treat a set of control sections with RNase to detect binding to non-mRNA components.

19.2.2.9 Interpretation of mRNA measurements

The methods described here are, under optimum conditions, both accurate and sensitive in measuring mRNA levels. However, the following considerations are important in placing the results in context.

- Sampling time may be critical. Maximal gene transcription and mRNA accumulation occurs at different times in different cell types and under different conditions. For example, mouse MT-1 mRNA reaches a maximum level between 4 and 6 h after cadmium induction in liver,[99] but after only 30 min in human monocytes *in vitro*.[66] There is no specific time following treatment that induced gene transcription and mRNA levels should be measured. Therefore, measurements at multiple time points should be considered.
- Methods should provide information on the specificity of hybridization of probes to adequately distinguish hybridization between target RNA and nonspecific sequences. Increased levels of immature mRNA may not result in increased production of functional protein, or multigene families may produce nontarget mRNAs that cross-hybridize to some degree with radiolabeled probes. Some methods (slot and dot blots, for example) sacrifice characterization of specificity in favor of speed and sensitivity, while others (Northern blots, ribonuclease protection, RT-PCR, and primer extension, for example) include an assessment of mRNA size and/or sequence to confirm identity.
- Increased transcription and mRNA level may not be reflected in enhanced protein activity. Changes in mRNA stability, processing, and "masking" of mRNA from translation by proteins or antisense RNA,[15,16,100,101] as well as posttranslational protein modification, can all affect subsequent protein level and function. Measurement of target protein expression (by Western blot, enzyme-linked immunosorbent assay [ELISA], or radioimmunoassay,[90] and function (by assay of altered enzymatic or other activity of target proteins, or altered cellular activity as a result of altered target gene expression) must be part of assessments of altered gene expression.

- Cell populations both *in vitro* and *in vivo* can be heterogeneous with respect to the expression of specific genes.[102] For example, MT mRNA in mouse placenta and trophoblast is low overall but high in specific cells when assessed by *in situ* hybridization to radiolabeled probes.[103]

19.3 Intervention in gene expression

The most widely used research tool to explore the function of genes is incorporation of foreign nucleic acids into isolated eukaryotic cells and germ-line and somatic cells of whole organisms. Foreign DNA incorporated into cultured somatic cells and directing production of foreign RNA was first described for virus-encoded genes in the early 1970s.[104] Today, transgenic cells and animals harbor a wide variety of foreign DNAs. A detailed description of protocols is available[34,35,105,106] and is not addressed here: it is assumed that readers will go to these sources for details. Cultured cell lines and animals with stably incorporated transgenes, however, are now widely available as test organisms by toxicologists whose expertise lies outside the specific molecular biological methods used to generate these organisms. Therefore, although they are of immense value to toxicologists, some cautions in interpreting data arising from their use must be recognized.

19.3.1 Transfection of structural genes

Structural genes encoding functional proteins — under the control of regulatory regions (including promoters and enhancers[107]) that direct transcription at a high level — can be introduced into individual cells by the process of gene transfection. There are many methods to transfer foreign genes into cells, including calcium phosphate-mediated gene transfer, electroporation, viral infection,[105] and cationic liposome-mediated gene transfer.[35] Their relative merits have been discussed in detail.[105]

Transfected genes may be heterologous (i.e., derived from organisms other than those into which they are introduced) or homologous (i.e., identical to or derived from structural genes already present in transfected cells). Genes of direct and obvious interest to toxicologists and involved in cellular response to toxic agents, including those encoding Cu,Zn superoxide dismutase (SOD–1),[108,109] genes important in programmed cell death (p53[110,111] and bcl-2[110,112]), enzymes important in cytochrome P450 activity,[113] DNA repair, and cell cycle-regulating proteins,[114-116] genes important in cellular drug resistance (*p*-glycoprotein,[117] mrp,[118] glutathione metabolism,[119] and others[120]) have been introduced as transgenes into somatic eukaryotic cells. Gene transfection can be either stable or transient.

19.3.1.1 Stable transfection

Stable transfection assumes incorporation of transgenes into cells such that the foreign DNA is heritably transferred to progeny cells and animals. This stability of incorporation and expression makes these the most readily available cells and organisms for dissemination among researchers not directly engaged in molecular transgenic methods. However, the frequency of stable transfection (i.e., the number of cells expressing the foreign gene after transfection followed by a period of cell proliferation) is relatively low, except in cases of gene transfer by high-titer infectious retrovirus.[105] Stable transfectants typically arise with a frequency of between one cell in 10^3 to one in 10^5. Therefore, enrichment for stable transfectants is required. To do this, a selectable marker gene conferring resistance to a toxic agent is included in the expression vector responsible for expression of the gene of interest. Commonly used selectable marker genes include the multiple drug resistance (mdr1) gene conferring resistance to colchicine and other toxic natural products,[121] the dihydrofolate reductase (dhfr) gene conferring resistance to methotrexate,[122] the metallothionein gene to confer resistance to cadmium salts,[123] and the aminoglycoside phosphotransferase (aph) gene (usually denoted *neo*) to confer resistance to G418 (Geneticin).[124] Other selectable markers are also available.[105] Control cells are transfected with the eukaryotic expression vector alone, either minus the transgene or containing a transgene incapable of directing production of active protein (i.e., inserted in reverse orientation in the vector or lacking transcription and/or translation initiation sequences).

In all cases of selection and enrichment for transfectants, lengthy exposure to toxic agents is required. This is an obvious disadvantage to toxicologists. Treatment with toxic agents may both induce and select for characteristics in test cells other than the presence of the transgene. For example, stable transfectant populations expressing metallothionein transgenes, selected on the basis of resistance to heavy metal toxicity,[125,126] must be used cautiously: exposure to metals can either induce or select cells with increased resistance to other toxic agents,[126] even in the absence of altered metallothionein expression.[127] These unknown and undetected characteristics could have profound implications in assessing the effect of toxicants, and a cautious approach should be taken in interpreting toxicant data from these cells and animals.

A second disadvantage of stable transfection arises from the possibility that incorporation of a foreign transgene may not have neutral consequences for the expression of constitutive genes. Transfected cells may alter the expression of their own genes as an adaptive response to the presence of the foreign DNA. If the constitutive genes with altered expression are of importance in the toxic conditions being investigated, then altered responses may not be directly attributable to the direct effects of the transgene. In interpreting results, the possibility that transgenes may have indirect effects that alter responses should be considered. Finally, stable transfection generally involves covalent linkage of foreign DNA into the genome of recipient cells, and the site of incorporation differs from cell to cell. Constitutive genes at the site of incorporation may potentially be inactivated or have their expression increased by placement in close proximity to powerful promoter/enhancer sequences present in eukaryotic expression vectors. Therefore, it is important to assess the consequences of transgene expression in several stable transfectants with different foreign DNA incorporation sites.

On the other hand, stable transfection has the advantage over transient transfection (Section 19.3.1.2) of allowing expression of foreign genes in virtually all test cells. In addition, the cell lines and transgenic animals generated by the process provide a permanent test organism available for long-term use in multiple laboratories.

19.3.1.2 Transient transfection

Transient transfection involves introduction of foreign DNA into cultured cells[105] in high copy number to generate a "burst" of expression for a defined period of time (generally hours or days). However, the DNA in most transfected cells is not incorporated into high molecular weight genomic DNA in the nucleus, is not effectively replicated during cell proliferation, and may be selectively degraded through the action of constitutive cellular enzymes: this results in the disappearance of the transgene and its products. Because of its temporary nature, transient transfection is not yet a practical method to alter gene expression in primary organ cells. However, there are several advantages of transient over stable transfection for single cells in culture.

- A larger number of foreign DNA copies can be introduced and assessed than in stable transfectants. Transient transfection generally results in 1000- to 10,000-fold more copies within cells than stable transfection.[68]
- Transfected cells can be assessed for the physiological consequences of foreign gene expression during progressive loss of transfected DNA copies and their expression. Therefore, very closely related populations of cells with and without the transgene can be compared. Stably transfected cells separated from control cells several

months or more before they are available for experimentation have an increased risk of differing from control cells in expression of genes other than the transgene.

- Some transfection methods (those using cationic liposomes, for example) allow transfection frequencies in some cell types that result in the majority of treated cells expressing the transgene.[68,128] Therefore, some of the advantages of stable transfection can be combined with those of transient transfection. However, variability in transfection efficiency among cell types makes it imperative that transfection frequency be measured, either by demonstrating altered expression target proteins by immunoassay, immunohistochemical detection, and altered physiological response[129,130] or by cotransfection of β-galactosidase expression vectors that introduce blue color in the presence of appropriate sugars.[130] The color can be used to assess the presence of foreign transgenes in individual cultured cells and cells in tissues, as a consequence of both transient and stable transfection, by visual microscopy or spectrometry.

19.3.2 Gene inactivation

Cells in culture and in whole animals can be induced to produce functional foreign proteins, and the effect of these gain-of-function manipulations can be assessed under subtoxic and toxic conditions. However loss-of-function events can also be induced in cells by either site-directed insertional mutagenesis (so-called gene knockout experiments) or by antisense nucleic acids (to selectively inactivate target mRNAs to down-regulate, but not eliminate, genes of interest). These experiments are designed to specifically inactivate genes of biological interest in order to observe the effect of lost function on a host of biological events. In addition, transgenic mice have been generated harboring foreign genes specifically designed to measure mutagenicity (transgenic mouse *lacI/Z* mutation assays). Thus, transgenic mice with specific deletions of functional genes and with marker genes for assessment of the mutation potential of toxic agents and conditions are available.

19.3.2.1 Transgenic mouse mutation assays

Some chemicals display both tissue and gene-specific mutagenic action.[131] To measure the genotoxicity of chemicals and physical conditions *in vivo*, transgenic mice containing the bacterial *lacZ* gene (Muta™Mouse)[132] or *lacI* (Big Blue™)[133] in every cell have been generated. The former (MutaMouse) have an incorporated lambda bacteriophage shuttle vector containing a target gene encoding bacterial β-galactosidase (β-gal). Damage to the foreign β-gal gene after treatment of mice with suspected mutagens is an indicator of overall genome damage. To assess β-gal gene damage induced in tissues *in situ*, DNA is isolated from tissues and cells of the transgenic mice, and the lambda shuttle vector "rescued" from genomic DNA in the presence of lambda packaging extract. Lambda bacteriophage harboring β-gal genes formerly in mouse cells are those used to infect bacteria: infected bacteria (in the presence of appropriate sugar substrate and inducer) produce a blue color if they contain active, undamaged β-gal genes and white color if they contain damaged, inactive β-gal genes. The frequency of white plaques against a blue background is a measure of mutation frequency. A modification of the assay to select for growth of *lacZ*$^-$ bacteria[132] has simplified the data-gathering process enormously, in that tedious analysis of large numbers of rescued vectors is eliminated, and some time-consuming manipulations and inductions are omitted.

The alternative assay system (Big Blue) is similar except that the foreign target gene is the bacteriophage *lacI* gene: mutations to *lacI* result in the formation of blue plaques, while undamaged, functional *lacI* results in white plaques.[133] Mutation frequency is assessed, in this case, as the number of blue plaques against a background of white plaques: an improvement in visibility that enhances data-gathering capacity.

The merits of both assays have been assessed.[131] In general, the techniques are too new to replace established *in vitro* mutagenicity assays, but offer great promise (pending further data and discussion) for assessing mutagenic potential and may eventually be part of routine assessment of chemicals and conditions for somatic and germ cell mutagenicity *in vivo*.

19.3.2.2 Site-directed insertional inactivation

Spontaneous mutations of interesting genes have been instrumental in determining the function of proteins. However, the random nature of such mutations makes them impractical for routine use in a systematic approach to exploring gene activity. Insertional inactivation is a process whereby specific constitutive genes in cultured cells or whole animals are inactivated or mutated in a systematic, targeted way.[134,135] In general, mutant mouse strains are produced by transfecting a DNA construct containing target gene sequences in combination with sequences containing a desired mutation into pluripotent mouse embryonic stem (ES) cells (derived from the inner cell mass of a blastocyst-stage embryo) or related embryonic carcinoma (EC or EK) in culture. A common technique is to transfect a drug resistance gene (usually *neo* for resistance to G418) flanked by two regions of homology to the target gene: through a homologous double crossover recombination event, target gene sequences are replaced by the replacement construct. *Neo* simultaneously disrupts the function of the gene sequence into which it inserts and confers resistance to G418 to allow selection of rare stable transfectant cells. However, only a small and variable fraction of recombination events are targeted to the gene of interest. The majority are random and of no use for homologous gene inactivation. Cells carrying them must be eliminated *in vitro* in order to end up with only targeted insertional mutants for use in producing appropriate transgenic "knockout" animals. A number of strategies to eliminate nontargeted insertional mutants have been described, including positive–negative selection[136] and use of endogenous promoters.[137] The types of mutations produced by insertional inactivation range from complete inactivation (knockout) to subtle changes in gene structure and activity through "hit and run" allele replacement techniques[138] originally developed in yeast.

Once target genes are inactivated or mutated in ES, EC, or EK cells *in vitro*, the powerful somatic genetic selection techniques described above can be employed (by drug and toxin resistance conferred by transgenes) to select appropriate cells for use in producing transgenic animals. Once cells are selected and characterized, they can give rise to a chimeric or mosaic mouse when introduced into a normal blastocyst isolated from a fertilized female, which is then transferred into the uterus of a "pseudopregnant" (hormonally-primed) foster mother. Chimeric animals contain cells with or without the transgene, depending on which adult tissues the ES cells (which have the capacity to contribute to all tissues, including the germ line[139]) have colonized. Chimeric animals are hemizygotic (they have only one copy) for transgenes or inactivated constitutive genes. To test for colonization of the germ line and to obtain larger numbers of hemizygotic mice, individual chimeric mice can be bred back to wild-type parental animals. Fifty percent of offspring will be hemizygotes, which are bred to each other to produce litters of which 25% will be homozygotic (with two copies, one on each member of paired chromosomes) for the transgene or altered constitutive gene. In cases where homozygosity is deleterious (i.e., the altered constitutive gene is essential, or high dosage of the transgene is damaging), it is often an advantage to maintain transgenic mouse lines as hemizygotes, with homozygotes obtained by appropriate breeding when required.

A list of the genes inactivated by targeted recombination, and the organisms in which they exist (including prokaryotes, yeast, nematodes, fruit flies, plants, and mice and other mammals) is large and growing. Transgenic mouse lines of interest to toxicologists include those with combined deleted expression of metallothionein isoforms 1 and 2, which result in animals with increased sensitivity to metal toxicity;[140,141] transgenic mice with deleted expression of genes important in programmed cell death and sensitivity to toxicant-induced apoptotic death (retinoblastoma [RB],[142] p53,[143] and bcl-2αβ[144]); and transgenic mice with deleted expression of cellular tumor-associated genes and transcription factors, including the Wilms' tumor suppressor gene (WT–1) and *N-myc*,[145] to name only a few.

19.3.3 *Antisense nucleic acids*

During the past two years, numerous experiments have demonstrated successful down-regulation of specific gene products by exposure to oligonucleotides.[146–152] These oligonucleotides are complementary DNA or RNA (antisense nucleic acids), which may interact with mRNA to inhibit translation and enhance degradation or with DNA to inhibit transcription. Antisense nucleic acids may be synthetic single-stranded DNA sequences transfected into cells, or they may be antisense RNA sequences transcribed from foreign DNA stably or transiently incorporated into transgenic cells. Similar to the gene knockout approach, synthetic antisense nucleic acids are intended to diminish constitutive gene expression: relative advantages and disadvantages are outlined in Section 19.4.2.

Run-on transcription of vectors directing expression of antisense RNA can also be measured, provided that unlabeled, immobilized driver DNA is single-stranded and complementary only to the antisense RNA transcripts: driver cDNAs are unsuitable for this purpose, since they are double-stranded and complementary to both mRNA transcribed from constitutive genes and transcripts antisense to those mRNA molecules. This approach has been successful in measuring transcription of both thymidylate synthase (TS) genes, and vectors expressing RNA antisense to TS, in human MCF-7 breast cancer cells (Figure 1) (DeMoor and Koropatnick, manuscript submitted).

Naturally occurring antisense nucleic acids as regulators of gene expression have been described in prokaryotes,[153] but have not yet been established as mediators of gene expression in eukaryotes. Methods for production and experimental use of antisense nucleic acids to down-regulate endogenous gene expression has been described.[154] With respect to stably incorporated antisense RNA expression vectors in transgenic animals, several model transgenic lines have been generated, including those expressing RNA antisense to interleukin-3 (IL-3) mRNA,[155] glucocorticoid receptor mRNA,[156] pancreatic β-cell glucokinase,[157] and the glucose transporter GLUT-2.[158] The generation of transgenic mice expressing antisense RNA to other genes important in enhancing and/or inhibiting the activity and effect of toxic agents is an exciting area for future development.

19.4 *Cellular responses to intervention in gene expression*

19.4.1 *Gain-of-function events*

As described above, foreign proteins can be expressed in cultured cells and whole organisms by transfecting functional foreign genes, which contribute mRNA and then foreign protein. Physiological changes in transgenic cell and animal populations can then be assessed and correlated with foreign gene/protein expression and activity. However, some cautions are in order in assessing effects.

- Increased mRNA and active protein production directed by transgenes may have deceptive consequences, depending on the context in which they are expressed. For example, metallothionein protein shows nuclear plus cytoplasmic, or only nuclear, localization, depending upon developmental stage or expression in some tumor cells.[159] The importance of nuclear vs. cytoplasmic localization in the physiological function of MT is unknown. Therefore, high-level expression of a transgene does not necessarily imply high-level appropriate gene product activity. The directed expression of transgene products within specific cellular compartments (by addition of nuclear localization signals, for example) might be considered under such circumstances.

- Highly related genes from one organism expressed in another may be utilized in unpredictable ways. For example, mouse MT-1 cDNA expressed in Chinese hamster ovary (CHO) cells leads to markedly decreased resistance to the chemotherapeutic agent cisplatin.[160] However, the same cDNA expressed in mouse B16F1 melanoma cells does not (J. Koropatnick, unpublished observations). Therefore, the genetic background in which the transgene is expressed is of vital importance in assessing function.
- Powerful viral and eukaryotic promoters in eukaryotic expression vectors induce transgene expression at high (and often nonphysiological levels). If proteins expressed from transgenes have concentration-dependent functions, then the physiological consequences of such abnormal expression must be interpreted cautiously.

19.4.2 Loss-of-function events

Difficulties in appropriate expression of functional transgenes makes gene knockout and antisense nucleic acid down-regulation strategies particularly attractive in assessing the function of constitutive genes. These two techniques have relative advantages and disadvantages.

- For genes that are members of families with the capacity to functionally complement each other, each family member must be disrupted one by one in the gene knockout strategy if complementation effects are to be eliminated. For example, the presence of at least four members of the metallothionein gene family (MT-1, MT-2, MT-3, and MT-4) in rodents[161] could potentially allow functional complementation after experimental diminishment of MT expression by gene knockout.[140,141] This can be laborious, especially when gene family members are widely separated on the same chromosome or are on separate chromosomes. On the other hand, antisense nucleic acids may have sufficient complementarity for several related mRNAs to down-regulate many members of the same protein family.[129]
- Alternatively, enhanced mRNA and protein expression of one transgenic isoform might be compensated for by decreased expression of a complementary constitutive isoform, or a constitutive protein of dissimilar sequence but similar function. Thus, it is possible that cells respond to manipulation of expression of specific genes (either up or down) by modulating expression of constitutive genes. That modulation may be difficult to detect and may contribute in an unknown way to induced physiological changes.
- Gene knockout reduces constitutive expression of a specific gene to zero. Complete loss of essential genes is lethal: these cells have diminished usefulness as test organisms. On the other hand, antisense nucleic acids tend to diminish, rather than abolish constitutive gene expression.[129,154] Diminished rather than eliminated expression of essential genes may allow cell and whole organism survival and facilitate assessment of the function of essential genes. However, the amount of essential gene product may not correlate well with function. For example, if a low threshold amount of gene expression is sufficient to carry out 100% of the physiological activity, then antisense diminution of expression to a level that is still above that threshold would fail to modify the function of the gene.

19.5 Summary

Powerful molecular genetic techniques are available to alter the genes directing expression of mRNA and protein within cultured cells and whole animals. These changes can be directed to altering the genetic response of cells to both programmed and extracellular signals, including those of importance to toxicology in general and renal toxicology in particular. Sensitive methods are also available to detect changes in expression of both foreign transgenes and constitutive genes. Despite their power, however, these techniques cannot stand alone as exclusive tools to explore the role of specific genes in toxicology and cellular homeostasis. Well-established biochemical, immunological, and cell biological methods are essential and must be part of an integrated approach to explore gene function.

19.6 Acknowledgment

Some of the studies reported here were supported by grants to J.K. from the Medical Research Council of Canada.

References

1. Lea, P.J. and Leegood, R.C., Eds., *Plant Biochemistry and Molecular Biology*, John Wiley & Sons, New York, 1993.
2. Glick, B.R. and Thompson, J.E., *Methods in Plant Molecular Biology*, CRC Press, Boca Raton, FL, 1993.
3. Ralston, D.M. and O'Halloran, T.V., Metalloregulatory proteins and molecular mechanisms of heavy metal signal transduction, *Adv. Inorg. Biochem.*, 8, 1, 1990.
4. Pawson, T., Signal transduction — a conserved pathway from the membrane to the nucleus, *Dev. Genet.*, 14, 333, 1993.
5. Imamoto, A., Soriano, P., and Stein, P.L., Genetics of signal transduction: tales from the mouse, *Curr. Opin. Genet. Dev.*, 4, 40, 1994.
6. Nishizuka, Y., Signal transduction: crosstalk, *Trends Biochem. Sci.*, 17, 367, 1992.
7. Vellanoweth, R.L., Suprakar, P.C., and Roy, A.K., Transcription factors in development, growth, and aging, *Lab. Invest.*, 70, 784, 1994.
8. Pabo, C.O. and Sauer, R.T., Transcription factors: structural families and principles of DNA recognition, *Annu. Rev. Biochem.*, 61, 1053, 1992.
9. Croston, G.E. and Kadonaga, J.T., Role of chromatin structure in the regulation of transcription by RNA polymerase II, *Curr. Opin. Cell. Biol.*, 5, 417, 1993.
10. Wolffe, A.P., The transcription of chromatin templates, *Curr. Opin. Genet. Dev.*, 4, 245, 1994.
11. Rio, D.C., RNA binding proteins, splice site selection, and alternative pre-mRNA splicing, *Gene Express.*, 2, 1, 1992.
12. Carte, K.C., Bowman, D., Carrington, W., Fogarty, K., McNeil, J.A., Fay, F.S., and Lawrence, J.B., A three-dimensional view of precursor messenger RNA metabolism within the mammalian nucleus, *Science*, 259, 1330, 1993.
13. Izzauralde, E. and Mattaj, I.W., Transport of RNA between nucleus and cytoplasm, *Semin. Cell. Biol.*, 3, 279, 1992.
14. Walden, W.E., Daniels McQueen, S., Brown, P.H., Gaffield, L., Russell, D.A., Gielser, D., Bailey, L.C., and Thach, R.E., Translational repression in eukaryotes: partial purification and characterization of a repressor of ferritin mRNA translation, *Proc. Natl. Acad. Sci. U.S.A.*, 85, 9503, 1988.
15. Sachs, A.B., Messenger RNA degradation in eukaryotes, *Cell*, 74, 413, 1993.
16. Ranjan, M., Tafuri, S.R., and Wolffe, A.P., Masking of mRNA from translation in somatic cells, *Genes Dev.*, 7, 1725, 1993.
17. Dix, D.J., Lin, P.N., Kimata, Y., and Theil, E.C., The iron regulatory region of ferritin mRNA is also a positive control element for iron-dependent translation, *Biochemistry*, 31, 2818, 1992.

18. Mizuno, T., Chou, M.-Y., and Inouye, M., A unique mechanism regulating gene expression: translational inhibition by a complementary RNA transcript (micRNA), *Proc. Natl. Acad. Sci. U.S.A.*, 81, 1966, 1983.
19. Raju, V.S. and Maines, M.D., Coordinated expression and mechanism of induction of HSP32 Cheme oxygenase-11 mRNA by hyperthermia in rat organs, *Biochim. Biophys. Acta*, 1217, 273, 1994.
20. Zalups, R.K., Fraser, J., and Koropatnick, J., Enhanced transcription of metallothionein genes in rat kidney: effect of uninephrectomy and compensatory renal growth, *Am. J. Physiol.*, 268, F643, 1995.
21. Tukey, R.H. and Okino, S.T., Quantitation of related gene products by nuclear run-on and Northern blot analysis, *Methods Enzymol.*, 206, 284, 1991.
22. Marzluff, W.F., Transcription of RNA in isolated nuclei, *Methods Cell Biol.*, 19, 317, 1978.
23. Marzluff, W.F. and Huang, R.C.C., in *Transcription and Translation: A Practical Approach*, Hames, B.D. and Higgins, S.J., Eds., IRL Press, Oxford, 1985, 89.
24. Greenberg, M.E. and Bender, T.P., Isolation of newly transcribed RNA, in *Current Protocols in Molecular Biology*, Ausubel, F.M., Brent, R., Kingston, R.E., Moore, D.D., Seidman, J.G., Smith, J.A., and Struhl, K., Eds., John Wiley & Sons, New York, 1994, 4.10.1.
25. Koropatnick, J., Amplified metallothionein-1 genes in adult mouse liver: induction of transcription and mRNA accumulation, *Proc. Soc. Exp. Biol. Med.*, 188, 287, 1988.
26. Kikuchi, K., Bichell, D.P., and Rotwein, P., Chromatin changes accompany the developmental activation of insulin-like growth factor 1 gene transcription, *J. Biol. Chem.*, 267, 21505, 1992.
27. Almendral, J.M., Sommer, D., HacDonald–Bravo, H., Burckhardt, J., Perera, J., and Bravo, R., Complexity of the early genetic response to growth factors in mouse fibroblasts, *Mol. Cell. Biol.*, 8, 2140, 1988.
28. Greenberg, M.E. and Bender, T.P., Isolation of newly transcribed RNA, in *Current Protocols in Molecular Biology*, Ausubel, F.M., Brent, R., Kingston, R.E., Moore, D.D., Seidman, J.G., Smith, J.A., and Struhl, K., Eds., John Wiley & Sons, New York, 1994, 4.10.1.
29. Almendral, J.M., Sommer, D., HacDonald–Bravo, H., Burckhardt, J., Perera, J., and Bravo, R., Complexity of the early genetic response to growth factors in mouse fibroblasts, *Mol. Cell. Biol.*, 2140, 1988.
30. Mulvihill, E.R. and Palmiter, R.D., Relationship of nuclear estrogen receptor levels to induction of ovalbumin and conalbumin mRNA in chick oviduct, *J. Biol. Chem.*, 252, 2060, 1977.
31. McKnight, G.S. and Palmiter, R.D., Transcriptional regulation of the ovalbumin and conalbumin genes by steroid hormones in chick oviduct, *J. Biol. Chem.*, 254, 9050, 1979.
32. Healy, A.M. and Gelehrter, T.D., Induction of plasminogen activator inhibitor-1 in HepG2 human hepatoma cells by mediators of the acute phase response, *J. Biol. Chem.*, 269, 19095, 1994.
33. McKnight, G.S., The induction of ovalbumin and conalbumin mRNA by estrogen and progesterone in chick oviduct explant cultures, *Cell*, 14, 403, 1979.
34. Sambrook, J., Fritsch, E.F., and Maniatis, T., *Molecular Cloning: A Laboratory Manual*, 2nd ed., Cold Spring Harbor Laboratory Press, Cold Spring Harbor, NY, 1989.
35. Ausubel, F.M., Brent, R., Kingston, R.E., Moore, D.D., Seidman, J.G., Smith, J.A., and Struhl, K., Eds., *Current Protocols in Molecular Biology*, John Wiley & Sons, New York, 1994.
36. Gilman, M., Preparation of RNA from eukaryotic and prokaryotic cells, in *Current Protocols in Molecular Biology*, Ausubel, F.M., Brent, R., Kingston, R.E., Moore, D.D., Seidman, J.G., Smith, J.A., and Struhl, K., Eds., John Wiley & Sons, New York, 1994, 4.1.1.
37. Fisher, D.E., Apoptosis in cancer therapy: crossing the threshold, *Cell*, 78, 539, 1994.
38. Chomczynski, P. and Sacchi, N., Single-step method of RNA isolation by acid guanidinium thiocyanate-phenol-chloroform extraction, *Anal. Biochem.*, 162, 156, 1987.
39. Birnboim, H.C., Rapid extraction of high molecular weight RNA from cultured cells and granulocytes for Northern analysis, *Nucleic Acids Res.*, 16, 1487, 1988.
40. Koropatnick, J. and Cherian, M.G., Exposure to different forms of cadmium in mice: differences in metallothionein and alphafetoprotein mRNA induction in liver and kidney, *J. Biochem. Toxicol.*, 3, 159, 1988.

41. Alberts, B., Bray, D., Lewis, J., Raff, M., Roberts, K., and Watson, J.D., *Molecular Biology of the Cell*, 2nd ed., Garland, Inc., New York, 1989, 531.
42. Moore, C.L. and Sharp, P.A., Site-specific polyadenylation in a cell-free reaction, *Cell*, 36, 581, 1984.
43. Kingston, R.E., Preparation of poly(A)$^+$ RNA, in *Current Protocols in Molecular Biology*, Ausubel, F.M., Brent, R., Kingston, R.E., Moore, D.D., Seidman, J.G., Smith, J.A., and Struhl, K., Eds., John Wiley & Sons, New York, 1994, 4.5.1.
44. Brown, T., Northern hybridization of RNA fractionated by agarose-formaldehyde gel electrophoresis, in *Current Protocols in Molecular Biology*, Ausubel, F.M., Brent, R., Kingston, R.E., Moore, D.D., Seidman, J.G., Smith, J.A., and Struhl, K., Eds., John Wiley & Sons, New York, 1994, 4.9.2.
45. Harris, J.F., Koropatnick, J., and Pearson, J., Spontaneous and radiation-induced genetic instability of heteromyeloma hybridoma cells, *Mol. Biol. Med.*, 7, 485, 1990.
46. Gait, M.T., Ed., *Oligonucleotide Synthesis: A Practical Approach*, IRL Press, Oxford, 1986.
47. Cherry, J.M., Computer analysis of DNA and protein sequences, in *Current Protocols in Molecular Biology*, Ausubel, F.M., Brent, R., Kingston, R.E., Moore, D.D., Seidman, J.G., Smith, J.A., and Struhl, K., Eds., John Wiley & Sons, New York, 1994, 7.7.1.
48. Albores, A., Koropatnick, J., and Cherian, M.G., Arsenic induces and enhances rat hepatic metallothionein production *in vivo*, *Chem. Biol. Interact.*, 85, 127, 1992.
49. Johnston, R.F., Pickett, S.C., and Barker, D.L., Autoradiography using storage phosphor technology, *Electrophoresis*, 2, 355, 1990.
50. Durnam, D.M. and Palmiter, R.D., A practical approach for quantitating specific mRNAs by solution hybridization, *Anal. Biochem.*, 131, 385, 1983.
51. Spanakis, E., Problems related to the interpretation of autoradiographic data on gene expression using common constitutive transcripts as controls, *Nucleic Acids Res.*, 21, 3809, 1993.
52. Spanakis, E. and Brouty–Boyé, D., Evaluation of quantitative variation in gene expression, *Nucleic Acids Res.*, 22, 799, 1994.
53. Berleth, E.S., Dolnick, B.J., Ehrke, M.J., and Mihich, E., RNA recovery efficiency for cultured cells and organ-derived cell suspensions, *Nucleic Acids Res.*, 22, 1925, 1994.
54. Harley, C.B., Normalization of RNA dot blots with oligo(dT), *Trends Genet.*, 4, 152, 1988.
55. Innis, M.A., Gelfand, D.H., Sninsky, J.J., and White, T.J., Eds., *PCR Protocols: A Guide to Methods and Applications*, Academic Press, New York, 1990.
56. Veres, G., Gibbs, R.A., Scherer, S.E., and Caskey, C.T., The molecular basis of the sparse fur mouse mutation, *Science*, 237, 415, 1987.
57. Gilliland, G., Perrin, S., and Bunn, H.F., Competitive PCR for quantitation of mRNA, in *PCR Protocols: A Guide to Methods and Applications*, Innis, M.A., Gelfand, D.H., Sninsky, J.J., and White, T.J., Eds., Academic Press, New York, 1990, 60.
58. Becker–André, M. and Hahlbrock, K., Absolute mRNA quantification using the polymerase chain reaction (PCR). A novel approach by a PCR aided transcript titration assay (PATTY), *Nucleic Acids Res.*, 17, 9437, 1989.
59. Wang, A.M., Doyle, M.V., and Mark, D.F., Quantitation of mRNA by the polymerase chain reaction, *Proc. Natl. Acad. Sci. U.S.A.*, 86, 9717, 1989.
60. Kawasaki, E.S., Sample preparation from blood, cells, and other fluids, in *PCR Protocols: A Guide to Methods and Applications*, Innis, M.I., Gelfand, D.H., Sninsky, J.J., and White, T.J., Eds., Academic Press, New York, 1990, 146.
61. Gilliland, G., Perrin, S., Blanchard, K., and Bunn, H.G., Analysis of cytokine mRNA and DNA: detection and quantitation by competitive polymerase chain reaction, *Proc. Natl. Acad. Sci. U.S.A.*, 87, 2725, 1990.
62. Baier, G., Telford, D., Gulbins, E., Yamada, N., Kawakami, T., and Altman, A., Improved specificity of RT-PCR amplifications using nested cDNA primers, *Nucleic Acids Res.*, 21, 1329, 1993.
63. Innis, M.A. and Gelfand, D.H., Optimization of PCRs, in *PCR Protocols: A Guide to Methods and Applications*, Innis, M.I., Gelfand, D.H., Sninsky, J.J., and White, T.J., Eds., Academic Press, New York, 1990, 3.
64. Frohman, M.A., Dush, M.K., and Martin, G.R., Rapid production of full-length cDNAs from rare transcripts: amplification using a single gene-specific oligonucleotide primer, *Proc. Natl. Acad. Sci. U.S.A.*, 85, 8998, 1988.

65. Noonan, K.E., Beck, C., Holzmayer, T.A., Chin, J.E., Wundere, J.S., Andrulis, I.L., Gazdar, A.F., Qillman, C.L., Griffith, B., Von Hoff, D.D., and Roninson, I.B., Quantitative analysis of MDR1 (multidrug resistance) gene expression in human tumors by polymerase chain reaction, *Proc. Natl Acad. Sci. U.S.A.*, 87, 7160, 1990.
66. Leibbrandt, M.E.I. and Koropatnick, J., Activation of human monocytes with endotoxin induces metallothionein expression and is diminished by zinc, *Toxicol. Appl. Pharmacol.*, 124, 72, 1994.
67. Wang, A.M. and Mark, D.F., Quantitative PCR, in *PCR Protocols: A Guide to Methods and Applications*, Innis, M.I., Gelfand, D.H., Sninsky, J.J., and White, T.J., Eds., Academic Press, New York, 1990, 70.
68. Leibbrandt, M.E.I., A Role for Metallothionein in Human Monocytes, Ph.D. thesis, University of Western Ontario, London, Ontario, Canada, 1994.
69. Tsai, C.Y., Wu, T.H., Huang, S.F., Sun, K.H., Hsieh, S.C., Han, S.H., Yu, H.S., and Yu, C.L., Abnormal splenic and thymic IL-4 and TNF-alpha expression in MRL-lpr/lpr mice, *Scand. J. Immunol.*, 41, 157, 1995.
70. Mori, K., Kobayashi, S., Inobe, M., Jia, W.Y., Tamakoshi, M., Miyazaki, T., and Uede, T., *In vivo* cytokine gene expression in various T cell subsets of the autoimmune MRL/Mp-lpr/lpr mouse, *Autoimmunity*, 17, 49, 1994.
71. Svoboda, M., Tastenoy, M., Vertongen, P., and Robberecht, P., Relative quantitative analysis of glucagon receptor mRNA in rat tissues, *Mol. Cell. Endocrinol.*, 105, 131, 1994.
72. Brandt, C.R., Pumfery, A.M., Micales, B., Bindley, C.D., Lyons, G.E., Sramek, S.J., and Wallow, I.H., Renin mRNA is synthesized locally in rat ocular tissues, *Curr. Eye Res.*, 13, 755, 1994.
73. Mohaupt, M.G., Elzie, J.L., Ahn, K.Y., Clapp, W.L., Wilcox, C.S., and Kone, B.C., Differential expression and induction of mRNAs encoding two inducible nitric oxide synthases in rat kidney, *Kidney Int.*, 46, 653, 1994.
74. Shankland, S.J., Scholey, J.W., Ly, H., and Thai, K., Expression of transforming growth factor-β1 during diabetic renal hypertrophy, *Kidney Int.* 46, 430, 1994.
75. Terada, Y., Tomita, K., Nonoguchi, H., Yang, T., and Marumo, F., PCR localization of C-type natriuretic peptide and B-type receptor mRNAs in rat nephron segments, *Am. J. Physiol.*, 267, F215, 1994.
76. Clapp, W.L., Bowman, P., Shaw, G.S., Patel, P., and Kone, B.C., Segmental localization of mRNAs encoding H^+/K^+-ATPase α and β subunit isoforms in rat kidney using RT-PCR, *Kidney Int.*, 46, 627, 1994.
77. Ahn, K.Y. and Kone, B.C., Expression and cellular localization of mRNA encoding the "gastric" isoform of H^+/K^+-ATPase α subunit in rat kidney, *Am. J. Physiol.*, 268, F99, 1995.
78. Rossi, G., Albertin, G., Belloni, A., Zanin, L., Biasolo, M.A., Prayer–Galetti, T., Bader, M., Nussdorfer, G.G., Palu, G., and Pessina, A.C., Gene expression, localization, and characterization of endothelin A and B receptors in the human adrenal cortex, *J. Clin. Invest.*, 94, 1226, 1994.
79. Melton, D.A., Krieg, P.A., Rebagliati, M.R., Maniatis, T., Zinn, K., and Green, M.R., Efficient *in vitro* synthesis of biologically active RNA and RNA hybridization probes from plasmids containing a bacteriophage SP6 promoter, *Nucleic Acids Res.*, 12, 7035, 1984.
80. Gilman, M., Ribonuclease protection assay, in *Current Protocols in Molecular Biology*, Ausubel, F.M., Brent, R., Kingston, R.E., Moore, D.D., Seidman, J.G., Smith, J.A., and Struhl, K., Eds., John Wiley & Sons, New York, 1994, 4.1.1.
81. Chamberlin, M. and Ryan, T., Bacteriophage DNA-dependent RNA polymerase, in *The Enzymes*, Vol. 15, Boyer, P., Ed., Academic Press, New York, 1982, 87.
82. McKnight, S.L. and Kingsbury, R., Transcription control signals of a eukaryotic protein-encoding gene, *Science*, 217, 316, 1982.
83. Triezenberg, S.J., Primer extension, in *Current Protocols in Molecular Biology*, Ausubel, F.M., Brent, R., Kingston, R.E., Moore, D.D., Seidman, J.G., Smith, J.A., and Struhl, K., Eds., John Wiley & Sons, New York, 1994, 4.8.1.
84. Toussaint, C., Bousquet–Lemercier, B., Garlatti, M., Hanoune, J., and Barouki, R., Testis-specific transcription start site in the aspartate aminotransferase housekeeping gene promoter, *J. Biol. Chem.*, 269, 13318, 1994.

85. Ilkbahar, Y.N., Wu, K., Thordarson, G., and Talamantes, F., Expression and distribution of messenger ribonucleic acids for growth hormone (GH) receptor and GH-binding protein in mice during pregnancy, *Endocrinology* 136, 386, 1995.
86. Menon, R.K., Stephan, D.A., Rao, R.H., Shen-Orr, Z., Downs, L.S., Jr., Roberts, C.T., Jr., LeRoith, D., and Sperling, M.A., Tissue-specific regulation of the growth hormone receptor gene in streptozocin-induced diabetes in the rat, *J. Endocrinol.*, 142, 453, 1994.
87. Berkowitz, D.E., Price, D.T., Bello, E.A., Page, S.O., and Schwinn, D.A., Localization of messenger RNA for three distinct α2 adrenergic receptor subtypes in human tissues. Evidence for species heterogeneity and implications for human pharmacology, *Anesthesiology*, 81, 1235, 1994.
88. Yamamoto, T., Feng, L., Mizuno, T., Hirose, S., Kawasaki, K., Yaoita, E., Kihara, I., and Wilson, C.B., Expression of mRNA for natriuretic peptide receptor subtypes in bovine kidney, *Am. J. Physiol.*, 267, F318, 1994.
89. Carver, L.A., Hogenesch, J.B., and Bradfield, C.A., Tissue specific expression of the rat Ah-receptor and ARNT mRNAs, *Nucleic Acids Res.*, 22, 3038, 1994.
90. Harlow, E. and Lane, D., *Antibodies: A Laboratory Manual*, Cold Spring Harbor Laboratory Press, Cold Spring Harbor, NY, 1988.
91. Gall, J.G. and Pardue, M.L., Nucleic acid hybridization in cytological preparations, *Methods Enzymol.*, 38, 470, 1971.
92. Berger, C.N., *In situ* hybridization of immunoglobulin-specific RNA in single cells of the β-lymphocyte lineage with radiolabeled DNA probes, *EMBO J.*, 5, 85, 1986.
93. Pardue, M.L., *In situ* hybridization, in *Nucleic Acid Hybridization: A Practical Approach*, Hames, B.D. and Higgins, S.J., Eds., IRL Press, Oxford, 1985, 179.
94. Zeller, R. and Rogers, M., *In situ* hybridization to cellular RNA, in *Current Protocols in Molecular Biology*, Ausubel, F.M., Brent, R., Kingston, R.E., Moore, D.D., Seidman, J.G., Smith, J.A., and Struhl, K., Eds., John Wiley & Sons, New York, 1994, 14.3.1.
95. Zeller, R. and Rogers, M., Counterstaining and mounting of autoradiographed *in situ* hybridization slides, in *Current Protocols in Molecular Biology*, Ausubel, F.M., Brent, R., Kingston, R.E., Moore, D.D., Seidman, J.G., Smith, J.A., and Struhl, K., Eds., John Wiley & Sons, New York, 1994, 14.5.1.
96. Rogers, M., Detection of hybridized probe, in *Current Protocols in Molecular Biology*, Ausubel, F.M., Brent, R., Kingston, R.E., Moore, D.D., Seidman, J.G., Smith, J.A., and Struhl, K., Eds., John Wiley & Sons, New York, 1994, 14.4.1.
97. Zeller, R., Fixation, embedding, and sectioning of tissues, embryos, and single cells, in *Current Protocols in Molecular Biology*, Ausubel, F.M., Brent, R., Kingston, R.E., Moore, D.D., Seidman, J.G., Smith, J.A., and Struhl, K., Eds., John Wiley & Sons, New York, 1994, 14.1.1.
98. Watkins, S., Cryosectioning, in *Current Protocols in Molecular Biology*, Ausubel, F.M., Brent, R., Kingston, R.E., Moore, D.D., Seidman, J.G., Smith, J.A., and Struhl, K., Eds., John Wiley & Sons, New York, 1994, 14.2.1.
99. Koropatnick, J., Andrews, G., Varshney, U., Gedamu, L., and Duerksen, J.D., Mouse hepatic metallothionein-1 gene cleavage by micrococcal nuclease is enhanced after induction by cadmium, *Nucleic Acids Res.*, 11, 3255, 1983.
100. Walden, W.E., Daniels McQueen, S., Brown, P.H., Gaffield, L., Russell, D.A., Gielser, D., Bailey, L.C., Thach, R.E., Translational repression in eukaryotes: partial purification and characterization of a repressor of ferritin mRNA translation, *Proc. Natl. Acad. Sci. U.S.A.*, 85, 9503, 1988.
101. Chu, E., Koeller, D.M., Casey, J.L., Drake, J.C., Chabner, B.A., Elwood, P.C., Zinn, S., and Allegra, C.J., Autoregulation of human thymidylate synthase messenger RNA translation by thymidylate synthase, *Proc. Natl. Acad. Sci. U.S.A.*, 88, 8977, 1991.
102. Poste, G., Pathogenesis of metastatic disease: implications for current therapy and for the development of new therapeutic strategies, *Cancer Treat. Rep.*, 70, 183, 1986.
103. De, S.K., Dey, S.K., and Andrews, G.K., Cadmium teratogenicity and its relationship with metallothionein gene expression in midgestation mouse embryos, *Toxicology*, 64, 89, 1990.
104. Pellicer, A., Robins, D., Wold, B., Sweet, R., Jackson, J., Lowy, I., Roberts, J.M., Sim, G.K., Silverstein, S., and Axel, R., Altering genotype and phenotype by DNA-mediated gene transfer, *Science*, 209, 1414, 1980.

105. Kriegler, M., *Gene Transfer and Expression: A Laboratory Manual*, Stockton Press, New York, 1990.
106. Pinkert, C.A. (Ed.), *Transgenic Animal Technology: A Laboratory Handbook*, Academic Press, San Diego, 1994.
107. Alberts, B., Bray, D., Lewis, J., Raff, M., Roberts, K., and Watson, J.D., *Molecular Biology of the Cell*, 3rd ed., Garland, New York, 1994.
108. Sakashita, A., Epstein, C.J., Carlson, E., and Koeffler, H.P., Hematopoietic progenitor cells of transgenic mice with increased copper/zinc-superoxide dismutase activity are resistant to tumor necrosis factor, *J. Cell Physiol.*, 160, 233, 1994.
109. Cadet, J.L., Kujirai, K., Carlson, E., and Epstein, C.J., Autoradiographic distribution of [3H]neurotensin receptors in the brains of superoxide dismutase transgenic mice, *Synapse*, 14, 24, 1993.
110. Merlino, G., Regulatory imbalances in cell proliferation and cell death during oncogenesis in transgenic mice, *Semin. Cancer Biol.*, 5, 13, 1994.
111. Tchang, F., Gusse, M., Soussi, T., and Mechali, M., Stabilization and expression of high levels of p53 during early development of *Xenopus laevis*, *Dev. Biol.*, 159, 163, 1993.
112. McDonnell, T.J., Marin, M.C., Hsu, B., Brisbay, S.M., McConnell, K., Tu, S.M., Campbell, M.L., and Rodriguez-Villanueva, J., The bcl-2 oncogene: apoptosis and neoplasia, *Radiat. Res.*, 136, 307, 1993.
113. Tiano, H.F., Hosokawa, M., Chulada, P.C., Smith, P.B., Wang, R.L., Gonzalez, F.J., Crespi, C.L., and Langenbach, R., Retroviral-mediated expression of human cytochrome P450 2a6 in C3H/10T½ cells confers transformability by 4-(methylnitrosamino)-1-(3-pyridyl)-1-butanone (NNK), *Carcinogenesis*, 14, 1421, 1993.
114. Koike, K., Moriya, K., Yotsuyanagi, H., Iino, S., and Kurokawa, K., Induction of cell cycle progression by hepatitis B virus HBx gene expression in quiescent mouse fibroblasts, *J. Clin. Invest.*, 94, 44, 1994.
115. Fausto, N. and Webber, E.M., Control of liver growth, *Crit. Rev. Eukaryot. Gene Expr.*, 3, 117, 1993.
116. Chandrasekaran, C. and Gordon, J.I., Cell lineage-specific and differentiation-dependent patterns of CCAAT/enhancer binding protein alpha expression in the gut epithelium of normal and transgenic mice, *Proc. Natl. Acad. Sci. U.S.A.*, 90, 8871, 1993.
117. Kane, S.E. and Gottesman, M.M., Use of multidrug resistance gene in mammalian expression vectors, *Methods Enzymol.*, 217, 34, 1993.
118. Grant, C.E., Valdimarsson, G., Hipfner, D.R., Almquist, K.C., Cole, S.P., and Deeley, R.G., Overexpression of multidrug resistance-associated protein (MRP) increases resistance to natural product drugs, *Cancer Res.*, 54, 357, 1994.
119. Connely, C.S., Fahl, W.E., Manoharan, T.H., and Iannaccone, P.M., Cell-specific expression of a recombinant rat glutathione S-transferase Ya gene in transgenic mice, *Pathobiology*, 61, 7, 1993.
120. Goldsworthy, T.L., Recio, L., Brown, K., Donehower, L.A., Mirsalis, J.C., Tennant, R.W., and Purchase, I.F., Transgenic animals in toxicology, *Fundam. Appl. Toxicol.*, 22, 8, 1994.
121. Kane, S., Troen, B., Gal, S., Ueda, K., Pastan, I., and Gottesman, M., Use of a cloned multidrug resistance gene for co-amplification and overproduction of major excreted protein, a transformation-regulated secreted acid protease, *Mol. Cell. Biol.*, 8, 3316, 1988.
122. Subramani, S., Mulligan, R., and Berg, P., Expression of the mouse dihydrofolate reductase complementary deoxyribonucleic acid in simian virus 40 vectors, *Mol. Cell. Biol.*, 1, 854, 1981.
123. Beach, L. and Palmiter, R., Amplification of the metallothionein-1 gene in cadmium-resistant mouse cells, *Proc. Natl. Acad. Sci. U.S.A.*, 78, 2110, 1981.
124. Southern, E.M., and Berg, P., Transformation of mammalian cells to antibiotic resistance with a bacterial gene under the control of the SV40 early region promoter, *J. Mol. Appl. Genet.*, 1, 327, 1982.
125. Kelley, S.L., Basu, A., Teicher, B.A., Hacker, M.P., Hamer, D.H., and Lazo, J.S., Overexpression of metallothionein confers resistance to anticancer drugs, *Science*, 241, 1813, 1988.
126. Kaina, B., Lohrer, H., Karin, M., and Herrlich, P., Overexpressed human MT-IIA gene protects CHO cells from killing by alkylating agents, *Proc. Natl. Acad. Sci. U.S.A.*, 87, 2710, 1990.

127. Koropatnick, J. and Pearson, J., Constitutive and inducible metallothionein expression and resistance to cisplatinum in mouse melanoma cells, *Somat. Cell Molec. Genet.*, 16, 529, 1990.
128. Ciccarone, V., Hawley–Nelson, P., and Jessee, J., Cationic liposome-mediated transfection: effect of serum on expression and efficiency, *Focus*, 15, 80, 1993.
129. Leibbrandt, M.E.I., Khokha, R., and Koropatnick, J., Antisense down-regulation of metallothionein in a human monocytic cell line alters adherence, invasion and the respiratory burst, *Cell Growth Differ.* 5, 17, 1994.
130. Sanes, J.R., Rubenstein, J.L.R., and Nicolas, J.F., Use of a recombinant retrovirus to study post-implantation cell lineage in mouse embryos, *EMBO J.*, 5, 3133, 1986.
131. Ashby, J. and Tinwell, H., Use of transgenic mouse *lacI/Z* mutation assays in genetic toxicology, *Mutagenesis*, 9, 179, 1994.
132. Gossen, J.A., Molijn, A.C., Douglas, G.R., and Vijg, J., Application of galactose-sensitive *E. coli* strains as selective hosts for *lacZ*⁻ plasmids, *Nucleic Acids Res.*, 20, 3254, 1992.
133. Kohler, S.W., Provost, G.S., Fiek, A., Kretz, P.L., Bullock, W.O., Sorge, J.A., Putman, D.L. and Short, J.M., Spectra of spontaneous and mutagen-induced mutations in *lacI* transgenic mice, *Proc. Natl. Acad. Sci. U.S.A.*, 88, 7958, 1991.
134. Mansour, S.L., Gene targeting in murine embryonic stem cells: introduction of specific alterations into the mammalian genome, *Genet. Anal. Tech. Appl.*, 7, 219, 1990.
135. Robertson, E.J., Using embryonic stem cells to introduce mutations into the mouse germ line, *Biol. Reprod.*, 44, 238, 1991.
136. Mansour, S.L., Thomas, K.R., and Capecchi, M.R., Disruption of the proto-oncogene int-2 in mouse embryo-derived stem cells: a general strategy for targeting mutations to nonselectable genes, *Nature (London)*, 336, 348, 1988.
137. Zimmer, A., Manipulating the genome by homologous recombination in embryonic stem cells, *Annu. Rev. Neurosci.*, 15, 115, 1992.
138. Hasty, P., Ramirez, S.R., Krumlauf, R., and Bradley, A., Introduction of a subtle mutation into the Hox-2.6 locus in embryonic stem cells [published erratum appears in *Nature*, 1991, 353, 94], *Nature (London)*, 350, 243, 1991.
139. Bradley, A., Evans, M., Kaufman, M.H., and Robertson, E., Formation of germ-line chimaeras from embryo-derived teratocarcinoma cell lines, *Nature (London)*, 309, 255, 1984.
140. Michalska, A.E. and Choo, K.H.A., Targeting and germ-line transmission of a null mutation at the metallothionein 1 and 2 loci in mouse, *Proc. Natl. Acad. Sci. U.S.A.*, 90, 8088, 1993.
141. Masters, B.A., Kelly, E.J., Quaife, C.J., Brinster, R.L., and Palmiter, R.D., Targeted disruption of metallothionein 1 and 2 genes increases sensitivity to cadmium, *Proc. Nat'l Acad. Sci. U.S.A.*, 91, 584, 1994.
142. Freund, R., Bauer, P.H., Crissman, H.A., Bradbury, E.M., and Benjamin, T.L., Host range and cell cycle activation properties of polyomavirus large T-antigen mutants defective in pRB binding, *J. Virol.*, 68, 7227, 1994.
143. Donehower, L.A., Harvey, M., Slagle, B.L., McArthur, M.J., Montgomery, C.A., Jr., Butel, J.S., and Bradley, A., Mice deficient for p53 are developmentally normal but susceptible to spontaneous tumors, *Nature (London)*, 356, 215, 1992.
144. Nakayama, K., Negishi, I., Kuida, K., Sawa, H., and Loh, K.Y., Targeted disruption of bcl-2 alpha beta in mice: occurrence of gray hair, polycystic kidney disease, and lymphocytopenia, *Proc. Natl. Acad. Sci. U.S.A.*, 91, 3700, 1994.
145. Igarashi, P., Transcription factors and apoptosis in kidney development, *Curr. Opin. Nephrol. Hypertens.*, 3, 308, 1994.
146. Izant, J.G. and Weintraub, H., Inhibition of thymidine kinase gene expression by anti-sense RNA: a molecular approach to genetic analysis, *Cell*, 36, 1007, 1984.
147. Izant, J.G. and Weintraub, H., Constitutive and conditional suppression of exogenous and endogenous genes by antisense RNA, *Science*, 229, 345, 1985.
148. Stout, J.T. and Caskey, C.T., Antisense RNA inhibition of endogenous genes, *Methods Enzymol.*, 151, 519, 1987.
149. Green, P.J., Pines, O., and Inouye, M., The role of antisense RNA in gene regulation, *Annu. Rev. Biochem.*, 55, 569, 1986.
150. Melton, D.A., Injected antisense RNAs specifically block messenger RNA translation *in vivo*, *Proc. Natl. Acad. Sci. U.S.A.*, 82, 144, 1985.

151. van der Krol, A.R., Lenting, P.E., Veenstra, J., Meer, I.M., van der Koes, R.E., Gerats, A.G.M., Mol, J.N.M., and Stuitje, A.R., Expression of an antisense CHS gene in transgenic plants inhibits flower pigmentation, *Nature (London)*, 333, 866, 1988.
152. Khokha, R., Waterhouse, P., Yagel, S., and Denhardt, D.T., Antisense RNA-induced reduction in murine TIMP levels confers oncogenicity on Swiss 3T3 cells, *Science*, 243, 947, 1989.
153. Tomizawa, J., Itoh, T., Selzer, G., and Som, T., Plasmid ColE1 incompatibility determined by interaction of RNA 1 with primary transcript, *Proc. Natl. Acad. Sci. U.S.A.*, 78, 6096, 1981.
154. Hélène, C. and Toulmé, J.J., Specific regulation of gene expression by antisense, sense, and antigene nucleic acids, *Biochim. Biophys. Acta*, 1049, 99, 1990.
155. Cockayne, D.A., Bodine, D.M., Cline, A., Nienhuis, A.W., and Dunbar, C.E., Transgenic mice expressing antisense interleukin-3 RNA develop a B-cell lymphoproliferative syndrome or neurologic dysfunction, *Blood*, 84, 2699, 1994.
156. Stec, I., Barden, N., Reul, J.M., and Holsboer, F., Dexamethasone nonsuppression in transgenic mice expressing antisense RNA to the glucocorticoid receptor, *J. Psychiatr. Res.*, 28, 1, 1994.
157. Efrat, S., Leiser, M., Wu, Y.J., Fusco–Demane, D., Emran, O.A., Surana, M., Jetton, T.L., Magnuson, M.A., Weir, G., and Fleischer, N., Ribozyme-mediated attenuation of pancreatic beta-cell glucokinase expression in transgenic mice results in impaired glucose-induced insulin secretion, *Proc. Natl. Acad. Sci. U.S.A.*, 91, 2051, 1994.
158. Valera, A., Solanes, G., Fernandez–Alvarex, J., Pujl, A., Ferrer, J., Asins, G., Gomis, G., and Bosch, F., Expression of GLUT-2 antisense RNA in beta cells of transgenic mice leads to diabetes, *J. Biol. Chem.*, 269, 28543, 1994.
159. Cherian, M.G., The significance of the nuclear and cytoplasmic localization of metallothionein in human liver and tumor cells, *Environ. Health Perspect.*, 102, 131, 1994.
160. Koropatnick, J. and Pearson, J., Altered cisplatin and cadmium resistance and cell survival in Chinese hamster ovary cells expressing mouse metallothionein, *Mol. Pharmacol.*, 44, 44, 1993.
161. Quaife, C.J., Findley, S.D., Erickson, J.C., Froelick, J., Kelly, E.J., Zambrowicz, B.P., and Palmiter, R.D., Induction of a new metallothionein isoform (MT-IV) occurs during differentiation of stratified squamous epithelia, *Biochemistry*, 33, 7250, 1994.

chapter twenty

Transgenic Animals

Siu-Pok Yee

20.1 Introduction....413
20.2 General methods for producing transgenic animals....414
20.2.1 Microinjection of DNA into pronucleus....415
20.2.2 Culture of early mouse embryo....416
20.2.3 Transgene design....417
20.2.3.1 Effects of prokaryotic sequences....417
20.2.3.2 Effects of intron sequences....417
20.2.3.3 Distinguishing transgenes from endogenous genes....417
20.2.3.4 Tissue-specific expression....418
20.2.3.5 Bicistronic transgenes....418
20.2.4 Applications....418
20.2.4.1 Gain-of-function....418
20.2.4.2 Loss-of-function....418
20.2.4.3 Transcription control....419
20.2.5 Identification and maintenance of transgenic mouse lines....419
20.2.6 Other considerations....420
20.2.6.1 Retrovirus-mediated transgenesis....420
20.2.6.2 Embryonic stem cell-mediated transgenesis....421
20.2.7 Targeting vectors....422
20.2.7.1 Application....422
20.2.7.2 Other considerations....423
20.2.8 Application to renal toxicology....423
20.3 Acknowledgment....423
References....423

20.1 Introduction

To function effectively, living organisms require a complex system involving mechanisms acting on effector molecules that carry out day-to-day cellular activities. The key regulatory events are mediated by cell-to-cell communications carried out by interactions among different biomolecules. These biomolecules include exocrine factors (e.g., hormones and growth factors); molecules that receive and process signals at the external cell membrane (e.g., hormone and growth factor receptors); molecules that transduce signals from the cytoplasm to the nucleus (e.g., steroid receptors); and molecules that act on DNA regulatory

0-8493-3341-5/96/$0.00+$.50

regions to modulate gene activity (transcription factors). Through this intricate system, a living organism can respond appropriately and effectively to different environmental cues (including treatment with toxic agents) by activating and/or repressing the expression of various genes responsible for producing regulatory biomolecules.

With advances in molecular biology that allow manipulating the genome of both single eukaryotic cells and multicellular organisms (transgenic animals), it is now possible to introduce foreign DNA into the mouse chromosome or inactivate endogenous genes by homologous recombination (gene targeting) to generate specific transgenic strains. Because of their well-defined genetic background and relative ease of manipulation and investigation, mice are the organism of choice. Transgenic mice provide an invaluable system to investigate the function of specific genes, including the effect of their absence, in mediating the response to different external challenges from the physiological environment of the whole animal. They also allow the study of the effect of the transgene on the normal development of organisms during embryogenesis and fetal maturation.

20.2 General methods for producing transgenic animals

There are three basic methods available to transfer genetic material into the mouse genome (Figure 1). They all involve the manipulation of preimplantation embryos to introduce foreign DNA into their chromosomes and identification of the transgenic animal and analysis of transgene expression. Each method has specific advantages and disadvantages. In all cases, a well-equipped and reasonably large vivarium is required to house the relatively large number of mice needed to provide the embryos for manipulation, pseudopregnant females as recipients of manipulated embryos, and maintenance of transgenic mouse strains. There are numerous review articles on the specifics of the subject,[1-6] and readers are referred to these for technical details.[7,8] This chapter describes the most commonly used methods to generate transgenic mice, highlights the advantages and limitations of each, and discusses factors relevant to the application of transgenic lines to toxicological analysis.

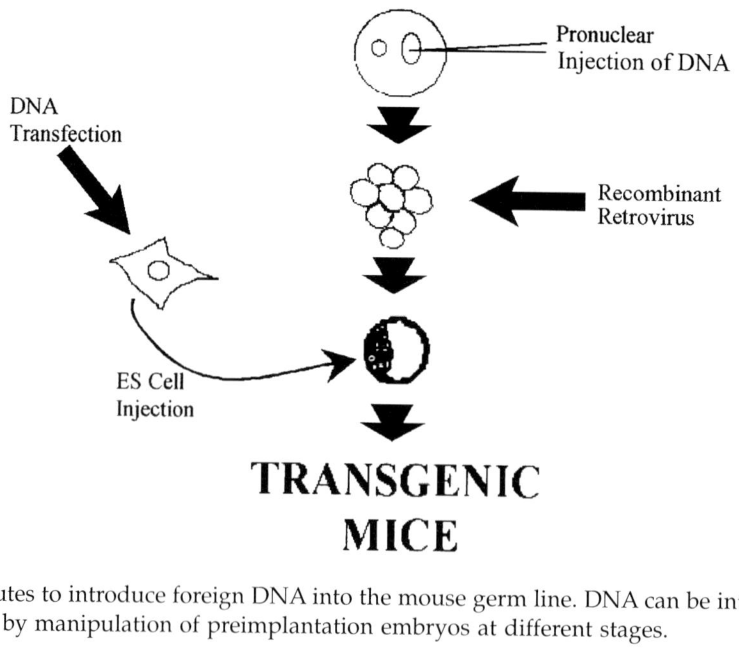

Figure 1 Routes to introduce foreign DNA into the mouse germ line. DNA can be introduced into the germ line by manipulation of preimplantation embryos at different stages.

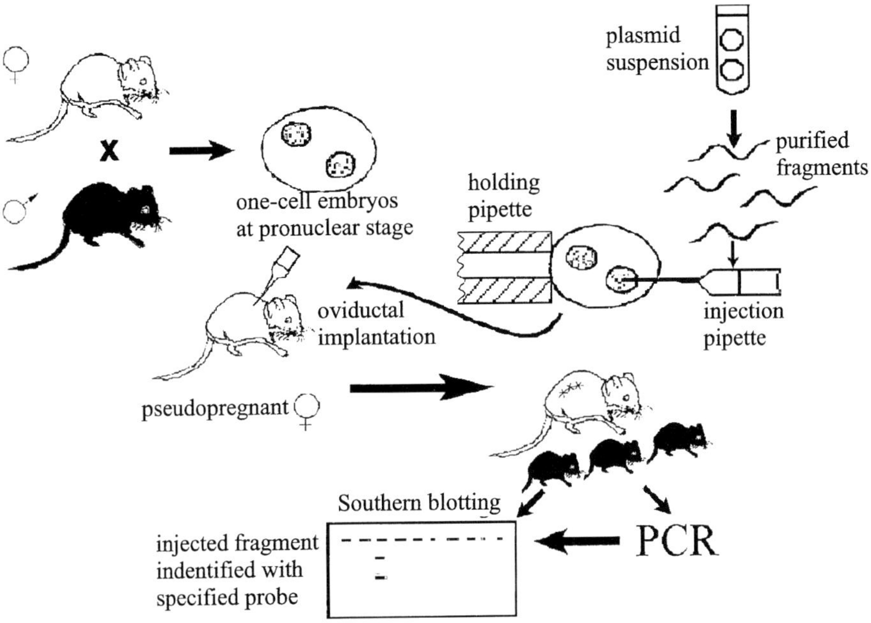

Figure 2 Production of transgenic mice by pronuclear microinjection. One-celled embryos are collected from superovulated donor females that have been mated with male studs. Purified DNA fragments containing the gene of interest are microinjected into the pronucleus of the embryos. The injected embryos are then returned to pseudopregnant females by oviduct transfer, and the resulting animals are screened for the presence of the transgene.

20.2.1 *Microinjection of DNA into pronucleus*

This is by far the most commonly used and successful procedure to generate transgenic mice. This method involves directly introducing DNA into the pronucleus of a one-celled embryo by microinjection. The conditions for the procedure have been well defined.[9] The process is shown schematically in Figure 2 and is summarized below:

1. Four- to six week old donor females are superovulated by the administration of gonadotropins to enhance the yield of mature eggs. The females are then mated with stud males.
2. Females with vaginal plugs are sacrificed 12 h *post coitum* (p.c.). Fertilized one-celled embryos are collected from the oviduct and maintained in M16 culture medium (see below) in an air/CO_2 incubator until use.
3. Purified DNA containing the gene of interest is then microinjected into the pronuclei of the one-celled embryos.
4. Embryos surviving the injection are implanted into the oviducts of 0.5 days p.c. pseudopregnant females for further development *in utero*. Pseudopregnant recipient surrogate females are generated by mating females in natural estrus with vasectomized sterile males. After mating with a sterile male, the female reproductive tract becomes receptive for transferred embryos, and her own unfertilized eggs will degenerate.
5. Only a fraction of animals that develop from microinjected embryos will successfully incorporate the foreign transgene. These transgenic animals directly derived by injection are termed "founder". All pups are marked by a unique pattern of ear punch holes or clipped toes, and a sample of tail tissue is taken. DNA prepared

from the tail biopsy of each animal is analyzed for the presence of the transgene by Southern blot to identify the founder animals.

6. Transgenic animals are then bred with wild-type, nontransgenic mice to generate a sufficient number of male and female "hemizygotes" (animals with only one copy of the transgene) to allow successful breeding to generate homozygotic transgenic mice. If the transgene is integrated into the sex chromosome, it will not be possible to generate a homozygotic transgenic line.
7. Stable transgenic mice can be characterized for transgene expression in different tissues and for phenotype changes.

This method is labor intensive and requires expensive specialized equipment. However, it is the most efficient way to generate transgenic mice expressing the gene of interest. The major pieces of equipment required to perform these procedures include inverted microscopes, micromanipulators to visualize and to manipulate the embryos, a pipette puller to produce glass injection needles, a microforge to prepare micropipettes to hold the embryo for injection, a stereomicroscope to isolate one-celled embryos and to implant injected embryos into the pseudopregnant females by oviduct transfer, and an air/CO_2 incubator to maintain the embryos.

20.2.2 *Culture of early mouse embryo*

Fertilized one-celled embryos must be maintained outside their natural environment in the process of producing transgenic mice. The one-celled embryos can be maintained in M16 medium in a 37°C incubator with 5% CO_2 for several days until they reach the blastocyst stage. They can be grown in M16 microdrops (approximately 50 µl) and covered by paraffin oil to prevent evaporation. During short periods of time (1 to 2 h) when they are manipulated outside the incubator, they can be maintained in M2 medium using HEPES buffer to maintain the proper pH. Although these media are now commercially available, it is often convenient to prepare concentrated stocks of components and make the medium when needed. The components of the concentrated stocks are listed below:

10× Stock A (g/100 ml)	NaCl	5.534
	KCl	0.356
	KH_2PO_4	0.162
	$MgSO_4 \cdot 7H_2O$	0.294
	Sodium lactate	2.608
	Glucose	1.000
	Penicillin	0.060 (10^5 units)
	Streptomycin	0.050
10× Stock B (g/100 ml)	$NaHCO_3$	2.101
	Phenol red	0.010
100× Stock C (g/10 ml)	Sodium pyruvate	0.036
100× Stock D (g/10 ml)	$CaCl_2 \cdot 2H_2O$	0.252
10× Stock E (g/100 ml)	HEPES	5.958
	Phenol red	0.010

All concentrated stocks should be filtered through 0.45-µm filters into sterile plastic tubes and stored frozen at –20°C. M2 and M16 medium can be prepared from stock solution as follows:

Stock	M2 (ml)	M16 (ml)
10×A	1.00	1.0
10×B	0.16	1.0
100×C	0.10	0.10
100×D	0.10	0.10
10×E	8.40	—
H_2O	7.40	7.40
BSA (100 mg/ml)	0.40	0.40
Total	10 ml	10 ml

Working medium should be made and sterilized by filtration before use and can be stored thereafter for up to one week at 4°C. Both media contain bovine serum albumin (BSA) that will reduce the stickiness of the embryos and aid in manipulation and also serve to absorb trace contaminants. However, some batches of BSA do not support early embryonic development. Stock solutions should be tested for their ability to sustain one-celled embryos through several divisions before use for microinjection.

20.2.3 *Transgene design*

It is now relatively common for investigators not directly engaged in production of transgenic mice to supply a construct containing the transgene, generated in their own laboratory, for production of transgenic animals by other laboratories or commercial transgenic services. Careful consideration in designing these DNA constructs is critical. The design of a transgene for microinjection is entirely dependent on the aim and nature of the specific experiment. A transgene should operate like any other gene in the mouse, and all the structural elements must be appropriately recognized by the regulatory machinery of the host. There are certain general roles that should be considered when designing a DNA construct for the generation of transgenic mice by microinjection.

20.2.3.1 *Effects of prokaryotic sequences*

Genes of interest are initially cloned in bacterial plasmids and will then be released from the prokaryotic cloning vector by restriction enzyme digestion. The DNA fragment will be purified prior to microinjection into embryos. Although it appears that prokaryotic vector sequences do not affect the ability of foreign DNA to integrate into the mouse genome, it has been reported that vector sequences can severely inhibit the expression of transduced genes in transgenic mice.[10–13] It is therefore advisable to remove all vector sequences from the cloned gene before microinjection to obtain optimal level of expression.

20.2.3.2 *Effects of intron sequences*

It has been reported that lower levels of transgene expression are obtained using cDNA-based constructs (i.e., those without intron sequences) compared to those using genomic sequences that include introns.[14] The addition of heterologous introns has also been shown to increase the level of cDNA-based transgene expression significantly without altering the tissue specificity of expression.[15,16] Therefore, care must be taken to ensure that appropriate intron sequences are included in the transgene construct.

20.2.3.3 *Distinguishing transgenes from endogenous genes*

It is important to distinguish the products of the transgene from endogenous RNAs or proteins. This may not be a problem when genes from heterologous species (human genes in mouse cells, for example) are used. However, when a mouse gene is used as a transgene in mouse cells, it may be necessary to "mark" the gene by insertion of a tag or an oligonucleotide into an untranslated exon[17] or construct a minigene encoding a shortened

RNA. For cDNA-based transgenes,[11] it may be possible to use intron and polyadenylation sequences from another gene or virus to serve both as a tag and to improve the level of expression.[18]

20.2.3.4 *Tissue-specific expression*

A variety of tissue-specific regulatory sequences have been studied in transgenic mice, and these regulatory sequences can be used to target the expression of the gene of interest both spatially within different cells and organs and temporally during development.[19-21] Since there is no single database dedicated to document tissue-specific regulatory sequences, it is advisable to search the literature for the appropriate sequences when designing a transgene for tissue-specific expression. In addition, there is the TBASE database, which has been established recently in Johns Hopkins University to organize information on transgenic animals and targeted mutations generated and analyzed worldwide and which could provide useful information. The address of the TBASE Web site is: htpp://www.gdb.org/Dan/tbase/tbase.html. One should also bear in mind that the 5′ upstream promoter might not necessarily contain all the tissue-specific regulatory sequences.[22] The internal ribosome entry site (IRES) sequence discussed below could provide an efficient way to track the tissue-specific and developmental stage-specific expression of the transgene.

20.2.3.5 *Bicistronic transgenes*

The initiation of translation in eukaryotic cells is generally dependent upon the binding of ribosomes to the 5′-cap structure of mRNA and scanning of the first AUG codon. The picornaviruses (including poliovirus and encephalomyocarditis virus (EMCV)) contain specific sequences within the untranslated region known as internal ribosome entry sites (IRES).[23,24] These sequences can act as a "ribosome landing pad" and allow internal cap-independent initiation of translation.[23] The identification and functional characterization of these sequences offers the possibility of designing transgenes that will generate bicistronic fusion mRNAs from the same promoter to produce two different proteins in the same cell at the same time. This strategy will also provide an efficient way to follow the expression of the transgene and also serve as a tag to distinguish it from the endogenous gene. For instance, a transgene containing a reporter gene such as *lacZ* could be coexpressed with the cDNA of interest using IRES sequences under the transcriptional control of the same promoter. The expression of the transgene can be detected by X-gal staining. The IRES-reporter gene sequence is also a convenient tag to distinguish the transgene from the endogenous gene.

20.2.4 *Applications*

20.2.4.1 *Gain-of-function*

One of the most common uses of transgenic mice is to study the phenotypic effect of transgene expression in order to evaluate the functional role of the gene of interest. The gene of interest can be expressed ubiquitously[25,26] or in a tissue-specific fashion[19-21] or can be inducible by other agents using a variety of regulatory sequences.[27-31]

20.2.4.2 *Loss-of-function*

Although complete loss-of-function mutant can be created only by gene targeting (see below), it is possible to generate partial loss-of-function transgenic mutant by microinjection. This can be achieved by expressing antisense constructs [32-34] or dominant negative mutant genes[35-39] to obtain partial inactivation of the gene of interest, as discussed in Chapter 19. Furthermore, using tissue-specific and developmental stage-specific regulatory sequences, it may be possible to inactivate a gene at a specific tissue and developmental stage and to allow it to function at earlier stages of development.

20.2.4.3 Transcription control

Another common use of transgenic mice is to study tissue-specific and developmental stage-specific gene regulation. "Reporter" genes (including those encoding chloramphenicol acetyltransferase, luciferase, or *lacZ*) under the control of regulatory sequences whose mode of control is under investigation can be introduced into mouse embryos.[11,40,41] Figure 3 shows that myogenin 5′ regulatory sequence can direct the expression of the *lacZ* reporter gene in a 13.5-day p.c. fetus.[41] This approach can provide a definitive way to analyze the ability of regulatory sequences to direct transcription to specific cells and organs during the development of the animal.

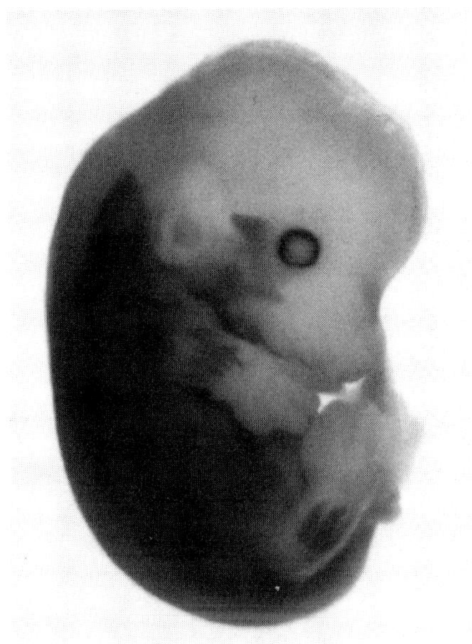

Figure 3 Using transgenic mice to define transcriptional regulatory sequenece. To direct the expression of lacZ reporter gene as the endogenous myogenin gene in a 13.5-day p.c. fetus, 1.1 kb 5′ upstream myogenin promoter sequence is sufficient.

20.2.5 Identification and maintenance of transgenic mouse lines

Choice of a parental mouse strain into which the transgene is to be introduced is important. It has been shown that a number of factors (including the yield of eggs and the overall rate of transgenesis) is strain dependent.[10] Furthermore, if the genetic background of the mouse strain is important to the nature of the experiments, one should ensure that the genetic background of the donor females and stud males are compatible with the design of the subsequent experiment using the resulting transgenic mice.

Injected DNA fragments generally arrange themselves in a head-to-tail array known as a concatamer before integration into the host chromosome.[42,43] However, it is not unusual for the injected DNA to undergo rearrangement or internal deletion leading to the inactivation of the transgene. The injected DNA fragments also often integrated into two different sites in the host genome.[44] Subsequent breeding will give rise to two genotypically different transgenic mouse lines from the same founder animal. It is therefore important to analyze the genomic DNA of the transgenic animals, usually obtained by Southern blot of DNA obtained by tail biopsy, to confirm the arrangement and integrity of the transgene. Polymerase chain reaction (PCR) can be used to screen the potential founder animals for the presence of the transgene before detailed Southern blot analyses are performed in positive animals to characterize the structure of the transgene (see Figure 1). After the structure of the transgene is established in a given transgenic mouse line, it is efficient, and advisable, to confirm the presence of the transgene in transgenic mice from time to time by PCR.

20.2.6 Other considerations

The efficiency of producing transgenic mice varies among experiments. Typically, under optimal conditions, 60 to 80% of the one-celled embryos will survive the injection, and 10 to 30% of the implanted embryos will survive and proceed through normal development. Among the mouse pups born, 10 to 40% will be transgenic and incorporate the transgene in their own chromosomes.

In most cases, the injected DNA will integrate into the chromosome at the one-cell stage. Every cell, including primordial germ cells, will harbor the transgene. However, in some cases the foreign DNA integrates at a later developmental stage, and not all cells in the animal will contain the foreign DNA. The resulting mice are "mosaic" for the transgene. The chromosomes of the progeny of these mosaic founders do not necessarily segregate according to Mendelian roles with respect to the transgene. Lengthy breeding may be necessary to obtain progeny harboring the transgene. Therefore, more time may be required to establish a transgenic line. If the expression of the transgene does not affect growth and development, transgenic mouse lines can be maintained as homozygotes (with respect to the transgene). However, the level of transgene expression might decrease after many generations of breeding.[45] The exact mechanism leading to the decreased level of transgene expression is not known, but it is speculated that accumulative methylation of the foreign incorporated DNA during breeding might be partly responsible. If the level of transgene expression is important for the experiment, it is advisable to check its level from time to time.

The injected foreign DNA integrates into the host genome randomly. The random integration could generate random insertional mutation by interruption of a normal gene. The integration of the transgene could also lead to rearrangement or deletion of the host flanking sequences. Approximately 5 to 15% of transgenic mouse lines generated by this method will harbor either recessive embryonic lethal or viable insertional mutations with visible, but unpredictable, phenotype. It is therefore important to ensure that the phenotypic alteration in the transgenic mice is due to the expression of the transgene. Furthermore, the level of transgene expression is generally independent of the transgene copy number except in the presence of locus controlling region (LCR).[22] However, the level of transgene expression could be affected by the flanking host sequences. It may be necessary to analyze two or more transgenic mouse lines for the effect of transgene expression on host mouse phenotype to control for such insertion site effects. Since the probability that the transgene will integrate into the same host site in two different founder mice is almost nil, analysis of at least two different mouse lines will eliminate the positional effect of host flanking sequences on the phenotypic change of the animal and the level of transgene expression.

20.2.6.1 Retrovirus-mediated transgenesis

This method involves cloning the gene of interest, usually cDNA, into a retrovirus vector. The vector will then be transfected into a helper cell line to produce high titer helper-free recombinant virus stocks and recombinant virus-producing cells for the infection of early embryos. The procedure is as follows:

1. Donor females are mated with stud males and eight-celled embryos to early morulae (2.5 days p.c.) are collected by flushing the oviducts with M2 medium. The zonae

are removed with acidic Tyrode solution, and the embryos are washed with M2 medium.
2. The embryos are then exposed to high titer helper-free recombinant virus stock [46] or are cocultivated with recombinant virus-producing cells.[47] These cells should be washed with alpha-modified MEM containing 10% fetal bovine serum to remove any selection medium. Zona-free embryos can be cocultivated with the virus-producing cells at 37°C for 24 h. The embryos will continue to divide and should be at the late morula–early blastocyst stage.
3. The infected embryos are then transferred to the uterus of 2.5 day p.c. pseudopregnant female mice for further development. Mice that proceed successfully to parturition can be screened for the presence of the transgene as described above.

The mechanism of retrovirus integration has been well characterized.[48] DNA is inserted into the host genome by a precisely defined mechanism. In most cases, only a single virus will infect each cell resulting in a single proviral genome being inserted into a single site of the host chromosome, with no rearrangement or deletion of the host genome. Since there are eight or more cells in the embryos during infection, this method will generate mosaic founder animals that do not contain the virus in each and every cell.

The main advantage of using recombinant retrovirus to generate transgenic mice is its technical ease and lack of requirement for expensive, specialized equipment. Since there is only one proviral genome inserted into the host chromosome without any rearrangement and deletion at the site of integration, it is much easier to identify and to retrieve host DNA flanking the insertion site. However, there are many disadvantages of this method that limit its usefulness. Among these are the extra steps required to produce high titer helper-free virus stock and virus-producing cell lines. There is also a high degree of resulting mosaicism, and it is not uncommon that there is no integration in the germ line. There is also a size limitation for the transduced DNA that can be encoded by retrovirus. Although the virus can express its genes well in differentiated cells, expression in early undifferentiated stem cells is often low.

20.2.6.2 Embryonic stem cell-mediated transgenesis

Embryonic stem (ES) cells are pluripotent cells derived from cultured blastocyst embryos. They can be maintained *in vitro* and still retain their normal karyotype. Foreign DNA can be introduced into these cells efficiently, and clonal cell populations can be selected for the presence of the DNA and other rare integration events. Thus, powerful somatic cellular genetic methods available for cultured cell lines can be applied to the ES cells that are available for production of transgenic mice. When the manipulated ES cells are injected into host blastocysts, they retain their potential to colonize the developing embryo and contribute to many cell lineages, including the germ cells of the resulting chimeric animal. Stable transgenic mice harboring the transduced DNA can then be produced through breeding of the chimeric animals. The procedure is illustrated in Figure 4. There are many different protocols to maintain and to manipulate ES cells, and the reader should refer to several excellent manuals for technical details.[7,8,49]

The most common use of ES cells today is to produce mouse strains with specific null mutations — that is, deletion or inactivation of target host genes. When cloned genomic DNA is introduced into cultured cells, it can locate its homologous sequences at specific chromosomal loci and undergo homologous recombination. The alteration of specific endogenous genes by homologous recombination is referred to as gene targeting. Our ability to perform gene targeting in ES cells provides us with a unique tool to introduce specific mutations into the mouse genome and to analyze the phenotypic consequences of specific genetic modification in the mouse.

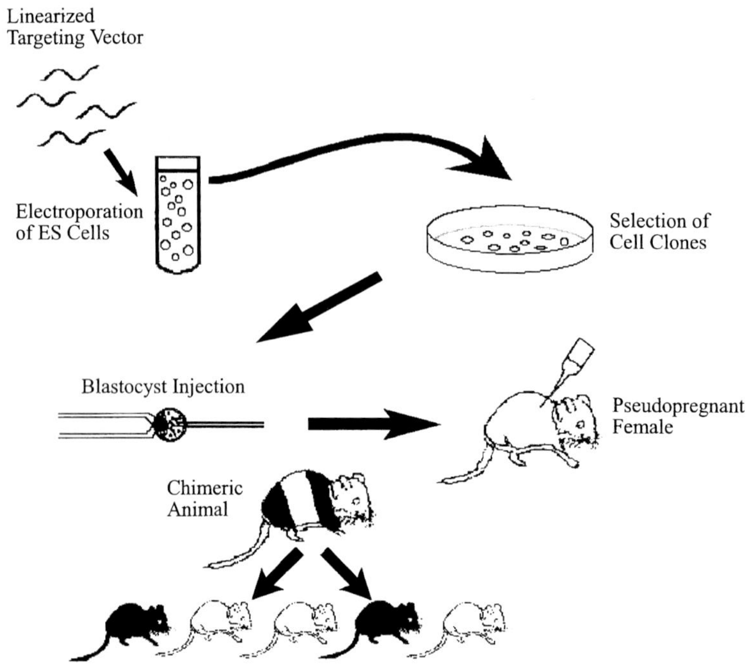

Figure 4 Embryonic stem cell-mediated transgenesis. Linearized targeting vector is introduced into ES cells and then subjected for selection. The cells are introduced back into blastocysts, and the manipulated blastocysts are returned to pseudopregnant females to produce a chimeric animal. Transgenic or knockout mice can then be obtained by breeding these chimeric animals with wild-type mice.

20.2.7 *Targeting vectors*

DNA sequences to inactivate host genes are referred to as targeting vectors. There are many different design strategies in producing targeting vectors, and they are dependent on the specific intended mutation and the nature of individual experiments. Readers should refer to recent reviews for detailed designs of different targeting vectors.[50]

All targeting vectors are designed to enhance homologous recombination and the subsequent selection of cells bearing the recombination product. There are several general considerations. Whenever possible, it is advisable to use isogenic DNA (genomic DNA isolated from the same mouse strain as the ES cells) for targeting. It has been shown that isogenic DNA sequences significantly improve homologous recombination frequency.[51] The overall length of homologous sequences is also important to improve the frequency of the targeting event, and a minimum region of homology of 1 kb is necessary for efficient targeting.[51,52] It is advisable to include positive and negative selection markers in the targeting vector to provide strong selection to isolate cells with the correct recombination products.

20.2.7.1 *Application*

Gene targeting in ES cells is the only method today to generate specific null mutations in the mouse genome and to produce loss-of-function mutant mouse strains. It has also proved useful in other applications (including the enhancer and gene trap methods)[53,54] to identify and isolate novel genes. The IRES sequence discussed above has been used successfully in ES cells.[56-57] Its application in gene targeting has been discussed in a recent review,[58] and it will undoubtedly expand the range of experiments using ES cells.

20.2.7.2 *Other considerations*

It is extremely important to ensure that the ES cells are maintained under optimal growth conditions at all times, and this requires constant attention to all details. Under suboptimal growth conditions, the cells will undergo chromosomal rearrangement and mutation to enhance their ability to grow *in vitro* and thereby decrease their ability to differentiate and to contribute to different cell lineages in the developing embryos. The growth conditions of ES cells have been well characterized, and readers are directed to other sources for detailed information.[59]

Production of transgenic mice using ES cells is expensive, labor intensive, and time consuming. It also requires expensive and specialized micromanipulators and microscopes to inject ES cells into blastocysts. ES cells can also be introduced back into the early developing mouse by aggregating them with cleavage stage embryos in culture dishes.[60] This method does not require expensive equipment, and the technique takes less time to master compared to microinjection.

20.2.8 *Application to renal toxicology*

Our knowledge of the function of a gene at the molecular and cellular level can now be expanded to the physiological level of the whole organism using special "designer" transgenic and knockout mice. Transgenic mice harboring genes that play important roles in renal function, development, and pathogenesis,[61-66] including renin[67,68] and Pax2,[69,70] have been produced, and they have provided us with valuable information about how they are regulated and function in the whole animal. With the advances in molecular biology, novel genes involved in renal function will be isolated. Our ability to manipulate the mouse genome will undoubtedly be invaluable to probe into their physiological function and will also allow us to produce mouse models for specific renal conditions and diseases.[70]

20.3 *Acknowledgment*

I would like to thank Jim Koropatnick for reading the manuscript and for his helpful comments, Clement Lo and Nick Lo for preparing the figures, and my sister, Louisa Chan, for helping to look after my newborn daughter while I was preparing this manuscript.

References

1. Jaenisch, R., Transgenic animals, *Science,* 240, 1468, 1988.
2. Gordon, J.W., Transgenic animals, *Int. Rev. Cytol.,* 115, 171, 1989.
3. Babinet, C., Morello, D., and Renard, J.P. Transgenic mice, *Genome,* 31, 938, 1989.
4. Hanahan, D., Transgenic mice as probes into complex systems, *Science,* 246, 1265, 1989.
5. Westphal, H., Transgenic mammals and biotechnology, *FASEB J.,* 3, 117, 1989.
6. Rossant, J. and Pedersen, R., Eds., *Experimental Approach to Mammalian Embryonic Development,* Cambridge University Press, 1986.
7. Hogan, B., Beddington, R., Costantini, F., and Lacy, E., *Manipulating the Mouse Embryo. A Laboratory Manual,* 2nd ed., Cold Spring Harbor Laboratory Press, Cold Spring Harbor, NY, 1994.
8. Wassarman, P.M. and DePamphilis, M.L., Eds., *Guide to Techniques in Mouse Development. Methods in Enzymology,* Vol. 225, Academic Press, New York, 1993.
9. Brinster, R.L., Chen, N.Y., Trumbauer, M.K., Yagler, M.K., and Palmiter, R.D., Factors affecting the efficiency of introducing foreign DNA into mice by microinjecting eggs, *Proc. Natl. Acad. Sci. U.S.A.,* 82, 4438, 1985.
10. Chada, K., Magram, K., Raphael, G., Lacy, E., and Costantini, F., Specific expression of a foreign beta-globin gene in erythroid cells of transgenic mice, *Nature,* 314, 377, 1985.

11. Krumlauf, R., Hammer, R.E., Tilghman, S.M., and Brinster, R.L., Developmental regulation of alpha-fetoprotein in transgenic mice, *Mol. Cell. Biol.*, 5, 2639, 1985.
12. Hammer, R.E., Krumlauf, R., Camper, S.A., Brinster, R.L., and Tilghman, S.M., Diversity of alpha-fetoprotein gene expression in mice generated by a combination of separate enhancer elements, *Science*, 235, 53, 1987.
13. Townes, T.M., Lingrel, J.B., Brinster, R.L., and Palmiter, R.D., Erythroid specific expression of human beta-globin genes in transgenic mice, *EMBO J.*, 4, 1715, 1985.
14. Brinster, R.L., Allen, J.M., Behringer, R.R., Gelina, R.E., and Palmiter, R.D., Introns increase transcriptional efficiency in transgenic mice, *Proc. Natl. Acad. Sci. U.S.A.*, 85, 836, 1988.
15. Palmiter, R.D., Sandgren, E.P., Avarbock, M.R., Allen, D.D., and Brinster, R.L., Heterologous introns can enhance expression of transgenes in mice, *Proc. Natl. Acad. Sci. U.S.A.*, 88, 478, 1991.
16. Choi, T.M., Huang, M., Gorman, C., and Jaenisch, R., A generic intron increases gene expression in transgenic mice, *Mol. Cell. Biol.*, 11, 3070, 1991.
17. Shi, Y., Son, H.J., Shahan, K., Rodriguez, M., Costantini, F., and Derman, E., Silent genes in the mouse major urinary protein gene family, *Proc. Natl. Acad. Sci. U.S.A.*, 86, 4584, 1989.
18. Balling, R., Mutter, G., Gruss, P., and Kessel, M., Craniofacial abnormalities induced by ectopic expression of the homeobox gene Hox1.1 in transgenic mice, *Cell*, 58, 337, 1989.
19. Muller, W.J., Sinn, E., Pattengale, P.K., Wallace, R., and Leder, P. Single-step induction of mammary adenocarcinoma in transgenic mice bearing the activated c-neu oncogene, *Cell*, 54, 105, 1988.
20. Sinn, E., Muller, W., Pattengale, P., Tepler, I., Wallace, R., and Leder, P., Coexpression of MMTV/v-Ha-ras and MMTV/c-myc genes in transgenic mice: synergistic action of oncogenes in vivo, *Cell*, 49, 465, 1987.
21. Jhappan, C., Geiser, A.G., Kordon, E.C, Bagheri, D., Hennighausen, L., Roberts, A.B., Smith, G.H., and Merlino, G., Targeting expression of a transforming growth factor beta 1 transgene to the pregnant mammary gland inhibits alveolar development and lactation, *EMBO J.*, 12, 1835, 1993.
22. Grovseld, F., van Assendelft, G.B., Greaves, D.R., and Kollis, G., Position-independent, high-level expression of the human beta-globin gene in transgenic mice, *Cell*, 51, 975, 1987.
23. Pelletier, J. and Sonenberg, N., Internal initiation of translation of eukaryotic mRNA directed by a sequence derived from poliovirus RNA, *Nature*, 334, 320, 1988.
24. Molla, A., Jang, S.K., Paul, A.V., Reuer, Q., and Wimmer, E., Cardioviral internal ribosomal entry site is functional in a genetically engineered dicistronic poliovirus, *Nature*, 356, 255, 1992.
25. Koopman, P., Povey, S., and Lovell–Badge, R.H., Widespread expression of human alpha 1-antitrypsin in transgenic mice revealed by in situ hybridization, *Genes Dev.*, 3, 16, 1989.
26. Tam, P.P. and Tan, S.S., The somatogenetic potential of cells in the primitive streak and the tail bud of the organogenesis-stage mouse embryo, *Development*, 115, 703, 1992.
27. Furth, P.A., St. Onge, L., Boger, H., Gruss, P., Gossen, M., Kistner, A., Bujard, H., and Hennighausen, L., Temporal control of gene expression in transgenic mice by a tetracycline-responsive promoter, *Proc. Natl. Acad. Sci. U.S.A.*, 91, 9302, 1994.
28. Kothary, R., Clapoff, S., Darling, S., Perry, M.D., Moran, L.A., and Rossant, J., Inducible expression of an hsp68-lacZ hybrid gene in transgenic mice, *Development*, 105, 707, 1989.
29. Ruther, U., Woodroofe, C., Fattori, E., and Ciliberto, G., Inducible formation of liver tumors in transgenic mice, *Oncogene*, 8, 87, 1993.
30. Semenza, G.L., Koury, S.T., Nejfelt, M.K., Gearhart, J.D., and Antonarakis, S.E., Cell-type-specific and hypoxia-inducible expression of the human erythropoietin gene in transgenic mice, *Proc. Natl. Acad. Sci. U.S.A.*, 88, 8725, 1991.
31. Wijnholds, J., Philipsen, S., Pruzina, S., Fraser, P., Grosveld, F., and Ab, G., Estrogen-inducible and liver-specific expression of the chicken Very Low Density Apolipoprotein II gene locus in transgenic mice, *Nucleic Acids Res.*, 21, 1629, 1993.
32. Matsumoto, K., Kakidani, H., Takahashi, A., Nakagata, N., Anzai, M., Matsuzaki, Y., Takahashi, Y., Miyata, K., Utsumi, K., and Iritani, A., Growth retardation in rats whose growth hormone gene expression was suppressed by antisense RNA transgene, *Mol. Reprod. Dev.*, 36, 53, 1993.

33. Moxham, C.M., Hod, Y., and Malbon, C.C., Gi alpha 2 mediates the inhibitory regulation of adenylylcyclase *in vivo*: analysis in transgenic mice with Gi alpha 2 suppressed by inducible antisense RNA, *Dev. Genet.*, 14, 266, 1993.
34. Cockayne, D.A., Bodine, D.M., Cline, A., Nienhuis, A.W., and Dunbar, C.E., Transgenic mice expressing antisense interleukin-3 RNA develop a B-cell lymphoproliferative syndrome or neurologic dysfunction, *Blood*, 84, 2699, 1994.
35. Dumont, D.J., Gradwohl, G., Fong, G.H., Puri, M.C., Gertsenstein, M., Auerbach, A., and Breitman, M.L., Dominant-negative and targeted null mutations in the endothelial receptor tyrosine kinase, tek, reveal a critical role in vasculogenesis of the embryo, *Genes Dev.*, 8, 18971, 1994.
36. Chang, P.Y., Benecke, H., Le Marchand–Brustel, Y., Lawitts, J., and Moller, D.E., Expression of a dominant-negative mutant human insulin receptor in the muscle of transgenic mice, *J. Biol. Chem.*, 269, 16034, 1994.
37. Werner, S., Weinberg, W., Liao, X., Peters, K.G., Blessing, M., Yuspa, S.H., Weiner, R.L., and Williams, L.T., Targeted expression of a dominant-negative FGF receptor mutant in the epidermis of transgenic mice reveals a role of FGF in keratinocyte organization and differentiation, *EMBO J.*, 12, 2635, 1993.
38. Saitou, M., Sugai, S., Tanaka, T., Shimouchi, K., Fuchs, E., Narumiya, S., and Kakizuka, A., Inhibition of skin development by targeted expression of a dominant-negative retinoic acid receptor, *Nature*, 374, 159, 1995.
39. Imakado, S., Bickenbach, J.R., Bundman, D.S., Rothnagel, J.A., Attar, P.S., Wang, X.J., Walczak, V.R., Wisniewski, S., Pote, J., Gordon, J.S., et al., Targeting expression of a dominant-negative retinoic acid receptor mutant in the epidermis of transgenic mice results in loss of barrier function, *Genes Dev.*, 9, 317, 1995.
40. Whiting, J., Marshall, H., Cook, M., Krumlauf, R., Rigby, P.W.J., Stott, D., and Allenmann, R.K., Multiple spatially specific enhancers are required to reconstruct the pattern of Hox-2.6 gene expression, *Genes Dev.*, 5, 2048, 1991.
41. Yee, S. and Rigby, P., The regulation of myognin gene expression during the embryonic development of the mouse, *Genes Dev.*, 7, 1277, 1993.
42. Brinster, R.L., Chen, H.Y., Trumbauer, M., Senear, A.W., Warren, R., and Palmiter, R.D., Somatic expression of herpes thymidine kinase in mice following injection of a fusion gene into eggs, *Cell*, 27, 223, 1981.
43. Costantini, F. and Lacy, E., Introduction of a rabbit beta-globin gene into the mouse germ line, *Nature*, 294, 92, 1981.
44. Lacy, E., Roberts, S., Evans, E.P., Burtenshaw, M.D., and Costantini, F., A foreign beta-globin gene in transgenic mice: integration at abnormal chromosomal positions and expression in inappropriate tissues, *Cell*, 34, 343, 1983.
45. Yee, S., Personal Communication.
46. Jaenisch, R., Germ line integration and Mendelian transmission of the exogenous Molony Leukemia virus, *Proc. Natl. Acad. Sci. U.S.A.*, 73, 1260, 1976.
47. Jaenisch, R., Jahner, D., Nobis, P., Simon, I., Lohler, J., Harbers, K., and Grotkopp, D., Chromosomal position and activation of retroviral genomes inserted into the germ line of mice, *Cell*, 24, 519, 1981.
48. Varmus, H., in *RNA Tumor Virus*, Weiss, R., Teich, N., Varmus, H., and Coffin, J., Eds., Cold Spring Harbor Laboratory Press, Cold Spring Harbor, NY, 1982.
49. Joyner, A.L., Ed., *Gene Targeting: A Practical Approach.*, IRL Press, Oxford, 1993.
50. Hasty, P. and Bradley, A., Gene targeting vectors for mammalian cells, in Joyner, A.L., Ed., *Gene Targeting: A Practical Approach*, IRL Press, Oxford, 1993, 1.
51. Deng, C. and Capecchi, M.R., Reexamination of gene targeting frequency as a function of the extent of homology between the targeting vector and the targeting locus, *Mol. Cell. Biol.*, 12, 3365, 1992.
52. Hasty, P., Rivera–Parez, J., and Bradley, A., The length of homology required for gene targeting in embryonic stem cells, *Mol. Cell. Biol.*, 11, 5586, 1991.
53. Gossler, A. and Zachgo, J., Gene and enhancer trap screens in ES cells chimeras, in Joyner, A.L., Ed., *Gene Targeting: A Practical Approach*, IRL Press, Oxford, 1993, 181.

54. Skarnes, W.C., Auerbach, B.A., and Joyner, A.L., A gene trap approach in mouse embryonic stem cells: the lacZ reporter is activated by splicing, reflects endogenous gene expression, and is mutagenic in mice, *Genes Devel.*, 6, 903, 1992.
55. Kim, D.G., Kang, H.M., Jang, S.K., and Sin, H.S., Construction of a bifunctional mRNA in the mouse by using the internal ribosomal entry site of the encephalomyocarditis virus, *Mol. Cell. Biol.*, 12, 3636, 1992.
56. Wu, H., Liu, X., and Jaenisch, R., Double replacement: strategy for efficient introduction of subtle mutations into the murine Col1a-1 gene by homologous recombination in embryonic stem cells, *Proc. Natl. Acad. Sci. U.S.A.*, 91, 2819, 1994.
57. Frey, S.O., Paielli, D.L., and Gilbert, J.D., Ectopic expression of the CCAAT/enhancer-binding protein promotes the adipogenic program in a variety of mouse fibroblastic cells, *Genes Dev.*, 8, 1654, 1994.
58. Mountford, P.S. and Smith, A.G., Internal ribosome entry sites and dicistronic RNAs in mammalian transgenesis, *Trends Genet.*, 11, 179, 1995.
59. Abbondanzo, S.J., Gadi, I., and Stewart, C.L., Derivation of embryonic stem cell lines, in Wassarman, P.M. and DePamphilis, M.L., Eds., *Guide to Techniques in Mouse Development. Methods in Enzymology*, Vol. 225, Academic Press, New York, 1993, 803.
60. Nagy, A. and Rossant, J., Production of completely ES cell-derived fetuses, in Joyner, A.L., Ed., *Gene Targeting: A Practical Approach*, IRL Press, Oxford, 1993, 147.
61. Trudel, M., D'Agati, V., and Costantini, F., C-myc as an inducer of polycystic kidney disease in transgenic mice, *Kidney Int.*, 39, 6656, 1991.
62. Fattori, E., Della Rocca, C., Costa, P., Giorgio, M., Dente, B., Pozzi, L., and Ciliberto, G., Development of progressive kidney damage and myeloma kidney in interleukin-6 transgenic mice, *Blood*, 83, 2570, 1994.
63. White, C.W., Nguyen, D.H., Suzuki, K., Taniguchi, N., Rusakow, L.S., Avraham, K.B., and Groner, Y., Expression of manganese superoxide dismutase is not altered in transgenic mice with elevated level of copper-zinc superoxide dismutase, *Free Radic. Biol. Med.*, 15, 629, 1993.
64. Semenza, G.L., Traystman, M.D., Gearhart, J.D., and Antonarakis, S.E., Polycythemia in transgenic mice expressing the human erythropoietin gene, *Proc. Natl. Acad. Sci. U.S.A.*, 86, 2301, 1989.
65. Moyer, J.H., Lee–Tischler, M.J., Kwon, H.Y., Schrick, J.J., Avner, E.D., Sweeney, W.E., Godfrey, V.L., Cacheiro, N.L., Wilkinson, J.E., and Woychik, R.P., Candidate gene associated with a mutation causing recessive polycystic kidney disease in mice, *Science*, 264, 1329, 1994.
66. Atala, A., Freeman, M.R., Mandell, J., and Beier, D.R., Juvenile cystic kidneys (jck): a new mouse mutation which causes polycystic kidneys, *Kidney Int.*, 43, 1081, 1993.
67. Sigmund, C.D., Expression of the human renin gene in transgenic mice throughout ontogeny, *Pediatr. Nephrol.*, 7, 639, 1993.
68. Sigmund, C.D., Jones, C.A., Kane, C.M., Wu, C., Lang, J.A., and Gross, K.W., Regulated tissue- and cell-specific expression of the human renin gene in transgenic mice, *Circ. Res.*, 70, 1070, 1992.
69. Dressler, G.R., Wilkinson, J.E., Rothenpieler, U.W., Patterson, L.T., Williams–Simons, L., and Westphal, H., Deregulation of Pax-2 expression in transgenic mice generates severe kidney abnormalities, *Nature*, 362, 65, 1993.
70. Keller, S.A., Jones, J.M., Boyle, A., Barrow, L.L., Killen, P.D., Green, D.G., Kapousta, N.V., Hitchcock, P.F., Swank, R.T., and Meisler, M.H., Kidney and retinal defects (Krd), a transgene-induced mutation with a deletion of mouse chromosome 19 that includes the Pax2 locus, *Genomics*, 23, 309, 1994.
71. Grandaliano, G., Choudhury, G.G., and Abboud, H.E., Transgenic animal models as a tool in the diagnosis of kidney diseases, *Semin. Nephrol.*, 15, 43, 1995.

Index

A

AAP (alanine aminopeptidase), as urinary marker, 20
ABT (1-aminobenzotriazole), 332
4-Acetamido-4'-isothiocyanostilbene-2,2'-disulfonic acid (SITS), 175
Acetaminophen, 334, 339
2-Acetylaminofluorene, 339
N-Acetyl-β-D-glucosaminidase (NAG), as urinary marker, 21–22
Acivicin (AT-125), 334
Acute renal failure (ARF), 283, 285
Acute tubular necrosis (ATN), 53
Adenine nucleotides, intracellular content, 158–159, 317–318
Adenocarcinoma, 240
Adenoma, 240
Adenovirus, 231
Alanine, kidney perfusion, 67
Alanine aminopeptidase (AAP), as urinary marker, 20
Alkaline phosphatase (AP), as urinary marker, 20, 164, 177, 200
Amiloride, 175
Amino acids, isolated kidney, 67
1-Aminobenzotriazole (ABT), 332
Aminoglycoside, toxicity, 179
p-Aminohippurate (PAH), 3, 92, 159, 175
Aminooxyacetic acid (AOAA), 334
Aminopeptidase M, 333, 334
Aminotriazole-inhibitable calatase assay, 260–263
Amphibian studies, isolated perfused kidney, 69
Amphotericin B, nephrotoxicity, 16
Analytic techniques, micropuncture and microperfusion, 91–92
Anesthesia, micropuncture, 81, 87–88
Antibiotics
  in cell culture, 205
  in tissue culture medium, 169
  toxicity, 119–120, 165, 180–181
Antigens, kidney-specific, 29
Antineoplastic agents, toxicity, 120, 180–181
Antioxidant enzymes, assay, 272–277
Antisense nucleic acids, 402
AP (alkaline phosphatase), as urinary marker, 20, 164, 177, 200
Apoptosis, 285, 293–295
Appearance flux rate, 138–139
Arachidonic acid, 333, 334
  oxidation, P450–dependent, 365
Arachidonic acid epoxygenases 2CAA, 358
Arginine, kidney perfusion, 67
Aromatic hydroxylation assay, 265–266
Arsenazo III, 302, 323–326
ARF (acute renal failure), 283, 285
Artifacts, renal histopathology, 54–55
Asymmetric PCR, 247
AT-125 (acivicin), 334
ATN (acute tubular necrosis), 53
ATP content, 116, 158–159, 317

B

Bath-to-lumen flux, 125, 139–144
Benzo[*a*]pyrene, 339
1-Benzylquinolinium, toxicity, 120
Bicistronic transgenes, 418
Biomarkers, see Markers
Biotransformation, nephrotoxicity, 331–344
Bleomycin-detectable iron assay, 270–272
Bradford protein assay, 341–342
Brendel-Vitron slicer, 110, 111
5-Bromo-2'-deoxyuridine (BrdU), as renal regeneration marker, 289–290
Brush border enzymes, 19–21, 164, 333–334
Bubble culture, 114
tert-Butylhydroperoxide (TBHP), cell injury by, 181

C

Calcium ions, mitochondria, 302–303, 322–326
Cannulation, isolated perfused kidney, 63–65
Carbapenem, toxicity, 165
Carboplatin, toxicity, 181
Carcinogenesis, see Renal carcinogenesis
Carcinogenicity bioassay, 238
Carcinogens, 241, 242
Carcinomas, 239
Catalase, measurement, 275
Catalase compound I, 260
Cathepsin B, as urinary marker, 22–23
Cavalieri principle, 47
CCD (cortical collecting ducts), 104, 131–137
cDNA, 389
CDNB (1-chloro-2,4-dinitrobenzene), 339, 343
Cefalozin, 223

Celiptium, toxicity, 120
Cell culture, 218–220, 226–227; see also Established cell lines; Immortalized cell lines
Cell culture techniques; see also Primary cell cultures
Cell immortalization, see Immortalized cell lines
Cell injury, 165, 166, 181, 257; see also Renal injury
Cell lines, 220
  established, 202
  293 human embryonic renal cell line, 229
  immortalized, 217–232
Cephaloridine, toxicity, 119, 165, 224
Cephalosporin, toxicity, 165
Cephalothin, 224
Chemical mismatch cleavage (CMC), 247
Chemiluminescence, 259–260, 366
Chimeric animals, 401
1-Chloro-2,4-dinitrobenzene (CDNB), 339, 343
Chlorzoxazone, 364
Chronic glomerular injury, 52
Cisplatin, toxicity, 120, 180–181
Cleaning pipette, 145
Clearance methods
  creatinine clearance, 12–14
  glomerular filtration rate, 8–9, 12–15
  inulin clearance, 1–7
  inulin in plasma and urine, 10–12
  renal clearance, 1–3, 15–17
Clearance ratio, 3
Clusterin, as marker, 292–293
CMC (chemical mismatch cleavage), 247
Collagenase treatment, 148
Collection pipette, 144, 145
Colloids, in perfusate, 67
Colorimetric detection, of inulin, 10–12
Computer-assisted reconstruction, nephrons, 52
Confocal microscopy, 52
Conjuganted dienes, 268–270
Constant volume pipette, 145
Coring, renal tissue, 112
Cortical collecting ducts (CCD), 104, 131–137
Cortical thick ascending limbs (CTAL), microdissection, 103
Creatinine clearance, determination of GFR using, 12–14
CTAL (cortical thick ascending limbs), microdissection, 103
Cycasin, 243
Cycle sequencing, 247
Cyclooxygenase, 333
CYP1A protein subfamily, 357, 363
CYP2A protein subfamily, 357
CYP2B protein subfamily, 357–258, 363
CYP2C protein subfamily, 358
CYP2E protein subfamily, 358–359, 363–364
CYP3A protein subfamily, 359, 364
CYP4A protein subfamily, 360, 364
Cysteine conjugate β-lyase, 333, 339, 344
Cysteinylglycine dipeptidase, 333, 334
Cytochrome *c* reduction assay, 258–259
  acetylated, 272–275
Cytochrome P450, 336, 354–355
  cellular metabolism, 165, 166
  detection
    immunochemical, 365–367
    RT-PCR, 367
  expression, 355–356
    enhancement, 361–362
  hybridization, 368–369
  inhibition, 362
  isozymes, 166, 332
  localization, 367–368
  measurement, 361
  monitoring, 338, 362–365
Cytokeratin filaments, 292
Cytosol, 341
Cytotoxicity; see also Nephrotoxicity; Toxicity studies
  in cultured cells, 164–165, 211–213
  renal proximal tubular cells, 176–181
Cytotoxicity assays; see also Toxicity studies
  acute cytotoxicity assay, 211–213
  adenine nucleotide intracellular content, 158–159
  lactase dehydrogenase release, 24, 116, 155–157
  markers, 19–31, 116, 156
  organic ion accumulation, 159–160
  oxygen consumption, 159
  potassium intracellular content, 157–158
  with renal proximal tubule suspensions, 155–160

D

DCT (distal convoluted tubules), microdissection, 103
DCVC (dichlorovinylcysteine), 119, 181, 303, 310
Denaturing gradient gel electrophoresis (DGGE), 245–246
Density gradient centrifugation, of renal tubular fragments, 195
3,7-Diamino-5-phenylphenazinium chloride, 313
2',7'-Dichlorofluorescein (DCF), 263
2',7'-Dichlorofluorescine diacetate (DCFH-DA), 263
N-(3,5-Dichlorophenyl)succinimide (NDPS), 339
Dichlorovinylcysteine (DCVC), 119, 181, 303, 310
DideoxyTTP (ddTTP), 247
Dienes, measurement of conjugated dienes, 268–270
Diethylnitrosamine (NDEA), 241, 242
Differentiation, regenerative renal cells, 292–293
Digitonin fractionation, of intact renal cells, 303–305
Digitonin/nagarse method, 305
Di-isopropanolamine, 242
Dimethylhydrazine, 243
Dimethylnitrosamine (NDMA), 241, 242
5,5-Dimethyloxazolidine-2,4-dione (DM), 316
Dioxetane, 259
Diphenylamine assay, inulin detection, 10–11
Direct immunofluorescence technique, 40–42
Direct sequencing, 247
Disappearance flux rate, 138
Disector, 46–47

Dissection, 129–135
microdissection, 97–105
Distal convoluted tubules (DCT), microdissection, 103
5,5'-Dithiobis(2-nitrobenzoic acid) (DNTB), 269
DM (5,5-dimethyloxazolidine-2,4-dione), 316
DNA
apoptosis, 293–295
bleomycin damage, 270
BrdU incorporation, 289
isolation, 249
renal mutagenesis, 244–249
sequencing, 247
stable transfection, 398–399
transient transfection, 399–400
DNTB (5,5-dithiobis(2-nitrobenzoic acid)), 269
Dog studies, clearance methods, 6, 7, 14
Dot blot analysis, 389
DTNB-GSSG reductase recycling assay, 269–270
Dynamic organ culture, 113–114

E

EETs (epoxyeicosatrienoic acids), 365
EGF (epidermal growth factor), 285
Electron microprobe analysis, 92
Electron microscopy, 42
apoptosis studies, 293
fixative, 37
tissue slices, 117
Electroporation, 225
Embryonic stem cell-mediated transgenesis, 421
Endoperoxide, 259
Enhanced chemiluminescence (ECL), 366
ENU (*N*-nitrosodimethylamine), 243
Enzymatic recycling assay, 320–321
Enzyme histochemistry, 43–44, 248–249
Enzyme-linked immunoabsorbance (ELISA), urinary RBP, 27–28
Enzymes
antioxidant enzyme assays, 272–277
distribution, 356
markers, 19–24, 116, 156
Epidermal growth factor (EGF), 285
Epithelial cells, see Renal epithelial cells
Epoxyeicosatrienoic acids (EETs), 365
Epoxygenase activity, 365
Erythrocytes, in perfusate, 61, 67–68
Erythromycin *N*-demethylation, 364
Established cell lines, 202
Ethoxyresorufin *O*-dealkylation assay, 363
N-Ethyl-*N*-hydroxyethylnitrosamine (EHEN), 241, 242
Ethyl methanesulfonate, 243

F

Famotidine, renal clearance, 15
Fast Garnet, 22
Fibrosarcoma, 239
Ficoll density-gradient centrifugation, 195
Fixation, 36–37, 54
Fluorescein isothiocyanate (FITC), 40
Fluorescent *in situ* hybridization (FISH), 244
(4'-Fluorobiphenyl)acetamide (FBPA), 241, 242
Fluorochromes, 40
Fluorometry, 86, 92, 263–265
Fluosol-DA, 68
Founder animals, 415
Fractionator principle, 49–51
Fura-2-acetoxymethyl ester, 323

G

G418, 222
Gain-of-function events, 380, 402–403, 418
Gene expression
deregulation, 380–381
in eukaryotes, 378–380
intervention, 398–403
Gene inactivation, 400–402
Gene knockout, 380, 400, 401, 403
Gene targeting, 422
Geneticin, 222
Gene transcription, 380–383, 419
Gentamicin
glomerular filtration rate, 15–16
toxicity, 119, 120, 179–180
GGT, see γ-Glutamyltranspeptidase
Glomerular filtration rate (GFR)
determination using creatinine clearance, 12–14
effects, toxicants, 15–16
in laboratory animals, 2
by plasma clearance of inulin, 8–9
single nephron, by micropuncture, 86
Glomerular lesions, histopathology, 52
Glomerular sclerosis, 52
Glomerular volume, 51, 55
Glomerulus
counting, 49–51
function, 218
microdissection, 103
Glucose, in primary cell culture, 174–175
γ-Glutamyltranspeptidase (GGT), 333
glutathione assay, 269
as urinary marker, 20–21, 164, 200–201
Glutathione (GSH), 266, 268–270, 320–322
Glutathione conjugates, 119, 333
Glutathione disulfide (GSSG), 266, 334
assay for, 320–322
measurement, 268–270
Glutathione peroxide (GSH-Px) assay, 275–277
Glutathione *S*-transferase (GST), 332–333, 343–344
Glycine, kidney perfusion, 67
Glycolytic metabolism, in primary cell cultures, 173
Gomori's silver-methenamine solution, 39–40
Growth factors, renal regeneration, 285–288
GSH-Px assay, see Glutathione peroxide assay
GSS, see Glutathione
GSSG, see Glutathione disulfide
GST, see Glutathione *S*-transferase

H

Haber-Weiss reaction, 257
Halogenated hydrocarbons, toxicity, 119
Harvesting, renal tissue, 129, 135–137
Heavy metals, 30, 117–118
Hematoxylin and eosin staining, 37
Hepatocyte growth factor (HGF), 285
HETEs (hydroxyeicosatetraenoic acids), 365
High-performance liquid chromatography (HPLC), 30–31, 137, 321–322
Histoautoradiography, with thymidine, 289
Histopathologic methods, 36, 52–55
  artifacts, 54–55
  computerized methods, 52
  confocal microscopy, 52
  electron microscopy, 37, 40, 117, 293
  enzyme histochemistry, 43–44
  fixation, 36–37
  immunofluorescence microscopy, 40–43
  immunohistochemistry, 43–44
  light microscopy, 37–40
  morphometric methods, 44, 51
  stereological methods, 44–51
  vascular lesions, 54
Holding pipette, 143–144
Housekeeping genes, 378–379
Human papilloma virus, for cell immortalization, 230
Hydrocarbons, toxicity, 119
Hydrogen peroxide, intracellular, 260–265
Hydroxyeicosatetraenoic acids (HETEs), 365
Hydroxyl radical, 257
  measurement, 265–266

I

IMCD (inner medullary collecting ducts), microdissection, 104
Immortalized cell lines, 217–232
Immunofluorescence microscopy, 40–43
Immunogold staining, 40
Immunohistochemistry, 43–44, 248–249
  localization of P450, 367–368
Immunostaining, 53
Incubation
  isolated epithelial cells, 340
  renal slices, 113–115
  subcellular fractions, 337–339
Indirect immunofluorescence technique, 40–43
Inner medullary collecting ducts (IMCD), microdissection, 104
Inorganic mercury, toxicity, 124–125, 178
In situ hybridization, 244, 368, 396–397
Insulin, in primary cell culture, 174–175
Insulin-like growth factor I (IGF I), 285
Internal ribosome entry sites (IRES), 418
Interstitial fibrosis, 53
Interstitial infiltrate, 53, 54
Interstitial lesions, histopathology, 53–54
Intracellular enzyme leakage, 116, 140–141
Intron sequences, 417
Inulin
  clearance methods, 2–7
  determination in plasma and urine, 10–12
  microanalytic techniques, 86, 92
  plasma clearance, 8–9
  single nephron filtration rate, 86
In vivo techniques
  microdissection, 97–105
  microperfusion and micropuncture, 79–92
IRES (internal ribosome entry sites), 418
Iron, 257–258
  bleomycin-detectable iron assay, 270–272
Iron-nitrilotriacetate complex (Fe-NaNTA), 242
Isolated nephron segments, 124–139
  calculations, 138–142
  pipettes, 142–146
  procedures
    dissection, 129–135
    harvesting, 129, 135–137
    perfusion, 135
    volume markers, 138
Isolated perfused kidney, 59–60
  advantages, 60–61
  amphibian, 69
  limitations, 61–62
  methods
    cannulation, 63–65
    isolation of kidney, 62–65
    perfusate, 61, 66–68
    perfusion apparatus, 65–66
  new developments, 68–71
  remnant kidneys, 69
  single-pass perfusion, 69
Isolated perfused renal tubule technique, 124
Isozymes, in renal tissue, 166, 332, 356–360

K

Kidney; see also entries under Renal
  anatomy, 238–239
  cannulation, 63–65
  function, 218, 331
  laparotomy, 62–65
  microdissection, 97–105
  micropuncture and microperfusion, 79–92
  necropsy, 248
Kidney-derived porphyrins, as urinary markers, 29–31
Kidney-specific antigens, 29
Kidney tissue, see Renal tissue
Krebs-Ringer-bicarbonate (KRB) solution, 66
Krumdieck slicer, 110, 111

L

Lactase dehydrogenase (LDH)
  assay, 155–157
  as marker, 24, 177–178, 199
Latex particle immunoagglutination (LIA), urinary markers, 24–26, 28

Lauric acid ω-hydroxylation, 364
Light microscopy, 37–40
Light mineral oil, tubule perfusion, 135
Lipoma, 239
Liposarcoma, 239
Liposomes, transfection, 235–236
LLC-PK_1 cell lines, 164–166, 220, 228–229
Locus controlling region (LCR), 420
Loop of Henle
  anatomy, 239
  microperfusion, 90
Loss-of-function events, 380, 403, 418
Low molecular weight proteins, as urinary markers, 24–29
Luciferin-luciferase assay, 116
Lucigenin, 259
Lumen-to-bath flux, 125, 134, 138–139
Luminol, 259
Lysozyme, as urinary marker, 23–24

M

Malondaldehyde (MDA), 266–267
Mammalian studies, 218
  microdissection and microanalysis, 97–105
  renal cortical slices, 110
Markers, 19, 177, 198–199
  p-aminohippurate, 92, 159
  enzymes, 19–24
  genes, 398–399
  kidney-derived porphyrins, 29–31
  kidney-specific antigens, 29
  proteins, 24–29, 116
  of renal differentiation, 292–293
  renal regeneration, 288–292
Masson's trichrome, 38, 52
Mass spectrometry, isolated perfused tubules, 137
3-MC (3-methylcholanthrene), 332
MDA (malondaldehyde), 266–267
MDCK cell line, 220, 227–228
Medullary thick ascending limbs (MTAL), microdissection, 103
Membrane permeability, 319
Membrane potential, mitochondria, 311–315
Membrane transport, nephrotoxicity, 344–348
Membrane vesicles, 346–348
Mercuric choloride, toxicity, 178
Mercury toxicity, 178, 224
  inorganic, 124–125, 178
  organic, 178–179
Mersalyl-Brij solution, 22
Metals, uptake and toxicity, renal cortical slices, 117–118
Methimazole, 333
3-Methylcholanthrene (3-MC), 332
Methylmercury, toxicity, 178–179
4-Methylpyrazole, 332
4-Methylumbelliferone (MUBF), 21
Metyrapone, 332
Microanalysis, 91–92, 97–98
  identification of nephron segments, 102–104
  microdissection, 91, 98–102
  microperfusion and micropuncture, 79–92
Microdissection, 91, 97–105, 147–148, 195
  identification of nephron segments, 102–104
  with molecular biology method, 104–105
  procedure, 102
  species difference, 100–101
  tissue preparation, 102
α_1-Microglobulin, 26–27
α_2-Microglobulin, 27
β_2-Microglobulin, 25–26, 394
Microinjection, pronuclear, 415
Micromanipulators, 84
Microperfusion techniques, 79–80
  equipment, 83–85
  microanalytic techniques, 91–92
  microdissection, 91
  preparation, 81–83
  procedure, 88–91
Micropipettes, 84–85
Micropuncture techniques, 79–80
  equipment, 83–85
  microanalytic techniques, 91–92
  microdissection, 91
  preparation, 81–83
  procedure, 85–88
Microscopy
  confocal microscopy, 52
  electron microscopy, 37, 42, 117, 293
  immunofluorescence microscopy, 40–43
  light microscopy, 37–40
  micropuncture and microperfusion, 84
  primary renal cell cultures, 208–209
  renal microvasculature during perfusion, 68–69
  scanning electron microscopy (SEM), 40
  tissue slices, 117
  transmission electron microscopy (TEM), 40
Microsomes, 341, 361
Mitochondria
  adenine and pyridine nucleotides, 317–318
  calcium ion distribution, 322–326
  energetic and redox status, 309–326
  function, 158, 317–322
  membrane integrity, 308–309
  membrane potential, 311–315
  model systems, 300–306
  permeability transition, 319
  pH gradient, 315–316
  respiration, 306–308
  thiol/disulfide status, 320–322
  toxicity in renal injury, 299–327
Molecular biology, with microdissection, 104–105
Molecular methods
  gene expression
    deregulation, 380
    in eukaryotes, 378–380
    intervention, 398–403
  genetic changes, 380–398
Morphometry, 44, 51, 52, 55
Mouse studies
  carcinogenesis and mutagenesis, 239–249

microdissection, 99, 101
transgenic animals, 400–401, 413–423
mRNA, 383–398
Mutations, 237, 244–248; see also Renal mutagenesis

N

NAG (*N*-acetyl-β-D-glucosaminidase), 21–22
Nagarse, 305
Naphthoflavone, 332
NDMA, (dimethylnitrosamine), 241, 242
NDPS (*N*-3,5–(dichlorophenyl)succinimide), 339
Necropsy, 248
Neoplastic lesions, see Renal carcinogenesis; Renal tumors
Nephroblastomas, 239, 243
Nephrogenic diabetes insipidus (NDI), 99
Nephrotoxicity, 378; see also Cytotoxicity assays; Renal toxicology; Toxicity studies
biotransformation, 331–344
cytochrome P450 as bioactivation system, 353–368
gene expression
deregulation, 380
in eukaryotes, 378–380
intervention, 398–403
gene transcription rate, 380–383
membrane transport, 344–348
mitochondria, 158, 299–327
mRNA, 393–398
Net fractional transport, 86–87
Nickel compounds, 243
N-[4-(5-Nitro-2-furyl)-2-thiazolyl]formamide, 242
p-Nitrophenol (PNP), 342–343
N-Nitrosodimethylamine (NDMA), 243
N-Nitrosodimethylamine *N*-demethylase (NDMAd), 363–364
N-Nitrosodimethylamine *N*-demethylation assay, 363–364
N-Nitrosoethylurea (ENU), 241, 242
N-Nitrosomethylurea (NMU), 242, 243
N-Nitrosomorpholine (NNM), 241, 242
NMR spectroscopy, isolated perfused kidney, 68
Northern blot analysis, 387–388
Nuclear run-on transcription (N-ROT), 381, 385, 386

O

Ochratoxin A, GFR, 16
Oil block, micropuncture, 88
OMCD (outer medullary collecting ducts), 104, 131
Oncogenes, 231
Optimization
immortalized cell lines, 224–227
primary cultures, 173–176
transfection, 224–226
of transfection, 225
Orbital suspension incubation, 114–115
Organic ions, accumulation, assay for, 159–160
Organic mercury, toxicity, 178–179
OSOM, 190–201, 239
Outer medullary collecting ducts (OMCD), 104, 131
Oxidative damage
lipid peroxidation measurement, 266–268
reduced glutathione and glutathione disulfide measurement, 268–270
Oxygen, 257; see also Oxidative damage; Reactive oxygen species
Oxygenation, in primary cell cultures, 173
Oxygen consumption, assay for determining, 159
Oxygen metabolites, 257

P

P450 inhibitors, 332
PAH (*p*-aminohippurate), 3, 92, 159, 175
Papillary micropuncture, 87
Papillomas, 239
Papilloma virus, 230
PCNA (proliferating cell nuclear antigen), as renal regeneration marker, 290–291
PCT (proximal convoluted tubules), microdissection, 103
S-(1,2,3,4,4'-Pentachloro-1,3-butadienyl)-L-cysteine (PCBC), toxicity, 164
Pentoxyresorufin *O*-dealkylation assay, 363
Percoll density-gradient centrifugation, 195–199
Perfusate, 61, 66–68, 133
Perfusion
apparatus, 65–66, 142
fixation, 37, 54
isolated nephron segments, 123–160
isolated perfused kidney, 59–71
microperfusion, 79–85, 88–92
species, 60
Perfusion pipette, 144, 145
Periodic acid-Schiff (PAS) method, 37–38
Permeability transition, mitochondria and, 319
1,10-Phenanthroline, 334
Phenol red, in tissue culture medium, 169
Phenylalanine, as detector molecule, 265–266
Phenylalanylglycine, 334
pH Gradient, mitochondria, 315–316
PHS (prostaglandin H synthase), 333, 336, 339
Pig studies, renal proximal tubular cells, 164–181
Pipette holders, 146
Pipettes, 142–146
PIXE analysis, 118
Plasma clearance, inulin, 8–9
Plasmids, 221–222, 229, 231–232
Polymerase chain reaction (PCR) technique, 244–247
Polyoma, 231
Ponceau-acid fucsin-orange G stain, 38
Porphyrins, kidney-derived, 29–31
Posttranscriptional controls, 379
Potassium, intracellular content, 157–158
Primary cell cultures, 202
renal proximal tubular cells, 163–181, 201–208
optimization studies, 173–176
toxicological studies, 176–181, 211–213
transfection, 221–222
Primer extension analysis, 395–396
Probes, 389–390

Prokaryotic sequences, 417
Proliferating cell nuclear antigen (PCNA), as renal regeneration marker, 290–291
Pronuclear microinjection, 415
Propylthiouracil, 333
Prostglandin H synthase (PHS), 333, 336, 339
Protein HC, 26–27
Proteins
  Bradford protein assay, 341–342
  enzymes, 116
  microsomal, 367
  renal regeneration markers, 290–292
  urinary markers, 24–29, 116
Proton induced X-ray emission (PIXE), 118–119
Protonmotive force, 310
Proximal convoluted tubules (PCT), microdissection, 103
Proximal straight tubules (PST), microdissection, 103
Proximal tubules, see Renal proximal tubules
Pyridine nucleotide, intracellular content, 317–318

R

Rabbit studies
  clearance methods, 5–7
  isolated nephron segments, 124–146
  microdissection, 99, 100–101
  primary cultures preparation, 220–221
  renal cortical slices, 110–120
  renal proximal tubular cells, 164–181
  suspensions of renal proximal tubules, 147–160
Radiochemical assay, inulin detection, 12
Rat studies
  carcinogenesis and mutagenesis, 239–249
  clearance methods, 4–7, 13–14, 16
  isolated, 59–71
  isozymes, 356–360
  microdissection and microanalysis, 97–105
  primary cultural of proximal and distal tubular cells, 201–214
  renal epithelial cells, 189–214
Reactive oxygen species, assays, 258–266
Redox status, mitochondria, 310–311
Relative volume, 45
Remnant kidneys, perfusion, 69
Renal carcinogenesis, 239–243; also Renal tumors
Renal clearance, 1–3, 15–17; see also Clearance methods
Renal cortex
  anatomy, 239
  epithelial cells, see Renal epithelial cells
  function, 116
  mitochondria, 326
Renal cortical slices, 110, 120
  incubation systems, 113–115
  membrane transport, 345–346
  metallic toxicant accumulation, 117–118
  proton induced X-ray emission (PIXE), 118–119
  slicers and slicing, 110–113
  toxicant studies, 119–120
  viability and toxicology assays, 115–117
Renal epithelial cells, 190–191
  assay methods, 209–211
  biochemical properties, 199–201
  immortalized cell lines, 217–232
    using plasmids with oncogenes, 231–232
    viral transformation, 229–231
  isolated cells, 339–340
  microscopy, 208–209
  primary cultures of proximal and distal tubular cells, 201–214
  purification, 195–199
  from renal cortex and OSOM, 191–195
Renal injury, 181, 283, 285
  adenine nucleotide intracellular content, 158–159
  apoptosis, 285, 293–295
  assay
    for antioxidant enzymes, 272–277
    bleomycin-detectable iron assay, 270–272
    for reactive oxygen species, 258–266
  lactase dehydrogenase release, 24, 116, 155, 157
  markers, 19–29
  measurement of oxidative damage, 266–270
  mitochondrial toxicity, 158, 299–327
  organic ion accumulation, 159–160
  oxygen consumption, 159
  potassium intracellular content, 157–158
  regeneration, 181
  repair mechanisms, 283–295
Renal medulla
  epithelial cells, 190–191
    biochemical properties, 199–201
    isolation, 191–195
    purification, 195–199
Renal mesenchymal tumors, 239, 241, 243
Renal metabolism, 331–335
  in vitro study, 335–344
  membrane transport, 344–348
Renal mutagenesis, 237–238, 244–248; see also Renal tumors
Renal papilla, 239
Renal pathology
  DNA and RNA isolation techniques, 219
  enzyme histochemistry/immunohistochemistry, 43–44, 248–249
  necropsy, 248
Renal proximal tubules (RPTs); see also Renal tubules
  anatomy, 239
  cells in primary culture, 163–166, 190–191, 203–208
    assay methods, 209–211
    cell culture, 203–208
    microscopy, 208–209
    optimization studies, 173–176
    toxicological studies, 176–181, 211–213
  cytotoxic assays, 155–160
  dissection, 130–131
  isolation, 147–155, 170–172
  microperfusion, 89–90
  regeneration, 181
  surface area, 48–49

suspensions, 147–160
toxicity studies, 124–125
volume fraction, 45
Renal regeneration, 283–286
growth factors, 285–288
markers, 288–292
Renal tissue, 218; see also Established cell lines; Immortalized cell lines; Primary cell cultures; Renal injury
assay
antioxidant enzymes, 272–277
bleomycin-detectable iron assay, 270–272
reactive oxygen species, 258–266
renal cortical slices, 115–117
cytochrome P450 expression, 355–360
harvesting, 129, 135–137
incubation, 113–115
intact renal cells, 301–305
isozymes in, 356–360
measurement of oxidative damage, 266–270
perfusion, 59–71, 79–85, 88–92, 123–160
slicing, 110–113
staining, 37–40
subcellular fractions, 335–339
viability, 115
Renal toxicology; see also Toxicity studies
antioxidants, 272–277
biotransformation, 331–348
carcinogenesis and mutagenesis, 237–249
clearance methods, 1–17
cytochrome P450, 165, 166, 353–369
histopathologic methods, 35–55
immortalized cell lines, 217–232
isolated perfused kidney, 59–71, 123–146
membrane transport, 331–348
microdissection, 97–105
micropuncture and microperfusion, 79–92
molecular methods, 377–404
oxidant metabolites, 255–277
renal cortical slices, 109–120
renal injury
mitochondrial toxicity, 158, 299–327
repair mechanisms, 283–295
renal proximal tubules
cell cultures, 163–181, 189–214
suspensions, 147–160
transgenic animals, 413–423
urinary markers, 19–31
Renal tubules
in vitro perfusion, 130–138
isolated perfused tubule technique, 124
lesions, 53
Renal tumors, 239–243; see also Renal carcinogenesis; Renal mutagenesis
Reporter genes, 419
Resorcinol assay, inulin detection, 11
Respiration
mitochondrial function, 306
toxicity indicator, 116
Respiratory control ratio (RCR), 308
Restriction fragment length polymorphism (RFLP) analysis, 244, 245
Retinol-binding protein (RBP), as urinary marker, 27–29
Retroviruses, for cell immortalization, 230–231
Retrovirus-mediated transgenesis, 420–421
Reverse transcription-polymerase chain reaction (RT-PCR)
microdissection, 99, 104–105
mRNA detection, 367, 391–395
Rhodamine, 123, 312–313
Ribonuclease protection assay, 395–396
RNA isolation, 249, 383–387
RNase A cleavage, 246
RPTs, see Renal proximal tubules

S

Safranine O, 313–315
Scanning electron microscopy (SEM), 40
Screening techniques, mutations, 244–248
SDS-PAGE, 367
Semiquantitative methods, 39–40, 54
Serial passaging, immortalized cells, 223
Signal transduction, 379
Silver-methenamine method, 39–40
Single-pass perfusion, isolated kidney, 69
Single radial immunodiffusion (SRI), urinary markers, 24, 26–27, 29
Single-strand conformation polymorphisms (SSCP), 245
SITS (4-acetamido-4'-isothiocyanostilbene-2,2'-disulfonic acid, 175
Slicers, renal cortical slices, 110, 111
Slot and dot blot analysis, 389
SOD (superoxide dismutase), assay for, 272–275
Sodium dodecyl sulfate-polyacrylamide gel electrophoresis (SDS-PAGE), 367
Southern blot-restriction fragment length polymorphism analysis, 244–245
SRI (single radial immunodiffusion, urinary markers, 24, 26–27, 29
Stable transfection, 398–399
Staining methods
hematoxylin and eosin staining, 37
immunogold staining, 40
Masson's trichrome, 38
periodic acid-Schiff (PAS) method, 37–38
silver-methenamine method, 39–40
Stains, light microscopy, 37–39
Stereological methods, unbiased, 44–51
Streptozotocin, 241, 242, 243
Structural genes, transfection, 398–400
Subcellular fractions, metabolism studies, 335–339
Submersion culture, 114
Sulfotransferase (ST), 332–333
Superoxide anion, 258–260
Superoxide dismutase (SOD), assay for, 272–275
SV40 transformation, 176, 231–232

T

Targeting vectors, 422
TBASE database, 418

TBHP (*tert*-butylhydroperoxide), cell injury by, 181
TEM (transmission electron microscopy), 40
Temperature-sensitive viruses, 229–230
Testosterone hydroxylation assay, 363
Tetraphenylphosphonium (TPP+), 311
Thiobarbituric acid reaction, 267
Thiol/disulfide status, intramitochondrial, 320–322
Thymidine, as renal regeneration marker, 288–289
Tissue fixation, 36–37
Toxicity studies, 219–220
  acute cytotoxicity assay, 211–213
  antibiotics, 119–120, 165, 179–180
  antineoplastics, 120, 180–181
  glomerular filtration rate, 15–16
  halogenated hydrocarbons, 119
  mercury compounds, 124–125, 178–179, 224
  renal clearance, 15
TPP+ (tetraphenylphosphonium), 311
Transcription, 380–383, 419
Transfection
  plasmid DNA, 221–222
  structural genes, 398–400
Transformation, 229
Transgenic animals, 413–414
  embryo culture, 416–417
  embryonic stem cell-mediated transgenesis, 421–423
  microinjection of DNA into pronucleus, 415–416
  mutation assays, 400–401
  retrovirus-mediated transgenesis, 420–421
  targeting vectors, 422–423
  transgene design, 417–418
Transient transfection, 399–400
Transitional cell tumors, 239, 242–243
Transmission electron microscopy (TEM), 40
Transplatin, toxicity, 181
Transport function, 86–87, 116–117
Triphenylmethylphosphonium (TPMP+), 311, 312
Trypsinization, 223

U

UDP-glucuronosyltransferase (UDPGT), 332–333, 338–339
  assay, 342–343
Ultramicroanalysis, 92
Uptake, 117
Urinary excretion rate, calculation, 1–2
Urinary markers, see Markers
UV spectrophotometry, conjugated dienes, 268

V

Vascular lesions, histopathology, 54
Vector sequences, 417
Vimentin, as marker, 292
2-Vinylpyridine, 270, 320–321
Viral transformation, 229–231
Volume fractions, 45
Volume markers, 138

W

Wax block, microperfusion, 89–90